" *A WONDERFUL COMBINATION OF COFFEE-TABLE BOOK,* *engaging and informative reading experience, and handy reference. It provides fascinating insight into the workings of the brain and their implications. Howard, like Carl Sagan, may be thought of as a popularizer who presents real science in an engaging and entertaining way.* "

BOOKLIST

" *I WAS SURPRISED TO FIND that what had started at ten at night as a quick scan ended about three the following morning. Simply put, this is good stuff. Complex subject matter is presented in a simple, straightforward, graphically appealing manner. And all of it is organized to help you deal not only with your role in business, but also your roles as spouse, parent, child, and friend.* "

Working Smart newsletter

" *IN BUSINESS TODAY, WE EITHER CHANGE OR DIE. To cope with change, we need a mind open to new ideas.* The Owner's Manual for the Brain *is for people who understand this: people who never stop learning, who want to improve themselves, who need to understand what motivates others.* "

Ed Crutchfield
Chairman and CEO
First Union Corporation

" *A VARIETY OF IDEAS AND PERSPECTIVES and some excellent reading lists for the general reader.* "

Library Journal

" *A PAINLESS AND FASCINATING WAY for everyone to understand the latest in brain research. But more important,* The Owner's Manual for the Brain *is a valuable resource for all of us who, as organizational change professionals, create change through people.* "

Joanne C. Preston, Ph.D.
Professor of Organization Development
Pepperdine University
Editor of *Organization Development Journal*

^{THE}
Owner's Manual FOR TheBrain

Everyday Applications from Mind-Brain Research

SECOND EDITION

Pierce J. Howard, Ph.D.

Bard Press

ATLANTA • AUSTIN

The Owner's Manual for the Brain
Everyday Applications from Mind-Brain Research

Bard Press
An imprint of Longstreet Press
2140 Newmarket Parkway, Suite 122
Marietta, GA 30067
770-690-1488 phone, 770-859-9894 fax
www.bardpress.com

ISBN 1-885167-41-5 paperback   ISBN 1-885167-38-5 hardcover

Library of Congress Cataloging-in-Publication Data

Howard, Pierce J.
    The owner's manual for the brain : everyday applications from mind
-brain research / Pierce J. Howard. – 2nd.
        p.   cm.
    Includes bibliographical references and index.
    ISBN 1-885167-38-5 (hc). – ISBN 1-885167-41-5 (pbk.)
    1. Brain.   2. Neuropsychology.   I. Title.   II. Title: Brain.
QP376.H76   199
6.12.8'2–dc21   99-41862
                                                                    CIP

The author may be contacted through
    *Cent*ACS Center for Applied Cognitive Studies
    1100 Harding Place
    Charlotte, North Carolina 28204
    704-331-0926 phone, 704-331-9408 fax
    info@centacs.com or www.centacs.com

A BARD PRESS BOOK

Copyediting: Helen Hyams
Proofreading: Helen Hyams, Deborah Costenbader, Letitia Blalock
Index: Kay K. Schlembach
Illustrations: Kim Allman, Round Rock Graphics
Text/Cover Design: Suzanne Pustejovsky
Composition: Round Rock Graphics

First Edition
    First printing: May 1994
    Second printing: May 1995
    Third printing: November 1996
    Fourth printing: November 1997

Second Edition
    First printing: November 1999
    Second printing: August 2000

Table of Contents

Quick Content Guide

Although everyone will find each chapter in this book relevant to his or her life in some way, those who fill special roles may find certain chapters of particular interest. Parts Two and Three deal with subjects like sleep, music, and sex that affect everybody every day; therefore, we suggest that all readers, regardless of their roles, would benefit from the materials in these chapters.

    Below are listed several role categories and the additional chapters that may be of special interest to people in these roles.

Doctors, lawyers, and others in professional practice	19–20, 23, 25, 28–30, 33–34
Human resource professionals	All
Managers	19–22, 29–34
Mental health professionals	All
Negotiators	19, 21, 29–31
Parents	All
Religious professionals	14, 19–22, 23–24, 32, 35–36
Research-and-development professionals	20, 29–31, 33–35
Salespeople	20–21, 32–34
Students	19–20, 22–30
Teachers, trainers, and coaches	19–31

> *There are two ways of spreading light: to be The candle or the mirror that reflects it.*
>
> —Edith Wharton

Preface

Why this book?

Tomes about the mind and brain pepper the shelves of airport kiosks and bookstores from Phoenix to Philly. This is the ninth year of the Decade of the Brain, but that is insufficient reason for yet another book, just as, for example, World Series time alone is not sufficient reason for another book on baseball.

The available books about the brain can be divided into two categories: research reports and practical applications. Neurobiology texts belong in the first category, and how-to books *(How to Increase Your Memory, How to Be More Creative)* belong in the second. This book serves to create an explicit overlap between these two categories. Research books generally decline to identify the everyday applicability of their findings—indeed, that is not their purpose. Practical books generally omit making the explicit connection between a piece of advice and its basis in research. The intention of this book is to yoke the two together as a team, by saying, "Here's what we know about memory storage in the brain, and here's how that knowledge can help us improve our recall of information."

Why me? I'm not an academic who must publish or perish, and I'm not a natural writer possessed with an irresistible urge to put pen to paper (or, more aptly, fingertips to keyboard). In fact, I'm a very extraverted guy for whom writing is the ultimate act of self-discipline—it doesn't come easy. Reading has traditionally been my introversive activity of choice. So why did I write this book? A story will explain.

All my life I had viewed myself as a dilettante. That changed in the spring of 1988, when I read *The Universe Within,* by Morton Hunt. Hunt, a science popularizer, introduced the English-reading world to cognitive science, the interdisciplinary approach to understanding the workings of the mind-brain. Each chapter of his book summarized research in an area that had been of interest to me: problem solving, creativity, learning theory, and so on. Voilà! I was no longer a dilettante, but a cognitive scientist. I began to read everything I could find dealing with this new field (which is described in Chapter One), and I found that the extensive scientific literature on brain research provided me with a basis for my applied interests.

In December 1988, I began serving a term on the program committee of the local chapter of the American Society for Training and Development (ASTD). The committee asked for program suggestions for monthly meetings in 1989, so I suggested that we bring in a speaker on the subject of cognitive science. After hearing my justification, they agreed that the chapter would benefit from such a program and asked me to find a speaker. I was able to find speakers who were expensive and practical in their approach or speakers who were inexpensive and theoretical in their approach, but I had to report that I was

> **"It is like the man who claimed to be selling Abraham Lincoln's ax—he explained that over the years the head had to be replaced twice and the handle three times."**
>
> —Stephen Pinker,
> *The Language Instinct*

unable to find anyone we could afford who was willing to present an application-oriented program to our group. I argued, and they agreed, that the more theoretical speakers would be hooted out of the hall. As a result, they asked, "Pierce, why don't you do a program?" I agreed.

I presented the program—"Brain Update"—in August 1989. After an encouraging reception, I presented the program in two other cities and then at the regional meeting in Gatlinburg, Tennessee, in the fall of 1990. After each of the four presentations, people came up to me and asked, "What have you written? Your content is fascinating, but we'd

like something written to consider in more depth." Responding to this encouragement as evidence of a genuine need, my wife and partner, Jane, and I decided that I should cut back on my consulting duties and write a book. That was in August 1991. I started writing and reading to fill in the gaps, closing in on fulfilling my commitment to provide you with written documentation of what I have enjoyed talking about from the front of the classroom. The result was the first edition of *The Owner's Manual for the Brain,* published in 1994. Five years later, I find that some, but not all, of the first edition has been replaced. Much has been added. Like Abe Lincoln's ax, the form remains the same.

How is this book unique? First, it stands with one foot in the research camp and the other in practice. Second, it reflects my twenty-plus years' experience as a management consultant. (I cannot apologize for the fact that this book reflects the part of the world with which I am familiar.) Third, I have included only brain research findings that have widespread practical applications. Findings that are interesting but not generally useful have not been included. Fourth, for the most part, the structure is aimed at those who will use the research, not the researchers themselves.

The basic structure of the book employs what I like to refer to as the "So what?" format. The typical response to reported research findings is "So what?" For example, research shows that the level of the hormone melatonin is directly related to the quality of our sleep. You may say, "So what?" Well, this book is designed with that question in mind. Every piece of research reported is followed by one or more specific suggestions for its application. Here is an example of what you will find.

TOPIC 7.4   Sleep and Exercise

Exercising tends to elicit cortical alertness, which is not what you want when going to sleep. Exercise relaxes you after experiencing stress, but good aerobic exercise generally puts your nervous system in a state of moderate arousal. In this condition, you are ideally suited for mental tasks. In order to sleep soon after a workout, you would need to consume carbohydrates and dairy products.

Applications

1 Exercise no later than several hours before bedtime.

2 If you must exercise just before retiring for the evening (I know a television sports announcer who exercises after a night game because he's so keyed up), try reading a relatively unemotional book in bed rather than an exciting one (Plato rather than Agatha Christie) to help you get to sleep.

The book is organized around these Topics (except for Chapters One, Two, Three, and Thirty-Seven). The numerical identifier refers to the chapter number and the sequence within that chapter. While most of the Application ideas are mine, several of my readers have suggested additional ideas. I have indicated their authorship following the suggestion. I look forward to including suggestions from other readers in subsequent editions of this book.

In its most general sense, this book is for people who want to use their heads. More specifically, it is for lifelong learners, professionals who value keeping up and/or ahead of the game, people developers, human resource professionals, leaders, consultants (internal and external), supervisors of teachers, training managers, educators of teachers, adult education professionals, train-the-trainer professionals, curriculum writers, curriculum designers, industrial and organizational psychologists, writers, and research-and-development professionals. I could summarize this list by reducing it to five types of readers: lifelong learners, educators, consultants, managers, and psychologists. You will gain insights into improving your personal effectiveness without having to wade through the tedium of academic detail (I've done that for you) or the fluff of wordy popularizers (I've cut away the padding).

This book *is not*

- A biology or medical text

- A psychology text

- An in-depth treatment of specific research findings

- A collection of esoteric findings that are interesting but not useful

- An in-depth treatment of general subjects (I only report the brain research findings that are relevant to the subject)

- A reference work for research scientists

This book *is*

- Application-oriented

- A reflection of my experiences as a management consultant

- Composed of findings that have practical applications

- A reference work for consumers

- Centered on the what and the why: what brain research suggests we could do for personal improvement and why we should do it

The book is designed to be something of an encyclopedia or resource book of application ideas. I suspect that a few people will read it from cover to cover, with most of you preferring to browse according to which sections are of the most current interest to you. Where the understanding of a chapter or Topic is particularly dependent on material that is covered elsewhere in the book, I have attempted to indicate that fact. In order to group the chapters for the convenience of most readers, I have divided the book into ten parts.

Part One serves as an introduction to the field of cognitive science. Chapter One provides an overview both of the field of cognitive science and of the book itself, as well as a look at current research on the nature-nurture controversy. Chapter Two reviews some of the basics of brain functions, while Chapter Three reviews major brain research technology. If you have a strong or recent background in cognitive science, you may choose to skim or skip these first three chapters. Part Two will prove to be of the greatest interest for most people, covering findings related to early development, diet, drugs, sleep, exercise, humor, music, and aging. Part Three covers matters of sex, gender, love, and relationships. Part Four discusses illness and injury. Part Five focuses on emotions, stress,

and motivation, while Part Six discusses aspects of personality such as personality traits and intelligence. This section will be particularly useful if you are interested in personnel selection, parenting, or similarities and differences in personal styles at work and at home. Part Seven is designed for the teacher in us all; it discusses how we learn and remember, facilitate learning, and develop language, with a special chapter on giftedness. Part Eight shows ways to maximize our creativity and problem-solving ability. Part Nine deals with workplace design and dealing with change and should be of particular interest if you are a people manager. The topics of Part Ten—epistemology and states of consciousness—may at first glance seem somewhat esoteric. However, epistemology is the ultimate domain of brain science. It is through appreciating the structure of knowledge that we develop peace in relationships, both in our homes and among nations. This final section should be of particular interest to those in peacemaking roles, such as preachers, diplomats, and negotiators.

My main purpose in writing this book is to help you discover ways to improve. By giving specific suggestions along with their research justifications, I hope to tweak your interest in opportunities for personal improvement. Because the scope is so inclusive, some of you may be frustrated by finding insufficient information on these pages to enable you to immediately implement an idea. To solve this problem, I would like to suggest several possible resources that could be helpful in leading you to further information or skill mastery:

- Talk with your public library's reference staff.

- Consult the continuing education department of a school of higher education near you.

- Consult officers in your local chapters of the ASTD or the National Society for Performance and Instruction (directories are available in your library).

- Write the authors of books mentioned in a specific Topic.

- Explore the Internet resources listed at the end of this book, and conduct your own Internet keyword searches.

- Read the materials listed at the end of each chapter and in the Resources at the end of the book that relate to ideas in which you are interested.

If, in your search to improve your skills, you seek out workshops on a particular subject mentioned in this book, be sure to evaluate the content of the workshop before attending. For example, don't just go to a "motivation" workshop. Find out whose theories or work the session is based on. Many workshops today use outmoded information. But that's a subject for another book.

I acknowledge debts to many in writing this book. To my readers, who've provided helpful suggestions and criticism: Mark Ardis, Rick Bradley, Susan Close, Bill Davis, Richard Furr, Janice Gamache, Vicki Halsey, Eric Jensen, John Kello, Shirley Lim, Deb Morris, Marselino Pangan, Dillon Robertson, Captain Eurydice Stanley (U.S. Army), and Malu Velazquez. To Gary John, the reader recruited by my publisher. To Chip Bell, who has encouraged me to write and who introduced me to Ray Bard. To Ray Bard, my publisher, for his wise counsel and constant support. To Suzanne Pustejovsky, who has visually transformed over eight hundred pages of words and numbers into a friendly yet sophisticated design. To Helen Hyams, my editor, for her insight and unflagging attention to detail. To my daughters, Allegra and Hilary, whose excitement in the process fueled me to return to the keyboard. To Jane, my wife and partner, for bearing the brunt of the emotional cost associated with writing a book. And to the staff at *Cent*ACS, who make my daily absence from home a time of joy and support— to them I dedicate this book.

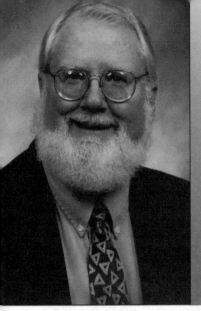

The Author

Pierce J. Howard, Ph.D. is director of research of the Center for Applied Cognitive Studies (*Cent*ACS), a research and dissemination firm headquartered in Charlotte, North Carolina. His wife, Jane, is managing director at *Cent*ACS. Together, they develop both public and organizational programs based on the most current research in cognitive science. These programs include workshops, breakfast seminars, speeches, retreats, a web site (www.centacs.com), custom-designed programs, and publications. Their special focus is on the Five-Factor Model of personality, for which they offer certification training and a wide range of support materials, software, services, advanced training programs, and annual learning conferences.

In addition, for the last twenty-five years, Dr. Howard has been an organization development consultant. His motivation and, hence, his own professional development stem from a deep-seated desire to help others learn how to overcome their obstacles. He has attended numerous workshops and professional meetings, read extensively in the field, conducted computer database searches, and created hundreds of workshop designs in an unrelenting effort to find the best ways to help people to solve problems, make decisions, create new approaches, and understand themselves and others—in effect, to take responsibility for their own growth and development both as individuals and as members of teams and organizations. Dr. Howard's skill and interest in debunking myths and finding the most effective ways to help others learn have served him well in the business community.

Dr. Howard grew up in Kinston, North Carolina. He received his B.A. degree in 1963 from Davidson College and his M.A. degree in 1967 from East Carolina University, both in English. In 1972, he received his Ph.D. degree in education with a special emphasis in curriculum and research from the University of North Carolina at Chapel Hill. His college years were interrupted by a three-year tour with the U.S. Army in Germany, where he served as an intelligence specialist.

In addition to his writing, research, and dissemination responsibilities, Dr. Howard serves as Adjunct Professor of Business and Psychology at Pfeiffer University–Charlotte and at the University of North Carolina at Charlotte. His professional affiliations include membership in the American Psychological Association, the International Society for the Study of Individual Differences, the American Society for Training and Development (ASTD), and the Organization Development Network. In 1992, the Charlotte Area ASTD Chapter recognized him with its Excellence in Service to the Profession Award. He has written and published numerous workbooks, tests, and other materials for clients. The first edition of his book, *The Owner's Manual for the Brain,* was published in 1994. Upon completion of this second edition, Pierce and Jane Howard will be hard at work writing a book on the Five-Factor Model of personality. For relaxation, they enjoy walking, cooking, chamber music, choral singing, reading, and camping. Their older daughter, Hilary, is an actress in New York, and their younger daughter, Allegra, is a medical risk specialist in Charlotte.

Part One

The Context for Using Your Owner's Manual

Forming a Foundation

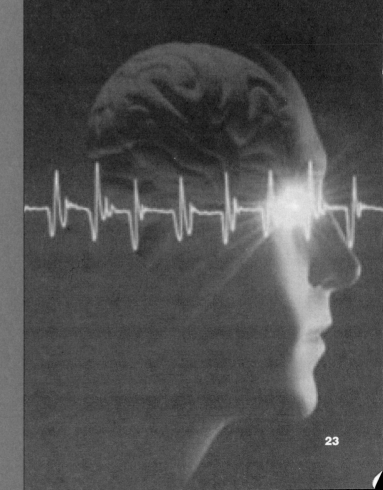

1

Getting Started

A Framework for Exploring Mind-Brain Concepts

World War II started something. The pain and tragedy of head injuries catapulted brain research into the foreground of scientific and pseudoscientific investigation. From the popular claims of split-brain research to the profound findings of neurotransmitter studies, discoveries by increasing numbers of researchers and readers have focused on learning how the brain works.

❝ Few minds wear out; more rust out. ❞

—*Christian Nestell Bovee*

This explosion of research has given birth to a new field of knowledge: cognitive science, also known as brain science. One feature that makes this field unique is that it is interdisciplinary—it is made up of more than one traditional field of study. The research has been conducted by investigators from seven broad fields, although some subdivisions of these fields are more germane to cognitive science than others; for example, psychopharmacology is more germane than social psychology. The fields are

1. Biology
2. Chemistry
3. Psychology
4. Information science
5. Philosophy
6. Anthropology
7. Linguistics

Prior to World War II, communication among scholars in these fields was minimal. But the momentum increased noticeably soon after the war ended. Most people seem to date the beginning of cognitive science as a formal interdisciplinary field of study from September 1948 (H. Gardner, 1985), when scientists assembled at the Hixon Symposium at the California Institute of Technology, which was titled "Cerebral Mechanisms of Behavior." Presenters included John von Neumann and Karl Lashley, representing mathematics and psychology. Many regard this meeting as the sounding of the death knell for the behaviorism of B. F. Skinner, Ivan Petrovich Pavlov, Edward Lee Thorndike, and John B. Watson, which had held sway until then. No more would strict stimulus-response explanations of human behavior be ascendant. With the rise of cognitive science came the doctrine that human behavior consisted of more than conditioned responses, that the human mind was indeed able to create, to choose, to reflect—in short, to explore the universe between stimulus and response. Stephen Covey (1990, p. 69) suggests that between stimulus and response, humans have the freedom to choose. Or, as Richard Restak (1991, p. 50) observes, we are moving from Socrates' "know thyself" to Kierkegaard's "choose thyself."

Emerging from over thirty years in the relative obscurity of academia, cognitive science had its coming-out with the publication in 1982 of Morton Hunt's *The Universe Within: A New Science Explores the Human Mind.* His highly readable volume introduced many to this new field. Drawing from examples in areas such as problem solving, creativity, decision science, epistemology, moral development, personality theory, artificial intelligence, logic, linguistics, learning theory, and memory, he showed how cognitive science has brought previously isolated fields together into one common alliance committed to describing how the mind works. He related how this alliance of scholars is collaborating to describe the mind's functioning from both the detailed, microscopic, bottom-up perspective, as in cellular neurobiology, and the big-picture, global, top-down perspective, as in discussions of primary personality traits. The excitement of this multipronged scientific movement lies in the moment when the bottom-up, or *molecular,* studies become recognized as equivalent to the top-down, or *molar,* studies.

An example of such a "meeting at the middle" can be found in Hans Eysenck's *The Biological Basis of Personality* (1967), in which he begins to establish the relationship between the reticular activating system (RAS) in the brain (a molecular structure) and the personality traits of extraversion and neuroticism (molar behaviors). Paul MacLean (1990) describes the bottom-up perspective as "objective" and the top-down approach as "subjective." The point where they meet defines the discipline of *epistemology* (see Chapter Thirty-Five). For an excellent and timely discussion of this molecular-molar relationship, see Cacioppo and Berntson (1992).

The Mind-Brain Dichotomy

As we slip into the content proper of this book, you will notice that the terms *brain* and *mind* are used interchangeably. IBMer E. Baird Smith has a comedy routine in which he asks, "Is your mind a part of your brain, or is your brain all in your mind?" In the nineteenth century, English scholar Thomas Hewitt Key played with this semantic difficulty by asking, "What is mind? No matter. What is matter? Never mind." This semantic puzzle needs attention! Dealing with the historical debate between mind and brain is beyond the purpose of this book. Understandable treatments are available in H. Gardner (1985) and Hunt (1982). In the seventeenth century, René Descartes argued for *dualism,* with "mind" a kind of software and "brain" a kind of hardware; he apparently developed this idea as a result of a rift with the church authorities, who allowed him to continue his work as long as he stuck to the body and let the church take care of the mind and spirit. Later, behaviorists like Skinner argued for *monism* (nothing exists other than cells), whereas current thinking argues for an *interactionist* approach. This approach describes the intimate, sensitive way in which mind (ideas and images) and body (cells, chemicals, and electricity) directly and immediately influence each other. As a simple example, we know that a joyful disposition (mind and spirit) can increase the number of "helper cells" in the immune system (brain and body) and that, conversely, a reduction in the number of helper cells can dampen a joyful disposition. We also know that using our memory and skills tends to preserve nerve cells ("use it or lose it") and that, conversely, losing nerve cells over time interferes with memory and skills.

To say "use your mind" or "use your brain" is to say the same thing. It is like saying "use your computer" versus "use your word-processing program." The features of one influence the features of the other. Ira Black (1991, p. 8) argues that our mental software and hardware are one and the same when he speaks of the "essential unity of structure and function." When the computer is turned off, the word-processing program cannot function. Yet just because the computer is turned on, that doesn't mean the program is being used, or being used to capacity. When the brain is dead, the mind cannot function. Yet just because the brain is alive, that doesn't mean the mind is being used, or being used to capacity. In a sense, then, the best definition of mind is that it is the state that occurs when the brain is alive and at work. Richard M. Restak, who wrote the books and television series *The Mind* (1988) and *The Brain* (1984), despaired of a crisp, clear definition that could distinguish between the two, concluding, "Mind is the astounding interplay of one hundred billion neurons. And more" (1988, p. 31). J. A. Hobson (1988, p. 230), in *The Dreaming Brain,* writes, "I believe that when we have truly adequate descriptions of brain and mind, dualism and all of its dilemmas will disappear. We will speak of the brain-mind as a unity, or invent some new word to describe it." To talk of the brain is to refer to the more molecular aspects of a phenomenon, while to talk of the mind is to refer to the more molar aspects.

Cognitive and *cognition* are our only words that refer to both brain and mind, and the public finds them smacking of the ivory tower. We do need a new word that the public will accept—perhaps something like *processor* or *reactor, main* or *brind.* Candace Pert, discoverer of the endorphin receptor, refers to the "bodymind," thus enlarging the discussion. She teaches that the brain and nervous system are so widely represented throughout the body with mutual receptors that it does not make sense to speak of them separately. Meanwhile, a good discussion of the nature of the mind and various states of consciousness is available in Daniel Dennett's *Kinds of Minds* (1996).

Human or Animal: What's the Difference?

Humorists, philosophers, scientists, theologians—all have made stabs at defining the difference between humans and animals. Consider:

> *"No animal admires another animal."*
> **—Blaise Pascal**

> *"Man is the only animal that blushes. Or needs to."*
> **—Mark Twain**

> *"The desire to take medicine is perhaps the greatest feature which distinguishes man from animals."*
> **—Sir William Osler**

The parade of quotes could quickly become tiring. I will, however, summarize both the popular and scientific efforts to describe this difference by one top-down and one bottom-up observation. The top-down observation: humans can learn to write, while animals can't. The bottom-up observation: humans have a proportionately greater area of uncommitted cerebral cortex, or cortex in which unused synapses are available to be committed to new learning (see Figure 1.1). The cerebral cortex (see Chapter Two for further discussion) is the part of the brain that houses the rational functions, such as problem solving, planning, and creativity. The comparison between a rat's brain and a human brain is dramatic. All but a sliver of the rat's brain is "committed" to motor, auditory, somatosensory, olfactory, and visual functions—that is, survival activities. These committed, or dedicated, areas can't be used for any other function, such as memory or problem solving, in much the same way that a word-processing machine can't be used for other computing functions. In contrast, well over half of the human brain is uncommitted and thus available for forming new synapses and networks in the service of creativity, problem solving, analysis, memory—in short, of civilization itself. In other words, we have a greater capacity for learning. (See the discussion of synapses in Chapter Two.)

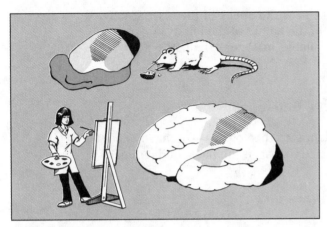

Figure 1.1. Cortical Commitment.
Note: A comparison of committed (shaded) and uncommitted (unshaded) regions of the cerebral cortex in rats (top) and humans (bottom).

Since the publication of the first edition of this book in 1994, a flurry of books has appeared on the subject of evolutionary psychology. These books are based on twenty years of assimilation of the monumental *Sociobiology,* by E. O. Wilson, which was published in 1975. Wilson's text has provided the major source of data for new Darwinists who are committed to the notion that a single human nature is deeply rooted in our primate ancestors and that this single human nature satisfactorily explains both the diversity and the commonality among us. This flurry of books includes J. Diamond, *The Third Chimpanzee: The Evolution and Future of the Human Animal* (1992) and *Guns, Germs, and Steel: The Fates of Human Societies* (1997a); J. L. Elman and others, *Rethinking Innateness: A Connectionist Perspective on Development* (1996); R. Wrangham and D. Peterson, *Demonic Males: Apes and the Origins of Human Violence* (1996); and R. Wright, *The Moral Animal: The New Science of Evolutionary Psychology* (1994). The net impact of these works is not so much to change the way we understand the mind-brain, but rather to deepen our understanding of how we got to be where we are. Specific points made by these new Darwinists will appear throughout this edition.

What Is the Mind-Brain?

Metaphors abound to explain the physical process that governs our behavior. Some explain it as a power plant, emphasizing the electro-chemical ionic transfers that culminate in the nervous system's capacity to supply enough power to illuminate a twenty-five-watt light bulb. Others explain it as a computer, using the analogy of RAM and ROM and bits and bytes and memory and storage to describe the brain's capacity to store 2.8×10^{20} bits of information. Still others see the brain as a library that can store ten million thousand-page books.

And some see the brain as a minigovernment that administers a vast array of bodily functions, from breathing and blood flow to meditation and stock market analysis.

May I have the envelope, please? The winner is—all of these and more. The closer we get to understanding the structure and function of the mind-brain, the more anomalies slip through the cracks of our descriptions. Should our goal be to have complete understanding? Probably. To settle for a lesser goal may blind us to new insights: if we are not expecting large gains in scientific progress, we are less likely to experience them. However, to the degree that we can humbly marvel in wonderment at the vast unexplained mystery of mind, brain, and behavior, we are more likely to live in peace with ourselves and our neighbors. With admitted imperfection of the self comes the humility that is necessary in order to develop satisfying relationships.

The Core Principles of Cognitive Science

In reflecting over the vast mind-brain literature, we see several patterns emerge. These patterns may best be described as the core principles of cognitive science—the concepts essential to making sense out of the thousands of pieces of research available to us. As an aid to browsing through this book, I will state here what I see as the core principles.

Nativism. The principle of nativism holds that we inherit our behavior and that our environment can either nurture it to develop naturally or distort it by withholding nurturance (food, shelter, warmth, touch, affection, attention, and so on).

Unity. The principle of unity holds that the body and the mind are one and the same, and that a change in one will result in a change in the other.

Connectivity. The principle of connectivity holds that the establishment of new connections between prior learnings is the essence of growth and development and that the condition of the connection points, like the condition of the gap in a spark plug, determines how well we function.

Interconnectivity. The principle of interconnectivity holds that each identifiable element in our vast storehouse of experiences and learnings is connected to each of the other elements, some more strongly or closely and others more loosely or distantly (thus, to remember a name, we silently say the alphabet until the name pops out).

Control. The principle of control holds that the health of the human (and animal) organism is a function of the degree to which the individual feels in control of his or her situation, with less perceived control resulting in poorer health and performance and greater perceived control resulting in better health and performance.

The Nature-Nurture Debate: The Pendulum Swings

In the first edition of this book (1994), I made a moderately strong statement about nature having drawn even with nurture in their power to account for the causes of individual differences. In the five years since that time, the overwhelming accumulation of research supporting the genetic basis of individual differences renders that statement obsolete. William Wright, in his excellent summary of behavioral genetics research, *Born That Way* (1998), concludes that genetics is the hands-down dominant determinant of who we are. Although the statistical concordance rates suggest that genetics, or nature, accounts for over 50 percent of individual differences, the remainder is not necessarily accounted for by the environment.

> "A devil, a born devil, on whose nature Nurture can never stick, on whom my pains, Humanely taken, all, all lost, quite lost . . ."
>
> —Prospero, of Caliban,
> in William Shakespeare's *The Tempest*

Environmental influences come in two forms: shared and nonshared. Shared influence includes the example of my mother having played the piano for all seven of us kids, while nonshared influence includes the example of my mother being forty-five when I was born (and no longer a tennis player, with all that entailed). Wright cites research that conclusively identifies nonshared influence as second in influence after genetics, with shared influence accounting for almost nothing. And Judith Rich Harris, in her paradigm-challenging book *The Nurture Assumption* (1998), points out that this nonshared influence comes primarily from the peer group, not the home. Rounding out the influence pattern is what has come to be known as the phenomenon of genetics choosing environment (rather than the old-school paradigm of environment shaping behavior). Examples of this include my having chosen to spend relatively more time with my mother, because my high-openness genes found more expression there than with the low-openness profile of my father. I could have chosen to go fishing with him, but that wasn't my cup of tea; I preferred experiencing arts and crafts and music and literature with my mother.

Furthermore, Wright and others (for example, Loehlin, 1992) have documented the phenomenon of the "certain transitoriness of environmental effects" (Loehlin, 1992, p. 84), which says that as we age, we tend to become more like the genetic blueprint with which we started life. Or, as Columbia University's Nathan Brody once commented in a speech, "Change is the process of becoming more like who we are." Loehlin points out that it is this transitoriness of environmental effects on personality that accounts for the variations in test-retest scores with personality instruments. Firmly rooted gene-based behaviors are constant, while episodic, environmentally influenced behaviors are more likely to come and go.

Consider the following cases, which show evidence of the heritability of behavior in organisms as simple as bees and as complex as humans.

Honeybees

"Foul brood" is an infectious disease of honeybees that afflicts larvae in the cells of their honeycomb. Certain hygienic strains of bees fight the disease by locating cells that have the disease, opening the wax cap, removing the larvae, and moving them out of the hive. W. C. Rothenbuhler (Dawkins, 1989) discovered that the behavior of the hygienic bees was governed by two distinct genes—one gene for uncapping the cell and a second gene for dragging out and disposing of the diseased larvae. Unless both genes were present in a worker bee, the hygienic behavior didn't happen. If a bee possessed only the uncapping gene, it would gleefully fill its day uncapping the disease-containing cells but would not remove the afflicted larvae. Alone, without any of the uncapping bees around, bees with the removal gene would do nothing. However, if Rothenbuhler himself removed the wax caps, the removal bees would gladly spend their days dragging diseased larvae out of the hive. (This reminds me of a friend who loved to wash dishes: when our Boy Scout troop went camping, I would always cook, and he would always wash. He didn't cook, and I didn't wash.)

Twins

Neubauer and Neubauer (1990, pp. 20–21) relate two striking examples of this persistence of genetic material:

1. Two monozygotic twin girls were separated at birth and placed in homes far apart. About four years later, researchers interviewed the adoptive parents of each girl. Shauna's mother said, "She is a terrible eater—won't cooperate, stubborn, strong-willed. I can't get her to eat anything unless I put cinnamon on it." Ellen's mother said, "Ellen is a lovely child—cooperative and outgoing." The researcher probed, asking, "How are her eating habits?" The response was: "Fantastic—she eats anything I put before her, as long as I put cinnamon on it!" (p. 20).

2. Two monozygotic twin boys were separated at birth and placed in homes far apart. They were interviewed twenty-seven years later. Both had turned out to be obsessive-compulsive neatniks, scrubbing their separate homes often and constantly picking up and making things neat and clean. When they were asked to explain their compulsion for neatness, one attributed it to his reaction to an adoptive parent who was a slob, while the other attributed it to his upbringing by an adoptive parent who was a neatnik!

Most researchers currently studying this nature-nurture relationship are calling it a fifty-fifty ratio, attributing half the variation in behavior to genetics and half to environmental influence. For example, if your IQ is 20 points above the mean, or about 120, then roughly 10 of the points are attributable to genetic influence and the other 10 to environmental influence. The general conclusion of most behavioral genetics researchers, however, is that environmental influence serves as an enhancer or preventer of genetic predispositions and, therefore, that environment can't create dispositions for which no genetic basis exists. This current research is a confirmation of the ancient saw that you can't make a silk purse from a sow's ear.

Just how do twin studies lead us to this conclusion? Monozygotic, or identical, twins, who develop from one single egg, have identical genetic coding. Some sets of twins are separated from one another at birth; for example, they may be given up for adoption, with one twin moving to California, the other to Georgia. Other pairs grow up together. To the degree that environmental influences shape behavior, identical twins reared together would be expected to be more similar than those reared apart. That, however, is not the case; the similarity between identical twins does not increase if they are reared together. Separated identical twins show strong similarities, even in their religious feelings and vocational preferences.

However, we must beware the temptation to think of specific traits or behaviors as purely innate. Elman states, "There is virtually no interesting aspect of development that is strictly 'genetic,' at least in the sense that it is exclusively a product of information contained within the genes" (Elman and others, 1996, p. xii). There is no sociability gene, no fat gene, no rape gene. But there are genes that will interact with the complex landscape of environment and inheritance to explain all manner of things. Elman comments: "Nature and nurture are like the Batman and Robin of developmental theory: They hang around waiting in the wings, swoop in and solve a problem, and then disappear before they can be unmasked" (p. xii).

Conclusions Regarding Nature and Nurture

According to Pinker (1994, p. 357), "It is not so easy to show that a trait is a product of selection. The trait has to be hereditary. It has to enhance the probability of reproduction of the organism, relative to organisms without the trait, in an environment like the one its ancestors lived in." So to the degree that all traits are hereditary, they are adaptive; they are helpful to survival. Every trait then, whether it be anger or reliability, solitude or defiance, has its survival value.

It is important to acknowledge the inherited component of individual differences. This does not mean that we must disavow the efficacy of environmental nurture, however. Wrangham and Peterson (1996, p. 106) underscore this point when they lament Margaret Mead's falsification of Samoan data in favor of her favorite theory: cultural determinism, the doctrine that culture, not inheritance, is the basis of behavior. They write, "Cultural determinism . . . leads us to hope . . . , but it can also bring us to oversimplify necessarily complex problems and to avoid examining hard realities. It can lead to denial, and the regressive creation of a mythical Arcadia." John Watson (1925) once wrote, "Give me a dozen healthy infants, well-formed, and my own specified world to bring them up in and I'll guarantee to take any one at random and train him to become any type of specialist I might select—doctor, lawyer, artist, merchant-chief, and yes, even beggar-man and thief, regardless of his talents, penchants, tendencies, and abilities, vocations, and race of his ancestors" (cited in Pinker, 1994, pp. 406–407). But today we know better. We owe our behavior to both our genes and our upbringing. They are inextricably interdependent, the weft and the warp of personality.

SUGGESTED RESOURCES

Dennett, D. C. (1996). *Kinds of Minds: Toward an Understanding of Consciousness.* New York: Basic Books.

Gardner, H. (1985). *The Mind's New Science: A History of the Cognitive Revolution.* New York: Basic Books.

Hunt, M. (1982). *The Universe Within: A New Science Explores the Human Mind.* New York: Simon & Schuster.

Neubauer, P. B., and Neubauer, A. (1990). *Nature's Thumbprint: The New Genetics of Personality.* Reading, Mass.: Addison-Wesley.

Pinker, S. (1997). *How the Mind Works.* New York: Norton.

Restak, R. M. (1984). *The Brain.* New York: Bantam Books.

Restak, R. M. (1988). *The Mind.* New York: Bantam Books.

Restak, R. M. (1991). *The Brain Has a Mind of Its Own.* New York: Harmony.

Wright, R. (1994). *The Moral Animal: The New Science of Evolutionary Psychology.* New York: Vintage Books.

Wright, W. (1998). *Born That Way: Genes, Behavior, Personality.* New York: Knopf.

Web Sites

National Center for Biotechnology Information (Human Genome Project information):
    http://www.ncbi.nlm.nih.gov

2

Brain Basics

A Refresher Course in Hardware and Hormones

66 *We need education in the obvious more than investigation of the obscure.* 99

—*Attributed to Oliver Wendell Holmes, Jr.*

Once upon a time there were only lizards and other such reptilian creatures. The *lizard brain* was simple, geared only to the maintenance of survival functions: respiration, digestion, circulation, and reproduction. Over evolutionary time, the leopard and other such mammalian creatures emerged. Extending out from the lizard brain stem, the *leopard brain* (now called the limbic system) added to animals' behavioral repertoire the capacity for emotion and coordination of movement. This second phase of brain evolution yielded the well-known general adaptation syndrome (GAS), or fight-or-flight response (Selye, 1952). The evolutionary advantages of this syndrome are attested to by the disappearance of many reptilian species. The third phase of evolution was the *learning brain*—the cerebral cortex. This third and most recent phase of brain evolution provided the ability to solve problems, use language and numbers, develop memory, and be creative. MacLean (1990) refers to the three stages of brain evolution as *protoreptilian, paleomammalian* (early mammal), and *neomammalian* (late mammal). Figure 2.1 contrasts the three brain stages.

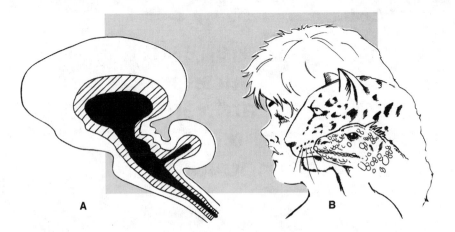

Figure 2.1. *Two Views of the Evolution of the Brain.*
Note: *(A)* The dark area represents the earliest appearance of the brain, the lizard or reptilian brain; the shaded area, the leopard or early mammalian brain; the light area, the learning or late mammalian brain. *(B)* Alternate illustration of these levels of brain development.

The millions of years of brain development from lizard to leopard to learner are repeated in each human embryo during the nine months in the womb. Thus, the development of an individual embryo (ontogeny) retraces (recapitulates) the evolutionary path of its ancestors (phylogeny). Scientists summarize this complex concept with those three words: ontogeny recapitulates phylogeny. The consequences of poisoning the brain with drugs or alcohol during pregnancy can be seen in infants whose development was arrested or thwarted at the lizard or leopard level. More complete yet highly readable treatments of brain development and function are available in Hunt (1982) and Restak (1984, 1988); a detailed encyclopedia of information is available in Gregory (1987).

Because this book is concerned with the day-to-day applications of brain science, I will not attempt to provide a complete physical description of the brain and all of its functions. It is not really important for you to know, for example, what the hypothalamus is or even what it does. I will dwell only on the physical aspects you should understand in order to apply the ideas presented here to everyday life. Two such physical aspects are the reticular activating system and the synaptic gap.

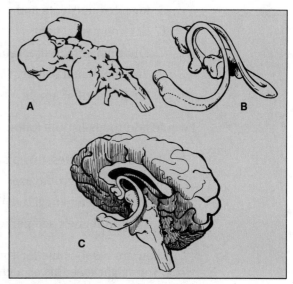

Two Key Features of the Brain: RAS and the Gap

A kind of "toggle switch" controls whether the leopard brain or the learning brain is currently in charge. This toggle, the *reticular activating system* (RAS), is located in an area beginning in the upper brain stem and continuing into the lower reaches of the cerebral cor-

Figure 2.2. Control Elements in the Brain.
Note: The reticular activating system *(A)* serves as a kind of toggle switch to allow either *(B)* the limbic system or *(C)* the cerebral cortex (shown with the RAS and limbic systems) to be in control of the brain at any one time.

tex (see Figure 2.2). RAS switching appears to occur at one of two times: when we become emotionally charged up or when we relax. When we become emotionally charged, as in the fight-or-flight response, the RAS shuts down the cerebral cortex, or learning brain. For all practical purposes, when the cortex is shut down, we proceed on "automatic pilot," where instinct and training take over. When the limbic system, or leopard brain, is shut down as a result of general bodily relaxation and removal of threat, the RAS switches the cortex back on and allows creativity and logic to return to center stage. The RAS is a large, diffuse neural process, and its effective functioning is important to both our personal survival and our ability to enjoy life.

Martin Moore-Ede, surgeon, physiologist, educator, researcher, consultant, and writer, talks about the nine "switches" that foster cortical alertness when activated (Moore-Ede, 1993):

1. A sense of danger, interest, or opportunity
2. Muscular activity
3. Time of day on the circadian clock
4. Sleep bank balance
5. Ingested nutrients and chemicals
6. Environmental light
7. Environmental temperature and humidity
8. Environmental sound
9. Environmental aroma

I would add to his list the following:

10. Recency of stressful episodes
11. Recency of aerobic exercise
12. Environmental negative ions
13. Degree of one's self-perception as being in control

If you are responsible for the overall effectiveness of a place of work, you might take this as a checklist for evaluating the degree to which that workplace fosters mental alertness. The overall effect of these switches is to influence our levels of alertness, described in Figure 2.3.

Another key feature of the brain is the *synapse*. The synapse is the point at which neurons, or nerve cells, connect with one another; its effective functioning is vital to our quality of life. A typical nerve cell is composed of a main cell body (with nucleus) and two branches, one outgoing and the other incoming, that serve as communication links with other nerve cells. The outgoing branch is called the axon, while the incoming branch is called the dendrite. The axon and the dendrite both have many connector points, so that a neuron can receive many messages through its dendritic terminals and send many different messages through its axonic terminals. The space where the axon of one neuron establishes a connection with the dendrite of another neuron is the synapse, or synaptic gap (see Figure 2.4).

Within each synapse, hundreds of receptors on the dendritic side wait for the proper chemical to be exuded from its dedicated

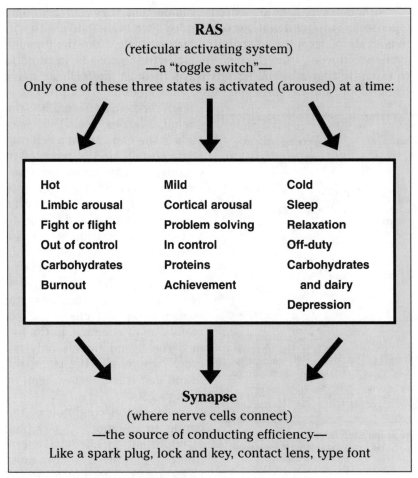

Figure 2.3. The Brain Process at a Glance.

axon. These chemicals are *ligands* or, as Candace Pert calls them, "informational substances"; they comprise three groups of chemicals: neurotransmitters, steroids, and peptides. These informational substances move from axon to dendritic receptor in a "lock-and-key" manner, in which one type of receptor and that type alone can admit its dedicated ligand. A given synaptic gap can contain multiple types of receptors, but each individual receptor can only admit its unique ligand. Only an endorphin can attach to an endorphin receptor, for example; dopamine would bounce off it.

Although synapses are extremely important, they represent only 2 percent of the total number of receptor sites in the body, with various kinds of receptors distributed far and wide, from the immune system to the gut, from the heart muscles to the gonads. In addition to synaptic transmission, ligands travel through intercellular space using blood and cerebrospinal fluid as a medium. This process is called *chemotaxis* (literally, "the chemical ferries itself"). Chemotaxis is the capacity of a cell that has a certain kind of receptor to detect, as if by radar, the presence of its ligands at some remote location within what Pert calls the bodymind. So, in addition to synaptic transmission, which is a direct form of intercellular connection, cells can connect, or communicate, by remote travel. The difference between synaptic transmission and chemotaxis is really one of distance. In the former, the ligand travels only microns, whereas in the latter, the ligand can travel inches, feet, or even meters.

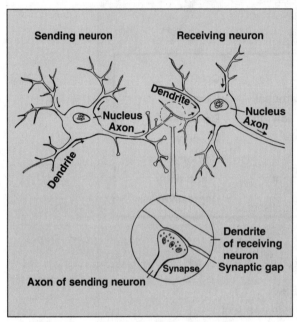

Figure 2.4. Basic Neuronal Structure.
Note: The lower, enlarged, area shows the synapse in some detail, while the upper area shows how it fits into the overall neuronal structure.

Just as the condition of the gap in an automotive spark plug is important to effective operation of a car, the receptors must be clean and in good condition for our nerves to work properly. You can clean the gap of a spark plug with a wire brush, and you can also clean the synaptic gap. Normal maintenance of the synapse is accomplished by the presence of *calpain,* a compound derived from calcium. Calpain acts as a kind of cleanser, dissolving protein buildup at the synaptic gap like a miniature PacPerson (remember the PacMan video game of the early 1980s in which a moving circular head gobbled a diet of dots?). The dietary source of the cleanser calpain is dairy products and leafy green vegetables. Too little calcium in the diet results in protein buildup at the synapse, with resulting loss of mental performance (for example, memory) as the buildup interferes with the ability of neural messengers to "jump" the synapse. On the other hand, if there is too much calcium in the diet, the excess calpain itself begins to interfere with neural transmissions. One drastic solution to remove protein from the synaptic gap is electric shock. Studies have shown that for aged patients with severe memory loss, improvements in memory lasted up to six months following shock treatment. Additional suggestions for caring for the synaptic gap appear in Table 2.1.

In a sense, RAS switching is the major determinant of our primary strategies from situation to situation (proactive-cortical versus reactive-limbic), whereas the condition of the synaptic gap and ligand receptors generally determines the effectiveness of the tactics we employ (memory, logic, creativity, movement, coordination, perception, and so on). The consequences of ineffective RAS switching are devastating. Recent studies have revealed tumors in the brains of some criminals. These tumors are hypothesized to have prevented

Table 2.1. The Care and Feeding of Synapses.

Sources	Work Examples
Environmental richness	Posters; sculpture; paintings; variation in paint, drapes, wallpaper; puzzles; games (mental and physical)
Diet	Follow National Research Council's Recommended Daily Allowances; do *not* eliminate fats, and avoid extremes of calcium (see Appendix A)
Snacks	For mentation: proteins and complex carbohydrates For relaxation: simple carbohydrates and fats
Exercise	Aerobic exercise 4 to 5 times per week
Atmosphere (such as ions)	Encourage fresh air for invigoration, not simple carbohydrates or caffeine; use air purifiers
Breaks	Encourage breaks after each learning episode (at least every 1½ hours)
Habits	Make new learning the organizational norm: skills, games, tapes, languages, names and faces; openly acknowledge and reward suggestions for improvement and new learning

RAS switching from the limbic system to the cortex, thus maintaining a level of rage behavior. In 1980, in Sacramento, California, a man turned himself in to authorities after repeated violent outbursts. His physician discovered that a tumor was causing pressure in a way that sustained limbic arousal. After surgical removal of the tumor, the pattern of rage disappeared. Apparently, the tumor had caused this man's RAS to lock up. Experimental efforts (Restak, 1984) to create the same type of uncontrollable rage have been carried out by implanting electrodes into the brains of bulls and cats. Activation of an electrode is the equivalent of constant pressure from a tumor. By simply turning a switch on or off, experimenters have turned rage and aggression on and off. An implanted cat in the middle of attacking a mouse would instantly turn friendly when the experimenter turned off the switch.

Neurotransmitters: The Alphabet of Personality

We are born with 100 billion brain cells, or neurons. It is not the number of neurons itself that determines our mental characteristics; it is how they are connected. Each cell reaches out to other cells through its axon (it "acts-on" other cells), with endpoints of the axon pairing up with receiving points on the dendrites ("end-right") of neighboring cells. Each neuron is connected to hundreds of other neurons by anywhere from one thousand to ten thousand synapses. Edelman (1992) estimates that it would take some thirty-two million years to count synapses in the cerebral cortex alone.

Learning is defined as the establishment of new neural networks composed of synaptic connections and their associated chemotaxic patterns. Gary Lynch of the University of California, Irvine, is one researcher who has confirmed that new synapses appear after learning. It is the density of the brain, as measured by the number of synapses, that distinguishes greater from lesser mental capacity. Ira Black (1991) defines knowledge as the "pattern of connectivity" between neurons, and learning as modifications to this pattern of connectivity. Only ten years ago, it was thought that learning consisted solely of the formation of new synapses. Today we regard the synapse as the structural center but acknowledge the vast intercellular movement through blood and cerebrospinal fluid as a coequal player in the learning process. The number of synapses and their condition, the circulatory system, and the cerebrospinal fluid form the stage upon which our electrochemical language plays out its drama. The alphabet of its physiological language is composed of over two hundred ligands.

The ligands are secreted by nerve cells, immune cells, and other cells that affect the formation, maintenance, activity, and longevity of synapses, neurons, and various organs. They are like the letters of the alphabet, with their "words" corresponding to behaviors. As words are composed of letters, with individual letters having predictable phonetic effects and groups of letters having predictable semantic effects, so behaviors are composed of ligand activity, with individual informational substances having predictable physiological effects and groups of them having predictable behavioral effects.

The ligands create two broad categories of effect: *excitation* (or *activation*) and *inhibition*. For example, one neurotransmitter will activate sleep and another will inhibit it. Drinking milk will trigger the release of melatonin, the neurotransmitter that activates sleep (and, along with the neurotransmitter serotonin, depression), but eating chocolate, which contains caffeine, will interfere with sleep. Still other chemicals serve as neuromodulators, affecting the intensity of excitation or inhibition. Intensity of transmission is measured by the *action potential,* an electrical charge with wave properties (see Figure 2.5). In the figure, Jane has a lower threshold for tasting salt (that is, she doesn't need as much for the same effect) compared to Janet. The *potential* for a "too much salt" response is not *activated* unless Jane's threshold is crossed.

The nature of the action potential is a key to understanding individual differences. Neurons don't even fire (react to a stimulus), for example, if the stimulus is too weak to cross the response threshold. The threshold for activation of a particular neuron is determined by a complex interplay of one's genetic code, physical condition (tired, pained, alert), and environment (noisy, light, cold, stimulating). Thus, although ligands constitute a kind of alphabet, other factors affect the nature of neural communication, in much the same way that volume, pitch, and speed affect how our spoken words are understood. I once counseled a young female manager who felt that she was being passed over unjustly for promotion to a field management position. Her manager declined her requests, saying that she was too valuable to be promoted. Her manner was so contrite that I speculated to her that her manager had most likely not heard her pleas for promotion; her voice and emotional level had not crossed his "threshold" for acknowledgment. She practiced a more forceful presentation, deliv-

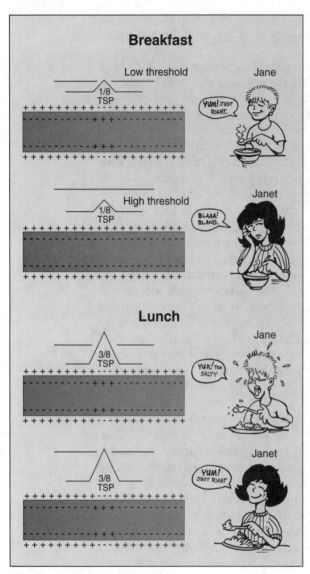

Figure 2.5. The Action Potential.

ered it to her manager, and was promoted within days!

Neurons average about three informational substances apiece: some may contain channels for only two, while others may have channels for five. Because each ligand can exist in a continuum of states—weak, medium, and strong—the types of information transmitted in one synapse can range from a dozen to a thousand. I have often thought of the human personality not as a computer but rather as something of a giant equalizer (see Chapter Twenty-One), the contraption stereo buffs use to modulate and transmit sound from their records, tapes, and CDs. Surely you've seen those electrical units with their levers and gauges hooked up to a stereo system. Well, the levers of the equalizer are analogous to the informational substances: one affects the quality of sound and the other the quality of behavior. A little less serotonin and more testosterone, a little less of the endorphins, the body's own tranquilizer—now we've got a real Bengal tiger on our hands! Add more serotonin—ah, now we're purring.

But this process is complex. Don't let my effort to simplify it obscure the vast interconnectedness of cells, chemicals, and systems. Black (1991, p. 37) writes: "Consideration of synaptic transmission has illustrated that the synapse is hardly a simple digital switch, enslaved to a few, simple physiological variables. Quite the opposite occurs. Synaptic communication is a remarkably flexible and changing process, subject to modification by intraneuronal, extraneuronal, local microenvironmental and even distant regulatory mechanisms."

Black goes on to describe the range of complexity of a single neuron. My summary of his description follows:

- Circuits of neurons are electrochemically coded.

- The circuits of a single neuron may use from two to five transmitters, or coded signal types.

- One transmitter may respond to stimuli independent of other transmitters.

- Each transmitter has multiple states (from two or three discrete states to a continuous state).

- So, for example, four transmitter types with three states each (weak, medium, and strong) would possess the potential for eighty-one distinct neuronal states.

- The number of neuronal states for a typical neuron may range from just under 100 to the thousands.

- Multiplying these numbers by 10^{11} neurons gives you some idea of the complexity of the system.

Following are some of the informational substances that appear frequently in the literature:

Norepinephrine (also called noradrenaline): This serves as a kind of "printer" that fixes information into long-term memory and helps to establish new synapses associated with memory. Rats deprived of norepinephrine can still learn but can't remember. The release of norepinephrine as a result of sympathetic arousal in the fight-or-flight syndrome explains why we so vividly remember information related to moments of shock, fright, or anger.

Calpain: This neurotransmitter serves as a cleanser when it is released by calcium into the synaptic gap.

Endorphins: Literally, this is the "morphine within" the brain, serving as a tranquilizer and analgesic. It is released in the presence of pain, relaxation exercises, vigorous exercise, and hot chili peppers.

Frank Etscorn, of the New Mexico Institute of Mining and Technology, injected endorphin blockers into the bloodstreams of jalapeño pepper eaters. The result was sheer agony. Hot chili peppers are not enjoyable without endorphin release.

Serotonin: Low levels are associated with depression, while increased levels are associated with sleep and relaxation. Serotonin is an amine that is metabolized from the amino acid tryptophan, which is produced in the pancreas by the hydrolyzing action of the enzyme trypsin on proteins. Serotonin constricts blood vessels and contracts smooth muscles; it and norepinephrine are both associated with the RAS switching mechanism: extreme levels prevent flexible switching. Serotonin is being closely observed in research on depression. While serotonin levels appear to be consistently related to depression, it cannot act alone in influencing depression. (In a 1983 UCLA study, a higher than average level of serotonin was found in dominant male vervet monkeys and in officers of college fraternities!)

GABA: GABA (gamma aminobutyric acid) is an inhibitor. Low levels of GABA in combination with low levels of serotonin are associated with violence and aggression. High levels of serotonin and GABA are associated with passive behavior. Franklin (1987) reported that levels of GABA drop while a person is watching violence in action, thus setting the stage for possible increased personal aggression.

Acetylcholine: Acetylcholine is a neurotransmitter that is metabolized from dietary fat (fat → lecithin → choline + cholinacetyltransferase → acetylcholine). It is absolutely essential to the health of the neuronal membrane: the cell wall becomes brittle without it. It is also necessary for activating REM (rapid-eye-movement) sleep, the stage of sleep in which we dream. That is why a minimum level of fat is necessary in our diet (see Chapter Five).

The Two Sides of the Brain

Volumes of research have documented the specialization of function in the two hemispheres of the brain, and this topic has captured the imagination of the reading public. Yet the practical, day-to-day implications are few. In addition, many of the findings are exaggerated, with fantastic conclusions drawn from scant data. We do know that the left brain is the seat of language, logic, interpretation, and arithmetic, while the right brain is the seat of geometry, nonverbal processes, visual pattern recognition (faces, lines), auditory discrimination, and spatial skills. We know that the left hemisphere governs activity on the right side of the body and the right hemisphere governs activity on the left side. We know that people of all ages inwardly exhibit measurable left-brain activity when they outwardly engage in approach behaviors, cheerfulness, and other such positive emotions. Avoidance behaviors and negative emotions, on the other hand, are associated with activity in the right brain (Fox, 1991). Many excellent summaries of this research are available (for example, Gazzaniga, 1985).

But while an abundance of literature is available on hemisphericity, the primary applications of its findings relate to medical and pharmaceutical research-and-development departments. Those of us out on the street can get little more than interesting poetry. A few everyday applications are available. For example, there is some evidence that talking, in and of itself, promotes positive emotions. If you know people who need cheering up, find ways to engage them in conversation, either actively or passively: go to a movie or carry on a conversation with a sick friend. There also is some evidence that artistic activity serves as a vehicle to express negative emotions. So if you know people who need to deal openly with negative emotions or experiences, try artistic, nonverbal modes of expression. However, to make a big deal, for example, out of "teaching to the right brain" makes appealing to one's creativity sound like something new. Hemisphere research has only confirmed that we have a more creative side and a more linear side.

SUGGESTED RESOURCES

Dennett, D. C. (1996). *Kinds of Minds: Toward an Understanding of Consciousness.* New York: Basic Books.

Gregory, R. L. (Ed.). (1987). *The Oxford Companion to the Mind.* New York: Oxford University Press.

MacLean, P. D. (1990). *The Triune Brain in Evolution.* New York: Plenum.

Pinker, S. (1997). *How the Mind Works.* New York: Norton.

Restak, R. M. (1994). *The Modular Brain.* New York: Scribner.

3

Tools of the Trade

Brain Imaging Technology and Other Research Methods

*T*wo popular resources enable current researchers to make progress in understanding the brain: imaging technology and animals. In this chapter, I will take a brief look at the options currently available and their unique capabilities. I will then summarize the reasons given for using animals to form conclusions about humans. Closing out the chapter, I will review the basic features of scientific method as they relate to brain research.

> ❝ *You cannot solve a problem with the same consciousness that created it.* ❞
> —*Albert Einstein*

Computerized Axial Tomography

Computerized axial tomography scans (also called CAT, or CT, scans) have been in use since the 1960s. The word *tomography* comes from the Greek *tomos,* or "section"; the word *tome* claims the same root. Tomography produces cross-sectional pictures of the brain that are like books, or tomes. When they are placed beside each other, they provide a 3-D image. CAT scans were first used in 1972. They combined X-ray technology and computer-imaging techniques to provide a more detailed image than X rays alone.

Positron-Emission Tomography

Positron-emission tomography (PET) catches the level of activity of specific areas of the brain at specific points in time. The mechanism consists of injecting very low level radioactive particles from a tracing solution directly into the brain's blood flow. The PET scanner monitors the emissions of these particles as they flow through the brain. When an area of the brain becomes active, it uses more blood and registers stronger signals on the scanner. The PET process has two drawbacks: first, because it uses radioactive material, it cannot be performed repeatedly on the same person, and second, it lacks speed. PET scans cannot be repeated rapidly enough to give a smooth depiction of a process or function.

Single-Photon Emission-Computed Tomography

Single-photon emission-computed tomography (SPECT) is a process similar to PET in that it uses radioactive particles. It is cheaper and easier to use than PET, but with a drop in its level of detail.

Magnetic Resonance Imaging

Magnetic resonance imaging (MRI) uses a machine in the shape of a huge tube that envelops the subject's whole body. Even with earplugs, the mighty racket is hard to eliminate. Regarded as the safest of the brain-imaging techniques, MRI has been around since the early 1980s, and its popularity is steadily growing. Basically, it provides a real-time image of blood-flow patterns, revealing what parts of the brain are active during particular tasks.

Researchers are able to view the way brain areas switch on and off as the subject performs different tasks. Rather than using radiation technology, MRI employs a complex interaction of radio waves and magnetic fields. Low-frequency radio waves (somewhat lower than FM radio waves) are emitted for the purpose of activating protons in brain tissue. Water molecules in different parts of the body respond differently to the presence of this wave-field. The resulting three-millimeter slices, or images, picked up by the superconducting electromagnet come together to form a 3-D portrait that tells the operator where surges in blood occur in relation to specific mental processes.

In 1991, Ken Kwong and Jack Belliveau of the Imaging Laboratory at Boston's Massachusetts General Hospital showed that MRI technology could be used to do more than take "still" pictures. Functional MRI (fMRI) was born; in fMRI, a series of pictures taken close in time actually portray a process, like a "moving" picture. The PET process is ineffective in taking such time-series shots because of its slowness: PET takes one minute to take the picture and nine minutes for the radioactive particles to dissipate. Thus, with PET, the steps of a function can only be described every ten minutes. With fMRI, a single shot takes from two to six seconds, and it can be repeated within seconds. The degree of faithfulness in portraying a process with PET and fMRI is like comparing the use of a thirty-five-millimeter still camera to that of a sixteen-millimeter movie camera.

Because it is both safe and noninvasive, fMRI can be used on any subjects, as long as they can handle the noise, the confinement, and the length of the session (up to one hour). Through 1997, the largest MRI machines were rated at 4 to 4.2 teslas, which are units of magnetic field strength. In 1998, The Ohio State University and the University of Minnesota each acquired machines rated at 7 to 8 teslas, a twentyfold increase in resolution, or clarity. Plans are under way for two 10-tesla machines to be installed, one on each coast of the United States. These larger-capacity imagers will permit giant steps in fields of research ranging from dyslexia to depression. But they don't come cheap. Researchers in early 1998 were charged an average of $439 per hour for using the fMRI setup, with the machine alone costing around $2 million. With the large price tag comes a good deal of flexibility: the fMRI machine can be programmed to perform a variety of analyses, including

- Classic structural scans

- Blood-oxygen-level scans

- Diffusion-weighted scans to detect the water level in damaged cells (used for stroke diagnosis)

- Perfusion-weighted scans to detect capillary blood flow

- Spectroscopy, for detecting levels of specific brain chemicals

Interpreting the output of a two-hour fMRI session is a mammoth undertaking. Approximately half a gigabyte of data is produced, the rough equivalent of four boxes of 3.5-inch computer disks. And the actual changes in blood flow that are measured are not huge swings; they typically represent around a 2 to 4 percent change. Multiple imaging technologies can be used in conjunction to provide complementary perspectives in order to improve diagnosis and understanding.

Optical Scanning

Currently under development, optical scanning is a device that attempts to use near infrared light to measure photons emerging through the skull. If successful, this technique could be used in the early detection of brain tumors.

The Use of Animals in Human Research

Both ethical and scientific questions surround the use of animals in human research. The benefits that humans derive from animal-based research continue to outweigh, in the eyes of most, concerns about the animals. The American Psychological Association (1992), along with other professional scientific associations, has established detailed ethical guidelines for the humane treatment of animal (as well as human) subjects. Professional researchers who do not adhere to these ethical guidelines are subject to disciplinary action.

Without animal research, the only way to test the effectiveness of pharmaceutical and surgical procedures would be with humans, or not at all. Without animals, experiments designed to identify the causes of human disorders would have to be done on humans, or not at all. Among the reasons neuroscientists feel comfortable using animals to test hypotheses about the human brain are the following:

- In rats, cats, dogs, monkeys, and humans, the brain consists of nerve cells and glial cells.
- All have equal numbers of neurons in their cortical columns.
- Neurons in all five have axons and dendrites.
- Synaptic complexity accounts for differences.
- All five communicate through the synapse.
- Neurotransmitters are similar in all five.
- Neurons all receive, store, and transmit impulses.
- Hormonal relationships are similar.
- The brains of all five are immature at birth.
- Brain development differs by sex for all five.
- Most of what we know about the human nervous system originated in animal research.

The Scientific Method: A Warning

Many of us tend to react to the reported results of scientific research as isolated fragments of absolute truth that identify predictable cause-and-effect relationships. The misery that can accompany such gullibility comes chiefly from two kinds of scientific report formats: the *correlation* and the *comparison of means.* A demonstration of the problems involved in accepting statistics without question is given in Figure 3.1. Helpful hints for detecting misleading presentations in statistical graphs and charts are also found in Darrell Huff's *How to Lie with Statistics* (1954), a classic still available in paperback.

The Correlation
Correlations are reported in statements such as "The more melatonin, the better you sleep" or "Melatonin is positively correlated with sleep" or "Melatonin and sleep are positively related" or "Melatonin and wakefulness are negatively related." We misunderstand these statements because they don't say that melatonin

A statement relating to the three boxes below might claim that one group scores higher than another. However, this statement does not, by itself, give you much information.

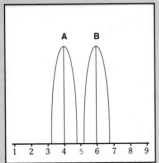 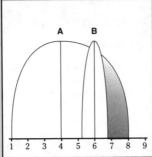 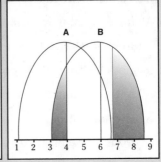

Why is this information incomplete?

- In all three examples, Group A scored an average of 4, while Group B scored an average of 6.
- In the left-hand box, however, *everyone* in Group B scored higher than anyone in Group A (this is very unusual).
- In the middle box, everyone in Group B outscored the average of Group A, but a substantial number in Group A outscored Group B altogether (shaded area).
- In the right-hand box, most of those in Group B outscored the average of Group A, but only a few outscored the highest scorers in Group A (right shaded area), and some scored below the average of Group A (left shaded area). Beware!

Why might a research finding not apply to you?

- Experiments conducted in clinics don't always apply to the everyday world.
- You may exhibit a particular feature that the research didn't account for, such as living in an unusual climate, having unusual dietary or exercise patterns, or being subject to environmental influences of which you may or may not be aware, such as gases or X rays.
- Your genetic code may render you resistant to the finding.
- You may be affected by medication you are taking, an illness you have or have had, or stress.
- Cultural differences may affect the findings.
- The statistics may be incompletely or misleadingly represented.
- The researchers may have made one of two basic errors:
  1. Saying that relationships or differences are present when in fact they are not
  2. Saying that relationships or differences are absent when in fact they are present

Figure 3.1. Why Statistics May Be Misleading.

causes good sleep, just that good sleep is more common among people who have more melatonin. The correlation doesn't mention, and probably doesn't take into account, other influences that might disrupt this relationship: daylight; other hormones; body weight; recency of eating a big meal, drinking alcoholic or caffeinated beverages, or consuming artificial sweeteners; high stress levels; the subject's age; the source of the melatonin; the environment (lab, airplane, bedroom, hotel) where the sleep was measured; and so on. It also doesn't specify whether the quality of the sleep was self-reported or was measured by an objective observer. All we know is that for some people, more melatonin means better sleep, but this may not be true for me or for you.

Recommendation: You must approach such conclusions with a cautious, experimental spirit. For example, try a warm cup of milk, which triggers melatonin production, before bedtime to see if you sleep better. If you don't, look for a possible influence that prevents the melatonin from "working," assuming that it really works. For example, don't drink alcohol close to bedtime.

The Comparison of Means

Comparisons of means are reported in statements such as "Males score higher on mathematics achievement tests, while females score higher on language achievement tests." We misunderstand this type of statement because it doesn't say how much higher each sex scores. The gender difference in math achievement scores is extremely small and is of little or no practical significance. The comparison also doesn't say which subtests are involved and whether the differences are true for all subtests. It doesn't say at what time of day the tests were administered; some evidence suggests that males' lower testosterone levels in the afternoon influence their achievement and females' lower estrogen-progesterone levels during the seven to fourteen days following ovulation influence theirs. In fact, if half the females in the sample took the tests during the two weeks following ovulation, which is a reasonable assumption, this could more than account for their lowered scores. In addition, we don't know whether the differences hold for all possible cultural groups—socioeconomic, ethnic, educational, and international. And the comparison doesn't say whether the range of scores of one group was similar to that of the other group. One group might score somewhat higher but with a very narrow range of scores, while the second group might score somewhat lower but with a wide range of scores.

In searching for the tallest person, for example, you would be more likely to find the tallest person in the second group (lower average height but with a wide range of heights) than in the first group (higher average height but with a narrow range of heights).

Recommendation: Realize that differences in average scores are differences in groups, not differences between individuals. Any individual may outscore or underscore members of another group, except in the rare circumstance when the ranges of scores do not overlap. The value of knowing about group differences is that it explains variations on some basis other than personal deficiency. For example, males tend to have better day vision, females better night vision, and this difference, where it is true, tends to increase with age. Here's how it applies to me: I typically do the laundry chores in our home, but if I do laundry in the evening, Jane sorts the socks. Acknowledging that this difference applies to us keeps her from accusing me of shirking!

The Caveat Box

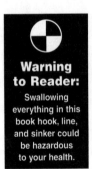

Warning to Reader: Swallowing everything in this book hook, line, and sinker could be hazardous to your health.

As a way of reminding you of the pitfalls of inappropriate reactions to scientific research results, I have come up with the Caveat Box. In the first edition, this message appeared throughout the book as a reminder to take statements with a grain of salt. We made the point emphatically! In this edition, we will show it only this one time. I hope you will view it both as a personal disclaimer—hey, I'm just passing on research reports—and as a consumer warning: life is not drawn in black and white, nor should our judgments be.

SUGGESTED RESOURCES

American Psychological Association. (1992). "Ethical Principles of Psychologists and Code of Conduct." *American Psychologist, 47,* 1597–1611.

Huff, D. (1954). *How to Lie with Statistics.* New York: Norton.

Shute, N. (1998, March 30). "The Ten–Minute Test for Strokes: New Breakthroughs in What MRIs Can See." *U.S. News & World Report,* pp. 69–72.

Part Two

*Getting
the Most
Out of
Every Day*

Wellness

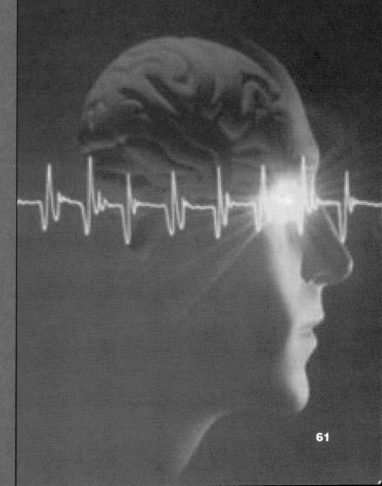

4

Starting Well

Windows of Opportunity

*T*raditional theories of child development, such as those of Jean Piaget, have emphasized stages, or steps. Accordingly, a child might be described as entering the "concrete operations stage." The mountain range of research data generated in child development centers around the world has wreaked havoc on this linear stage model, however, and a new, nonlinear, model is emerging. Robert Siegler, a psychology professor at Carnegie-Mellon

66 *Reckless youth makes rueful age.* 99

—*Thomas Moore*

University, has named it the "wave" model, implying that children might begin using a particular task or scheme earlier than was once thought and that at any given point in his or her development, a child might use as many as seven strategies that were formerly thought to appear at different stages. In any specific period of development, according to Siegler (1996), only one or two strategies typically predominate.

TOPIC 4.1   The Pregnant Brain: An Up-Front Note to Moms and Dads

I sometimes teach a module called "Gender Implications of Brain Research" for a local Women in Management seminar. On several occasions, women have asked me to explain their apparent (no, not apparent—real!) absent-mindedness and forgetfulness during late pregnancy and also in the postpartum period (during which memory maladies are joined by depression). Until now, my answer has been a combination of "We don't know" and "It's probably due to being awash in a sea of hormones." New findings from London's Royal Postgraduate Medical School, reported in the July 17, 1997, *Montreal Gazette,* help to clarify this. Anita Holdcroft, an anesthetist with the research team, reported that brain shrinkage of 3 to 5 percent during pregnancy is normal. Compare that to shrinkage of around 10 percent in Alzheimer's patients. Six months after delivery, the brains of all the women studied had returned to normal size. The shrinkage was found in all areas of the brain except for the pituitary, which in fact increased (this increase is related to the hormone bath). This finding helps to explain my students' concerns, as well as the finding of a research team at the University of Southern California. There, researchers administered cognitive functioning tests and found that 70 percent of the women in the ninth month of pregnancy exhibited difficulty in learning new information, with an average that was 15 to 20 percent worse than after delivery.

Application

When you experience an increase in absent-mindedness or some other decrease in mental effectiveness during late maternity and the early postpartum period, be amused at yourself and don't take it seriously. Know that your body is allocating resources elsewhere, and that all will be back to normal within six months after delivery.

TOPIC 4.2 Effects of Various Agents on the Embryo

During the first four months of pregnancy, brain cells in the embryo migrate from their original position to their ultimate destinations by way of glial cells, a type of supportive tissue. Alcohol appears to extend these migrations (the cells travel too far), whereas radiation appears to shorten them (they don't travel far enough). As a result, cells end up in the wrong location. The consequence is unpredictable malformation and dysfunction in the newborn infant. Heavier alcohol consumption during pregnancy may lead to mental retardation and abnormal physical development, whereas smaller amounts result in more subtle consequences. David Earnest led a Texas A&M University team that discovered that high doses of alcohol during the last trimester of pregnancy (actually, its equivalent period in rats) resulted in symptoms of advanced aging (*Houston Chronicle,* October 27, 1997, p. A5). The symptoms were those of a disrupted circadian rhythm, in which the rats' sleep was severely disturbed and erratic. Sleep disturbances are the second leading cause of institutionalization of seniors. Fetal alcohol syndrome, which was only discovered in 1973, is associated with a plethora of problems in adulthood: 90 percent of those born with this syndrome later have mental health problems, 60 percent have trouble with the law, 50 percent are involuntarily confined, and 50 percent are accused of inappropriate sexual behavior.

The effects of cocaine on the embryo are well documented in most daily newspapers, with lower birth weights, newborn withdrawal, smaller head sizes, and developmental delays among the consequences. Marijuana use during pregnancy appears to be associated with lower birth weights. Pregnant women who consume multivitamins have children with a 25 percent greater incidence of spinal-column defects. Prescription drugs can also have damaging effects on the embryo; double- and triple-check a prescribed drug before exposing an embryo to it. The effects of nicotine are mentioned in Topic 6.6.

Applications

1   Make no assumptions about what is safe to consume while pregnant. Instead, consult your obstetrician. If you are not sure of the advice you are given, consult a neuropharmacologist; if you are still not sure, do your own library research.

2   The first four months of pregnancy are especially critical. If you think there's a chance you are pregnant, assume you are and consume accordingly.

3   Pregnancy is a good time for mommy and daddy alike to have a nine-month moratorium on alcohol, tobacco, and other drugs. Find benign but acceptable substitutes, such as exotic juices, exercise, and snacks.

4   According to the National Institute on Drug Abuse, 25 percent of the four million babies born annually in the United States have been exposed to some legal or illegal drug and have thereby been placed at risk. Don't let your baby, or the baby of someone close to you, be one of these statistics.

TOPIC 4.3   Prenatal Learning

Increasing research (see Lecanuet, 1995) points to the fetal environment as crucial in the formation of personality, tastes, and even ability. Garlic in the amniotic fluid, for example, appears to predispose a child to accept garlic later in breast milk. Gestating infants learn to prefer their mother's voice patterns and heartbeat and recognize them after birth in contrast to those of strangers. The fetus can also learn to habituate to a stimulus (pay less attention to it over time), a precursor of later ability. The heart rate of the mother varies with the heart rate of the fetus: the mother's heart starts beating faster, then the baby's follows suit. Stress for the mother equates to stress for the fetus: higher cortisol in the mother is accompanied by higher cortisol in the fetus.

Application

Don't underestimate the value of the nine months of pregnancy as a time to begin providing the optimum environment for your child. Introduce different tastes, your favorite music, dance steps, and other experiences you enjoy.

| TOPIC 4.4 | **Temperament and the Prediction of Adult Personality** |

The term *temperament* refers to neurological processes that are (1) inherited and (2) observable as behaviors from infancy, even, in some cases, "observable" in the womb. Such examples of temperament are

- *Activity:* The number of times the infant moves her or his head, arms, hands, legs, or feet per unit of time

- *Adaptability (anger):* How quickly an infant adjusts, for example, to the disappearance of a parent

- *Approach/withdrawal:* The tendency to examine a novel object or person or back away

- *Attentiveness/persistence:* How long an infant persists in focusing his or her attention on a particular object or person

- *Rhythmicity:* The regularity or irregularity with which an infant defecates, urinates, gets hungry, and goes to sleep

- *Sensory sensitivity:* How much sensory stimulation (light, heat, touch, smell, noise) an infant is comfortable being around

These infant behaviors, known as the temperament of the child, foreshadow later adult personality. While temperament is inherited, adult personality is based on inheritance plus what is learned from the environment. But what is learned must form around the core of these inherited neurological processes (Halverson, Kohnstamm, and Martin, 1994).

Adult personality (see Chapter Twenty-One for a more complete treatment) is currently described in terms of the "Big Five" traits, and each of these traits has at its core one or more of the infant temperaments:

- The adult trait of Negative Emotionality concerns one's capacity for dealing with stress: rhythmicity predicts it.

- The adult trait of Extraversion concerns one's capacity for sensory stimulation: activity level and sensory sensitivity predict it. Very active infants who are comfortable with lots of stimulation tend to become more extraverted.

- The adult trait of Openness concerns one's breadth of interests: approach/withdrawal predicts it. Infants who approach and examine tend to be more innovative and creative.

- The adult trait of Agreeableness concerns one's tendency to submit to or defy others: adaptability predicts it. Infants who get angry when a parent departs tend to become challenging and egocentric as adults.

- The adult trait of Conscientiousness concerns the degree to which one is self-disciplined and focused on goals: attentiveness/persistence predicts it. Infants who spend longer periods of time focused on a single object or person tend to be more ambitious and self-disciplined as adults.

Application

While these infant precursors of adult personality are not 100 percent predictive, they are strong indicators. Begin at a child's earliest age to appreciate her or his individuality. Understand that attempts to suppress or change these inherited neurological processes can result in unhealthy development on the child's part. Rather than wishing a child were more still (that is, less active), celebrate her or his activity level and don't expect the child to be a retiring introvert as an adult.

TOPIC 4.5   Breast-Feeding

In *Early Development and Parenting,* Virginia Polytechnic Institute psychologist Philip Zeskind reports on an experiment with fourteen breast-fed babies and fourteen bottle-fed babies (Zeskind, Marshall, and Goss, 1992). He describes the nervous systems of bottle-fed babies as "engines out of tune," and those of breast-fed babies as well tuned and efficient. Breast-fed babies have overall lower heart rates and are more alert. They are also somewhat more irritable and sleep less, but Zeskind sees this as a desirable trade-off. In a larger study published in *The Lancet,* Dutch scientists followed 526 children for nine years. The findings: children who had breast-fed for at least three weeks were half as likely to suffer from neurological abnormalities as formula-fed children.

In a study conducted in New Zealand with more than one thousand children followed from birth to age eighteen, David Fergusson and John Horwood of Christchurch School of Medicine reported that breast-milk-fed babies scored consistently higher on a variety of cognitive measures, including standardized math and reading tests, teachers' ratings, and high school course grades (*New York Times,* January 6, 1998, p. F4). The longer a child was nursed, the greater the cognitive gains. Incidentally, in December 1997, the American Academy of Pediatrics changed its minimum recommended period of breast-feeding from six months to twelve months.

Applications

1 If you are the mother of a newborn, do what you need to do to breast-feed your baby as long as you can.

2 Many states have laws that make public breast-feeding a crime. Florida struck down its statute in March 1993. Help your state do the same if it has such a law.

TOPIC 4.6   Infant Feeding: Schedule Versus On-Demand

Gary and Anne Marie Ezzo have developed a "Preparation for Parenting" course aimed at a conservative Christian market. The course is supported by the book *On Becoming Baby Wise,* coauthored with pediatrician Robert Bucknam (Ezzo and Bucknam, 1998). The course recommends parent-controlled feedings on a three-hour schedule, rather than feeding on demand, which they say leads to kids becoming undisciplined, whining, demanding brats. Doctors say that there is no scientific basis for parent-controlled feeding. Some infants need to eat on shorter cycles, as little as ninety minutes apart. Doctors fear (and see evidence) that parent-controlled feeding can lead to nutritional deficiencies, dehydration, insufficient weight gain, and developmental abnormalities. Babies go through growth spurts, and their nutritional needs can change from day to day. The American Academy of Pediatrics guidebook recommends: "Your baby lets you know when he's hungry. Whenever possible, use [the baby's signals] rather than the clock to decide when to nurse him. Your baby's feeding needs are unique. No book can tell you precisely how much or how often he needs to be fed, or exactly how you should handle him during feedings. You will discover these things for yourself as you and your baby get to know each other" (Dietz and Stern, 1999).

Application

Do not let ideology interfere with the natural process of becoming attuned to your child's needs. Kids as well as adults do not all follow the same daily cycle of feedings. When a forty-year-old feels stomach pains, it's time for a carbohydrate snack. This doesn't show a lack of discipline. The car's running out of gas, and if it wants to get to its destination, you had better put something in the tank. Just because the car can't make it all the way without a little something extra doesn't mean it's a spoiled brat.

TOPIC 4.7 The Critical Early Years (Ages One to Three)

A growing body of research suggests that the first three years of life are critical to brain development. During this period, the infant has twice as many neurons *and* twice as many synapses as adults. By puberty, a radical pruning occurs that leaves the child on a more even playing field with adults.

William Staso, a school psychologist in Orcutt, California, in his book *What Stimulation Your Baby Needs to Become Smart* (1995), recommends seven critical periods to address:

1. *Month 1:* Eliminate background distraction (radio, television, washing machine) so your baby is optimally relaxed and attentive to your talking, singing, or other foreground activity.

2. *Months 1–3:* For proper neural articulation, emphasize contrasts (light versus dark colors, low versus high pitch, simple versus complex timbre, rough versus smooth textures). Parenthetically, it is interesting to note that children whose fathers were actively involved in the first six months of their care scored higher on subsequent measures of intellectual and motor development.

3. *Months 3–5:* For visual development, use pictures of baby's real-world objects (spoons, cups, wagons) as part of play activity.

4. *Months 6–7:* Emphasize cause and effect (turn the knob and the door opens), locations of various objects ("Where's the kitty? There she is!"), and functions of environmental objects ("What does the ball do? Bounce! See!").

5. *Months 7–8:* Emphasize sound as a signal of impending events (running water and a bath, car in the driveway and "Fonzy's back!").

6. *Months 9–12:* Explore motor and sensory skills and how they combine (turn the faucet and feel the water). Twelve-month-olds can remember behaviors they have observed for thirty seconds for up to one week. By around twelve months of age,

infants typically learn one or two new behaviors daily simply by observing people in their environment.

7. *Months 13–18:* Explore objects in the environment; this is the time to make the environment especially diverse and rich. Explore sequences and relationships (build towers of diverse shapes, make trains of different sizes—bigger, smaller, bigger, smaller, . . .). Psychologist Harlene Hayne finds that eighteen-month-olds can remember observed behaviors for up to one month.

Recent research has established parental nurture, specifically touching and stroking, as essential not only for healthy development in animals and humans but also for normal neuronal growth. Mark Smith, of the Du Pont Merck Research Laboratories, Wilmington, Delaware, found that laboratory animal infants deprived of maternal care lost brain cells at twice the rate of those who were left with their moms. Stroking stimulates the production of chemicals that inhibit the stress hormones—including cortisol—that kill neurons. In fact, Ron de Kloet, a neurobiologist at the University of Leiden in the Netherlands, reported at the October 1997 meeting of the Society for Neuroscience in New Orleans that even substitute parenting helps to avoid the chemical damage resulting from maternal deprivation. By stroking newborn mice who were deprived of their mothers with a moist brush (which simulated mom's licking) for one minute three times a day (sound like a prescription?), researchers were able to eliminate most of the neuronal damage that typically results from maternal deprivation. Mary Carlson of Harvard Medical School studied two- to three-year-old Romanian infants raised in orphanages or sent to poor-quality day care centers. She found that the orphans had abnormally high and lasting levels of cortisol, and that the day care children had abnormally high cortisol levels on weekdays; however, when they returned home for the weekend, their levels returned to normal (*Los Angeles Times,* October 28, 1997, p. 1A). High levels of cortisol are associated both with the destruction of brain cells and with learning and memory problems.

Craig Ramey, a psychologist at the University of Alabama in Birmingham, cites evidence that disadvantaged children benefit from a rich educational curriculum and a loving environment. Infants enrolled in such educational programs five days a week had IQs fifteen points higher than those of similar children who were not helped; the difference was first observed at the age of two.

Applications

1 Support early childhood interventions such as Head Start and an expanded Family and Medical Leave Act.

2 Expect and work toward the highest quality in day care programs. The U.S. Department of Defense has been cited for exemplary quality in its day care programs.

3 Make a poster of the seven periods identified above by William Staso. Use it as an aid in remembering what to emphasize in your play with your (and others') infants.

4 Ensure that the infants in your life receive touches and stroking from birth and throughout every day of their lives.

5 If you (as a nurse, aide, teacher, social worker) are around infants and have an idle moment, pick them up and hold or stroke them. In a recent trip to visit a friend in a hospital, I saw two nurses at the reception area of the floor I visited who were holding babies from the nursery, cooing, stroking, cradling, singing, laughing—generally giving pleasure and enjoying it. I don't know if they knew the research, but they were certainly engaged in behavior that the research strongly encourages.

6 For more details, obtain a copy of the Carnegie Corporation of New York's 1994 report, *The Early Brain,* by visiting its web site at www.carnegie.org.

TOPIC 4.8 Maturation and the Brain (Ages Two, Six, and Twelve)

The supplies of minerals inside our bodies are critical to the formation of new synapses. Without these raw materials, we could not build new connections between neurons, which means that we could learn nothing new. Eric Lenneberg (1967), a psycholinguist, has demonstrated that we experience three spurts of mineral production as we mature: (1) around age two, when we learn to walk and talk; (2) around age six, when we start to read, do math, and write; and (3) around age twelve, when we begin to reason abstractly. After the third spurt, which is associated with puberty, no more occur. Lenneberg reasons that after this third spurt, major new learnings become much more difficult. That is why, for example, it becomes harder to learn foreign languages after elementary school.

Applications

1 One reason some children learn to walk, talk, read, and so on earlier than others is that they begin their spurt of internal mineral production earlier. Without the minerals, they simply aren't ready. When they are ready, they will learn. Don't push children before they are ready, and don't fret or reprimand a child who appears to lag behind others. It doesn't signal that the child is lacking in ability; it just demonstrates his or her unique biological timetable.

2 The more varieties of experience children have before puberty, the more resources they have to build on as adults. Childhood experiences become the building blocks for adult accomplishments.

TOPIC 4.9 Irreversible Damage (Age Eight)

Generally, studies point to eight years of age as the point after which brain damage is irreversible. While neurons can be replaced, the current evidence is that replacement is slow and meager. However, in young children, other parts of the brain can pick up functions lost due to brain damage. The story is frequently told of a five-year-old who lost one entire hemisphere; this individual is now fifty years old and possesses an above-average IQ. After the age of eight, such recovery appears to be impossible.

On the other hand, loss of brain function is different from loss of brain cells. If the cells remain and only function is lost, growing evidence of the brain's plasticity suggests that dramatic recoveries are possible. Richard Restak (1997, pp. 50–51) tells the story of a seventy-eight-year-old woman who suffered a four-year worsening loss of mental function. When it was finally diagnosed as an obstructed cerebrospinal flow, doctors inserted a shunt and, to their surprise, found that she experienced significant recovery of mental function.

Applications

❶ Every time you put your children in an automobile, buckle them up with seat belts and car seats.

❷ Have high expectations for children younger than eight years of age who are recovering from brain damage.

❸ Be prepared for the possibility of permanent loss of function from brain damage that occurs after eight years of age.

TOPIC 4.10 Adverse Conditions and the Resilient Child

In a special issue of the *American Psychologist,* Ann Masten and Douglas Coatsworth (1998, pp. 205–220) conclude that two factors are associated most with the tendency of some children in unfavorable, adverse environments to emerge with competence in meeting the developmental tasks of growing up, from language development and self-control to the ability to form close friendships and succeed in both academic and extracurricular performance. The first factor is the child's relationships with *prosocial* (as opposed to antisocial) adults, whether they are within the immediate family or outside the family. The second factor is the possession of good intellectual functioning, including problem-solving ability, language comprehension and vocabulary, and logical-mathematical ability. Apparently a lack of sufficient brainpower reduces some children's ability to be clever in resisting and escaping antisocial influences.

Applications

❶ Focus on the schoolwork of at-risk children and help them to develop the cognitive skills that foster quick thinking; creative, out-of-the-box solutions; and patience in problem solving, so that they can take the time to understand the causes of problems and generate multiple possible solutions.

2 Focus on the social development of at-risk children, helping them to build long-term relationships with adults who are making ongoing, positive contributions to society, whether they are teachers, coaches, Big Brothers or Big Sisters, internship sponsors, career mentors, family members, neighbors, public safety officers, employers, co-workers, club advisers, social workers, or the members or staff of religious organizations.

TOPIC 4.11 Memory in Early Childhood (Infancy to Ages Seven to Ten)

The formation of memory involves both storage and recall. Infants appear to have an unusually high incidence of failure to store new memories. According to a panel of early childhood researchers at the April 1995 meeting of the Society for Research in Child Development (reported in the *APA Monitor,* June 1995, pp. 1 ff.), the storage failure rate begins to decline around age seven and reaches a normal rate at about age ten. However, under the proper circumstances, children can store memories permanently starting at the age of two. The panel described the proper circumstances as events having to do with the personal values, goals, and pleasures of the two-year-old.

Application

If you would like your two-year-old or older child to especially remember a particular experience, you must periodically assist the child in recalling the event.

TOPIC 4.12 The Adolescent Brain

Deborah Yurgen-Todd, director of neuropsychology and cognitive neuroimaging at McLean Psychiatric Hospital, Belmont, Massachusetts, has found that teenagers process emotions and instructions differently from adults. Functional MRI images that compared young people aged nine to seventeen with adults aged twenty to forty revealed that the young people processed emotions, instructions, and procedures much more consistently in the amygdala (the seat of emotions), while adults processed the same activities more consistently in the frontal lobe (the seat of rationality). In addition to processing these activities in an emotion-ridden manner—as if normal conversation were being passed through an emotional filter—the young people found it more difficult to accurately identify emotions expressed in the faces of other people. Part of the explanation for these phenomena relates to the continuing development of white matter necessary for complete communication. The frontal area of the brain does not appear to be fully mature until around the age of thirty.

Applications

1 When young people respond emotionally, understand that the storm is natural and not to be taken personally. Let it pass like a summer shower and get on with life.

2 Take care to educate your young people over time in the correct identification of the emotions of others in their lives. Accurately identifying emotions is a development-related skill.

3 When young people follow directions imperfectly, understand that internally, the directions had to pass through a tempest-tossed sea. Supplement the original instructions or directions with spoken or written reminders or crutches. And be kind. Expect incomplete reception of your original message. Don't be blameful; be patient. And be glad when they've grown out of it!

SUGGESTED RESOURCES

Alkon, D. L. (1992). *Memory's Voice: Deciphering the Brain-Mind Code.* New York: HarperCollins.

Caplan, T., and Caplan, F. (1982). *The Second Twelve Months of Life.* New York: Bantam Books.

Caplan, T., and Caplan, F. (1984). *The Early Childhood Years: The Two to Six Year Old.* New York: Bantam Books.

Caplan, T., and Caplan, F. (1995). *The First Twelve Months of Life* (rev. ed.). New York: Bantam Books.

Halverson, C. F., Jr., Kohnstamm, G. A., and Martin, R. P. (Eds.). (1994). *The Developing Structure of Temperament and Personality from Infancy to Adulthood.* Hillsdale, N.J.: Erlbaum.

Leach, P. (1997). *Your Baby and Child: From Birth to Age Five* (rev. ed.). New York: Knopf.

Lecanuet, J. P. (1995). *Fetal Development: A Psychobiological Perspective.* Hillsdale, N.J.: Erlbaum.

Sears, W., and Sears, M. (1993). *The Baby Book.* New York: Little, Brown.

Shelov, S. P. (1998). *Caring for Your Baby and Young Child* (rev. ed.). New York: Bantam Books.

5

Nourishment

Food for the Body, Fuel for the Brain

66 *The best doctors in the world are Doctor Diet, Doctor Quiet, and Doctor Merryman.* **99**

—Jonathan Swift

*A*s recently as World War II, scientists as well as the general public considered diet to have little or no influence on mental functioning. Research over the last forty years, however, has revealed a close relationship between diet and the brain—so much so, in fact, that trendy brain bars are popping up that specialize in juices and foods considered to improve mentation, or mental activity. It is becoming clearer that our brain influences what and how we eat, and that what and how we eat influences our brain. This chapter identifies various specific findings in this arena of the food-brain connection.

| TOPIC 5.1 | **Recommended Food Balance** |

The National Research Council, after reviewing more than five thousand studies, published a thirteen-hundred-page report in 1989 entitled *Diet and Health: Implications for Reducing Chronic Disease Risk*. A popular version of the report was published later (Woteki and Thomas, 1992). For a detailed summary of the report, see Appendix A (for a current version, check the home page of the USDA Center for Nutrition Policy and Promotion at www.usda.gov/fcs/cnpp). In general, the researchers found that Americans eat excessive amounts of fat, simple carbohydrates, and protein and insufficient amounts of complex carbohydrates (see Table 5.1). In addition, they found that dietary supplements, especially if they are taken beyond the recommended daily allowance, have no benefits and may be toxic. Exceptions exist; consult your physician if you are in doubt.

Table 5.1. Imbalance in American Diets.

Type of Food	Today's Menus	Better Menu
Fat	36% of calories	30% or less of calories
Cholesterol	Men: 435 mg daily Women: 304 mg daily	Less than 300 mg daily
Carbohydrates	45% of calories	At least 55% of calories
Protein	Men: 1.75 times the RDA[a] Women: 1.44 times the RDA	No more than twice the RDA

Source: Adapted from "The Latest Word on What to Eat" by Anastasia Toufexis, March 13, 1989, *Time*, 133(11), pp. 51–52.
[a]RDA = recommended daily allowance.

Applications

Note: All of the following recommendations assume that you engage in a reasonably active lifestyle.

❶ Emphasize fish, skinless poultry, lean meats, low-fat or non-fat dairy products, and complex carbohydrates (fruits, vegetables, and starches). Complex carbohydrates should comprise more than half the daily allowance of calories.

❷ Limit egg yolks, organ meats, fried foods, fatty foods (pastries, spreads, dressings), animal fat (it has no known benefits and may cause cancer), alcohol, and most shellfish (there is some debate over which; scallops are apparently okay).

❸ Eliminate dietary supplements, such as vitamins and minerals, except as recommended by a reputable doctor. Megadoses, unless specifically prescribed by a physician, have questionable benefits and may be toxic. Calcium supplements, fish oil capsules, and fiber supplements provide no established benefits; these ingredients must be consumed in their normal state, in food. Consult a neuropharmacologist if you are in doubt about the effects of supplements and megadoses. Vitamin megadoses taken by expectant mothers have shown adverse effects on the spinal columns of their newborns.

The subject of dietary supplements is both a huge industry and a raging debate. Richard Restak (1997, p. 37) says, "No one is certain, with most experts now favoring an increased intake of fruits and vegetables rather than of vitamin supplements," while Robert Haas (1994) encourages a variety of supplements. Restak concludes that vitamins and minerals are best utilized in interaction with the joint effect of other plant chemicals (in other words, vitamins should be taken in plant form, not pill form). Hedge your bets by eating right and taking a modest supplement, like one daily multivitamin. Many of the so-called 100 percent safe and mind-healthy supplements do not withstand the test of time and research. Recently, the Federal Trade Commission required the makers of Herbal Ecstasy, who claimed "absolutely safe natural highs," to include a warning label concerning the risk of damage to the heart and central nervous system. And a ten-year, $43 million study of beta-carotene reported in the May 5, 1997, *New England Journal of Medicine* found that megadoses of beta-carotene (ten times the U.S. Recommended Daily Allowance) among 29,133 older male smokers resulted in 18 percent more lung cancer in the experimental group than in the controls. See also the discussion in Topic 5.11.

4 Fat should comprise no more than 30 percent of your daily calories. As a general guide, one tablespoon of peanut butter has eight grams of fat, or ninety calories, so a daily allowance of 2,100 calories translates to the equivalent of no more than seven table-spoons of peanut butter per day. (Much debate centers around the recommended level of fat in the daily diet. Those with cardiovascular disease should follow a guideline that allows a maximum of 10 per-cent of the daily calorie allowance for fat rather than 30 percent.)

5 Of the fat maximum (the equivalent of seven tablespoons of peanut butter a day), no more than 10 percent (that's less than the equivalent of one tablespoon of peanut butter) should be saturated fat, such as coconut oil or animal fat.

6 Limit alcohol to the equivalent of two regular cans of beer per day or two small glasses of wine (that is, no more than one ounce of alcohol daily). *Exception:* Expectant mothers should consume no alcohol.

7 Limit protein to eight grams per kilogram of body weight a day. For a 180-pound person, that would be one 8.4-ounce hamburger patty per day; for a 120-pound person, one 5.6-ounce hamburger per day.

8 Limit salt to about a teaspoon per day.

9 I could recite a litany of the effects of various vitamin and mineral deficiencies, such as thiamine deficiency, which causes memory loss, and iron deficiency in expectant mothers, which results in brain slow-down in their children. Suffice it to say that failure to consume a balanced diet will take its toll on brain function. If you are in doubt, consult your physician or take a reputable multivitamin (not a megavitamin!).

TOPIC 5.2 Daily Calorie Allowance

Russell Wilder, senior physician at the Mayo Clinic, found that any diet of under 2,100 calories per day is deficient in some vitamin, mineral, or trace element, unless it is tailored by a physician for a patient. Of course, this 2,100-calorie target is based on a nonexistent "average" person. Adjustments are required to allow for an individual's gender, body type, and lifestyle. After three months on an excessively low-calorie diet, people exhibit faulty memories, increased error rates, inattentiveness, clumsiness, panic, nightmares, feelings of persecution, anxiety, hostility, and quarrelsomeness (Minninger, 1984).

Regularity is also helpful. University of Arizona neuropsychologist Gary Wenk cautions that stuffing at holidays (yourself, not the turkey!), for example, results in memory loss because less oxygen reaches the brain (it diverts to the tummy), as well as raising other health risks. Wenk's research recommends a daily allowance of 1,200 calories for optimum longevity and mental function. I have seen no corroboration of Wenk's findings, but they are consistent with other studies (mostly on mice) that associate minimal calories with maximal longevity.

Applications

1 Do not limit yourself to fewer than 2,100 calories (adjusted for gender, body type, and age) for a sustained period without being monitored by a physician.

2 If you wish to follow Wenk's recommendation of 1,200 calories, do so under a physician's supervision. Monitor vitamin and mineral levels periodically.

TOPIC 5.3   Appetite Control

Two primary chemical actors head the complex cast of characters in the tense drama of appetite control: chemicals that trigger hunger and chemicals that trigger satiety. If these are in good order, much of the rest of one's chemical makeup will have a minimal effect on appetite and weight control. Significant discoveries have entered the scene in the last five years, and huge pharmaceutical product development research efforts currently focus on finding acceptable exogenous (externally administered) ways to optimize a person's hunger-satiety balance. Current estimates based on twin studies consider the genetic influence on weight to be extremely high—around 60 to 70 percent. Combined with the meager 5 percent success rate of diets, this paints a bleak picture for the role of self-control in weight management. Authorities suggest that we'd be better off changing the environment than trying to change the individual. Do we hear a movement afoot to abolish fatty fast food? The environmentalists formed the Sierra Club. How about the Soybean Club for the nutritionists!

Sarah Leibowitz, a neurobiologist at Rockefeller University in New York City, has identified the area of the brain in which this drama plays out: the paraventricular nucleus (PVN) of the hypothalamus. Chemical players that trigger appetite include galanin (discovered by Leibowitz, this is a neuropeptide that craves fat), norepinephrine, neuropeptide Y, and cortisol. Chemical players that shut down appetite include enterostatin (produced by the stomach and pancreas in response to the ingestion of fat), serotonin, dopamine, cholecystokinin (CCK), and leptin (from the Greek *leptos*, "thin"), a protein produced by the newly discovered "obesity gene" on chromosome 6. In addition, a research team led by Masashi Yanigasawa at the Howard Hughes Medical Institute at the University of Texas Southwestern Medical Center in Dallas has reported the discovery of two hormones that send a hunger message (*Cell*, February 20, 1998). Yanigasawa calls these hormones orexin-A and orexin-B. The orexins have their own receptor network in the hunger section of the hypothalamus and have been found to send an extremely strong hunger signal in mice. Development is under way for use with humans as both a stimulant and a suppressant of appetite.

David York, of the Pennington Biomedical Research Center at Louisiana State University, learned that enterostatin shuts off the pleasure system of the brain (see Topic 19.7), which is activated in ecstasy as a response to fat consumption. Fat loses its appeal when enterostatin levels are sufficiently high. Low galanin levels are associated with low fat intake, and high galanin levels are associated with high fat intake, *unless* enterostatin levels are also high, when fat intake will be limited (because fat satiety is reached more quickly). If enterostatin levels are low, then fat satiety will be delayed, *unless* galanin is also low, when little fat will be ingested. More recently, Stephen Bloom, an endocrinologist at the Royal Postgraduate Medical School in London, announced in *Nature* the discovery of a suppressor similar to enterostatin named GLP-1 (glucagon-like peptide-1), whose receptors are located in the hypothalamus.

The 1997 spring issue of *On the Brain* (Harvard Mahoney Neuroscience Institute Letter) announced the identification of leptin receptors in the hypothalamus. Leptin is secreted by adipose tissue (fat cells) as a messenger to the hypothalamus with information about whether it wants more fat, less fat, or is just fine, thank you. Obese mice lose their excess fat when injected with leptin. Roger Unger of the University of Texas Southwestern Medical Center at Dallas reported in the April 29, 1997, *Proceedings of the National Academy of Sciences* that leptin is also active in burning up fat inside the adipose tissue. So leptin performs at least two functions: it metabolizes fat within fat cells and it sends messages to the hypothalamus. Apparently, although I haven't seen this reported, leptin is the instigator of the hypothalamic secretion of galanin. The overall process (see Figure 5.1), then, is something like this: fat cells send leptin to the hypothalamus, which interprets the information and decides when to send out galanin to fish for fat, which results in the release of enterostatin when the fat hits the pancreas.

In a recent and related discovery, researchers at the University of California, Davis, announced in *Nature Genetics* (March 1997) the discovery of a gene that governs what one does with excess calories: whether one converts it into normal body heat or stores it as fat to "get through winter or famine." The protein associated with this gene, UCP2, occurs at high levels in animals who do not gain weight from high-fat diets. With the discovery of this process, and of leptin receptors in particular, great strides will surely be made in carrying this new knowledge closer to a harmless drug for appetite control.

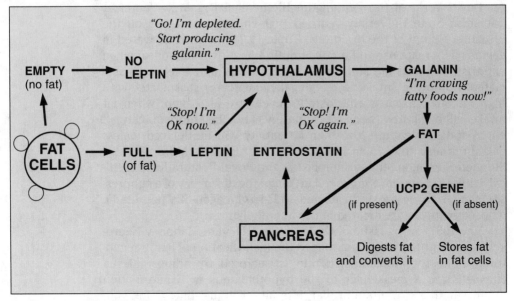

Figure 5.1. How Fat Cells Work.

Current drugs for appetite control treat symptoms, not causes. One such symptom is the increase in dopamine and serotonin levels produced by fat consumption—a kind of reward system first discovered by Bartley Hoebel of Princeton University. The triggers and suppressants listed above relate to the causes of good and poor appetite control. Drugs like phentermine (increases dopamine), Prozac (increases serotonin), Orlistat (blocks fat absorption), fenfluramine (increases serotonin), and dexfenfluramine (a component of fenfluramine known commercially as Redux) do not address the root causes of craving and satiety, but rather provide the effect of pleasure from having eaten, thereby covering up the cravings. Recent warnings suggest that only the morbidly obese should use the powerful "Fen-phen" combination of fenfluramine and phentermine; studies show ill effects on the heart, lungs, and brain in both animals and humans. Even the drugs prescribed singly, like Redux (dexfenfluramine by itself), are oversubscribed, according to Mark Molliver of Johns Hopkins University School of Medicine. Molliver was quoted in the March 17, 1997, *Dallas Morning News* as saying, "I've gotten calls from patients all over the country. They are 20 pounds overweight and were given Redux. I think it's being used to a degree that's completely inconsistent with medical ethics." Part of the question has been resolved: in September 1997, the Food and Drug Administration pulled both dexfenfluramine (Redux) and fenfluramine (Pondimin, half of the Fen-phen combination) off the market because of their link to serious heart problems.

Sarah Leibowitz has identified the chemical sources of urges for specific food groups, as well as the time of day during which the urges are strongest (Collin, 1992, p. 74). A summary is shown in Table 5.2.

Yale University researchers reported at a spring 1998 meeting of the Society of Behavioral Medicine in New Orleans that high cortisol levels are associated with high cravings for fatty snacks. When they are given a choice, high-cortisol snackers head for the nachos, while low-cortisol snackers head for lower-fat snacks. Cortisol levels are increased by stressful experiences.

Another line of research has identified three levels of body chemistry: *nontasters, tasters,* and *supertasters.* One's level is determined by two genes: the gene for tasting PROP (6-n-propylthiouracil) and the gene for determining the density, or number per unit area, of fungiform papillae on the tongue. Fungiform papillae are the housings for taste buds. Nontasters cannot taste PROP (it tastes just like water or paper) and have fewer papillae. Tasters can taste PROP; it tastes bitter to them. Supertasters can taste PROP and have denser concentrations of papillae; to them PROP tastes extremely bitter. Not

Table 5.2. The Chemistry of Food Urges.

Food Group	Chemical Basis of Desire	When Desire Is Strongest
Carbohydrates	Turned on by norepinephrine, neuropeptide Y, cortisol; turned off by serotonin	On waking and early morning; desire decreases as the day goes on
Protein	Turned on by serotonin, opiates; turned off by neuropeptide Y, norepinephrine, dopamine, galanin	Alternates with carbohydrates in morning; rises gradually toward middle of day; peaks at dinner and evening
Fat	Turned on by galanin, opiates, aldosterone; turned off by dopamine	Desire increases during middle of day and predominates in evening

Source: Adapted from "Sarah Leibowitz (Interview)" by Fran Collin, May 1992, *Omni, 14*(8), p. 74.

only does the intensity of taste increase as the number of papillae rises; the number of pain receptors also increases. Roughly 25 percent of people in the United States are nontasters and 25 percent are supertasters, with tasters making up 50 percent of the population.

Nontasters eat a wider variety of foods than the other two groups. A higher proportion of females, Asians, and blacks are supertasters. Supertasters tend to have lower cholesterol and to be less obese. To the supertaster, bitter tastes more bitter, sweet tastes more sweet, fat tastes more creamy, and salty tastes more salty. Ginger, alcohol, carbonated beverages, and chili's capsaicin all create a greater sensation of burning on the supertaster's tongue. Supertasters are more likely to reject bitter foods such as green tea, soy products, grapefruit, coffee, cabbage, broccoli, mustard greens, saccharine, Brussels sprouts, and spinach. The University of Michigan's Adam Drewnowski, a professor of environmental and industrial health, is using a National Cancer Institute grant to determine if such taste preferences are causing women with breast cancer to reject foods high in antioxidants. Supertasters appear to experience an advantage in the battle of the bulge. Some research suggests that they find fatty and sugary foods too intense and avoid them (reported in the *American Psychological Monitor,* January 1998, p. 13). Because the aversion to bitter foods in supertasting women increases significantly during the first trimester of pregnancy (when toxins can do the most damage to a fetus), researchers suspect that the supertaster status prevalent among women is an evolutionary advantage.

Understand that preferences and aversions in regard to certain foods are not imaginary; they are genetic. To find out how you stack up, do two things. First, get some phenylthiocarbamide (PTC) paper from your local chemical supply store. Tasting these paper strips will let you know if you can taste PROP. If they just taste like paper, you are 50 percent on your way to being a nontaster. Second, swab your tongue with some blue food coloring. Then find one of the small, circular, lifesaver-like stickers used for reinforcing the holes in notebook paper. Place it in the center of your tongue, toward the tip. Near a mirror, shine a flashlight on the circumscribed area and count the number of papillary bumps (the blue sticks to everything but the bumps). The more bumps you have, the more of a taster you are. Nontasters tend to have around five bumps, while supertasters can have thirty or more.

Applications

1 If you have a problem with being overweight, have your doctor look for products that either limit galanin production, bind galanin receptors, or increase enterostatin or leptin levels.

2 If you have a problem with being underweight, have your doctor look for products that boost galanin production, stimulate galanin receptors, bind enterostatin or leptin receptors, or use some combination of these techniques.

3 Until better medical intervention based on recent discoveries becomes available, your best help for appetite control is to exercise regularly and to manage your environment so that fatty, sugary alternatives are not available.

4 Save fat consumption for evenings, when desire is strongest for most of us.

5 When eating an early-evening meal, minimize carbohydrate consumption and maximize protein. When eating very late, minimize protein to avoid interference with sleep.

6 When possible, after a stressful episode, dissipate cortisol with exercise before subjecting yourself to the temptations of fatty snacks. For example, during a break, rather than heading for the snacks, try taking a ten-minute brief walk first.

TOPIC 5.4 Taste

The tongue recognizes different tastes differently. Sweet is identified on the tip of the tongue, sour on the sides, bitter on the back of the tongue (hence the gagging that often accompanies bitter tastes), and salt all over, but especially in the front (Ackerman, 1990).

Applications

1 If you are tasting an unpleasantly sour substance, try to avoid having the substance touch the sides of your tongue.

2 If you are tasting something to determine if it is bitter, understand that you are not getting an accurate reading until the substance hits the back of your tongue. It is then natural to gag it up and out, as that is the only way to bypass the back of your tongue if you don't want further experience with the substance.

3 If you are eating something too sweet or salty and you must continue, avoid placing the substance on the front of your tongue.

4 For information on nontasters, tasters, and supertasters (and chili peppers), see Topic 5.3.

TOPIC 5.5   Metabolism

Paul Moe, research leader in the Energy and Protein Nutrition Laboratory of the U.S. Department of Agriculture, reports that in their human experiments in the calorimeter (a nine-by-ten-foot chamber that measures oxygen input and carbon dioxide output with eighty thousand sensors to determine total energy expenditure), they found no differences in the efficiency with which different people metabolize food. Their conclusion was that differences in weight can't be blamed on differences in metabolism; they result from excess eating and/or deficient exercise.

William Bennett (1991) argues, however, that each body has its own "set point," or genetically programmed level of body fat. It would be a lifelong battle to attempt to maintain a lower set point. For example, if a woman's set point is 150 pounds and she decides to drop 10 pounds, her body will forever be trying to recover the lost fat. Bennett argues that to minimize fat, we should avoid the two things that tend to raise our set point: inadequate exercise and excessive fat consumption. He's convinced that simple overeating in and of itself is not the culprit. In a study where subjects were overfed 900 calories a day for fourteen weeks, identical twins gained weight at about the same rate, while gains from 9½ to 29 pounds were reported for unrelated people. Bennett maintains that the metabolisms of any two people at their set point would appear normal. Hence, his findings seem compatible with Moe's.

More recently, a team of scientists from New York's Rockefeller University determined that metabolism maintains a tenacious hold on weight. After losing 10 percent of their body weight, patients expended 15 percent less energy than expected for someone of their newly acquired reduced size. Reporting in the *New England Journal of Medicine,* Kassirer and Angell (1998) explained that the body resists weight change, struggling to return to its former weight. This has been explained as an evolutionary boon to more primitive peoples subject to famine and spartan winters, but a bane to modern folk plagued with daily abundance. This regulatory system appears to keep everyone at her or his normal weight, whether slim or heavy. In a 1997 Harris poll of overweight adults who dieted, two out of three reached their target, while only one in nine kept the weight off (the average loss was thirty-four pounds, the average rebound gain, thirty-one). There is evidence that this set point can be adjusted over a substantial length of time: sustained high-fat diets can raise it and sustained exercise programs can lower it.

How seriously should you fight the metabolic tug-of-war? The current indicator among nutrition experts is the BMI, or body mass index. A BMI of 30 or higher (some say 25) is cause for concern and indicates a need to get one's weight down by lowering fat intake and increasing exercise. A BMI of 40 or higher is considered morbidly obese and strongly suggests a need to take pharmaceuticals, whose risks are outweighed by the risks resulting from obesity. Here is how you compute your BMI (from Gibbs, 1996, p. 90):

$$BMI = w/h^2$$

w = weight in kilograms (pounds divided by 2.2)

h = height in meters (inches divided by 39.4)

Applications

1 When there's a choice, walk; don't ride.

2 When there's a choice, stand; don't sit.

3 When there's a choice, exercise or escape; don't snack.

4 Serve smaller portions. A couple in our neighborhood maintain trim profiles without exercising, yet without giving up any favorite foods. We've sworn they had to have God-given metabolisms that allowed this indulgence. A while ago, we had them over for dinner. Because the serving dish was in front of the woman, she served the stew in bowls to the rest of us. To my consternation, I noticed that my portion barely covered the bottom inch of a bowl with a three-inch wall! I looked at my wife, who knowingly smiled back at me. Later that night, we agreed: it isn't just metabolism; it's portion size. We both grew up in homes where large portions were served. If we didn't eat large portions and ask for seconds, our mothers took it as rejection. We have to rescript ourselves to feel all right about eating smaller portions. The task is clear—and uphill!

5 When you are hungry between meals, avoid fatty snacks.

6 If you are confident that your exercise and diet levels are appropriate for you, learn to accept your set point and not feel guilty.

7 A thorough review of dieting issues is available in Brownell and Rodin (1994).

TOPIC 5.6   The Role of Fat

Fat is the dietary source of acetylcholine, a neurotransmitter that is crucial to maintaining the condition of neural cell membranes. While too much fat is unhealthy, too little fat is also unhealthy: with too little acetylcholine, the neural cell membranes will become brittle and deteriorate over time. The result of this deterioration is memory loss and a general decrease in brain function. Dietary fat metabolizes into lecithin, which further metabolizes into choline, which then, with the help of the catalyst cholinacetyltransferase, metabolizes into acetylcholine. Some research indicates that doses of choline can improve the problem of severe memory loss.

A series of meta-analyses (DeAngelis, 1992) suggests that low-fat diets, while improving death rates from heart disease, increase death rates that result from suicides, homicides, and accidents. This apparent relationship between low-fat diets and negative affect adds emphasis to the potential dangers to the human system of too little fat.

Application

Do not eliminate fat from your diet! Aim for the recommended daily allowance (see Topic 5.1, Application 4).

TOPIC 5.7 Food and Mood: The Role of Carbohydrates, Proteins, Fats, and Sugars

The four food groups act on mood and the brain in the following ways:

Protein (in flesh, legumes, tofu): Contains an abundance of the amino acid L-tyrosine, which produces norepinephrine and dopamine (leading to elevated alertness and stable memory)

Complex carbohydrates (in vegetables, grains, fruits): Contain an abundance of the amino acid L-tryptophan, which is necessary to produce serotonin (leading to a sense of satiety and relaxation)

Fats (in dairy, meat, oils): Important for the production of acetylcholine, which is crucial for memory formation and general neural integrity (an absence of acetylcholine leads to the breakdown of neural membranes and advanced aging)

Simple carbohydrates (sugars): A quick energy booster, but without the "time-release" quality of complex carbohydrates, which provide glucose for longer periods (sugars alone lead to sluggishness)

The brain needs 180 grams of carbohydrates per day. Complex carbohydrates (grains, seeds, beans, fruits, and vegetables) metabolize more gradually and provide a steadier release of glucose for use by the body. Simple carbohydrates such as sugar, on the other hand, provide a quick rise in blood sugar followed by a letdown. To give you a rough idea of how much food is required to ingest 180 grams of carbohydrates, a small banana contains 21 grams.

Haas (1994) points out that the sequencing of proteins and carbohydrates is important. If you're having a "California"-style salad for lunch and want to be alert after lunch, eat the chicken (protein) first, so that the L-tyrosine gets to your brain first. Then eat the rest of the salad, with L-tryptophan lagging. Eating in this order ensures that you get the energy from the carbohydrates without the sleepiness. If you eat the carbohydrates first or simultaneously with the protein, the tryptophan will dominate and reach the brain first, thus establishing lower arousal and higher relaxation.

A Hebrew University research team led by Nachum Vaisman learned that children aged eleven to thirteen showed improved performance on cognitive tests when they consumed milk and cereal within thirty minutes of the test. Children who had eaten breakfast at home two hours before the test showed no improvement in cognitive performance over children who hadn't eaten breakfast at all. Apparently the boost in brain sugar levels just preceding the test also boosted performance.

Applications

1 Serve mainly carbohydrates and fats prior to an event where you want people relaxed and easy to please, such as a sales presentation.

2 Serve mainly proteins prior to an event where you want people alert and analytical, such as a staff meeting. Or put protein out first, carbohydrates later.

3 Save fats for the evening, when you crave them most and when you have the least need for alertness.

4 Time snacks to just precede a time of day when you need a boost in mental performance (a test, a presentation, a meeting, a new learning challenge, an important new sales call).

5 Follow this recommended daily meal and snack content:

> *Breakfast:* Complex carbohydrates + protein (skim milk + cereal)
>
> *Mid- to late-morning snack:* Complex carbohydrates (fruits or grains)
>
> *Lunch:* Protein first (chicken or shrimp cocktail), then complex carbohydrates
>
> *Afternoon snack:* Complex carbohydrates (fruits, vegetable juice, or grains)
>
> *Dinner:* Complex carbohydrates, fats, minimal protein
>
> *Bedtime snack:* Complex carbohydrates, sugar, fats (at last, banana ice cream!)

TOPIC 5.8   Breakfast

Ernesto Pollitt of the University of Texas Health Science Center at Houston compared the school performance of children who skipped breakfast to the performance of those who ate a good breakfast (Pollitt, Leibel, and Greenfield, 1981). Those who ate breakfast made measurably fewer errors as the morning wore on. Other studies of both children and adults have confirmed this finding.

Application

Don't skip breakfast. If you must eat on the fly, at least grab a piece of bread that's not dredged in fat and sugar, or a banana, or a glass of milk.

TOPIC 5.9   **Violence and Sugar**

Many studies report drops in violent acts when, for example, residents of detention centers are fed low- or no-sugar diets. Stephen Schoenthaler (1983), of the Social Justice Program at California State College, Stanislaus, reports from a 1980 study at the Tidewater Detention Center in Chesapeake, Virginia, that high-sugar diets promote violence in this way: whenever the limbic system and the cerebral cortex have to vie for scant supplies of glucose, the limbic system always wins. With a high-sugar diet, the body is left depleted of blood sugar when a hit of dietary sugar wears off because insulin is released to shut down the body's production of glucose; the limbic part of the brain then gobbles up all of the available glucose, starving the cerebral cortex and making emotional behavior dominant (the limbic system is in control) and pushing rational behavior into the background.

When I taught high school, I once had a violent student in my eleventh-grade homeroom. I called his parents in for a conference. The mother (the father was on the road) described a typical day. I noticed that the boy was rising at 5:30 A.M. in order to catch a 6:15 A.M. bus to school. Meanwhile, the mother stayed in bed. The son left the house without human contact or food intake, stopped by a convenience store on the way to the bus stop, grabbed a grape soda and a pack of doughnuts or cookies, and caught the bus. When he arrived at school, therefore, he was on a sugar high and was affable and demonstrative for about one hour; then, after the sugar wore off, he started hitting people. Why didn't his mother fix breakfast? Because he didn't like her breakfasts. I asked what he'd eat if she fixed it. We agreed on a hamburger and a glass of milk, of all things. Within two weeks, his old pattern had changed, succumbing to that of a reasonably likable seventeen-year-old. I'm sure that he benefited not only from the substantial breakfast, but from having some contact with his mother before leaving home.

The February 3, 1994, *New England Journal of Medicine* reported a blind study with forty-eight children aged three through ten who were given diets high in sucrose, aspartame, or saccharin. Behavior and mental performance remained similar among all groups. In another study reported in the January 1994 issue of *Pediatrics,* fifteen children with attention deficit disorder received ten times the normal daily amount of aspartame; they didn't act any differently from those taking a placebo.

Applications

1 Ensure that sugary foods do not replace healthy foods; at most they should only supplement them.

2 Look for other causes of behavioral problems than sugar and sweeteners.

TOPIC 5.10 Sodium

Sodium is not just bad for hypertension and the heart. Overconsuming sodium can also lead to electrolyte imbalances and accompanying mental dysfunction. The typical body requires about 1,000 milligrams of sodium daily and about five times that much potassium. (The balance between sodium and potassium is important for effective neural transmission.) To give you a rough idea of how easy it is to overconsume sodium, one tablespoon of soy sauce contains about 1,000 milligrams, or the recommended daily allowance.

Applications

1 Don't salt your food, or at least limit yourself to one shake or pinch.

2 Use a variety of spices and peppers to compensate tastewise for lessened salt intake.

TOPIC 5.11 Vitamin and Mineral Deficiencies

Vitamin and mineral deficiencies result from either insufficient intake or inadequate absorption. The first can be fixed by a varied and balanced diet composed primarily of fresh or frozen foods. The second can be fixed by appropriate injections administered by a physician. The consequences of a sustained deficiency are fatigue, loss of appetite, poor concentration, failing memory, depression, and insomnia. You can confirm and specify a suspected deficiency through a blood test at a laboratory qualified to test for vitamin and mineral content.

Now that I have said that, consider what Jane E. Brody describes as "Vitamania" (*New York Times,* October 26, 1997). From 1990 to 1997, spending on vitamin and mineral products more than doubled, from roughly $3 billion to $6.5 billion, according to the Council for Responsible Nutrition in Washington, D.C. Yet this buying pattern is not based on any clear results. The notion that vitamin and mineral supplements benefit healthy people who consume a balanced diet is supported by meager evidence. And even for those who need more vitamins and minerals—the elderly, smokers, the undernourished, the sick, pregnant women—the research findings are uncertain. Interestingly, most of the consumers of supplements are active nonsmokers who do not drink alcohol heavily, eat more fruits and vegetables and are better educated than the norm, and have comfortable incomes. One thing is clear: vitamin takers do not live longer or die less frequently from cancer, based on a thirteen-year study of over ten thousand Americans by Atlanta's Centers for Disease Control and Prevention, and this 1993 report (available from their web site at www.cdc.gov) also found no support for the notion that vitamin and mineral supplements can compensate for slack eating habits.

Brody concludes that consumers are, in essence, voluntary subjects in a national marketing-driven experiment. Enough good, long-term studies on the effects of vitamin and mineral supplements are simply not available, and the jury is still out on their relative helpfulness and harmfulness. A few bits of good news are available: supplements can remedy the deficiencies that cause such diseases as scurvy and rickets. But nothing is available that addresses cancer, heart disease, osteoporosis, longevity, and overall well-being. In addition, a considerable list of dangers is emerging, including the following:

- Vitamin E megadoses (a relative term, but suggesting more than the USRDA) can interfere with Vitamin K (which affects blood clotting).

- Calcium megadoses limit the absorption of iron and perhaps that of other trace elements.

- Although taking 500 milligrams of vitamin C daily does have an antioxidant effect, British doctors at the University of Leicester reported in *Nature* (April 1998) that it also has a pro-oxidant effect, attacking DNA. They join Victor Herbert of Mount Sinai School of Medicine in New York, who has been arguing for decades that extra vitamin C promotes free radicals (unlike the vitamin C in orange juice, which is an antioxidant).

- Zinc megadoses can reduce the body's copper levels, interfere with immune responses, and decrease levels of high-density lipoproteins (the "good" cholesterol).

- Folic acid megadoses can mask Vitamin B-12 deficiency and adversely affect anticonvulsant medications.

The one certainty that emerges from these studies is the benefit of eating a variety of foods, minimizing fat, and maximizing fruits, vegetables, and complex carbohydrates. And to hedge your bets, take a daily multivitamin. In fact, on April 7, 1998, reversing a trend of discouraging vitamin supplements, the National Academy of Sciences recommended for the first time that members of the following two groups take specific supplements:

1. Women of childbearing age need 400 micrograms of folic acid daily. That amount is guaranteed in most multivitamins and is difficult to get through a normal diet. Insufficient folic acid in these women increases the chance of birth defects in their offspring.

2. Adults over age fifty need 2.4 micrograms of Vitamin B-12 daily in order to minimize the chance of developing anemia. Between 10 and 30 percent of people over the age of fifty lose the ability to absorb B-12 from food.

Applications

1 Vitamin supplements are best absorbed when taken with other foods. Caffeine, however, obstructs absorption, so take your multivitamins with a meal that does not include coffee, tea, or caffeinated sodas.

2 Mineral supplements are best absorbed between meals.

3 If you think that you have some of the symptoms of a deficiency, take a blood test to determine your vitamin and mineral content.

4 To get the most nutrition from your foods:

- Replace canned food with fresh or frozen food.
- If you use canned food, retain and use the juices in other dishes, unless you detest high sodium.
- Keep milk and bread in opaque containers.
- Don't leave food in the freezer too long.
- Use fresh juice immediately, preferably the same day it is squeezed.
- Avoid soaking vegetables.
- Choose pressure cooking, steaming, microwaving, or boiling to cook vegetables, using minimum water, leaving skins on, and cooking the vegetables the shortest amount of time possible.

5 Factors that obstruct absorption, destroy nutrients, or both include the following:

- An excessively low calorie count
- Alcohol
- Nicotine
- Tannin
- Aspirin
- High fiber in the diet
- Medications
- Cooking

6 Hedge your bets and take a multivitamin! I do.

TOPIC 5.12 Food Additives

Ben Feingold of the Feingold Association has found that people, especially children, react to food additives that interact with the natural salicylates in good food (A. Winter and R. Winter, 1988). Food additives include artificial sweeteners such as aspartame, flavor enhancers such as monosodium glutamate, preservatives such as nitrites, artificial colors, and artificial flavors. Aluminum-based additives (found in antacids and double-acting baking powder) appear to have especially adverse effects on the nervous system. Reactions include poor concentration, short attention span, fidgeting, aggressiveness, excitability, impulsivity, a low frustration threshold, clumsiness, and insomnia.

Applications

1 Avoid foods with additives for yourself, your loved ones, friends, and co-workers. Just don't make them available. While this subject is still being hotly debated, it would seem wise to minimize or eliminate additives in the diet, especially for expectant mothers and children exhibiting the symptoms described above.

2 Read food labels to check for additives, especially aluminum.

3 Candace Pert (1997) cautions us not to eat any food that is not six thousand years old! In other words, let the test of time guide food selection.

TOPIC 5.13 Diet and Peak Physical Performance

At the request of the U.S. Army Research Laboratory's Military Nutrition Division, the National Academy of Sciences' Committee on Military Nutrition Research looked at the contribution of six food groups to various aspects of military performance. The goal: to improve soldiers' physical and mental performance through nutrition by 10–15 percent by fiscal 1998. Their recommendations are listed here as Applications.

Applications

1 Use carbohydrates (found in cereals, grains, vegetables, and fruits) to increase your capacity for physical work and reduce anxiety. A special Kool-Aid type of brew boosted with powdered carbohydrates has been found to enhance performance.

2 Use caffeine to increase mental alertness and physical endurance. (For proper dosage, see Topic 6.3.)

3 Use tyrosine (this amino acid is found in proteins, especially nuts, and is particularly high in cashews and sesame seeds) to better withstand extreme cold and to better adjust to high altitudes. The army uses a powdered supplement in a food such as applesauce.

4 Use choline (found in egg yolks, liver, and soybeans) to increase mental clarity. Choline also has been shown to take five minutes off a marathoner's time.

5 Use carnitine (found in red meat, liver, and heart) to increase physical performance over a long period of time.

6 Use structured lipids (a manufactured product used in hospitals to boost the caloric intake of some patients) to strengthen immune responses and to decrease susceptibility to disease and infection.

TOPIC 5.14 Undernourishment and Performance

In the February 1996 issue of *Scientific American,* Larry Brown, of the Tufts University Center on Hunger, Poverty and Nutrition Policy, and Ernesto Pollitt, of the University of California, Davis, School of Medicine, reported on a major study involving over two thousand children in Central America. By providing calories, protein, vitamins, and minerals, researchers observed reverses in poor academic performance that had been attributed to poverty. Other research has demonstrated that a major effect of undernourishment is significantly lessened social interaction, adding lack of exposure to lack of mental energy.

Application

For children in poverty, academic intervention alone is not enough to improve performance. They need protein and calories as well as instruction and caring. Support programs in your region and elsewhere that provide nutritional supplements for children in poverty.

SUGGESTED RESOURCES

Bouchard, C., and Bray, G. A. (Eds.). (1996). *Regulation of Body Weight: Biological and Behavioral Mechanisms.* New York: Wiley.

Brownell, K. D., and Rodin, J. (1994, September). "The Dieting Maelstrom: Is It Possible and Advisable to Lose Weight?" *American Psychologist, 49*(9), 781–791.

Gibbs, W. W. (1996, August). "Gaining on Fat." *Scientific American,* pp. 88–94.

Haas, R. (1994). *Eat Smart, Think Smart.* New York: HarperCollins.

Katahn, M. (1991). *One Meal at a Time.* New York: Norton.

Somer, E. (1995). *Food and Mood.* New York: Henry Holt.

Thomas, P. R. (Ed.). (1995). *Weighing the Options: Criteria for Evaluating Weight-Management Programs.* Washington, D.C.: National Academy of Sciences Press.

Winter, A., and Winter, R. (1988). *Eat Right, Be Bright.* New York: St. Martin's Press.

Winter, R. (1995). *A Consumer's Guide to Medicines in Food.* New York: Crown Trade Paperbacks.

Yepsen, R. B., Jr. (1987). *How to Boost Your Brain Power: Achieving Peak Intelligence, Memory and Creativity.* Emmaus, Pa.: Rodale.

6

Powders and Elixirs

Mind-Altering Agents

*66 Our body
is a well-set clock,
which keeps good
time, but if it
be too much or
indiscreetly
tampered with,
the alarm runs
out before
the hour. 99*

—Joseph Hall

*L*eo Tolstoy included in his ethic of love an injunction against consuming anything that detracted from one's normal state of full alertness. Thus, he declined coffee as well as alcohol. This chapter does not make such a demand of its readers; its purpose is to summarize findings related to the impact of various kinds of drug intake on the brain.

The word *drug* comes from the Middle English *drogge* (as well as French and German forms), which means "dry." It refers to the various powders (that is, the dried forms) we know as chemicals, or drugs. I use this word to refer to any consumable substance taken for the purpose of intervening with the normal functioning of the mind-brain. Expectant mothers should read this chapter carefully. According to a 1994 survey by the National Institute on Drug Abuse, among 2,613 mothers giving birth at fifty-two hospitals, 5.5 percent had used an illegal drug (marijuana or cocaine) during pregnancy, 18.8 percent had used alcohol, and 20.4 percent had used cigarettes.

Drugs act on our bodies in the same way that ligands do. Typically, a drug acts on the same "lock and key" receptor as a corresponding neurotransmitter or peptide. Sylwester and Hasegawa (1989) summarize this in "How to Explain Drugs to Your Students":

- Amphetamines block dopamine and norepinephrine reuptake channels.

- Alcohol mimics and decreases gamma amniobutyric acid (GABA).

- Opiates mimic endorphins.

- Mescaline mimics norepinephrine.

- Phencyclidine (PCP) increases dopamine levels.

- Lysergic acid diethylamide (LSD) mimics serotonin.

- Nicotine mimics acetylcholine.

- Muscarine mimics acetylcholine.

- Barbiturates mimic GABA.

- Valium enhances GABA's ability to bind to its inhibitory receptors.

- Antipsychotic drugs such as haloperidol block dopamine receptors.

- Atropine blocks acetylcholine receptors.

- Scopolamine blocks acetylcholine receptors.

- Cocaine blocks dopamine and norepinephrine reuptake channels.

- Tricyclic antidepressants block reuptake channels for norepinephrine and serotonin.

- Antidepressants inactivate monoamine oxidase (MAO) enzymes.

- Caffeine extends the stimulant action of cyclic AMP.

- Lithium modulates extreme cyclic AMP effects.

- Tetrahydrocannabinol (THC), the active ingredient in marijuana, mimics anandamide, one of the body's naturally recurring pleasure chemicals (see Topic 6.5).

- Gamma hydroxybutyrate (GHB), aka "Georgia Home Boy" and "Goop," increases levels of dopamine.

TOPIC 6.1 | Alcohol

Alcohol serves as a disinhibitor; that is, it "unlocks" normal inhibitions. It also serves as a depressant, or downer (often combined with coffee, whose caffeine serves as an upper). Alcohol destroys brain cells, primarily in the left hemisphere, the seat of language and logic. The number of cells killed varies according to the amount of alcohol consumed. Alcoholics and heavy drinkers kill off about sixty thousand more neurons per day than their light-drinking and teetotaling friends. A Reuters release reported that people who drink heavily for thirty to forty years die with brains that weigh 105 grams less than the brains of their light-drinking friends (1,315 grams versus 1,420 grams). If you must drink alcohol, limit the amount to one ounce per day (the equivalent of two regular beers or two small glasses of wine).

Scott Swartzwelder, a psychiatrist at Duke University Medical Center, has found that the equivalent of up to two drinks daily appears to be benign in the adult brain, but the same amount for young people appears to depress NMDA (N-methyl-D-aspartate) receptors, thus interfering with learning and memory. Although the research was performed with rats, parallel results in humans have been confirmed.

Ernest Noble, of the UCLA School of Medicine, has found that two to three drinks a day, four days a week, have an adverse effect on brain function, especially for those over forty. This level of alcohol consumption also causes premature aging. Studies of the brains of alcoholic men show reduced blood flow in the frontal lobe, the seat of memory formation, creativity, and problem solving. Alcohol makes the nerve membrane more fluid and less viscous than normal, which results in structural instability and increased susceptibility to structural changes and damage. Swartzwelder and Richard Morrisett, of Omaha's Nebraska Medical Center, have identified a major cause of alcoholics' faulty memory: in research on rats, they found that alcohol blocks NMDA receptors in the hippocampus, thus interfering with the passing of messages in this memory "center" in the brain.

Elizabeth Ginsburg, a gynecologist at Brigham and Women's Hospital in Boston, examined the effect of alcohol consumption on women taking estrogen replacement therapy (ERT). Women who consumed the equivalent of three to five drinks a day showed levels of estradiol (the most potent form of estrogen) that were three times the intended level. Because of the unknown effects of these elevated levels of estradiol (and because of suspected links between long-term ERT and breast cancer), Ginsburg cautions women on ERT to go light on social drinking until more is known.

A 1992 University of Minnesota report (cited in Rose, 1998), based on data from 356 twin pairs, suggests that the causes of alcoholism are genetic only when it occurs in adolescent males. When alcoholism develops in adult males or in women, the evidence points to environmental causes. Franklin (1987) reports that Japanese researchers have identified two genes that control different alcohol-related enzymes: a slow-acting enzyme that breaks down alcohol slowly, giving its bearer a low tolerance for alcohol and a proneness to get sick before excessive consumption, and a fast-acting enzyme that breaks down alcohol quickly, giving its bearer a high tolerance for alcohol and a proneness to drink large quantities, with an attendant reputation for "being able to hold liquor." The Japanese found that although the two genes were divided 50-50 among the general population, only 2 percent of alcoholics have the slow gene; the other 98 percent are "sitting ducks for alcoholism" (pp. 166–167). This finding is supported by a U.S. study by Marc Schuckit and Tom Smith, who reported in the March 1996 *Archives of General Psychiatry* that in a father-son study of 358 pairs of men, the best predictor in twenty-year-olds of eventual alcoholism, after having an alcoholic father, is having a low physiological and psychological sensitivity to alcohol (the fast-acting gene).

Like heart disease, alcoholism is not one disease, but a complex of diseases: the fast enzyme, a low pain threshold, chemical malformations, depression, brain wave abnormalities, and low levels of MAO. When treating alcoholism, more than one of these issues may need to be addressed. For example, low levels of MAO are associated with impulsivity, short attention span, pleasure seeking, and a low pain threshold. Alcoholics who have low MAO tend to exhibit more violent forms of alcoholism. Also, to the degree that an alcoholic has a low pain threshold, treating the source of pain would also partially address the need to drink as a form of self-treatment for disease and/or pain. I remember consuming alcohol to relieve low back pain. When it was finally diagnosed as gout, I discovered that the alcohol was in fact exacerbating the gout. When the gout was treated, the need for daily "medication" disappeared. Depression is another application of the self-medicating quality of alcohol. Barbara Mason reports in the March 13, 1996, *Journal of the American Medical Association* that the tricyclic antidepressant desipramine relieves alcohol-associated depression and that it also lowers the chances of relapse.

The demographics of alcoholism are changing. The number of women diagnosed with alcoholism has risen to almost four million; over the 1970s, the elderly showed an increase of over 50 percent in their incidence of alcoholism. In fact, upward of 20 percent of seniors over the age of sixty-five have problems with alcohol, with an estimated three million diagnosed as alcoholics. More seniors are hospitalized for problems with alcohol than for heart problems; of those hospitalized over the age of sixty, about 25 percent are diagnosed as alcoholics. That's one-quarter of Medicare costs going to treat alcohol abuse. And that proportion will increase.

Applications

1 In planning a cocktail party or reception, do not allow for more than the equivalent of two beers per person. If individuals want to drink more, you may have it available, but make them pay for it. Don't put yourself in the position of making it easy for a person to consume more than one ounce of alcohol daily.

2 If you run a bar and are having a "happy hour" (illegal in some states), cut off special prices after the second drink. Have customers pay full price for third and subsequent drinks.

3 Provide information (posters, notices on menus, placards on tables, and so on) cautioning against consumption of more than two alcoholic drinks per day.

4 Consider medical intervention for male adolescents who show alcoholic tendencies. Counseling alone is not sufficient to counterbalance a genetic predisposition.

5 If you're pregnant, ideally you should not drink at all, but especially during the first four months (see Topic 4.2).

6 If you're on ERT, limit yourself to a couple of drinks a day until more is known.

7 The National Council on Alcoholism and Drug Dependence has information on treatment programs around the country. Contact them through their web site at www.ncadd.com.

8 The National Drug and Alcohol Abuse and Treatment Referral service is available through their web site at www.drughelp.org and through their twenty-four-hour help line at 800-378-4435.

9 Consuming alcohol suppresses REM sleep, so for a better night's sleep, quit drinking early enough to rehydrate your body with several glasses of water. For a vivid description of the effect of alcohol on sleep, see Hobson (1994, chapter 15, especially pages 270–276).

TOPIC 6.2 Aspirin

Much has been written recently about the ability of aspirin (acetylsalicylic acid) to thin blood and about its potential positive effects on blood pressure and the associated lower risk of heart attack and stroke. In addition, the right amount of aspirin can ameliorate dementia (general deterioration of mental ability):

one aspirin a day will improve dementia, but two a day worsen it. After one year on one aspirin a day, demented patients showed a 17 percent improvement in tests of cognitive ability; after two years, they showed a 21 percent improvement. (See the additional discussion of pain medications in Topic 14.3.)

Application

If you have a friend or family member who is suffering from dementia and the aspirin treatment has not been suggested, you might arrange to consult with the patient's physician about its appropriateness. Be aware of possible side effects, such as stomach upset.

TOPIC 6.3   **Caffeine**

Caffeine is a stimulant, or upper, that exists naturally in around sixty plants, the most familiar being kola nuts, tea leaves, cacao and coffee beans, maté leaves, and guarana paste. Its effect is heightened physiological arousal, which is similar to arousal caused by stress in that it results in the release of cortisol. Chemically, caffeine belongs to a class of compounds called methylxanthines, along with theophylline and theobromine, all of which have the ability to trick the brain into thinking they are the neurotransmitter adenosine. Adenosine (see Chapter Twenty) is a relaxant that is required to restore the central nervous system from sympathetic to parasympathetic arousal, or from stress to relaxation. By binding adenosine receptor sites, caffeine blocks the relaxing effects of adenosine and maintains high arousal.

In a National Academy of Sciences study of military nutrition, caffeine's arousing properties were found to be associated not only with mental alertness, but also with physical endurance. James Lane, Research Professor of Behavioral Medicine at Duke University, has determined that people who drink caffeine and have stressful jobs experience more health problems than those who have stressful jobs and don't consume caffeine. This is because of the double-whammy effect of having cortisol coming from two sources: stress and caffeine (see Topic 20.5 for a description of how cortisol works).

Roger Spealman of Harvard Medical School has identified another specific action caused by caffeine (he also identified its adenosine-blocking action): it inhibits phosphodiesterase (PDE). PDE is an enzyme that breaks down adenosine, so inhibiting PDE makes more adenosine available. This results in psychomotor stimulation, increased alertness, faster heart rate, and faster breathing. Excessive arousal appears to result in errors of commission (for example, typographical errors), whereas deficient arousal appears to result in errors of omission (for example, skipping a paragraph while typing). Routine tasks are less affected by excess arousal, while more complex, unfamiliar tasks appear to suffer under high-arousal conditions, which can make concentration difficult (see the discussion of the Yerkes-Dodson law in Topic 20.5). Caffeine consumption can also trigger panic attacks.

Interestingly, the less impulsive personality generally wakes up in a higher state of cortical arousal. If the less impulsive person consumes caffeinated beverages upon waking, he or she will tend to perform poorly on complex mental tasks. If the more impulsive person tries a complex mental task upon waking before consuming a caffeinated beverage, he or she will tend to perform poorly. Toward the end of the day, this pattern switches: in the evening, less impulsive people perform complex mental tasks better with a hit of caffeine; more impulsive people perform complex tasks better without it.

Takayuki Shibamoto, an environmental toxicologist at the University of California, Davis, reports that coffee beans contain over one thousand chemical compounds. Some of these compounds are antioxidants, the chemicals that disarm (or bind) free radicals and inhibit their insatiable appetite for vital cell membranes. This is true of coffee beans in their solid state. After being brewed, regular or decaffeinated coffee produces another three hundred chemical compounds that are all antioxidants.

The normal effective dose of caffeine is generally estimated at 100 milligrams or, more precisely, at 2 milligrams per kilogram of body weight (roughly 1 milligram of caffeine per pound of weight). Ten grams is a lethal dose, while for small children 35 milligrams per kilogram of body weight is toxic (that's about 500 milligrams of caffeine for a thirty-pound child). Table 6.1 shows some common caffeine levels. Note that the figures for coffee and tea are averages and represent a wide variation in actual amounts of caffeine.

Some have touted ginseng supplements as a natural way to boost one's energy. Interestingly, researchers at the Rochester Institute of Technology in New York have discovered that caffeine and caffeine-like substances have been added to many ginseng supplements. If you're a ginseng user, check your product out carefully to ensure that you're not getting caffeine instead of active ginseng.

Consumption of 400 to 500 milligrams of caffeine per day is associated with dependence (A. Winter and R. Winter, 1988). Symptoms of caffeine dependence are diarrhea, nausea, light-headedness, irregular heartbeat, irritability, and insomnia. One dramatic warning sign of caffeine dependence is a feeling of dizziness upon standing after having been prone (normal people experience a rise in blood pressure, while caffeine addicts experience a drop). Another symptom is the so-called Yom Kippur headache associated with fasting (and abstaining from coffee) for twelve to sixteen hours.

The arousal effects of one cup of caffeinated coffee last approximately six hours but vary according to the individual. I'm 6 feet 1½ inches tall, weigh 250 pounds, and am fifty-seven years old. If I drink caffeinated coffee after 5:00 P.M., I have trouble getting to sleep that night. If I drink more than two cups of strongly caffeinated coffee in a short time, I get jittery and have trouble concentrating. My limit is one cup of strong, two cups of moderate, or three cups of weak caffeinated brew.

Table 6.1. Common Caffeine Levels.

Substance	Amount in Milligrams
Drip coffee (5 ounces)	150
Percolated coffee (5 ounces)	100
Espresso (2 ounces)	100
Instant coffee (5 ounces)	50
Decaffeinated coffee (5 ounces)	2
Tea (5 ounces, brewed 1 minute)	10–30
Tea (5 ounces, brewed 5 minutes)	20–50
Iced tea (12 ounces)	70
Cocoa (6 ounces)	5–10
Chocolate syrup (2 tablespoons)	5
Milk chocolate (1 ounce)	6
Baking chocolate (1 ounce)	8–35
Chocolate powder mix (3 heaping tablespoons)	8
Soft drinks (12 ounces)	50[a]
Guarana "Magic Power" (15 milliliters of alcohol with 5 grams of guarana seeds)	250
NoDoz, Vivarin	200
Excedrin	130
Midol, Anacin	65
Dristan, other cold remedies	20–35

Source: Columbia University School of Public Health, *Health and Nutrition Newsletter, 2*(2), 1986; National Soft Drink Association; *Journal of American Diet, 74,* 28–32, 1979; *Bowes and Church's Food Values of Portions Commonly Used* by A. D. Bowes, Philadelphia: Lippincott, 1989.

[a]The actual range is from about 30 milligrams in Canada Dry Cola to about 59 milligrams in Sugar-Free Mr. Pibb.

While coffee usually produces feelings of energy and motivation (women who drink coffee are less likely to commit suicide than those who don't, according to a report in the *Archives of Internal Medicine*), coffee has a dark side: the *Diagnostic and Statistical Manual of Mental Disorders* (DSM-IV) (American Psychiatric Association, 1994) includes four caffeine-related diagnoses: caffeine intoxication, caffeine-related anxiety disorder, caffeine-related sleep disorder, and (in the appendix) caffeine withdrawal. In addition to these problems, caffeine, a stimulant, can wreak havoc with calming prescription drugs such as antidepressants, antianxiety medication, and neuroleptic tranquilizers. Initially suspecting panic disorder and agoraphobia for a woman who came into the Center for Stress and Anxiety Disorders in Albany, New York, doctors were surprised to find that she was on a steady daily diet of thirty cups of coffee!

In addition to the foregoing disorders, studies in which megadoses of caffeine were given to pregnant rats have produced mixed results regarding birth defects. One reason: studies in the early 1980s force-fed rats through a tube directly into the stomach, while later studies have simply added caffeine to the rats' drinking water. The Food and Drug Administration has concluded that the evidence is not conclusive regarding the danger to human reproduction, but hedging its bets, it recommends that expectant mothers consume caffeine in moderation. Caffeine also makes its way into breast milk.

The myth that a cup of coffee for the road counteracts the effects of alcohol after a night of drinking is just that—a myth. At Hull University, students who had consumed vodka were given two cups of coffee. Those who were given caffeinated coffee made twice as many psychomotor errors as those who drank decaffeinated coffee or no coffee at all. In addition, in a study of fifteen hundred college students, higher caffeine consumption was found to be correlated with lower academic performance.

As with most so-called laws of nature, exceptions abound.

Applications

❶ Know your limit. If you are in doubt, limit yourself to one cup of strong caffeinated brew (or two moderate or three weak cups) every six hours. More physically active people can have somewhat more caffeine and have it more often.

2 Make noncaffeinated alternatives available to guests, especially for introverts in the morning and extraverts in the evening.

3 If you are responsible for a meeting, do not provide more than the equivalent of two moderately caffeinated cups of brew per person. If people ask for more, let them purchase it on their own. Don't be responsible for providing them with an excuse for less than effective mental activity. Switch to noncaffeinated alternatives (coffee, tea, bottled water, soft drinks, juice) after the initial allotment runs out. Ideally, people should have a choice between caffeine (green tea is ideal), a complex carbohydrate (for example, V-8 juice), or bottled water.

4 I've found some hotels and restaurants to be unconcerned about supplying noncaffeinated beverages for breaks. You must be specific in asking for them when you order.

5 If you're pregnant, consult your physician about your proper dose of caffeine. Better yet, give it up during your pregnancy. During the months when you're nursing your infant, take care that your caffeine consumption is moderate and occurs shortly after nursing, not before. Caffeine that you consume before nursing will enter your breast milk and provide unnecessary stimulation for your nursing child.

6 Check the newsgroup alt.drugs.caffeine on the Internet for further information and discussion. A FAQ (frequently asked questions) file is available. It is maintained by Alex Lopez-Ortiz at the University of Waterloo, Ontario, Canada. E-mail him at alopez-o@neumann.UWaterloo.ca.

TOPIC 6.4 Cocaine

When an endorphin neurotransmitter jumps a synapse and lands on a receptor site, a pleasurable sensation ensues. Normally, the endorphins then detach from the receptor site and return to their presynaptic location. Cocaine attaches itself to the endorphins at the receptor site and prevents their return to the presynaptic site. Thus, (1) the pleasurable effect is maintained and

(2) there is a shortage of endorphins when the cocaine is metabolized, resulting in a strong letdown and the urge to use more of the drug. Cocaine constricts blood vessels in the brain. The more cocaine, the more constricted the brain's blood vessels. This constriction leads at a minimum to impaired mental function and at the maximum to brain damage.

As reported in *Science* (Lester, 1998), in an analysis of eight studies of children exposed to cocaine when their mothers used it during their pregnancy, Brown University researchers found that

- Cocaine-exposed children averaged 3.26 IQ points lower than nonexposed children.

- The damage is more subtle than was once supposed. There appears to be no severely crippling brain damage.

- The cocaine-exposed children's loss in the ability to understand, or "receive," language was more severe than their IQ loss.

- The annual cost to society of these cocaine-related impairments could be as high as $352 million; it appears in the form of special education requirements for these children in school.

The Brown researchers observed that a three-point IQ deficit is less noticeable for a high-IQ child than for a borderline child. This loss serves as a double whammy for poor children who suffer decreased mental performance as well as socioeconomic disadvantages. Barry Lester, the lead author, avers that some mental impairments can be partially eradicated by early intervention in the form of specific therapies soon after birth.

Applications

1 Don't!

2 Maximize the use of natural highs provided by the body. Aerobic exercise and laughter are two good sources of natural highs.

❸ Do whatever is in your power to prevent pregnant women from using cocaine.

❹ In cases where newborns are known to have been exposed to cocaine through their mothers' use, advocate immediate intervention to stimulate language reception skills.

TOPIC 6.5 Marijuana

Roy Matthew, director of the Duke Alcoholism and Addictions Program, affiliated with Duke University in Durham, North Carolina, reports that steady users of marijuana (ten joints a week for three years) showed a dramatically lower (and permanent) baseline level of cerebral blood flow than nonusers. Cerebral blood flow is a measure of brain activity. Those who smoked once or twice during a three-year period showed no measurable drop in baseline cerebral flow over time. However, the same nonusers and infrequent users showed an immediate measurable drop in cerebral blood flow right after smoking one joint. Continued steady use of marijuana resulted in what Matthew calls the "amotivational syndrome"—lethargic, self-defeating behavior resulting in loss of interest in work or school, abandonment of long-term plans, and loss of pleasure in normal activity.

The active ingredient in marijuana—tetrahydrocannabinol, or THC—has a naturally occurring equivalent in the human body. This substance, called anandamide, from the Sanskrit for "internal bliss," was discovered by William Devane and Raphael Mechoulam of Hebrew University of Jerusalem. Researchers are looking for other THC-like substances that occur in the body naturally, with the hope that safe pharmaceutical applications for the control of mood without marijuana's undesirable side effects will be available in the near future. At an October 26, 1997, presentation in New Orleans for the Society for Neuroscience, researchers from the University of California, San Francisco; the University of Michigan; and Brown University reported that animal research demonstrates the effectiveness of cannabinoids (a family of drugs that include THC as a primary ingredient) as a nonaddictive painkiller.

Application

If effective use of your mind is important to you, don't use marijuana. Legal and controlled uses of its active ingredients are just around the corner.

TOPIC 6.6 Nicotine

Nicotine interrupts the flow of oxygen to the brain, particularly in the right hemisphere. The resulting oxygen deprivation is accompanied by decreased metabolism of glucose, which translates into sluggish and faulty memory, ineffective problem solving, and lower mental output in general. In addition, nicotine elevates levels of cortisol, the stress hormone. On a different front, nicotine appears to release a flood of beta-endorphins and dopamine, which together serve to enhance mood. This finding relates to the work of Caryn Lerman, a psychologist with Georgetown University in Washington, D.C., who has found that upward of 40 percent of smokers entering smoking-cessation programs are depressed. This level of depression is triple that found among nonsmokers. Lerman and others have concluded that these depressed smokers are, in effect, self-medicating for depression with nicotine. Smokers who report depressed moods at the beginning of smoking-cessation programs are the most likely to relapse, and depressed smokers who treat their depression with both talk and pharmaceutical therapy are much more likely to quit smoking and remain nicotine-free. Effective antidepressant and smoking-cessation drugs include Zyban, or buproprion, and nortriptyline. Neal Benowitz, a professor at the University of San Francisco's Department of Medicine, says that they both work as well as the nicotine patch or gum (*New England Journal of Medicine,* October 23, 1997).

Interestingly, some current twin studies are pointing toward the possibility that depression and nicotine addiction share a common gene. In fact, Margaret Spitz and her colleagues at the M. D. Anderson Cancer Center in Houston have identified a genetic constellation, including a variant of the dopamine-related DRD2 gene, that is common to smokers. They hypothesize that smokers, and possibly other stimulus seekers such as overeaters and alcohol abusers, have a brain pleasure center that is underactive. For them, stimulants are required to generate the endorphins that nonsmokers (or people who do not use stimulants) produce normally. Both the findings and their implications, however, are far from universally agreed upon. Specific preventive and treatment options are still in the future. In the meantime, the use of dopamine-releasing drugs such as bromocriptine and buproprion (and even some drugs used in treating Parkinson's disease) may be helpful in addressing the smoking urge.

We've all heard that women should not smoke during pregnancy. Researchers at Cornell University and the University of Rochester, for example, report that children whose mothers smoked while pregnant have significantly lower IQs; this is attributed to reduced oxygen flow and the effect of some four thousand chemical components in tobacco smoke that can damage a child's neural development. But recent research suggests that stopping during pregnancy may not be enough. Michael Weitzman of the Rochester (New York) School of Medicine, in a study of the mothers of 2,256 youngsters aged four to eleven, found that when mothers smoked after delivery, their children had twice as many behavioral problems and alterations in brain function as children whose mothers did not smoke. In another study, Denise Kandel of Columbia University reported in the *American Journal of Public Health* in 1983 that daughters (but not sons) of mothers who smoked during pregnancy are from three to six times more likely to smoke (depending on the sample observed) than daughters of mothers who did not smoke during pregnancy.

As part of a study of osteoporosis, for which white women are at highest risk, Heidi Nelson of the Oregon Health Sciences University School of Medicine reported that white women over sixty-five years old who smoked ($n = 9,704$) performed more poorly on eleven out of twelve tasks, including strength, agility, and balance (Nelson, Nevitt, and Scott, 1994). The overall effect of smoking for these women was to add five years to their age.

Jack Henningfield, a National Institute on Drug Abuse Research Center psychologist, reports that within four hours after smoking their last cigarette, smokers' accuracy and speed decreases in logical decision making, arithmetic, and short-term memory tasks. This decline in cognitive processing is attributed to changes in the brain's electrical activity. In addition, smokers who've succeeded in quitting permanently show a similar degradation in performance for one to two months after quitting. The latter finding varies widely for individuals, but all apparently recover eventually.

A comment on passive smoke. Mounting evidence, much of it provided by the Environmental Protection Agency and disseminated in a 1993 report (with continuing supplements, available on-line at www.oehha.org), points to scientific agreement over the following associations with tobacco smoke in one's environment:

- It increases the risk of asthma, bronchitis, and pneumonia.

- It increases the risk of heart disease and heart attack.

- It raises levels of carbon monoxide in the bloodstream, thereby reducing oxygen flow to the heart, brain, and other organs.

- It increases the frequency and duration of ear infections in young children.

- It increases the risk of sudden infant death.

Applications

1 If you have excess brainpower that you don't want or need, then enjoy smoking. It's a good way to cut your brain down to a more humble performance level. Otherwise, don't smoke.

2 If you are a parent or you live or work around children, know that smoking around children has a high likelihood of causing behavioral and mental dysfunction.

3 If you are involved with a smoking-cessation program, ensure that you screen for depression and treat clients accordingly. If you are a smoker who wants to quit, have yourself evaluated for possible depression and accept appropriate treatment. In either case, nicotine used as a mood elevator must be replaced by other, healthier mood elevators, such as the endorphin rush provided by aerobic exercise.

4 If you are a smoker who operates machinery, don't do so when you need your next nicotine hit. If you've quit smoking recently, be aware that your performance will be inferior until you've recovered completely. Airplane pilots and other high-performance drivers should be particularly aware of this.

5 Insist on your rights as a nonsmoker to live, work, and play in a smoke-free environment. Don't live with a smoker who insists on smoking around you, and insist that your employer provide smoke-free work areas.

6 For a review of treatment guidelines in smoking cessation, see Wetter and others (June 1998).

7 Obtain the excellent booklet *Tobacco Biology, and Politics,* by Stanton A. Glantz, published in 1992 by Health Edco; P.O. Box 21207; Waco, Texas 76702-1207; phone: 800-299-3366. *(Contributed by Glenda Davenport-Cook)*

TOPIC 6.7 Prescription Drugs

Nervous system depressants affect brain function. Sleeping pills, tranquilizers, muscle relaxers, and antianxiety drugs all affect the quality of brain function, as do cortisone and arthritis drugs. Valium (diazepam), in particular, affects the ability to drive safely, including staying in one's lane, maintaining a constant speed, braking in a reasonable distance, recognizing signs quickly, and having peripheral awareness (A. Winter and R. Winter, 1988). Matthew Muldoon of the University of Pittsburgh reported on a study of the effects of cholesterol-lowering drugs at the November 10, 1997, meeting of the American Heart Association. In a double-blind study of 194 men and women, half got lovastatin (Mevacor), a popularly prescribed cholesterol-lowering drug; the other half got placebos. The scores on attention and mental dexterity were 10 percent lower for the lovastatin group, while memory scores were about equal. This difference in attention and dexterity could have a significant effect, for example, on the ability to operate vehicles and equipment in "heavy traffic" situations.

Merrell Dow Pharmaceuticals identified the following drugs as tending to impair performance in operating machinery (A. Winter and R. Winter, 1988): painkillers, antidepressants, antihistamines, tranquilizers, sedatives, antipsychotics, stimulants, some antihypertensives, and anticholinergics. The effects of these drugs are typically worsened when they are taken along with alcohol. In addition, certain combinations of these drugs can produce unpleasant or even lethal side effects.

Recently a new agency was formed to study differences in body chemistry between ethnic groups. The Center on the Psychobiology of Ethnicity, located in Torrance, California, at the Harbor–University of California at Los Angeles Medical Center, presented its initial research reports in 1992. For further information, contact Dr. Keh-Ming Lin, Director; The Center on the Psychobiology of Ethnicity; Harbor-UCLA Medical Center; 1124 West Carson Street, B-4 South; Torrance, California 90502; phone: 310-222-4266.

Applications

1 Try to find a nonpharmaceutical alternative to the prescription drugs listed in this Topic. Confer with your physician about how to identify nonpharmaceutical treatments.

2 Just as unions are sometimes considered an antidote to bad organizational management, so are pharmaceuticals an antidote to poor self-management. Ensure that you have taken charge of your life with diet, exercise, and stress elimination or reduction before you allow yourself to become drug-dependent. Read Covey (1990) and Sternberg (1988). And read on!

3 Be a "reluctant chemist," to use J. Allan Hobson's expression (1994, pp. 280–281). He writes:

> Even if . . . individuals have serious problems, their doctors should prescribe drugs only as a temporary means to jolt them out of their state and should then turn to scientific humanism for the long-term cure. These individuals may need a drug for a few days or weeks to break their cycles, but then they must use volition to keep themselves healthy. *Only volition can cure them.* [Italics mine.] That's why groups like Alcoholics Anonymous work; there is a collection of people who mutually support each other. There is a collective will. Once the individuals in the group feel the power of their own volition, they can control their states, and the natural healing power of the mind and body will kick in.

TOPIC 6.8 Brain Nutrient Drugs

Dean and Morgenthaler (1990) make dramatic claims for a new family of drugs—*nootropics* (from the Greek *noos,* or "mind," and *tropos,* or "change"). According to their research, nootropic drugs can improve mental function and arrest or even reverse some brain diseases. Most of the so-called nootropics are chemical efforts to duplicate various neurotransmitters and neuro-modulators. Many of these drugs have not been approved for use in the United States.

Richard Restak (1997) advises generally that nondietary sources of brain nutrients "cannot substitute for a diet rich in fruits and vege-tables" (p. 37). (See the extended discussion in Topics 5.1 and 5.11.) A much-publicized brain nutrient is the "human growth hormone" (HGH). Restak points to HGH research as an example of the difficulty in interpreting results. Daniel Rudman, an endocrinologist at the Medical College of Wisconsin in Milwaukee, was trying to find a way to reverse the pituitary gland's decreasing production of growth hor-mone as we age, with sixty-year-olds having on average a 90 percent lower level of growth hormone than forty-year-olds. Rudman, working in the 1980s, injected synthesized HGH into elderly subjects and found a virtual "fountain of youth" effect—increased muscle mass, increased sex drive, and so on. But when the research was repeated in the 1990s by physicians at the University of California, San Francisco, the results were not remarkable. What was the dif-ference? Observers, including Rudman's widow, have concluded that the study in the 1980s, in which the subjects knew what they were being given, fell victim to the "self-fulfilling prophecy," whereas the San Francisco study was a blind study in which subjects did not know what the injections contained. Concludes Restak, "I encourage you to cultivate a healthy skepticism and remember this growth-hormone study later . . . when we [look at] other drugs and chemi-cals that are reputed to extend the life span" (p. 44).

Applications

1   As a general rule, for the normal healthy person with no evidence of dementia, I recommend nonpharmaceutical methods for improving brain function (diet, exercise, and training in the many areas described in this book).

2   For exceptional cases where deterioration of brain function does not respond to available interventions, Dean and Morgenthaler (1990) can help in identifying a doctor who is willing to prescribe nootropic drugs. Their book itself will tell you how to become a part of the nootropic network.

TOPIC 6.9   **The Effects of Chemicals on the Elderly**

Steffie Woolhandler, of Cambridge Hospital and Harvard Medical School, warned against improper prescriptions for people over sixty-five. Table 6.2 shows some of her findings.

Application

If you or someone close to you is over sixty-five years of age, be certain that any prescription drugs you and/or they have been pre-scribed satisfy Woolhandler's guidelines. Get a copy of her article if your doctor is not familiar with it. Be confident that the prescrip-tions have minimal or no undesirable side effects. Find the least problematic alternative.

A Final Word on Drugs

Deborah Mash, director of the University of Miami Medical School's Brain Endowment Bank, in an April 18, 1994, Knight-Ridder release, concluded that over the long term, the amphetamines and cocaine are extremely toxic to the brain. Specifically, early use of these drugs winds up later revealing shrunken and distorted neurons in the

Table 6.2. Potential Problems with Drugs for the Elderly.

Drug	Potential Problems
Sleeping Aids and Tranquilizers	
Diazepam (Valium)	Addictive, too long-acting, drowsiness, falls, confusion
Chlordiazepoxide (Librium, Librax)	Too long-acting, falls
Flurazepam (Dalmane)	Too long-acting, falls
Meprobamate (Miltown, Deprol, Equagesic, Equanil)	Addictive, too long-acting, falls
Pentobarbitol (Nembutal)	Addictive, too long-acting
Secobarbitol (Seconal)	Addictive, too long-acting
Antidepressants	
Amitriptyline (Elavil, Endep, Etrafon, Limbitrol, Triavil)	Dizziness, drowsiness, inability to urinate
Pain Relievers	
Propoxyphene (Darvon Compound, Darvocet, Wygesic)	Addictive, little better than aspirin, more side effects than morphine, seizures, heart problems
Pentazocine (Talwin)	Addictive, seizures, heart problems
Dementia Treatments	
Cyclandelate	Not effective
Isoxsuprine	Not effective

Source: Adapted from "Inappropriate Drug Prescribing for the Community-Dwelling Elderly" by S. M. Wilcox, D. U. Himmelstein, and S. Woolhandler, *Journal of the American Medical Association, 272*(4), July 27, 1994, pp. 292–296.

nigrastriatal pathway, affecting motor coordination and often presaging the onset of Parkinson's disease. Interestingly, marijuana and LSD, often thought to have long-term toxic effects, do not show ill effects over the long haul, according to Mash. On the other hand, Roy Matthew of Duke University (see Topic 6.5) has found that heavy marijuana use results in permanent, reduced cerebral blood flow.

SUGGESTED RESOURCES

Sylwester, R., and Hasegawa, C. (1989, January). "How to Explain Drugs to Your Students." *Middle School,* pp. 8–11.

Wilcox, S. M., Himmelstein, D. U., and Woolhandler, S. (1994, July 27). "Inappropriate Drug Prescribing for the Community-Dwelling Elderly." *Journal of the American Medical Association, 272*(4), 292–296.

Winter, A., and Winter, R. (1988). *Eat Right, Be Bright.* New York: St. Martin's Press.

Yepsen, R. B., Jr. (1987). *How to Boost Your Brain Power: Achieving Peak Intelligence, Memory and Creativity.* Emmaus, Pa.: Rodale.

Web Sites

National Clearinghouse for Alcohol and Drug Information, Research and Statistics page:
   www.health.org/survey.htm

7

A Good Night's Sleep

Cycles, Dreams, Naps, and Nightmares

66 *What a delightful thing rest is! The bed has become a place of luxury to me. I would not exchange it for all the thrones in the world.* **99**

—*Napoléon Bonaparte*

A good night's sleep should be declared a basic human right. Research is growing nearer to establishing the purpose of sleep. For example, Robert Stickgold (1998) has reviewed the research on sleep and memory and points out that among rats, sleep deprivation prevents memory formation. This chapter reviews research findings that may be helpful in understanding both what a good night's sleep is and how we can manage to get one.

127

TOPIC 7.1   The Sleep Cycle

The infant averages 14 hours of sleep, the mature adult averages 7.5 hours, and the senior adult (over seventy-five) averages 6. Before the invention of electric lights, typical adults slept for 9 hours. When all cues to time of day are removed, typical adults will sleep for an average of 10.3 hours out of each 24, similar to their cousins, apes and monkeys. However, studies show that the length of sleep is not what causes us to be refreshed upon waking. The key factor is the number of complete sleep cycles we enjoy. Each sleep cycle contains five distinct phases, which exhibit different brain wave patterns. For a complete description, see *The Mind in Sleep* (Arkin, Antrobus, and Ellman, 1978) or *Sleep: The Gentle Tyrant* (Webb, 1992). For our purposes, it suffices to say that one sleep cycle lasts an average of 90 minutes. See Figure 7.1 for details.

If we were to sleep completely naturally, with no alarm clocks or other sleep disturbances, we would wake up, on the average, after a multiple of 90 minutes—for example, after 4.5 hours, 6 hours, 7.5 hours, or 9 hours, but not after 7 or 8 hours, which are not multiples of 90 minutes. In the period between cycles we are not actually sleeping; this is a sort of twilight zone from which, if we are not disturbed

---

Average cycle = 1 hour, 30 minutes

Non-REM = 65 min.	REM = 20 min.	Non-REM = 5 min.
"Normal sleep"	*"Dream"*	*"Normal sleep"*

REM phase begins as shorter (< 20 minutes), ends as longer (> 20 minutes).

Alcohol, stuffing oneself, and medication shorten REM phase.

One individual's cycles can vary by as much as 60 minutes from the shortest to the longest (for example, shortest may be 60 minutes and longest 120 minutes, for an average of 90 minutes).

Between cycles, one is not asleep ("twilight zone").

Figure 7.1. The Sleep Cycle.

(by light, cold, a full bladder, noise), we move into another 90-minute cycle. A person who sleeps only four cycles (6 hours) will feel more rested than someone who has slept for 8 to 10 hours but who has not been allowed to complete any one cycle because of being awakened before it was completed. Within a single individual, cycles can vary by as much as 60 minutes from the shortest cycle to the longest one. For example, someone whose cycles average 90 minutes might experience cycles that vary in length from 60 to 120 minutes. The standard deviation for adult length of sleep is 1 hour, which means that roughly two-thirds of all adults will sleep between 6.5 and 8.5 hours, based on an average of 7.5 hours.

A friend once told me, "All this stuff about cycles is a bunch of bunk. I wake up every morning when the sun rises." After talking about his sleep patterns, he discovered that he was self-disciplined in such a way that his bedtime was consistently about 7.5 hours before sunrise. He was waking between cycles, and the song of a bird, the cry of a baby, or the pressing of a full bladder could have been equally as effective as the sunrise in waking him. All it takes to awaken someone between cycles, especially if she or he has had sufficient sleep, is a gentle stimulus.

When my alarm goes off during the last half of my cycle, for a few hours I feel as if a truck has hit me. When it goes off during the first half of my cycle, it is like waking after a 15- to 20-minute nap, and I feel refreshed. Our motor output system from the brain is completely shut down during REM sleep; that is why we dream we are moving but don't actually move and why we feel so lifeless when we wake during REM sleep. Our motor output system hasn't kicked back in yet!

Applications

1 Keep a sleep journal. Record the beginning and waking times for each natural sleep episode that is uninterrupted by an alarm or any other disturbance. Find the common multiple. For example, if your recorded sleep periods were 400, 500, 400, 200, and 700 minutes, you would conclude that your personal sleep cycle typically lasts for 100 minutes, or about 1.6 hours.

2 Once you know the length of your typical sleep cycle (if you haven't kept a journal, you might assume 90 minutes), then, where possible, plan your waking accordingly. For example, my cycle is 90 minutes. If I am ready for bed at 11:00 P.M. and I know that I must rise at 6:00 A.M. in order to make a 7:00 breakfast meeting, I read for about 45 minutes to avoid having the alarm go off during the last half of my cycle. Conversely, if I go to bed at midnight, I set my alarm for 6:30 A.M. and rush to get ready, rather than being interrupted toward the end of my fourth cycle.

3 In support of waking naturally, William Moorcroft of the Luther College sleep laboratory reports that if we get the same amount of sleep each night, we don't really need an alarm clock, except as a backup (*Sleep,* January 1997). Subjects who were asked to visualize their time of waking on an imaginary clock face were generally able to rise at the desired time without an alarm. The key techniques: get the same amount of sleep nightly, choose your own time, visualize before sleep onset, and use a backup (a clock set 15 minutes later than your target rising time).

TOPIC 7.2   The Circadian Rhythm

From the Latin *circa* ("about") and *dies* ("day"), the term *circadian* simply means "about a day." Researchers have located the part of the brain that runs our body clock—the suprachiasmatic nucleus (SCN). We have assumed for centuries that our bodies' circadian rhythm has a twenty-four-hour cycle. Thus, we should be renewed and refreshed after every twenty-four-hour period. Recent research by Charles Czeisler of Harvard University and the Center for Circadian and Sleep Disorders at Brigham and Women's Hospital in Boston, as well as research by others, suggests that in fact, many of us have a body clock set for a twenty-five-hour day and most of us have a natural tendency to stay up later and wake later than we do. That's why so many people play catch-up with their sleep on the weekend.

Czeisler has discovered that when twenty-four-hour shift work is necessary, there is an optimum schedule based on this twenty-five-hour rhythm. The shifts should progress from day to evening to night, each lasting several weeks, with workers going to sleep progressively later. In this manner, when workers who have worked up to an 11:00 P.M. bedtime end a day shift, they start an evening shift;

they keep the 11:00 P.M. bedtime for several days and move to a mid-night bedtime, then, after several days, to a 1:00 A.M. bedtime, and so on, until several weeks later they are going to bed at 7:00 A.M. and rising to start an evening shift at 4:00 P.M. This schedule takes advantage of the body's natural tendency to go to bed later and rise later—that is, to live a twenty-five-hour day. (Table 7.1 illustrates how we may take advantage of this twenty-five-hour circadian rhythm while working shifts.)

Table 7.1. An Ideal Sleep-Shift Progression.

Day	Shift Starts	Shift Ends	Bedtime	Waking Time
1	12:00 midnight	8:00 A.M.	1:30 P.M.	9:00 P.M.
2	(Off)		2:30 P.M.	10:00 P.M.
3	(Off)		3:30 P.M.	11:00 P.M.
4	8:00 A.M.	4:00 P.M.	4:30 P.M.	12:00 midnight
5	8:00 A.M.	4:00 P.M.	5:30 P.M.	1:00 A.M.
6	8:00 A.M.	4:00 P.M.	6:30 P.M.	2:00 A.M.
7	8:00 A.M.	4:00 P.M.	7:30 P.M.	2:30 A.M.
8	8:00 A.M.	4:00 P.M.	9:30 P.M.	5:00 A.M.
9	(Off)		10:30 P.M.	6:00 A.M.
10	(Off)		11:30 P.M.	7:00 A.M.
11	4:00 P.M.	12:00 midnight	1:00 A.M.	8:30 A.M.
12	4:00 P.M.	12:00 midnight	2:00 A.M.	9:30 A.M.
13	4:00 P.M.	12:00 midnight	3:00 A.M.	10:30 A.M.
14	4:00 P.M.	12:00 midnight	4:00 A.M.	11:30 A.M.
15	4:00 P.M.	12:00 midnight	5:00 A.M.	12:30 P.M.
16	(Off)		6:30 A.M.	2:00 P.M.
17	(Off)		7:30 A.M.	3:00 P.M.
18	12:00 midnight	8:00 A.M.	9:00 A.M.	4:30 P.M.
19	12:00 midnight	8:00 A.M.	10:00 A.M.	5:30 P.M.
20	12:00 midnight	8:00 A.M.	11:00 A.M.	6:30 P.M.
21	12:00 midnight	8:00 A.M.	12:00 noon	7:30 P.M.

For a person working normal days, the body clock seems to be set as follows:

Time	Effect on Body
6:00 P.M. to midnight	Stomach acid is high; hormone levels drop; blood pressure, pulse rate, and body temperature drop.
Midnight to 6:00 A.M.	Lowest body temperature is between 2:00 and 3:00 A.M. Body is at its lowest level of efficiency between 4:00 and 6:00 A.M. (3:00 to 5:00 A.M. for early birds, 5:00 to 7:00 A.M. for night owls). This is a highly accident-prone period, characterized by low body temperature and low kidney, heart, respiratory, and mental functions.
6:00 A.M. to noon	Upon waking, pulse rate and blood pressure rise sharply; body temperature rises; blood clotting activity is high. Rote memory is at its sharpest.
Noon to 6:00 P.M.	The sense of smell is better. Body temperature is at its highest between 2:00 and 3:00 P.M., then dips in mid- to late afternoon. Grip strength is at its highest. Tolerance for alcohol peaks around 5:00 P.M.

Research is discovering increasingly more hormones and other body chemicals whose levels rise and fall with circadian regularity, so much so, in fact, that a new term, *chronotherapy,* has arisen to describe the practice of coordinating pharmaceutical and other treatments with time of day. William Hrushesky (1994), of Albany Medical College in New York, summarizes the circadian aspects of several major illnesses:

Rheumatoid arthritis: Worst in morning

Nonrheumatoid arthritis: Worst in evening

Asthma: Worst in early morning (2:00 to 6:00 A.M.)

Cardiovascular disease: Highest risk in morning

Various cancers: Optimal times for treatment are highly rhythmic

See Hrushesky (1994) for a more detailed discussion.

The body's clock can get thrown out of kilter by disease, aging, travel, and other factors. Because the clock seems to be triggered by the daily pattern of sunrise and sunset, it can be reset by the use of bright lights. (Light treatments have also been found effective in relieving winter depression; see Topic 18.5.) Czeisler reported in a May 3, 1990, press release that looking into a four-foot-square array of sixteen forty-watt bulbs according to his schedule can successfully reset the body clock up to ten hours in two days. To set a person's clock back, light treatment should be administered after the body's low-temperature point (4:00 to 6:00 A.M.); to set the body clock forward, light treatment should be administered before the low point.

Light inhibits the body's release of melatonin, a neurotransmitter associated with sleep, while darkness triggers its release. Czeisler's light treatment apparently resets the body's time for shutting down melatonin release. He also recommends lightproofing the sleeping quarters of someone who must sleep during the day or in a lighted room, including use of a face mask. Sleeping in total darkness maximizes the chance of obtaining sufficient melatonin release. Recent research by Scott Campbell of Cornell University Medical College, White Plains, New York, indicates that the light does not have to enter the body through the optic nerve. In his research, Campbell aimed lights behind the knee and achieved the same circadian changes as those achieved through eye-borne light.

In a recent line of research reported in the *New York Times,* December 27, 1995 (see also Wolfson and Carskadon, 1996), developmental psychologists have discovered an apparent anomaly in the circadian rhythm of teenagers. Sleep studies have shown that adolescents have higher levels of melatonin later in the morning than people who are younger or older. As a result, teenagers who start school at 7:30 A.M. typically live with a constant sleep deficit and engage in microsleep throughout the day. John Allen of Johns Hopkins University's Sleep Disorder Center found that adolescents who started school at 9:30 A.M. performed better academically than their peers who started at 7:30 A.M.

On early risers versus those who sleep into the morning, Sydney Harris once commented in his daily syndicated newspaper column, "Some say there are morning people and night people—it isn't so— night people are just teenagers who've never grown up!" Recent research, however, has shown that there really is such a thing as "morningness," or the tendency to awaken up to two hours before those who don't have morningness. Researchers at Stanford University and the University of Wisconsin report that morningness is genetically controlled (*Sleep,* October 1998). They have identified a specific gene whose variations from individual to individual appear to be associated with whether one is an early bird or a night owl.

Applications

1 Don't get up early (4:00 to 6:00 A.M.) to finish a project; stay up later if you must. Research documents the futility of getting up early. You're fighting your natural tendency to sleep later as well as working during the period of your body's lowest efficiency.

2 As 4:00 A.M. approaches, go to sleep. If you must stay awake and safety is an issue (for example, if you are driving or operating other equipment), then try to have someone to talk to. Social inter-action appears to be the best stimulant. Caffeine also helps. Take breaks. Keep cool. Avoid heavy carbohydrate or fatty snacks; stick to proteins and light complex carbohydrates. Bright lights help, as does your attitude; think about something that excites you. If you know ahead of time that you will have to be up and alert during these early-morning hours, take a nap the afternoon before. David Dinges, a sleep researcher on the faculty of the University of Pennsylvania, has done research that shows that people who nap before staying up all night perform better than those who don't (Dinges and Broughton, 1989).

3 With around two hundred sleep clinics in the United States and many others spread throughout the world, don't accept what you perceive as a problem with sleep. Check yourself in for observation. For information on various sleep programs, contact the Association of Professional Sleep Societies; 1610 14th Street, NW, Suite 300; Rochester, Minnesota 55901.

4 See the Applications for Topic 7.3.

5 If you must sleep during daylight hours, use a face mask and earplugs to better simulate the darkness and quiet of night.

6 Dark places are associated with depression for a reason: they have insufficient light to shut down melatonin production. If you or a friend have a tendency toward depression, avoid dairy products and choose bright, well-lighted, sunny environments.

7 Avoid setting your alarm for earlier than 6:00 A.M. Prepare the night before if getting up at 6:00 A.M. will be a rush for you: lay out your clothes; prepare breakfast, such as a bagel or yogurt; and put coffee on a timer or premake it and zap it in the microwave at 6:00 A.M. Take a nap the afternoon before if you must set the alarm before 6:00.

8 If you must regularly get up before 6:00 A.M., reset your body clock by ensuring darkness and quiet for an early-to-bed schedule and waking up to bright lights. Remember, sunrise is the trigger for the typical body clock.

9 Teenagers ideally should not begin school before 9:30 A.M. If they must and you are responsible for their performance, help them to compensate for their accumulated sleep deprivation: wake them up to bright lights, permit naps, have them exercise in the early morning just before beginning class work, avoid breakfasts that are full of fats and simple carbohydrates and choose breakfasts with protein and complex carbohydrates, and make caffeinated beverages available in the morning.

10 For extended information on sleep and adolescents, consult the *School Start Time Study: Final Report Summary,* available on-line at www.coled.umn.edu/CAREIwww/General/sstbiblio.htm.

11 If you or someone close to you suffers from a major illness, ask your physician about the optimal time of day for medication and other forms of treatment. If your doctor is unfamiliar with chronotherapy and the circadian aspects of treatment, you should ask elsewhere. Start with Hrushesky (1994).

12 For current sleep information and research results, visit the "Searle healthnet: sleep" web site at www.searlehealthnet.com/sleep/dateline. The site features highlights of recent sleep news and is updated every couple of weeks.

TOPIC 7.3 **Time-Zone Changes**

Extraverts adapt more quickly to time-zone and shift changes, while the physiology of introverts resists time changes. The principal problem is resetting the body's clock; introverts need more help in doing this. The major factors in resetting the body clock are the neurotransmitters serotonin and melatonin. Serotonin can be controlled by diet, and melatonin can be controlled both by diet and by the use of available light. Carbohydrates, fats, and dairy products in general tend to increase serotonin, and total darkness hastens the flow of melatonin. Incidentally, melatonin is a metabolite of serotonin.

Applications

1 If you have a more introverted personality, make an extra effort when you must travel through different time zones or change shifts. Light therapy helps (see Topic 34.2); in addition, avoid caffeine, alcohol, artificial sweeteners, and food additives for six hours before you try to sleep after a time-zone change. Consume dairy products, carbohydrates, and fats for maximum facilitation of sleep (milk and cookies, cheese and bread).

2 If you are responsible for managing shift schedules, remember that more extraverted personalities are less disrupted by time-zone or shift changes. This doesn't mean that introverts can't be called on to work night shifts, but you should (a) be sure that they know the precautions to take for minimum disruption and (b) accept their bodily resistance to time changes as normal and not as an attitude problem.

3 Try the following pattern, or something like it, if traveling across time zones gets you down. This pattern assumes a 6:00 P.M. departure in the United States from the East Coast and an 8:00 A.M. (local time) arrival in Europe or Africa, with your body operating as though it were actually 2:00 A.M. You are, in essence, being asked to skip one night's sleep. The solution is to sleep once you arrive or on the plane. Sleeping once you arrive is best, if you can arrange it. Remember, consume no caffeine or other stimulants for six hours before the flight, and use an eye mask and earplugs. In order to sleep on the plane, however, you must trick your body into thinking it's bedtime shortly after you take off. Following this schedule the week before you leave can help (assume a 6:00 P.M. Saturday departure):

Day	Rising Time	Bedtime
Sunday	7:00 A.M.	11:00 P.M.
Monday	6:30 A.M.	10:30 P.M.
Tuesday	6:00 A.M.	10:00 P.M.
Wednesday	5:30 A.M.	9:30 P.M.
Thursday	5:00 A.M.	9:00 P.M.
Friday	4:30 A.M.	8:30 P.M.
Saturday	4:00 A.M.	8:00 P.M. (airborne)

If you can manage this schedule, you should get at least a few ninety-minute cycles of sleep and you will feel much better for it. Remember, use an eye mask and earplugs, and consume no caffeine, alcohol, or artificial sweeteners after 1:00 P.M. on the day of departure. Your body will then feel as if it's early morning instead of the middle of the night when you land. And when 10:00 P.M. (local time overseas) rolls around on Sunday, your body clock will feel as if it's about 1:30 A.M. (since, if you were following the above pattern at home, you'd go to sleep about 7:30 P.M., or 1:30 A.M. local time). If you don't follow this pattern, when it's 10:00 P.M. on Sunday night, your body will feel as if it's 4:00 A.M. Clear? It won't work for everyone, but give it a try if eastward overseas flights really bother you. Westward flights don't bother most people because it's just like staying up later but being able to have a normal night's sleep, in accordance with the body's naturally advancing rhythms.

4 Charles F. Ehret of the Argonne (Illinois) National Laboratory recommends the anti-jet-lag diet (Yepsen, 1987), an alternating pattern of fasting and feasting that proceeds as follows:

- Three days before the flight, have high-protein feasts at breakfast and lunch and consume only complex carbohydrates for supper; take caffeine only between 3:00 and 5:00 P.M.

- Two days before the flight, fast on broth soups, salad, and fruit; follow the same caffeine rule.

- One day before the flight, follow the same pattern and the same caffeine rule as three days before (feast).

- Flight day is fast day: for east-west flights, fast only half a day, with caffeine in the morning; for west-east flights, fast all day, with caffeine between 6:00 and 11:00 P.M.
- Upon arrival, sleep until breakfast; all three meals on the day of arrival are feasts. Begin and continue on the day of arrival with all the lights turned on and remain active.

5 If you live on the East Coast of the United States and must fly to the West Coast, decide if you will actually be there long enough to justify going through a change of body clock. Jane Howard says, "Often I will go to a two-day meeting in the West, go to bed on Eastern time, and pretend I'm still in the East with respect to meals and caffeine. I go to bed around 9:00 P.M. West Coast time and wake up around 4:30 A.M. Reentry to the East Coast is a breeze; my body clock remains unchanged. I miss out on night life with this plan, but marrieds should feel okay about that."

TOPIC 7.4 Sleep and Exercise

Exercising tends to elicit cortical alertness, which is not what you want when going to sleep. Exercise relaxes you after experiencing stress, but good aerobic exercise generally puts your nervous system in a state of moderate arousal. In this condition, you are ideally suited for mental tasks. In order to sleep soon after a workout, you would need to consume carbohydrates and dairy products.

Applications

1 Exercise no later than several hours before bedtime.

2 If you must exercise just before retiring for the evening (I know a television sports announcer who exercises after a night game because he's so keyed up), try reading a relatively unemotional book in bed rather than an exciting one (for example, Plato rather than Agatha Christie) to help you get to sleep.

TOPIC 7.5   Sleep and Diet

Milk products stimulate melatonin production, which improves sleep. Whether skim or fat, milk (like complex carbohydrates) contains L-tryptophan, the amino acid that is a precursor of melatonin (and serotonin).

Simple sugars and fats decrease the oxygen supply to the brain, which decreases alertness and makes you sleepy.

Alcohol consumption reduces the relative amount of time spent in REM sleep; therefore, sleep following alcohol consumption is not as restful as alcohol-free sleep. The more alcohol we consume, the less REM sleep we get and the less rested we are in the morning.

Food additives in general and artificial sweeteners in particular tend to increase alertness, which interferes with sleep. Eating a large meal in the evening also interferes with sleep.

Applications

1 To maximize the chances of a good night's sleep, avoid snacks with additives or artificial sweeteners before bedtime and eat moderately.

2 To increase your chances of a good night's sleep, have a milk product or light carbohydrate snack shortly before bedtime. *Warning:* If you have the classic "warm milk," don't sweeten it with artificial sweetener. Have it plain or with honey, sugar, or some other natural flavoring.

3 If you drink alcohol in the evening, plan to allow at least one hour for the alcohol to metabolize before you go to sleep; allow more time for more consumption. Also, alcohol dehydrates and water rehydrates, so it helps to drink water between the time you stop drinking alcohol and the time you go to bed. For example, if you've been drinking alcohol throughout an evening dinner party at your home, clean up that night, not the next day, as a way of giving the alcohol time to metabolize, and drink water while you're cleaning. Or go for a gentle walk or stroll before retiring, then read for a while—and drink water. If you want a restful night's sleep, switch to a nonalcoholic beverage before the evening is over.

4 When flying across time zones, avoid drinking caffeine and alcohol in favor of milk.

TOPIC 7.6 Sleep and Weight

The amount of sleep we require is directly related to our body weight—that is, skinnier people require less sleep; heavier people sleep more.

Application

If you would like to require less sleep, get trim.

TOPIC 7.7 The Effect of Odors on Sleep

Peter Badia, of Bowling Green State University in Ohio, reports from his sleep lab research that most odors disrupt sleep; the heart rate increases and brain waves quicken. One odor, heliotropine, which has a vanilla-almond fragrance, does not disrupt sleep and may help (Kallan, 1991).

Applications

1 Try Amaretto liqueur or almond extract in your hot milk before going to sleep. Or try a few drops of vanilla extract in your bedtime milk.

2 Eliminate strong odors before going to sleep. Sleeping with an open window can help to diffuse odors.

TOPIC 7.8   The Effect of Sleep Deprivation

People who are significantly deprived of sufficient sleep engage in microsleep, a brief period in which they lose consciousness. Microsleep is not restorative; it is a warning that you have lost control. A person who has begun to microsleep is a safety hazard. It is possible to drift in and out of microsleep and not be aware of it. Torbjorn Akerstedt, who conducts sleep research at the Karolinska Institute in Stockholm, connected eleven railroad operators to wire monitors. He found that six exhibited microsleep (that is, they dozed at the helm according to the electrode measurements), yet only four were aware that they had dozed. Two plowed through warning signals while asleep (Long, 1987).

In the September 11, 1997, issue of the *New England Journal of Medicine,* the same phenomenon was reported for long-haul truck drivers, with half of the drivers studied exhibiting signs of drowsiness for at least six minutes during a week on the road. Drivers in the United States get eight hours off after driving ten. The study shows, however, that they average only four hours forty-seven minutes of sleep, with the other three hours devoted to a variety of unwinding activities. Understandably, the drivers don't want to spend all of their off time sleeping. Some researchers recommend expanding the off time to ten hours.

Eve Van Cauter, a sleep researcher at the University of Chicago, has studied the chemical effects of sleep deprivation. She has found that the loss of even an hour or so of sleep for two or three nights in a row results in attendant increases in cortisol (see Topic 20.5) and decreases in growth hormone and prolactin. All three of these changes are the opposite of those that occur during a normal good night's sleep (around 7.5 to 8 hours for most people). Typically, following a normal night's sleep, prolactin and growth hormone increase while cortisol decreases. Another chemical change involves the reduced production of adenosine triphosphate (ATP). During sleep, the body produces ATP to replace what was burned up during the previous waking episode as a source of energy. A by-product of burning ATP is adenosine, which, as it accumulates throughout the waking episode, ultimately signals the brain that fatigue is coming on. Failure to get a good night's sleep results in (1) an inadequate supply of ATP for the next waking episode and (2) an excess of fatigue-signaling adenosine.

The consequences of all these chemical changes include depletion of the immune system, the growth of fat rather than muscle, possible harming of brain cells, acceleration of the aging process, memory impairment, and an increasing risk of depression. Van Cauter warns that a good night's sleep should be as high a priority for fitness buffs as aerobic exercise and proper nutrition. Many cultures, however, praise those who "need" less sleep and refer to those desirous of a good night's sleep as "wimps" or "wusses."

Amy Wolfson, a psychology professor at the College of Holy Cross, Worcester, Massachusetts, reported at the American Psychological Association's Women's Health Conference in 1996 that women working forty-hour weeks averaged about one hour's less sleep a night than they needed. The deprivation is greater when children under eighteen are at home. Thomas Roth, head of the Sleep Disorders and Research Center at Detroit's Henry Ford Hospital, proposes a simple test for sleep debt: if you fall asleep in less than six minutes, the chances are that you are sleep-deprived. People typically take more than six minutes and upward of fifteen minutes to fall asleep. Of course, exceptions occur.

June Pilcher and Allen Huffcutt, psychologists at Bradley University, Peoria, Illinois, reviewed nineteen studies of sleep deprivation, with a total of 1,932 subjects (*Sleep,* June 1996). Their conclusion was that sleep deprivation has the largest effect on mood (it fosters a more negative mood), with a somewhat smaller effect on cognitive tasks and an even smaller effect on physical tasks. Overall, the average performance of sleep-deprived individuals was around the ninth percentile among the 1,932 total subjects.

The safety hazards of severe sleep deprivation—several days without sleep—can be eliminated by one night of natural, uninterrupted sleep (typically nine to ten hours).

Applications

1 If you must experience severe sleep deprivation, nap whenever possible.

2 If you have experienced severe sleep deprivation and are engaging in a safety-related activity such as driving or operating large machinery, take appropriate safety precautions: alert a backup, take frequent breaks and move around, take deep breaths, or sip a caffeine drink.

3 The maximum sleep deprivation possible without posing a major safety hazard is either (a) two to three days on no sleep, (b) six days with 1.5 hours' sleep each day, or (c) nine days with 3 hours' sleep each day (Webb, 1982).

4 Support naps and extended sleep periods for operators of long-haul vehicles.

5 Stand up for your rights. Don't let your peers sneer at you for getting proper sleep. They're the losers. Don't wake up early to have your workout; the stress from sleep loss cancels the benefits of the exercise.

TOPIC 7.9 Sleep and Medication

In the first edition of this book, I pointed out that European research on melatonin as the sleep neurotransmitter was far ahead of research in the United States. Of course, the United States has now caught up. The production of melatonin, a naturally occurring hormone, is triggered by the pineal gland in the absence of sunlight; sunlight's reappearance suppresses the production of melatonin (even for the blind). Melatonin is produced by the protein AA-NAT. As the brain perceives darkness, AA-NAT levels rise and so do melatonin levels. When the lights come back on, AA-NAT levels fall, and melatonin falls. Researchers call melatonin the "Dracula hormone" because it simulates the effect of nighttime. Melatonin is available from most health food stores, drugstores, and even supermarkets. The most common dosages range from 0.5 milligram to 10 milligrams. Although no harmful side effects have been reported (people do dream more vividly), most folks are taking too much. Dosage should begin at 0.5 milligram and increase by 0.5-milligram increments until the optimum level is found. A friend of ours, deprived of melatonin by lactose intolerance (melatonin is also a metabolite of dairy products), started out with a 3-milligram capsule and found himself getting a good night's sleep for the first time in years. I encouraged him to cut back and find the lowest possible dosage, which he has done. He's settled in at 1.5 milligrams.

Caution: Just to be on the safe side with melatonin, purchase only pills synthesized in the laboratory and avoid pills extracted from animals. Animal-derived melatonin carries a small chance of bringing along viruses and who knows what else. Check the label and/or consult with your pharmacist. Also, be aware that not everyone has endorsed melatonin as a sleep medication. Clifford Saper (1996), Putnam Professor of Neurology and Neuroscience at Harvard Medical School, writes, "At present, taking melatonin for sleep is both without sound basis and potentially dangerous, as the long term effects of it have never been studied adequately" (p. 3). He is especially concerned about lack of certification that the pills contain no contaminants.

The sleeping pills Dalmane and Halcion, while inducing sleep, have a negative effect on brain function, causing memory loss, withdrawal symptoms, and loss of coordination.

Steve Henriksen, of the Scripps Research Institute in La Jolla, California, reported in *Science,* June 9, 1995, that a compound identified as cis-9,10-octadecenoamide, dubbed oleamide, when injected into rats, even well-rested ones, results in a quick, deep sleep. The sleep appears to exhibit the features of natural sleep, including the lowering of body temperature. The compound occurs naturally in the cerebrospinal fluid of cats, rats, and humans. The substance, which is a lipid, is found at higher levels in sleep-deprived cats, lower levels in rested cats. When injected animals were roused from a deep sleep, they showed no apparent ill ("hangover") effects from the injections. The Scripps laboratory has successfully synthesized oleamide. Eventually, treatment will be available for humans either in the form of oleamide-based pills, which increase levels of oleamide, or oleamide hydrolase inhibitors, agents that prevent the breakdown of naturally occurring oleamide, thus optimizing one's natural supply.

Applications

1 People in their twenties should take melatonin infrequently and only for insomnia.

2 Those in their thirties to fifties may take it more frequently for insomnia.

3 Those over sixty should take it daily for insomnia.

4 Begin with 0.5 milligram two hours before desired sleep onset, and increase by 0.5 milligram until desired sleep quality is attained.

5 For jet lag associated with travel involving time-zone changes, try 1 milligram for each time zone crossed. Take your dosage a few hours before bedtime at your destination and again when you return.

6 Consult your physician if you are taking other medications, or if your dosage exceeds 10 milligrams.

7 Take melatonin only in the evenings, unless you are taking it for help with sleep problems associated with changing work shifts. In that case, take your dosage two hours before desired sleep onset, regardless of the time of day.

8 Try natural sleep inducers (see the summary at the end of this chapter) before developing a dependency on medication. If nothing works for you, consult your physician.

9 Blind people should continue to have eye checkups to ensure that they retain the capacity to register light. Otherwise, they lose the regularity of their biorhythms. In particular, they should not replace their natural eyes with artificial eyes that may be more pleasing for others to look at; again, that amounts to cutting off the receptors that tell the pineal gland to stop producing melatonin.

TOPIC 7.10 Naps

People who consistently nap live longer and show a 30 percent lower incidence of heart disease. My eighty-nine-year-old father-in-law (now deceased) took a nap after lunch for seventy years and outlived all the men in his family. The ideal time for a nap, according to David Dinges, a University of Pennsylvania sleep researcher, seems to be twelve hours after the midpoint of one's previous night's sleep. So if I sleep from 11:00 P.M. to 6:00 A.M., my nap urge should be around 2:30 P.M. The ideal length seems to be thirty minutes. Evening naps appear to interfere with sleep. The worst time to nap is at the bottom of the circadian rhythm, between 3:00 and 6:00 A.M. (Webb, 1982).

Rossi and Nimmons (1991) talk of "ultradian breaks" and recommend two or three twenty-minute naps a day. The urge to nap occurs in a natural rhythm and denying this urge has a negative effect on health, productivity, and general well-being. This denial occurs most commonly among office workers who stoically resist throughout the day. The result is chronic mild arousal.

Psychologists Mark Rosekind, of the NASA Fatigue Counter-measures Program, and David Dinges, of the University of Pennsylvania Medical School, have teamed to measure fatigue in pilots crossing multiple time zones (transmeridian flights). They found that pilots who were allowed a planned forty-minute rest period including a nap never lapsed in their performance, yet both rested and unrested pilots showed physiological measures of fatigue during the last ninety minutes of flight. The unrested group had twice as many measurably sleepy episodes as the rested group. The pilots' performance was measured by a timed response to a visual cue (*APA Monitor,* May 1996).

Lydia Dotto (1990) points out that the effects of napping are different for the sleep-deprived and the nondeprived. She found that for the sleep-deprived, napping improves performance but not mood; for normal sleepers, napping improves mood but not performance.

Applications

1 When possible, take a fifteen- to thirty-minute nap in early to midafternoon to get recharged. Some people practice meditation to achieve the same effect. Minimize your reliance on caffeine for recharging. *Viva la siesta!*

2 Although naps are generally recommended, they are crucial for people who do not get an uninterrupted night's sleep. The First Napper, President Bill Clinton, reportedly sleeps four to six hours, then naps at least once daily, anywhere from five to thirty minutes, and awakes refreshed. He claims to be able to nap leaning against a wall.

3 Provide a "nap room" at work. *(Contributed by Vicki Halsey of Blanchard Training)*

TOPIC 7.11 Dreams

Everybody dreams. Dreaming takes place during REM sleep, which first begins around the fourteenth to sixteenth week in the womb. The REM sleep of infants occupies about 45 to 60 percent of their total sleep time, while mature and senior adults engage in REM sleep about 20 to 25 percent of their sleep time. During REM, the nervous system's sensory output, external sensory input, and inhibition or control are blocked. Physiologically, this is accompanied by a drastic drop in production of the neurotransmitters serotonin and norepinephrine. Meanwhile, as the inhibiting effect of the serotonin and norepinephrine disappears, the neurotransmitter acetylcholine increases in the brain stem and activates a flood of internal memories and perceptions. The fact that we exert no management of these internal perceptions results in an often bizarre collage of whatever comes to the big screen during this central core dump.

Recent research by Allan Braun of the National Institutes of Health and Thomas Balkin of Walter Reed Army Institute of Research revealed that brain scans of dreaming subjects contained no activity in the frontal area of the brain, which is involved in planning and higher reasoning, thereby confirming the "unmanaged" nature of dreams. Interestingly, and in additional partial confirmation of the "unmanaged" theory, David Maurice, a professor of ocular biology at New York's Columbia-Presbyterian Medical Center, says that the primary purpose of rapid eye movement is to restore levels of oxygen to the cornea.

Hobson (1988) has defined a theory of dreams he calls the *activation-synthesis model,* which states that dreams are made (synthesized) out of the uncontrolled internal images and perceptions that bounce off each other (are activated) during REM sleep. He argues, accordingly, that "the meaning of dreams . . . is thus transparent rather than opaque. The content of most dreams can be read directly, without decoding. Since the dream state is open-ended, individual dreams are likely to reveal specific cognitive styles, specific aspects of an individual's projective view of the world, and specific historical experiences" (p. 219). Hobson points out that the physiology and content of dreams are similar to those of mental illness. The difference, he says, is that in dreaming we don't expect to have control of our minds, whereas the mentally ill have poor or no control of their memories and images where we would expect control to exist. He also presents a highly readable, recent review of dream research, including its history, a neurobiological description of dreaming, and a discussion of the interpretation of dreams.

Applications

1 Regard your dreams as a form of brainstorming, in which a flood of unevaluated and unmanaged images and ideas piggyback off each other and merge in often bizarre ways.

2 Understand that the search for latent, hidden meanings in dreams is a game with a potential for inappropriate results. I had a dream last night about trying to destroy a toy train before a Japanese woman prevented me; my wife was setting the charge as I kicked off on my bicycle. Each of these images represents something I read about recently: major rail accidents in Manhattan and South Carolina and an article in *Time* magazine about a Japanese executive who was forced to take a vacation. Don't ask why these images occur in your dreams; more appropriately, ask where they come from. Remember that bizarre combinations can result from zero management control.

TOPIC 7.12 Nightmares

Visualization techniques have proved to be a big help in reducing or eliminating nightmares. They consist of re-creating a visual scene or episode with one's eyes closed and can include actual physical movements; watch Olympic skiers visualize a run with movements before starting. These techniques can be self-taught and self-administered, or they can be learned with the help of a therapist or dream specialist.

Applications

1 If you want to try teaching yourself visualization techniques for nightmare reduction, try the following:

- Recall your most recent nightmare in full detail.
- Alter a significant detail in the nightmare (change a tiger to a cat, a man to a woman, a knife to a feather).
- Play through the complete nightmare, substituting this new detail throughout.
- Continue this sequence until the nightmare stops or becomes acceptable.

2 Visit a sleep clinic for professional help.

TOPIC 7.13 Sleep Differences Between the Sexes

The National Sleep Foundation published a report, available on their web site at http://206.215.227.10/nsf/publications/women.html, on October 22, 1998, that stated that women are 50 percent more likely to have disturbed sleep than men. Women's insomnia stems from menstruation, pregnancy, and menopause. An average of 2.5 nights of sleep disturbance are associated with the early stage of menstruation in 71 percent of women, totaling 30 days of poor sleep annually; disturbed sleep is reported by 79 percent of pregnant women; and menopause disrupts an average of five nights monthly in 56 percent of women. For the latter group, estrogen replacement therapy appears to ease insomnia.

Applications

1 Don't be one of the 7 percent of pregnant women who drink alcohol to help them sleep. It not only doesn't help you sleep; it also puts the fetus at risk.

② Be aware of the normal tendency for menstruation, menopause, and pregnancy to disrupt normal sleep. Try the specific recommendations listed in this chapter for help in getting to sleep, and see the summary list at the end of this chapter. When sleep disruption persists, reserve the right to take a nap to counter the effects of sleep deprivation.

TOPIC 7.14 **Getting Back to Sleep**

If you've awakened in the middle of the night and can't get back to sleep, it's a good bet that you've somehow become aroused. What you need to do is shut down your aroused state. Several of the strategies mentioned earlier in this chapter will minimize the chance of your waking. However, if the worst happens and you become wakeful, there are several ways to lower your level of arousal.

Applications

① Often, we can't get to sleep because thoughts are racing around in our heads trying to keep from being forgotten. Keep a pad and pen beside your bed and take a mental dump by writing down all those thoughts that are bumping into each other. You can then sleep peacefully and deal with them tomorrow.

② Sometimes our sleep is disturbed by an emotionally arousing disturbance, such as a phone call or a surprise intrusion. You need to come down from this state of limbic arousal—in other words, you need to get bored again. Try reading the most sleep-inducing book you can think of.

③ Get out of bed, leave the bedroom, and engage in a constructive but boring activity in subdued light. Getting up to a large dose of bright light will suppress melatonin production, which you don't want to happen. Associate your bed only with sleep.

④ Drink a cup of warm milk with honey.

5 Take a melatonin pill.

6 Check to make sure that your room is pitch-black; use wide, long, opaque shades that block out all light, or an eye mask.

7 Meditate.

8 If you can, simply enjoy resting.

TOPIC 7.15 Sleep and Aging

The senior adult's sleep episodes (which can include more than one sleep cycle) are 20 percent shorter than those of younger people (6 versus 7.5 hours), and the total time awake between initially going to sleep and getting up for good in the morning progresses gradually from around 1 percent in infancy to around 6 percent in seniors.

Applications

1 Although some shortening of sleep requirements and some increase in sleep-time wakefulness are normal in senior adults, drastic changes are not. Look for pharmaceuticals, diet, illness, or lack of exercise as probable culprits.

2 Understand that you probably will not sleep as long and as continually at age seventy-five as you did at age twenty-five. Build a nap into your schedule and simply get up and do something constructive if you cannot sleep.

TOPIC 7.16 Stability in Sleep Patterns

A study that related pilot error in landings to the interval between sleep periods (Webb, 1992) found that the more variable the interval between sleep periods, the more likely a pilot is to make an error in landing. In other words, for a five-day period, if pilot A is up for seventeen hours the first day, twelve the second, twenty the third, fifteen the fourth, and twenty-one the fifth, and pilot B is up for sixteen, eighteen, seventeen, eighteen, and sixteen hours on the same five days, pilot A will be more likely to make an error in landing (or other similar errors) than pilot B, whose intervals between sleep periods showed less variation from day to day.

Cross-cultural studies by Sara Harkness, an associate professor of human development and anthropology at Pennsylvania State University, found that quality of sleep in infants was related to lifestyle issues. For example, Harkness found that Dutch parents tend to pick up infants less during the day, encourage less stimulating activities during the day (for example, they do not appear to take infants to shopping malls), and put them to bed nightly at the same time. This preference for rest and regularity, according to Harkness, results in Dutch babies sleeping longer than American babies and sleeping through the night at an earlier age than American babies (reported by the Associated Press, February 21, 1995).

Applications

1 Pilots, and others in jobs with major safety implications that require continuing alertness, should minimize day-to-day variations in the number of hours between getting up and going to sleep.

2 Be aware that your infant's sleep patterns may reflect your lifestyle. For more regular sleep, prefer a more routine and less stimulating lifestyle.

TOPIC 7.17 A Note on Yawning

Yawning isn't what it's cracked up to be. Monica Greco, a psychologist at Rowan College in Philadelphia, and Temple University psychologist Roy Baenninger have spent years observing yawning in humans and animals. They have concluded that predators yawn much more than herbivores. Herbivores have less need to stay aroused, because their diet is a stationary target, whereas predators must stay very alert in order to capture prey and to avoid being captured. Compare the relatively laid back plant-eating giraffe, who doesn't yawn at all, to the frequently yawning and ever-active lion. In a November 22, 1994, Knight-Ridder release, Greco and Baenninger describe yawning as a method of self-arousal, and not as a sign of sleepiness. The yawning response appears to be triggered when dopamine falls below acceptable levels in the brain. The yawn exercises jaw muscles that affect the flow of blood to the brain. A good yawn reoxygenates the brain, leading to increased arousal and alertness. Evolutionarily, yawning is nature's way of priming the brain out of low arousal when things are boring but it's dangerous to be inattentive to what's going on.

Application

Enjoy your yawns, and don't be embarrassed that people may think you're sleepy. Consider a yawn to be nothing more than your (and others') right to a jolt of fresh air. Others should, in fact, consider your yawns as a compliment—after all, you're trying to remain maximally alert for them!

A Final Word on Sleep

Here are some of the major principles associated with good sleep:

Getting to Sleep

Consume dairy products (the warmer the better).

Avoid artificial sweeteners.

Avoid food additives.

Avoid caffeine within six hours of bedtime.

Keep to a regular bedtime.

Consume carbohydrates and fats.

Avoid protein.

Read or view unexciting material.

Avoid exercise within four hours of bedtime.

Sleep in absolute darkness (use a mask if necessary).

Maintain quiet (use earplugs if necessary).

Do not take naps after 3:00 P.M.

Meditate.

Avoid beans, raw onions, cruciferous vegetables (broccoli, cauliflower, cabbage), and spicy foods before bedtime.

Take melatonin pills.

Getting Quality Sleep

Lose weight.

Avoid alcohol within four hours of bedtime.

Drink water after alcohol consumption.

Plan sleep according to sleep cycles and circadian rhythms.

Do aerobic exercise regularly, but not close to bedtime.

Getting Back to Sleep

Write down what's on your mind.

Read something unexciting.

Drink warm milk with honey.

SUGGESTED RESOURCES

Arkin, A. M., Antrobus, J. S., and Ellman, S. J. (Eds.). (1978). *The Mind in Sleep.* Hillsdale, N.J.: Erlbaum.

Coren, S. (1996). *Sleep Thieves.* New York: Free Press.

Hobson, J. A. (1988). *The Dreaming Brain.* New York: Basic Books.

Sahelian, R. (1997). *Melatonin: Nature's Sleeping Pill* (2nd ed.). Garden City Park, N.Y.: Avery Publishing Group.

Webb, W. B. (1992). *Sleep: The Gentle Tyrant* (2nd ed.). Bolton, Mass.: Anker.

Web Sites

National Sleep Foundation:
   www.sleepfoundation.org

8

The Body Cognitive

The Effects of Exercise

R esearch is catching up with folk wisdom. From Homer ("Too much rest itself becomes a pain") to Shakespeare ("The labor we delight in physics pain"), the contributions of physical activity to mental performance have been touted. But not until recently have research findings supported these claims. This chapter visits some of these findings.

> **Strength of mind is Exercise, not Rest.**
>
> —Alexander Pope

TOPIC 8.1 Physical Activity

Jean Pierre Changeux (1997), of the Pasteur Institute in Paris, and Christopher Henderson, a researcher at the Developmental Biology Institute of Marseilles, have found that simple movement of the muscles stimulates the growth of axons, which carry messages between neurons. The number of axons is directly related to intelligence, and people (infants as well as adults) who move about more benefit from greater axonal development. Less movement results in fewer axons. Hence, the couch-potato syndrome is associated with lesser intelligence.

Applications

1 Move it or lose it.

2 Encourage physical activity from the cradle to the grave. Even people confined to wheelchairs or with limited mobility should move whatever they can. *(Contributed by Jane Howard)*

TOPIC 8.2 Aerobics

Covert Bailey (1991) applies the term *aerobic* to exercise that meets four criteria:

1. It must be nonstop.
2. It must last for a minimum of twelve minutes.
3. It must proceed at a comfortable pace.
4. It must exercise the muscles of the lower body.

He defines "comfortable pace" with a formula: at the conclusion of exercising, your pulse should be 220 minus your age, times 0.65 (or 0.8 for athletes). For me, that would mean a pulse of about 110. This formula is intended for the average person (about two-thirds of the population). For a more personal application of the formula, check pages 41–45 in Bailey (1991).

Mentally, aerobic exercise has at least six effects:

1. It clearly improves speed of recall, and much research points to an effect on the quality of mental functioning and the amount of recall.

2. It releases endorphins, the neurotransmitters that relax us into a state of cortical alertness. This is not the only way to reach cortical alertness (other relaxation methods will work as well), but it is certainly one way.

3. As reported in a National Institute of Mental Health study of over nineteen hundred individuals, people with little or no recreational activity are twice as likely to have depressive symptoms as people who regularly do aerobic exercise.

> "One of the first lessons one learns . . . is that the mind is a powerful factor in everything you do, including those exercises that seem to require a maximum of physical strength."
>
> —Joe Hyams,
> *Zen in the Martial Arts*

4. Aerobic exercise increases the number of neurotrophins (nerve growth factor), agents that stimulate the growth of nerve cells, that are available to the brain and nervous system, according to the work of Carl Cotman, director of the Institute for Brain Aging and Dementia at the University of California, Irvine. Cotman says that there is an optimum amount of exercise; rats who run five miles, for example, have no more neurotrophins than those who run only two. Kenneth Cooper (H. Thompson, 1995) underscores this point. Cooper, who started the aerobics craze with the publication of his book, *Aerobics* (1968), is concerned that overly vigorous exercising releases excess free radicals. He recommends the equivalent of walking two miles in under forty minutes, five times a week. In fact, he remarks, "If you are running more than fifteen miles a week, you are running for some other reason than your health" (quoted in H. Thompson, 1995, p. 136).

5. William Greenough, a professor at the University of Illinois' Beckman Institute, has determined that aerobic exercise results in an increase in capillaries around the neurons in the brain, causing more blood and oxygen to reach the brain.

6. Arthur Kramer, a research psychologist who is also with the Beckman Institute, has established that a forty-five-minute

water aerobics class three times a week, lasting for ten weeks, in people sixty-three to eighty-two years old, results in improved, faster reaction times. He further avows that declines in reaction time appear to be related to declines in fitness more than to aging. (The last three studies were summarized in Brink, 1995.)

Interestingly, Edwin Boyle, Jr., director of research at the Miami Heart Institute, found that arteriosclerotic patients with memory loss improved their memory after breathing pure oxygen, with effects lasting up to six months! Aerobic exercise, of course, heightens oxygen intake.

Another series of studies has concluded that hunger is inhibited when (1) the brain contains high levels of glucose and serotonin and (2) the blood contains high levels of epinephrine, norepinephrine, and dopamine. Exercise tends to raise levels of all five of these neurotransmitters.

A few words of caution. First, exercise appears to be more effective in preserving mental function that could decline with aging, rather than in improving function among people who have always been sedentary and who, later in life, try to make up for lost time. Second, the benefits of exercise are associated with long-term exercising, rather than brief episodes of several months' duration. And we lose the benefits of having exercised when we stop.

Applications

1 For maximum benefit, exercise after the most stressful part of the day is over and before a period in which mental alertness is required or desired. For some of us, this may have to be an either-or situation. High stress nullifies the effect of aerobic exercise. You must exercise again after a stressful episode. (Stress releases the toxin cortisol, and aerobic exercise dissipates it. For more discussion of this relationship, see Topic 20.4.)

2 Avoid exercising before bedtime. It tends to interfere with sleep.

3 Don't ride when you can walk; don't sit when you can stand.

4 Learn deep-breathing exercises (breathe in for six counts, hold for four counts, expel for six counts) and isometric exercises for times when you must be sedentary for long periods.

5 Ensure that you and all your family members get aerobic exercise (brisk walking or its equivalent) for thirty to forty-five minutes a day, at least five days per week.

6 Exercise your influence to ensure that your local schools are providing daily aerobic exercise for students. According to the President's Council on Physical Fitness and Sports, only 36 percent of kids in grades 1–12 get a daily thirty-minute aerobic workout. (Forty percent of five-year-olds already show at least one heart disease risk factor!)

TOPIC 8.3   The Importance of Choice

Norman Cousins (1989) wrote of studies that emphasize how choice influences the degree of health benefits of exercise. If an individual is forced to engage in an exercise against his or her will, the health benefits tend to be lessened. Cousins cited the ineffectiveness of his having been assigned to walk on a treadmill versus his dramatic improvement after he changed, by his choice, to walking on a track. Apparently the stress of engaging in exercise that is not of our choosing can outweigh its health benefits. As another example of this, my wife's first husband loved playing tennis, especially during hot summer afternoons. She hated it and often sustained headaches when she was pressured into playing with him. She still avoids tennis eighteen years later. (See Chapter Twenty for further discussion of the importance of personal control in managing stress.)

James Gavin, director of the graduate program in applied human sciences at Concordia University in Montreal, has developed a model for prescribing exercise regimens based on personality characteristics. This is related to Cousins's notion of choice in that Gavin maintains that some kind of exercise will appeal to everyone. In his book *The Exercise Habit* (1992), he includes a seven-dimension psychosocial scale to assist in relating exercise to personality.

Applications

1 Avoid engaging in an exercise for its health benefits if you don't really have a positive attitude toward it. Choose an exercise that appeals to you. I've had many friends try to encourage me to take aerobics classes. For me, personally, that is a distasteful proposition—I don't like the music many aerobics instructors use to motivate their participants. Instead, I walk. I love to walk. I could write an essay on why I like walking, but I'd better resist . . .

2 Read Gavin's *The Exercise Habit* (1992).

TOPIC 8.4   Altering Mood and Cravings

In a study of sixteen addicted smokers and eighteen regular snackers, Robert Thayer (1989) reported that brisk ten-minute walks reduced their cravings and improved their mood. The walking smokers reported an average increase of 50 percent in the time before they craved a smoke over the control subjects. Those in a poor mood who walked instead of having a snack reported significantly higher and longer elevations of mood over nonwalking snackers. In subsequent studies, Thayer and others have found that an intensive workout (a forty-five-minute jog) has no more effect on mood than a ten-minute brisk walk.

Gregory Mondin, of the Department of Counseling Psychology, University of Wisconsin–Madison, tested ten volunteers who were accustomed to working out six days a week. After skipping two workouts, all experienced one or more of various mood swings, including anxiety, depression, confusion, and that "blah" feeling. Resuming their exercise routine fixed things right up.

Michael Gallagher, vice-dean of the School of Osteopathic Medicine at the University of Medicine and Dentistry of New Jersey in Newark, has found that participating in regular, nonjarring (that is, not jogging) aerobic exercise, such as swimming, using a stationary bicycle, or walking, improves the chances of avoiding migraine headaches among those prone to suffer from them. Apparently, one precursor of migraines is muscle tension, and the endorphins released by aerobic exercise decrease that tension.

One explanation of exercise's benefits comes from the research of the University of Georgia's Rod Dishman, a professor of exercise science, who has identified an increase in epinephrine levels as a result of sustained exercise. Epinephrine permeates the locus coeruleus, which is a kind of junction box for the several brain functions associated with mood and emotion. As a result, Dishman theorizes, exercise-increased levels of epinephrine serve to lubricate the individual's mechanism for coping with stress. Interestingly, he points out, several of the antidepressant drugs are associated with elevated levels of epinephrine. Mark Sothman, dean of the School of Allied Health at the Indiana University School of Medicine, says that aerobic exercise, in effect, provides a workout for the body's internal communication system so that when stress occurs, one's physical coping mechanisms are in good order. Both Sothman and Dishman have confirmed these relationships in animal and human experiments (they are summarized in the July 1996 *APA Monitor*).

Applications

1 During prolonged sedentary periods or periods of stress, take a brisk ten-minute walk every couple of hours—outdoors, if possible.

2 During coffee breaks, try taking a ten-minute walk outside instead. The resulting natural arousal will equal or better the arousal you would get from more caffeine and stale office air. Walk by yourself or with a group, whichever pleases you.

3 If not even a ten-minute walk is possible, at least do a few jumping jacks, sit-ups, push-ups, isometric exercises, or stretches, or just simply meditate, as a way to release the tension build-up accompanying lack of exercise.

TOPIC 8.5   Extreme Exercise and the Staleness Syndrome

John Raglin, an Indiana University sports psychologist and kinesiologist (raglinj@indiana.edu), has tagged a condition resulting from continuing high athletic performance and workouts as the "staleness syndrome" (*APA Monitor,* April 1996; see also his "Overtraining and Staleness" in Singer, Murphey, and Tennant, 1993). Around 5 to 10 percent of athletes who train intensely develop a pattern of irritability, tension, anger, lack of desire to train, sleep disturbance, muscle soreness, decrease in immune function (and accompanying susceptibility to infectious diseases), depression, perceptual changes (for example, routines may suddenly seem harder), and general mental instability. The result is an abrupt halt in the ability to perform. Even short breaks or reduced workout schedules don't relieve the pattern. Only complete rest for several months appears to restore the prior performance level, yet the prior levels are not always regained. About 60 percent of elite long-distance runners will suffer from staleness at some point. Staleness also affects about 30 percent of sub-Olympic athletes, as well as some recreational athletes, who train seriously.

Raglin has found that staleness can be avoided by monitoring athletes' moods. In an experiment with swimmers, researchers administered a mood test, the Profile of Mood States (POMS) (McNair, Lorr, and Droppleman, 1971), and varied the swimmers' workout schedules in a way that kept their moods within an optimum range. For the first time in ten years, no team member developed staleness. Raglin (personal correspondence) reports that scores on the POMS correlate nicely with relevant biological changes, such as muscle glycogen, cortisol, and neuromuscular function, suggesting that the psychological mood changes are symptoms of physical changes. Unfortunately, many athletes misinterpret the symptoms and mistakenly choose to work out harder (with even worse results) rather than to lighten up.

Applications

1 If you train intensely or are associated with athletes who train intensely, contact Raglin for specific suggestions. Begin by visiting his web site at www.indiana.edu/~kines/raglin.htm.

② Raglin suggests that because athletes in intense training tend to be honest about physical symptoms and mood states, a simple seven-point scale that measures soreness, general well-being, and perceived exertion can serve as well for self-monitoring as the seventy-two-item, five-minute POMS.

③ Staleness in exercise bears a remarkable similarity to burnout at work. See the discussion of burnout in Topic 20.4 for further understanding and recommendations concerning this phenomenon.

TOPIC 8.6 Exercise and Testosterone

Jim Morrison, a psychologist at Iona University in New York, has established that the traditional vigorous workout dramatically increases testosterone levels in men but, interestingly, not in women. As a result, men who return to the stress of work immediately after a workout are more likely to experience emotional outbursts and acts of aggression. Men who cool off for fifteen to twenty minutes do not experience such outbursts. The effect is greater after a competitive, nonaerobic workout like handball than after a noncompetitive, aerobic workout like brisk walking.

Applications

① Men should allow a twenty-minute "chill" after working out and before entering a stressful setting. Otherwise, be prepared to deal with the consequences of a possible outburst.

② When a twenty-minute cooldown is not possible, engage in meditation, deep breathing, isometrics, or some other process that assists in refocusing and relaxing.

TOPIC 8.7 Exercise and Smoking

The Cleveland Clinic's Michael Lauer studied three thousand people and reported in *Circulation* (as cited in the September 27, 1997, *Chicago Tribune*) that the heart rates of a certain category of smokers fail to increase with exercise. Normally, one's body produces epinephrine during exercise, which increases the heartbeat. Nicotine produces a similar effect, and Lauer attributes the lack of rate increase in some smokers to a kind of tolerance their system builds up toward exercise-induced epinephrine. Because of the constant signals from nicotine, the heart ignores the exercise-induced epinephrine signals. These smoking exercisers without rate increases are five times more likely to have a heart attack than are nonsmokers with normal heart-rate reactions to exercise.

Application

This is simply another reason to quit smoking. If you are a smoker and you think your exercise is offsetting the effects of smoking, you might check your actual rate before and after exercising to see if you're really getting any circulatory system benefit from the exercise.

TOPIC 8.8 Soccer Headers

Adrienne Witol, an inpatient psychologist at the Medical College of Virginia, and Frank M. Webbe, a professor in Florida Institute of Technology's School of Psychology, studied sixty male soccer players who were at least fifteen years of age and who played five times per week. They determined that players who engaged in "heading" the ball more frequently performed less well on tests of visual searching, attention, mental flexibility, general IQ, and facial recognition than did players who headed the ball infrequently or never. Because the study was not longitudinal, the researchers do not know if the loss of mental function associated with heading the ball is reversible once the players no longer participate in soccer.

Application

If you are a soccer player or associate with soccer players, support the practice of "heading" on an extremely limited basis, if at all. Why take such a risk? Heads are not made for bashing.

TOPIC 8.9   Peak Athletic Performance

Charles Garfield (1984) has described a process that guides athletes into superior performance using mental training. In fact, he reports that one can reduce one's physical training (for example, running laps) and, by replacing physical training with mental training, increase levels of performance. Garfield's process includes visualization, mental rehearsal techniques, goal setting, and volitional self-awareness.

Applications

1 If you desire to be a peak athletic performer, read and digest Garfield's book.

2 Another "mental training" approach to peak athletic performance has been developed by Carol Ann Erickson and Arlene Berkman of the Brain-Body Center for Performance Enhancement; Scarsdale, New York; phone: 914-725-2458.

SUGGESTED RESOURCES

Bailey, C. (1991). *The New Fit or Fat.* Boston: Houghton Mifflin.

Brink, S. (1995, May 15). "Smart Moves." *U.S. News & World Report,* pp. 76–85.

Changeux, J.-P. (1997). *Neuronal Man: The Biology of Mind* (L. Garey, trans.). Princeton, N.J.: Princeton University Press.

Coop, R. H. (1993). *Mind over Golf: Play Your Best by Thinking Smart.* Old Tappan, N.J.: Macmillan.

Garfield, C. A. (1984). *Peak Performance: Mental Training Techniques of the World's Greatest Athletes.* Los Angeles: Tarcher.

Gavin, J. (1992). *The Exercise Habit.* Champaign, Ill.: Human Kinetics.

Morgan, W. P. (Ed.). (1997). *Physical Activity and Mental Health.* Washington, D.C.: Taylor & Francis.

Neeper, S. A., Gomez-Pinilla, F., Choi, J., and Cotman, C. W. (1995). "Exercise Raises Brain Neurotrophins." *Nature, 373,* 109.

Singer, R. B., Murphey, M., and Tennant, L. K. (Eds.). (1993). *Handbook of Research on Sport Psychology.* Old Tappan, N.J.: Macmillan.

9

Humoring the Mind

Laughter as Free (or Cheap) Medicine

> **Strange, when you come to think of it, that of all the countless folk who have lived before our time on this planet not one is known in history or in legend as having died of laughter.**
>
> —Sir Max Beerbohm

Twenty years ago, humor would not have made its way into a book about brain research. However, we have discovered a dramatic relationship between laughter, a sense of humor, levels of neuro-chemicals such as endorphins, and the function of the immune system—such a dramatic relationship, in fact, that Norman Cousins used slapstick comedy as a "sleeping pill." Today, increasingly, researchers are trying to get a handle on the nature of humor, and on who benefits from different kinds of humor.

TOPIC 9.1 The Structure of Humor

Willibald Ruch, who teaches in the psychology department of Heinrich Heine University in Düsseldorf, Germany, challenged the psychological research community in 1991 to develop a universal taxonomy of humor. Countries that have validated the ensuing model, called the 3WD model ("WD" for "Witz Dimensionen," German for "humor dimensions"), include Austria, France, Italy, Turkey, and the United States. The model of humor appreciation has two modes: the stimulus (the joke) and the response (amused or not amused).

The stimulus, or joke, will fall into one of two *structure* categories plus a *content* category. The content category describes a joke as either *sexual* or *not sexual,* independent of the structure of the joke: the content overrides the structure. The two structure categories are *incongruity resolution* and *nonsense*. In incongruity resolution, the punch line reveals information that clarifies earlier incongruities. Example: A priest asks the bishop, "Is it permissible to smoke while praying?" The bishop replies, "Certainly not!" Later, a fellow priest, hearing of the first priest's embarrassment at the hands of the bishop, advises: "Next time, ask if it is permissible to pray while smoking." In the nonsense category, the punch line does not clarify earlier incongruities; rather it confounds them by making no resolution at all, by making only a partial resolution, or by introducing even more absurdity or incongruity. Example: Question: "How many psychologists does it take to screw in a lightbulb?" Answer: "Only one, but the light bulb must really want to change."

> "With the fearful strain that is on me night and day, if I did not laugh I should die."
>
> —Abraham Lincoln

The response has two conditions: funny or not funny and aversive or not aversive. So a joke may be funny yet aversive, funny and not aversive, not funny and aversive, or not funny and not aversive. A funny and aversive joke would be one in which the respondent dislikes, say, a reference to her or his religion but appreciates the good punch line. Maximum joke appreciation is defined as a judgment of funny and not aversive, while minimum appreciation is defined as aversive and not funny. Thus, a joke can be evaluated with the 3WD model and receive scores on six categories. These categories are presented in Table 9.1.

Table 9.1. The Six Dimensions of Humor Appreciation.		
Categories	**Funny**	**Aversive**
Incongruity resolution (structure)	Funny and incongruity-resolving	Aversive and incongruity-resolving
Nonsense (structure)	Funny and nonsensical	Aversive and nonsensical
Sexual (content)	Funny and sexual	Aversive and sexual

Forabosco and Ruch (1994) report that personality traits (see Chapter Twenty-One for complete definitions of personality traits) are associated clearly with appreciation (funny and not aversive) of the three structure and content categories:

- People low in Extraversion and low in Openness prefer incongruity resolution humor.

- People high in Extraversion and high in Openness prefer nonsense humor.

- People high in Negative Emotionality, Extraversion, and Openness and low in Agreeableness enjoy sexual humor.

They also reported that older subjects preferred incongruity resolution humor, while younger subjects preferred nonsense humor.

Application

If you are preparing jokes for a presentation, public or private, and the stakes are high, you might try managing your risk in joke telling by assessing the audience with respect to Extraversion (sales representatives are usually higher, engineers lower, for example) and Openness (people with high Openness are usually more liberal; those with low Openness are more conservative). Emphasize incongruity resolution humor with older, more conservative, less outgoing groups. Emphasize nonsense humor with younger, more liberal, more outgoing groups. If your audience has a mixture of these characteristics, then mix up the humor structure.

TOPIC 9.2 Humor and the Immune System

Norman Cousins (1979, 1989) is known as the founder of psychoneuroimmunology (PNI) (see Topic 14.2). Originally he called the concept of mentally influencing the immune system "hardiness." One of the four critical ingredients of hardiness is positive emotions, which Cousins defines as maintaining a sense of humor and general joyfulness. He refers to laughter as "internal jogging." Laughter is healthy. Laughter appears to be an especially important ingredient in recovering from life-threatening illnesses. Cousins (1989) found that even a few moments of laughter can reduce the sedimentation rate, which is a measure of inflammation. Specifically, according to research by Lee S. Berk, a professor at the Schools of Medicine and Public Health at Loma Linda University in California (*APA Monitor,* September 1997, p. 18), laughter results in

- Enhanced respiration

- An increased number of immune cells

- An increase in immune-cell proliferation

- A decrease in cortisol

- An increase in endorphins

- An increase in salivary immunoglobulin type A concentrations

Tests of problem-solving ability yield better results when they are preceded by laughter. Laughter has a way of turning off posterior hypothalamic activity and allowing the cerebral cortex to carry on stress-free activity. Cousins reports that ten minutes of laughter can provide a person who is in pain with at least two hours of good sleep. David McClelland (1986) has confirmed that salivary immunoglobulin type A is significantly higher among people with a stronger sense of humor.

Michelle G. Newman, a psychologist at Pennsylvania State University, reports from her research that people can learn to use humor as a coping device and that this learned humor has marked effects (*APA Monitor,* September 1997, p. 18). She asked people who normally did not use coping humor to make up, impromptu, a comedic monologue to accompany the videotape of a gruesome industrial accident. Those who made up a nonhumorous monologue to accompany the video showed a measurably higher stress response (measured by blood pressure, skin conductance, and skin temperature) than the humorous commentators.

While Newman shows that one can learn to use humor as a coping device, Lee Berk and some associates have developed a computer program that analyzes people's humor preferences, so that a kind of humor prescription can be written for them. He calls the program SMILE (Subjective Multidimensional Interactive Laughter Evaluation). After ten minutes, using a question-and-answer format, SMILE prints out a humor profile for an individual along with a detailed list of books, videos, comic personalities, and other resources especially chosen to match her or his profile.

Applications

1   Check out the bibliography on laughter in the back of Cousins (1989). Cousins made the "humor cart" famous. Today many hospital oncology departments have a wide variety of laughter-producing materials available for patients and their families, from comic books to videos, audiotapes, and humorous books and magazines.

2   Give yourself permission to perform the whole range of laughs— from the gut-massaging belly laugh to the social titter.

3   Consciously develop your sense of humor, both as an originator of humor and as someone who appreciates and reacts to humor. Here are some suggestions for developing your sense of humor:

- Whenever you hear something funny that you like, try telling it three times within twenty-four hours. Then you're likely to remember it.

- Keep a list of the key words and phrases of your favorite jokes, riddles, and humorous stories (I keep mine on a piece of paper in the black leather folder I carry to meetings and appointments). When you anticipate a need for one of them, pull out your list ahead of time and select one or more that are appropriate for the occasion. If you don't trust your judgment, confer with your spouse or a colleague.

- Keep a humor file, both on your computer and in your paper file cabinet. Bring out some of your humor pages for friends to enjoy from time to time.
- Explore Internet humor resources; there are plenty of "joke-of-the-day" mail lists.
- Read the biographies and autobiographies of your favorite humorists. Pick up techniques from their lives, and share amusing episodes from their lives with your associates.

❹ Order your personal humor profile based on Lee Berk's SMILE software for $9.95 by calling 800-759-1294 or by visiting SMILE's web site at www.touchstarpro.com/smile-software.html. Or go ahead and order the software!

TOPIC 9.3 Humor and Gender

John Martellaro of the *Kansas City Star* reported on an informal survey among stand-up comics. Although the findings reflect a trend and not a clear-cut gender difference, generally these folks who live by their audience savvy agree on certain tendencies toward gender differences with respect to humor. Men have the following preferences:

- The humor doesn't have to be quite so intelligent.

- They appreciate silly or slapstick humor more.

- They typically respond better to dirtier or cruder humor laced with profanities.

- They typically don't laugh at jokes about themselves or about men in general but will laugh about women or about other specific men; that is, they are more likely to laugh at jokes at other people's expense.

- They are more reactive and tend to be less patient with longer prologues.

- They like anything physical and aggressive.

- Specifically, they like the Three Stooges, Tim Allen ("Home Improvement"), cartoons (especially "The Simpsons," "Ren and Stimpy," and "Road Runner"), films with Mel Brooks and Chevy Chase, Jackie Gleason's "The Honeymooners," "Monty Python," and John Cleese.

Women have the following preferences:

- They enjoy jokes that involve childbirth and raising children.

- They have a generally "dry" sense of humor.

- They laugh at jokes about themselves and other women as well as jokes about men; that is, they are more likely to laugh at jokes at their own expense.

- They like jokes about relationship stuff and the battle of the sexes.

- They like the person telling a joke to set up a scenario, not just go for the quick punch.

- They like the cute, romantic, sugar-coated stuff.

- They are turned off by the graphically dirty.

- Specifically, they like Jerry Seinfeld, Jay Leno, "Cheers," John Candy, films with Doris Day and Rock Hudson, "The Andy Griffith Show," "Family Ties," and W. C. Fields.

The comics agreed that "family, food, and sex" are, for the most part, good common ground.

In partial confirmation of this "folk" approach to humor research, Herbert M. Lefcourt, a psychologist at the University of Waterloo, Ontario, Canada, has reported that males and females who use humor to cope with stress will tend to experience different results: females' systolic blood pressure falls, while that of males elevates. Females who joke about their stress have lower blood pressure than those who don't, while males who joke about their stress have higher blood pressure than those who don't. Lefcourt blames this difference on their two distinctly different kinds of humor: females laugh at themselves and males laugh at others. For example, when they make a social blunder, females tend to say something self-deprecating (such as referring to their clumsiness), while males tend to say something aggressive. Upon dropping a glass of milk, a female might say, "My, my, oh what a clumsy klutz I am!" A male might say, "Did I drown that cockroach yet? At least maybe I knocked him out!" As a result, the female restores "social closeness," while the male, in effect, tries to maintain his dominant position in the "social hierarchy." The former lowers blood pressure; the latter raises blood pressure (*APA Monitor,* September 1997, pp. 18 ff.).

In addition to Lefcourt's work, Robert Provine, director of the neuroscience program at the University of Maryland Baltimore County; Glenn Weisfeld, a psychology professor at Wayne State University in Detroit; and Richard Alexander, Hubbell Professor of Evolutionary Biology at the University of Michigan at Ann Arbor, report on their various research efforts on gender differences in humor (*APA Monitor,* September 1997, p. 16). Provine reports that while the average speaker laughs 46 percent more than the audience, women laugh 127 percent more than their male audiences and males laugh 7 percent *less* than their female audiences. Provine concludes that the trend is for men to be humor producers, women to be laughers. Alexander expands on this trend by theorizing that humor production (jokes and puns, for example) serves to establish the humorist's status, while the laugher signals acceptance of, and frequently submission to, the humorist. Laughter creates the social perception of granting status to the humorist. It's dominance and submission all over again.

Applications

❶ To fully develop your sense of humor, allow yourself to explore all ranges of humor content. If you fit the stereotypically male or female humor profile, consciously expect humor from heretofore unhumorous sources. Don't just say you don't like Jay Leno; if you find yourself watching Jay Leno involuntarily, allow yourself to be surprised with something really laughter-provoking. Minimize preconceptions about humor.

❷ If some of your humor doesn't work around members of the opposite gender (or members of your own gender, for that matter), realize that the problem may not be your style. They may not like certain humor content regardless of who's telling it!

3 If you are a male, understand that using aggressive humor as a way of coping with stressful situations does not help your stress. Practice a more self-deprecating approach: learn stock lines, such as "If only Mommy and Daddy could see me now," or "Well, nobody can accuse me of batting a thousand!" or "That's not the first time and it won't be the last! Blast!" Observe other males who make aggressive, attacking jokes when they are under stress, and practice rewording or reframing their comments to be self-deprecating. Realize that aggressive, combative humor in stressful situations is not heart-healthy.

4 If you are a woman who does not use humor to cope in stressful situations, learn some good self-deprecating lines to use as needed, such as "Well, I sure get the klutz prize today!" or "Infamy, infamy, somebody's got it in-for-me" (from the Broadway musical *Me and My Girl*) or "I'm just a girl who can't say no!" Realize that using such self-deprecating humor lessens your feeling of stress.

5 If you see yourself as more of a humorist than a laugher, consider the possibility that you hold back laughter as a nonverbal way of refusing to confer status on another person. Be aware of the power of appreciative laughter to make other people feel good about themselves, as well as to lower your own stress level.

SUGGESTED RESOURCES

Cousins, N. (1979). *Anatomy of an Illness.* New York: Norton.

Cousins, N. (1989). *Head First: The Biology of Hope.* New York: NAL/Dutton.

Forabosco, G., and Ruch, W. (1994). "Sensation Seeking, Social Attitudes and Humor Appreciation in Italy." *Personality and Individual Differences, 16*(4), 515–528.

Ruch, W. (1988). "Sensation Seeking and the Enjoyment of Structure and Content of Humour: Stability of Findings Across Four Samples." *Personality and Individual Differences, 9,* 861–871.

10

Music

As a Means and as an End

> **Music has charms to soothe a savage breast, To soften rocks, or bend a knotted oak.**
>
> —William Congreve, The Mourning Bride

Historically, music has been mostly entertainment and, to a lesser degree, a communication tool. From the chamber music of aristocrats to the bugle calls of soldiers, music has cut through the normal channels of words with a stirring directness and immediacy. Increasingly, music has acquired new roles—medicinal, facilitative, and mood-altering. This chapter will explore some of these more recent musical functions.

TOPIC 10.1   Learning Music

Researchers at the University of Konstanz in Germany have determined through magnetic resonance imaging that the area of the somatosensory cortex allocated to the fingers of the left hand is larger for string players than for nonplayers. The size of the enlarged area is not related to the number of hours of practice daily, but it is related to the number of years spent playing the instrument. The window for learning musical instruments appears to be from three to ten years of age. It is harder to learn after ten years of age, and concert-quality players generally begin their instrumental study before the age of ten.

Looking for the secret of perfect pitch (the ability to sing a pitch without a preceding musical point of reference, as in "Can you hum an 'A' for me?"), Gottfried Schlaug, then a neurological fellow with the Heinrich Heine University in Düsseldorf, Germany (now with Beth Israel Hospital in Boston), took magnetic resonance images of the brains of thirty musicians, eleven of whom had perfect pitch, and thirty nonmusicians. The eleven musicians with perfect pitch had a planum temporale in the left hemisphere that was 40 percent larger than the planum temporale in the right hemisphere. The nineteen musicians without perfect pitch had only a slightly enlarged planum temporale, which was not significantly different from that area in the nonmusicians (*Science,* February 3, 1995).

Schlaug reported that the evidence pointed to perfect pitch occurring only among musicians who had been exposed to music before age seven, with the likelihood of acquiring perfect pitch extremely unlikely when initial exposure to music came after ten years of age. Some people without perfect pitch do have the 40 percent enlarged area, so Schlaug concludes that nature and nurture both play a role. The enlargement is necessary but not sufficient for perfect pitch; one must also be exposed to music in a timely manner.

In related research at Montreal's McGill University, brain scans of musicians with perfect pitch showed greater activation in the left posterior dorsolateral frontal cortex while listening to musical tones; people who did not have perfect pitch, but who did have relative pitch, only showed greater activation in this area when they were comparing notes. Research team leader Robert Zatorre (1998) concluded that this area of the brain is activated when naming notes, and that it is activated spontaneously for people with perfect pitch.

Applications

1   Encourage young children to sing; sing with them and encourage them to sing with others.

2   If your child shows an interest, get an instrument early. Suzuki violin, piano, and flute instruction begins before school age, and instruments are available in appropriate sizes for young children.

3   Expose your child to musical training before the age of seven and continue for the best chance of developing perfect pitch.

TOPIC 10.2 Musical Training and Spatial Ability: The Mozart Effect

Frances Rauscher, who at the time was at the University of California, Irvine; along with Gordon Shaw, Linda Levine, and Katherine Ky, all of UC Irvine; and Eric Wright, of the Irvine Conservatory of Music, gave twice-weekly keyboard lessons of twelve minutes each, provided daily thirty-minute group singing lessons, and supervised daily practice with twenty-two three-year-olds for as long as the students desired. The tunes included children's songs and folk melodies. Three control groups were monitored: one with group singing alone, one with computer keyboard training, and a third with no lessons. This program extended over eight months in two Los Angeles preschools. Measuring spatial reasoning by manipulating various objects, Rauscher found that spatial-reasoning tests administered after four months and again after eight months showed a 35 percent improvement in spatial reasoning among the experimental group. None of the control groups showed pretest to post-test improvement in spatial ability (*APA Monitor*, October 1994, p. 5). At a presentation given as part of the Learning Brain Expo in San Diego, California, October 30, 1998, Gordon Shaw pointed out that the entire experimental group showed improvement, the low-scoring students as well as the high scorers. In other words, if you can visualize the distribution of scores as a normal curve, the entire curve moved to the right about 35 percent.

The preschool study was an extension of earlier research conducted by Rauscher in which thirty-six college students listened to Mozart's *Sonata for Two Pianos in D Major* (K. 448) for ten minutes just before taking an intelligence test. The students who listened to the Mozart piano music scored, on average, 60 percent higher (equivalent to eight to nine points) than students who had listened to relaxation tapes with Philip Glass's "minimalist" music or who had just meditated silently. However, the benefits disappeared after about ten to fifteen minutes (*Nature,* October 1993). Researchers see this phenomenon as a kind of warm-up effect, in which the complexity and regularity of classical music activates the neural circuitry of the brain associated with spatial reasoning. Apparently, the effect of music instruction on young children, in whom neural circuitry is relatively more plastic, or changeable, is significantly more long term than the effect of music listening among older learners. In a follow-up study with second graders, two Los Angeles classrooms received four months of piano keyboard training (three hours of training weekly with no practice). Afterward, they showed a 27 percent increase in scores on fractions and proportional math (the results will be published in the spring of 1999).

Rauscher, who is now an assistant professor of child development at the University of Wisconsin–Oshkosh, also played music to groups of rats for twelve hours a day, using a repeating-loop audiotape. One group heard Mozart (the same K. 448!), one listened to Philip Glass, and a third got silence. These lab rats had been performing in mazes on a daily basis. With music added, things changed. The Mozart rats began executing their mazes significantly faster, but the Glass and silent-treatment rats showed no increase in speed. The effect lasted for about four hours after the tapes ended.

One final note. Why Mozart? Why not Brahms, Beethoven, or Stravinsky? In planning the original research, Rauscher and her colleagues reasoned that Mozart is unique in that he exhibits three remarkable characteristics: everybody seems to like his music, he began composing at an early age (four to five years old), and throughout his prolific output there doesn't seem to be a dud. The conclusion drawn from this is that Mozart's brain was probably ideally suited for musical composition and that he can be regarded as the purest exemplar of satisfying musical composition.

Applications

❶　Consider encouraging all child care providers in your area to include appropriate periods of music listening. Although intensive research continues to be done with music, some implications are beginning to emerge. In fact, the states of Georgia and Florida have already begun mandating Mozart for tots, with Florida requiring music in day care centers and Georgia handing out free tapes.

❷　Encourage young children to learn piano keyboarding.

❸　Encourage young children to learn the instruments of their choice in addition to piano keyboarding.

❹　Encourage people to play Mozart and similarly uncomplicated baroque and classical music as a brain organizer.

❺　Visit the Music Intelligence Neural Development project's web site at www.mindinst.org for more information on music and neural development. The web manager will respond to requests for reprints.

❻　Look for Gordon Shaw's book, *Music Enhances Learning,* soon to be published by Academic Press.

TOPIC 10.3 **When Music Interferes with Learning**

Proponents of "accelerated learning" (see the beginning of Chapter Twenty-Three) have long argued that learners remember more material when it is taught to the accompaniment of music such as Vivaldi's and Mozart's. The research, however, does not support this claim. In a study by M. J. Wagner and G. Tilney (1983), the accelerated-learning students in two German courses of equal length learned 50 percent less. And in a study

> "Music oft hath such a charm
> To make bad good, and good provoke to harm."
>
> —William Shakespeare, *Measure for Measure*

by B. J. Bush (1986) at the Defense Language Institute in Monterey, California, a ten-week accelerated-learning course in Russian was compared to a fifteen-week traditional course; the music-accompanied accelerated learners mastered 40 percent less information than those using traditional pedagogy. Part of the explanation must be that the music competes for the attentional focus of the learner. (See the discussion of attention in Topic 23.9.)

H. J. Crawford and C. H. Strapp (1994) studied the effects of listening to music on verbal and visual-spatial performance, with the following conclusions:

1. Those who choose to use music to accompany study are much more extraverted.

2. Extraverts in general report that they are less bothered by noise and music.

3. People's self-perception of the degree to which music and noise bother them is unreliable.

4. Vocal music is more bothersome than instrumental music.

5. Music interferes more with complex tasks than it does with simpler tasks and more with verbal tasks than with visual-spatial tasks.

Applications

❶ Limit music to transitional uses in a learning environment. Don't allow it to compete for attention with the material to be learned.

❷ If you insist on using music to accompany rote learning, use melodies that are universally known by your learners, such as "Twinkle, Twinkle, Little Star." If the melody is a well-established schema for the learner, it is less likely to compete and more likely to support the learning.

TOPIC 10.4 | Music and Mathematical Ability

Martin Gardiner, a researcher at the Music School in Providence, Rhode Island, reports in *Nature* (May 23, 1996) on first and second graders who took seven months of weekly one-hour Kodály instruction. Twenty-five percent more of these students were at grade level or higher in math aptitude than were fellow students who had not taken the course. The Kodály method involves a structured, sequential learning approach (similar to mathematics instruction) in which one skill is mastered before the next is learned. Apparently it is not just the music and visual arts and group singing that account for the advantage; it's the sequential method itself.

Application

Call the Kodály Center of America at 401-521-7006 for the Kodály program nearest you.

TOPIC 10.5 | Music and the Injured Brain

Michael Rohrbacher, director of music therapy at Shenandoah University, Winchester, Virginia, and consultant to the National Institutes of Health (NIH), reports the preliminary results of an NIH Office of Alternative Medicine study on the effects of music on the emotions of patients with injured brains. By listening to music of their own choosing, especially music they grew up with, brain-injured patients showed an increased ability in emotional empathy, increased lucidity if they were confused, and improved recovery and rehabilitation time. Modern music, especially of the pounding, heavy-metal persuasion, appeared to be less effective.

In a related experiment, John Hughes, of the University of Illinois, played Mozart (K. 448 again!) for epileptic patients and found that twenty-nine out of thirty-six showed a statistically significant decrease in epileptic spiking while listening. Popular piano music of the 1940s did not yield the same effect. In a similar vein, physician Gordon Shaw of the University of California, Irvine, reported in an address to the 1998 Jensen Learning Conference in San Diego on an experiment by Johnson and Cotman in which Alzheimer's patients improved on a paper-folding task while listening to Mozart.

Applications

1 Provide music from a patient's youth (and of her or his choosing) to enhance recovery. Ah, to convalesce with Little Richard and the Brandenburg Concerti!

2 Obtain material from these two organizations:

American Music Therapy Association (AMTA); 8455 Colesville Road, Suite 1000; Silver Spring, Maryland 20910; phone: 301-589-3300.

International Society for Music in Medicine (ISMIM); Sportkrankenhaus Hellersen; D-5880 Ludenscheid; Germany; phone: 02351 434219. This organization copublishes the *International Journal of Arts Medicine.*

TOPIC 10.6   The Effect of Music on Mood

Here are some general guidelines on the human response to various aspects of music:

- The higher the pitch, the more positive the effect generated.

- Slower, minor keys warm the brain, which fosters both cortical and limbic alertness.

- Faster, major keys cool the brain, which fosters better moods.

- Classical composers (for example, Mozart, Haydn, and Beethoven) and mid- to late Baroque composers except for Bach (for example, Vivaldi, Scarlatti, Handel, and Corelli) are considered universal donors in the musical world—that is, they tend to offend the fewest listeners.

Carl Charnetski, chair of the psychology department at Wilkes University in Wilkes-Barre, Pennsylvania, measured the immunoglobulin A (IgA) production of college students who listened to either smooth jazz, regular jazz, alternating clicks and tones, or nothing. Smooth jazz was associated with a 14 percent increase in IgA, regular jazz with a 7 percent increase, clicks and tones with a 19 percent decrease, and nothing with nothing! I'm not sure what to make of this, other than to say that mellow music appears to enhance immune function, and that Wilkes University students find smooth jazz (the Muzak variety) mellow. I suspect that those of us who find Mozart or Vivaldi mellow could expect similar benefits!

Glenn Wilson (1994) has found the following:

- Repetitive rhythms, such as Ravel's "Bolero" and the minimalist music of Philip Glass, induce a trancelike state that occasionally borders on ecstasy.

- Musical rhythms liberate the mind from ordinary states, hence the popularity of music in religious and military settings.

- Music that slows gradually has a gradual relaxing effect.

- Lullabies in many cultures imitate the breathing rhythms that occur in sleep.

- The body's rhythms will adapt to the rhythms of live, close-up music.

- In all cultures, observers are able to correctly identify the music of other cultures that is intended to convey specific human moods and needs, such as war, mourning, love, hunting, and sleep inducement (that is, lullabies!). Wilson's findings are summarized in Table 10.1.

Table 10.1.
Musical Elements Associated Cross-Culturally with Specific Moods.

Element	Joy	Sadness	Excitement
Frequency	High	Low	Varied
Melodic variation	Strong	Slight	Strong
Tonal course	Moderate, first up, then down	Down	Strongly up, then down
Tonal color	Many overtones	Fewer overtones	Barely any overtones
Tempo	Rapid	Slow	Medium
Volume	Loud	Soft	Highly varied
Rhythm	Irregular	Regular	Very irregular

Source: Adapted from *Psychology for Performing Artists: Butterflies and Bouquets* by G. D. Wilson, 1994, London: Jessica Kingsley.

Application

Following are some appropriate workplace uses of music:

- *Retail stores:* Faster, higher-pitched music in a major key (for example, Vivaldi's *The Four Seasons*)
- *Waiting rooms:* No vocal music or TV, please (so people like me can read)
- *Workplaces where routine work is done:* Slower, lower-pitched music in a minor key (for example, Barber's "Adagio for Strings")

TOPIC 10.7 Music and Personality

Glenn Wilson (1994) reports studies by Glasgow, Little, Zuckerman, Davies, Konecni, and others that begin to build a profile of how people with different personalities respond differently to various aspects of music. Among the findings are these:

- People who score as being "conservative" on personality tests tend to prefer music that is simpler and more familiar, while "liberals" tend to find greater pleasure in more complex and unfamiliar music.

- People who score high on "sensation seeking" tend to prefer more complex and unfamiliar music.

In a survey conducted by Glenn Wilson in 1984, several interesting associations between singers' voices and their personalities emerged (G. D. Wilson, 1994, pp. 137 ff.):

- The higher the voice, the greater the singer's emotionality.

- The higher the voice, the more stage fright and variability the singer has from performance to performance.

- Basses have higher testosterone and, along with it, more affairs and greater ambition.

- Tenors miss the most cues, sopranos the fewest.

- Compared with singers, nonsingers as a group are less extraverted, less conceited, more intelligent, more faithful, and more considerate.

Instrumental musicians have been the subject of several studies by Kemp, Piparek, Eysenck, Davies, Wills, Cooper, and Marchant-Haycox. Glenn Wilson (1994, pp. 176 ff.) summarizes these studies:

- Instrumentalists are more introverted and more anxious than nonmusicians.

- Brass players are less neurotic, more extraverted, less agreeable, and less conscientious than other instrumentalists (see Topic 4.4 and Chapter Twenty-One for definitions of these personality traits).

- String players are higher in Negative Emotionality than other instrumentalists.

- Jazz musicians are more neurotic, higher in Openness, less agreeable, and less conscientious.

Application

Incorporate personality qualities associated with specific musical interests when entertaining or planning events for musicians. For example, because brass players and singers are more extraverted, plan for lots of party time!

TOPIC 10.8 | Music as Psychotherapy

Is evidence available that music is veritably able to "soothe a savage breast," as William Congreve suggests? Glenn Wilson (1994, pp. 218–221) reviews the evidence and reports that music cures in a variety of ways, some more short-lived and others longer-lasting:

- Music provides a nonverbal means of communication for people who have lost the ability to communicate verbally.

- Among the elderly, music, whether in a live concert or in some form of electronic media, has the capacity to promote positive reminiscences. The results include positive mood, improved communication, pain relief, improved rates of healing, and generally better health and dispositions.

- Among a variety of patients, music can unleash verbal communication that for various reasons was previously suppressed.

- Ample stories abound of music's ability to moderate pain, such as Pablo Casals's testimony that although he was crippled by arthritis in his later years, playing the cello released him from the pain and stiffness.

- Music appropriate to the patient can calm schizophrenics and depressives.

- "Vibroacoustic therapy," which surrounds patients with speakers and vibrators, has shown success in alleviating symptoms in patients with arthritis, cerebral palsy, asthma, back pain, and circulatory disorders. In addition, vibroacoustic therapy has been used as a postevent relaxant for skiers, runners, and business executives.

- In one-on-one music therapy, a musician improvises accompaniment to the work of a co-therapist, providing rhythmic, harmonic, and melodic support for the therapist's work with profoundly disabled and/or disturbed children.

Application

Begin a service in your community such as the Music in Hospitals project in England, in which professional singers and instrumentalists donate their time to communicating with patients in hospitals, hospices, and nursing homes.

SUGGESTED RESOURCES

Campbell, D. (1997). *The Mozart Effect.* New York: Avon.

Jourdain, R. (1997). *Music, the Brain, and Ecstasy: How Music Captures Our Imagination.* New York: Morrow.

Ortiz, J. M. (1997). *The Tao of Music: Sound Psychology.* York Beach, Maine: Samuel Weiser.

Tomatis, A. (1991). *The Conscious Ear.* Barrytown, N.Y.: Station Hill Press.

Wilson, G. D. (1994). *Psychology for Performing Artists: Butterflies and Bouquets.* London: Jessica Kingsley.

Web Sites

American Music Therapy Association home page. Contains a wide variety of resources, including publications and links to other web sites:
www.musictherapy.org

Mozart Effect Resource Center:
www.mozarteffect.com

Music and mind site, with a variety of links, including the *International Journal of Arts Medicine* and the Mozart Effect Resource Center:
www.mmbmusic.com

Music Intelligence Neural Development project:
www.mindinst.org

National Association for Music Therapy home page:
www.namt.com

11

Finishing Well

Use It or Lose It

Although not all of us will be blessed with the opportunity to know the perspective of old age, certainly all of us have an interest in knowing what cognitive science research has discovered about the effect of aging on mental structure and ability. This chapter focuses on findings that can help us to age with maximum effectiveness and to better understand those who are preceding us into the Golden Age.

> **Do not go gentle into that good night.**
>
> —*Dylan Thomas*

First, one note. Much of what we know about adult development is coming out of the Baltimore Longitudinal Study of Aging, in which 2,400 volunteers of all ages travel annually (at their own expense) to Johns Hopkins' Bayview Medical Center for three days of examination. Begun in 1958, it is the longest-running study of its kind. In the first twenty years, only white men were studied, with women and African Americans added to the study in 1978. Blacks are still under-represented at 13 percent (compared to the target of 20 percent). The study continues to recruit volunteers in specific age, race, and sex categories. If you are interested in joining, call 800-225-2572. Among their findings: personality doesn't change essentially from age thirty on, vocabulary continues to grow into later life, problem-solving and reasoning skills continue into old age, and people age at different rates.

Another adult development study that is just beginning to bear research fruit is the Nun Study, which was initiated by graduate student David Snowden in 1986 through his contact with the School Sisters in Mankato, Minnesota. His study, housed at the Sanders-Brown Center on Aging at the University of Kentucky, expanded to include other nuns from School Sisters convents in Chicago, Milwaukee, St. Louis, Baltimore, Dallas, and Wilton, Connecticut. The study began with 3,926 Notre Dame sisters born between 1886 and 1916, most of whom had joined the order in their twenties. Autopsies are beginning to reveal new knowledge, particularly about Alzheimer's disease. Results from this study are of particular interest because of the relative similarity of the lifestyles among the nuns.

> **"To add life to years, not just years to life."**
> —Motto of the Gerontological Society of America

One promising line of research was reported by Marsel Mesulam, then of Harvard Medical School, now a psychiatry professor at Northwestern University. While at Harvard, Mesulam and other researchers identified a chemical, acetylcholinesterase, that is present at higher levels in people over ninety who have better mental abilities. The Harvard researchers have isolated a kind of cell in the brain that makes this chemical; it is hoped that in time, drugs will be able to regulate acetylcholinesterase.

TOPIC 11.1 General Effects of Aging

We are born with roughly 100 billion neurons. By establishing connections between neurons, or making new synapses, the brain increases its mass threefold until the early twenties. Conventional wisdom has decreed that some 100,000 neurons die each day of our lives. This is not the case. Individual rates of brain cell loss vary widely. Proportionately more are lost in the frontal and temporal cortex, especially the motor cortex, which contains the long axons from the spine necessary for balance. Alcohol consumption increases the daily destruction in proportion to the quantity consumed (around 60,000 neurons per day for a heavy drinker or alcoholic). Sickness, medication, and untold other assailants can also increase the rate of neuronal loss. The average person loses about 10 percent of his or her brain weight in a lifetime. This loss in brain weight used to be interpreted as the result of deceased neurons, but today it is interpreted as the result of shrunken neurons. Men lose more than women, and men lose more in the left hemisphere, which controls language, than in the right, which controls visual-spatial skills. Females experience about a two-ounce drop in brain mass around menopause, while males experience their accelerated loss beginning somewhere around age sixty.

Experts caution that we should take extra care of our brains, for, unlike other organs and body systems, neurons are not thought to divide and duplicate themselves. However, recent research by Fred Gage, a professor at the Salk Institute for Biological Studies in La Jolla, California, has revealed that mice who live in enriched environments and exercise their minds and bodies more show 15 percent increases in brain cells compared to fellow rodents in more mundane surroundings. In October 1998, Gage, along with Swedish researchers, reported the first observed regenerated brain cells in humans. In partial confirmation of the applicability of Gage's results to humans, Marian Diamond, a professor of integrative biology with the University of California, Berkeley, has found a higher proportion of *glial cells* (structural cells, also called "helper" cells, which provide nutrition for other neurons), not only in these enriched-environment rats, but also in the brain of Albert Einstein. His brain, preserved by Princeton University scientists in 1955 when he died at age seventy-five, shows a clearly higher ratio of glial cells to normal neurons in comparison to the brains of eleven men of average intelligence. In the meantime, why not play it safe and encourage everyone to keep body and mind active? Certainly this is a modest proposal.

As a general rule, aging itself does not have a large impact on deterioration of brain function. Although a debate continues to rage on this issue, following are a baker's dozen of what are accepted to be the most significant assailants on neurons:

- Medication
- Chronic disease (especially heart disease)
- Extended grief over personal loss
- Alcohol
- The absence of a stimulating partner
- An unfavorable living environment
- An inflexible personality style
- A sedentary lifestyle
- High blood pressure, especially in middle age
- Lack of stimulation
- A low educational level and absence of curiosity or a desire to learn
- Malnutrition
- Depression

The lesson of all this is: *Use it or lose it!* As neurologist David Krech says, "They who live by their wit die with their wit." Dean Keith Simonton, who teaches psychology at the University of California, Davis, has studied the creative careers of composers, writers, and artists. He found that the degree of creativity does not diminish with age, but the kind of creative energy sometimes changes. Igor Stravinsky, for example, switched in later life from a more traditional tonality to the "twelve-tone row," or music written "in series." Thomas Edison, Johann Wolfgang von Goethe, Victor Hugo, Claude Monet, and Titian did some of their best work in their seventies and eighties. George Bernard Shaw, Pablo Picasso, Arthur Rubinstein, Albert Schweitzer, and Pablo Casals were still active in their nineties. Also:

- David Ray of Franklin, Tennessee, learned to read at ninety-nine.

- Armand Hammer actively headed Occidental Petroleum at ninety-one.

- At ninety-two, Paul Spangler completed his fourteenth marathon, while at ninety-one, Hulda Crooks climbed Mount Whitney (the highest mountain in the continental United States).

- George Burns performed in Proctor's Theater, Schenectady, New York, first at age thirty-one and again sixty-three years later at age ninety-four.

- Kathrine Everett was still practicing law in North Carolina at age ninety-six.

- The classical pianist Mieczyslaw Horszowski recorded a new album at the age of ninety-nine.

- Martha Graham still choreographed in her nineties.

- Photographer Imogen Cunningham worked in her nineties.

- Grandma Moses retired from crocheting with arthritis around age seventy and started a new career in painting.

At age seventy-six, my mother-in-law moved to North Carolina from Alabama. A long-time church organist, she found a new service niche. She was in high demand for after-dinner music and music therapy classes at her retirement home, and she played frequently in the musical interlude just before her church's Sunday morning service. Seven years later and eighty-three, she has moved to a nursing home, where she still tries on her better days to entertain her friends and fellow residents on an electronic keyboard, where she has been known to experiment with some unfamiliar rhythms and timbres provided by Sony! She is well respected for her talent.

The more we use our brains as we age, the higher our performance level stays and the higher is our ratio of synapses to neurons—that is, our brains stay denser the more we use them. Nerve growth factor (NGF) is one of many trophic, or nutritional, agents that stimulate and support growth of the myelin sheath—the coating of the neural fiber—and of new synapses. NGF is released by neural transmission itself. Exercise also produces extra NGF (see Topic 8.2). In other words, by using our nervous system, we grow it.

Applications

1   Make it a personal goal to continually learn something new. Once you've mastered it to the point where it is routine, it's time to learn something new.

2   Disuse breeds disuse. Use what you know and have. Fight idleness and boredom with all your energy. If you can't think of anything to do, offer yourself as a volunteer; there are plenty of organizations waiting for you to help out. You can be helpful to others either from the confines of your own home (for example, by telephoning, addressing, sewing, or mending) or at another site, such as an office park or hospital.

3   Strive to maintain a balanced diet from this point on. See Topic 5.1 and Appendix A.

4   Exercise caution when changing physical positions after age fifty. Be especially careful when using ladders or stools to gain height; most people's sense of balance just isn't what it used to be. Leave the shower, tub, and car with a little more caution. And be sure to exercise regularly.

5   Assume that you will retain your full mental powers forever. Just because we slow down doesn't mean we have to stop! We will always have a contribution to make!

TOPIC 11.2   Old Age and Mental Ability

Two clear trends have been found to be associated with the aging brain:

1. Between the ages of twenty and sixty, reaction time doubles; that is, we slow down.

2. The ratio of synapses to neurons increases for those who continue to use their brains and decreases for those who stop using their brains (see Figure 11.1). Learning means new synapses, and new synapses mean higher density, which counterbalances the normal brain weight loss. Accordingly,

performance continues to improve with age among those who use their brains, while it declines among those whose brains retire when they retire from their jobs.

In a Harvard Medical School study of over one thousand physicians, Dean Whitla and Sandra Weintraub found that the ten physicians over age sixty-five with the highest performance scores on the Assessment of Cognitive Skills, an unpublished computer-administered test developed by Harvard's Douglas Powell (see Allison, 1991), were still actively working as physicians, while the ten with the lowest performance scores were not working any longer. The working and non-working physicians showed similar patterns of medication and illness, so the difference in performance cannot be attributed to those factors. In other words, their Physical Health and Mental Health scores were independent. I know that "Use it or lose it" sounds like an oversimplification, but . . .

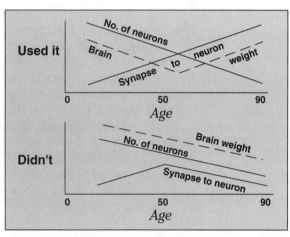

Figure 11.1. The Effect of Inactivity and Disuse on the Brain.

Many reports show mental abilities declining in old age, but these reports typically fail to control for degree of brain use. Apparently the nonusers are bringing down the scores of the users! Referencing the Seattle Longitudinal Study, Warner Shaie of the Pennsylvania State University Gerontology Center finds that measurable loss in mental performance (for example, loss in spatial reasoning) can be reversed with training, except for performance loss caused by brain damage from drug use, disease, or trauma.

In a project funded by the University of California at Los Angeles Task Force on Psychoneuroimmunology, George Solomon and John Morley found that age does not uniformly affect the immune system (Cousins, 1989). Older healthy people show immune levels of white blood cells, lymphocytes, granulocytes, and so on that are somewhat higher than those of comparable younger people. In addition, older adults with "hardy" attitudes (those who maintain their commitment, positive emotion, self-control, and exercise) show an even higher level of immune cells as well as of endorphins.

Applications

❶ Plan for retirement. Don't become a television addict without hobbies or interests.

❷ Beware, as you age, of depending on speedy performance in order to feel good about yourself. If you feel that you are over-extending yourself, begin to move toward activities that are compatible with slower reaction times. You might move from driving cars and riding motorcycles to walking, riding bicycles or tricycles, and taking buses. Move from power tools to hand tools, from debate to dialogue, from reading stories to storytelling. One of the reasons that bridge, canasta, checkers, chess, Go, and many other such games are successful as intergenerational activities is that they are highly tolerant of varying speeds of individual play. Develop increasing pride in the quality of your accomplishments, decreasing pride in the speed of their execution.

❸ As you age, maintain high expectations for yourself, keep developing your sense of humor, take control of stress, and continue to exercise and eat right.

❹ In the face of disease, "Accept the diagnosis but defy the verdict," as Norman Cousins says (Cousins, 1989). Examples of recovery from "terminal" illnesses are numerous and increasing. The limits of the mind's ability to positively influence health are unknown.

TOPIC 11.3 Maintaining Control and Optimism

The principles elaborated later in Topic 20.5 concerning the effect of control on stress apply equally to seniors. Specifically, Judith Rodin of Yale University (Keeton, 1992) has demonstrated that nursing home residents aged sixty-five to ninety who are allowed to take a direct planning and decision-making role in their programming (1) live longer, (2) are sick less, (3) are happier, (4) are more alert, and (5) have less of the stress hormone cortisol.

Psychology professors Christopher Peterson of the University of Michigan and Martin Seligman of the University of Pennsylvania (see Topic 20.1) found that baseball players who were more optimistic at age twenty-five lived significantly longer. In another vein, William Strawbridge of the California Public Health Foundation found that in a study of five thousand people over twenty-eight years of age, people who attended religious services had a 36 percent lower death rate. However, reporting in the June 1997 *American Journal of Public Health,* Strawbridge qualified the findings, cautioning that the lower rate could be related to improved health practices, higher social contacts, and more stable marriages, each of which is associated with, but not limited to, religious participation.

Now, there is control, and then there is control. Having some control over one's destiny is one thing, but being a control freak is another. Michael Babyak, an assistant clinical professor of medical psychology at Duke University, in a twenty-two-year longitudinal study of 750 white, middle-class men, has found that men who always need to be in control (monopolizing conversations, frequently interrupting, having a compulsive need to be number one, and exhibiting other forms of social dominance) tend to die younger than men whose social behavior is calmer and more accepting of the ascendancy of others.

Applications

① If you are responsible for the care of older adults, do everything you can to include them in planning, decision making, and problem solving. Share responsibility and control with them. If you are on the staff of a community for older adults, establish committees, consult with the residents, and empower them by responding to their ideas, requests, and needs.

② If you are an older adult, whether you are living alone or in a community, continue to be involved in planning your life; if you live in a community for older adults, establish committees, create suggestion boxes, ask those charged with your care to consider your ideas, and pool your resources for trips and other big-ticket items, such as lawyers, entertainment, transportation, or equipment.

TOPIC 11.4 Diet and Aging

Evidence points toward the significant effects on longevity of restricted diets. In other words, the less you eat, the longer you live. Roderick Bronson and Ruth Lipman of the Human Nutrition Research Center at Tufts University in Boston report that reducing patients' normal food intake by 40 percent results in a 20 percent longer life span. Their report (Raloff, 1991) argues that diet restriction (1) limits deoxyribonucleic acid (DNA) damage, (2) increases enzyme-mediated repair of DNA, and (3) reduces expression of proto-oncogenes (cancer-causing genes). Richard Weindruch of the Institute on Aging at the University of Wisconsin–Madison recommends daily consumption of 1 gram of protein and 0.5 gram of fat for each kilogram (2.2 pounds) of weight for longevity. Back in the 1930s, Clive McCay of Cornell University found that rats whose diets had 35 percent fewer calories lived 35 percent longer. However, while excessive consumption clearly affects longevity, current research reveals that people naturally gain weight as they age. The new weight charts, such as the one devised by Reubin Andres, clinical director at the National Institute on Aging, allow for considerably more weight than the more traditional charts developed by Metropolitan Life Insurance Company.

Restak (1997) cautions about generalizing animal research results to humans. He does, however, find promise in a line of research by Denham Harman of the University of Nebraska Medical School. Harman worked with free radicals, molecules containing one unpaired electron. Such molecules are unstable, grabbing at available unpaired electrons like starving creatures and indiscriminately foraging. A negative outcome: free radicals consume available electrons in the mitochondria of the cell nuclei and destroy DNA, with the effect of accelerated aging. A positive outcome: free radicals are bound by the available electrons in antioxidants such as vitamin C and beta-carotene. Restak warns that people should not rely on pills as a source of antioxidants, preferring that they consume them in their natural form, in fresh fruits and vegetables.

Applications

1 If living longer is more important to you than eating a lot, consider cutting back your consumption by about one-third. For more information, contact the Human Nutrition Research Center; Tufts University; Boston, Massachusetts 02111; phone: 617-556-3000. Be aware, however, of the Mayo Clinic finding (Minninger, 1984) that a diet of less than 2,100 calories daily—unless it is personally monitored by a physician—typically results in less than ideal mental functioning (see Topic 5.2).

2 To keep free radicals from chomping down on you, provide antioxidants to keep them at bay. Feed them, or they'll feed on you. Sample recommendation for one day's worth of food for free radicals: ½ cup of broccoli, 6 ounces of cranberry juice, ½ cup of strawberries, ½ cup of orange juice, and a kiwi.

TOPIC 11.5 Exercise and Aging

According to research reported in Folkins and Sime (1981), exercise programs can at least arrest and often reverse many of the degenerative physical effects of aging in older patients. One explanation of this phenomenon is that exercise promotes increased absorption of oxygen. William Greenough, a neuroscientist at the University of Illinois, identified an increase in capillaries around neurons in the brain as a result of aerobic exercise. Carl Cotman, a neurology professor at the Institute for Brain, Aging and Dementia at the University of California, Irvine, found that aerobic exercise produces an increase in neurotrophins. Neurotrophins are nerve growth agents—a "fertilizer" for nerve cells.

Arthur Kramer, a psychology professor with the University of Illinois' Beckman Institute, established that aerobic exercise (a forty-five-minute water aerobics class, three times a week, lasting for ten weeks) in sixty-three- to eighty-two-year-olds resulted in improved, faster reaction times. He avers that declines in reaction time are generally more attributable to declines in fitness than to aging. Aerobic exercise is best. In a study conducted by researchers at the Salt Lake City Veterans Administration Hospital, three out-of-shape groups were followed: one was put on a walking regimen, another lifted weights, and the third carried on business as usual with no exercise of any kind. The walkers showed significantly higher scores on eight tests of mental ability, the weight lifters showed a little improvement, and the others showed no improvement.

Applications

1 Keep walking, briskly.

2 Inquire about organized and medically supervised exercise programs for seniors and join up. Senior centers have taken the lead in this area.

3 Don't stop exercising because you think you're too old. There's an aerobic exercise that's safe and beneficial for you.

4 Ensure that you and all your family members get aerobic exercise for thirty to forty-five minutes at least five days per week.

TOPIC 11.6 Combining Diet and Exercise

In a study reported in Merzbacher (1979), individuals with cardiovascular disease and an average age of sixty were placed on the Pritikin diet, which includes more complex carbohydrates and fewer proteins and fats, and were assigned six to ten miles per day of jogging or walking. After completing this twenty-six-day program, subjects scored higher on intelligence tests and had measurably improved their circulatory system.

Application

Don't just exercise: eat right.

TOPIC 11.7 Night Vision

The quality of our night vision decreases with age. At fifty-seven, I am already aware of poorer distance vision when driving at night. Also, men tend to have better day vision (note that more women wear sun-protective glasses), and women tend to have better night vision (Moir and Jessel, 1991).

Manley West, a University of West Indies pharmacology professor, researched the rumor that marijuana improved night vision. He discovered that a nonpsychoactive ingredient in marijuana, canasil, caused a significant improvement in night vision. At the time of this writing, canasil, which is the same ingredient in marijuana that relieves glaucoma, is not yet available in the United States.

Applications

❶ As you age, take extra precautions when you drive at night, especially if you are a man. Allow extra distance between you and vehicles in front of you, drive more slowly, and take more breaks. Let a younger person or a woman drive when possible.

❷ All other things being equal (driving skill, physical condition, road familiarity, and so on), a woman will be a safer driver at night because of generally superior night vision. During the day, men will tend to be safer because they are less subject to fatigue from the sun. Women will generally desire or require more breaks to avoid eye fatigue during the day, with men requiring more during the night.

❸ Understand that these differences exist, and don't interpret people who are different from you as weak, malingering, or inferior.

TOPIC 11.8 Memory and Aging

Although the memory processes slow down as we age, the accuracy of our memories improves. When he administered recall-and-recognition tests to youths and seniors in church fellowship halls, Paul Foos, of the psychology department at the

University of North Carolina at Charlotte, found that the seniors, with an average age of sixty-five, consistently beat the youths. As we age, the number of items we can associate to a particular memory chunk dramatically increases. So while we may take longer, the likelihood of accurate recall increases. In fact, there is some evidence that the rich associative network of seniors is one factor in the slowdown of their memory processes.

My eighty-two-year-old brother-in-law and I were riding through eastern North Carolina in 1993 to a family reunion. Making small talk, I referred to a basketball player from our hometown of Kinston who had recently signed to play basketball at the University of North Carolina, calling him Shackleford. My brother-in-law commented that I didn't have the name right. I agreed and we both started searching our minds for the right name. He won the race. I asked him how he'd remembered. He said that he got an image in his mind of a furniture store in Goldsboro (on his route for many trips from Chapel Hill to Kinston) called Stackhouse Furniture, flipped from that image to one of a retired professor friend in California named Stackhouse, and came up with "Stackhouse," the right name. (Alas! How memory is fickle. After reading this passage, my brother-in-law corrected me: his friend Stackhouse was not a professor, but a businessman, and the Goldsboro store was not a furniture store, but a lumber business!) My effort to describe this process is captured in Kim Allman's illustration in Figure 11.2. Apparently, my brother-in-law's network of isolated memories connected in something like the following manner to give him the right answer (follow along with Figure 11.2):

1. He heard "Shackleford," a relatively new auditory memory gained around age seventy, based on a well-known Kinston athlete who attended North Carolina State University, not the University of North Carolina at Chapel Hill.

2. He associated the name Shackleford to basketball and Kinston.

3. He unconsciously and instantaneously relived his frequent trips from Chapel Hill to Kinston to visit his parents and his in-laws.

4. A prominent building halfway between the two towns, Stackhouse Furniture (correction: Lumberyard), popped up ever so briefly into his consciousness.

5. This submerged memory of the furniture (lumber) store, firmly entrenched from about the age of seventeen,

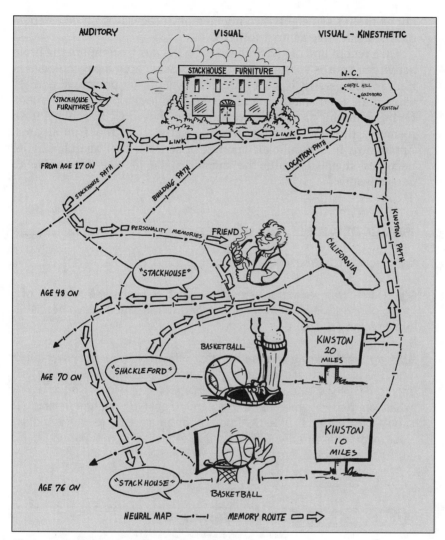

Figure 11.2. My Brother-in-Law's Memory Process.

connected to another strong memory of his long-standing friendship, from about the age of forty-eight on, with a California professor (correction: businessman) named Stackhouse.

6. By the time he envisioned his California friend, he became conscious that the name "Stackhouse" was the one he was looking for.

I hope that at age eighty-two my memory processes will be as abundant and effective as my brother-in-law's.

In a recent line of research using PET scans to compare the brain activity of youths versus seniors, Daniel Schachter, a psychologist at Harvard University, has found equal levels of hippocampal activity when both youths and seniors are engaged in the process of remembering something easily. However, when they are "searching" for a memory, the youths show greater activity in the frontal area. Apparently, in a significant number of seniors, the "search engine" becomes sluggish, while the memories lie in wait for a rise to consciousness.

Applications

1 Slow is OK. You'll get there.

2 Don't push seniors to remember more quickly; the frustration of being pushed will interfere with the effort to remember. Give people the time they need.

3 Try the "I knew it all the time" test. Harvard University psychiatry and neurology professor Marilyn Albert suggests that when your memory fails you and you subsequently recall, or are reminded of, what you tried to remember originally, you should have the feeling: "Yes—I knew that all along." A more appropriate time to worry about your memory is when you recall or are reminded of a memory and it does not feel familiar to you.

TOPIC 11.9 Aging, Versatility, and Creative Genius

Vincent Cassandro observed that certain creative artists appear to die earlier than their peers (Mozart at thirty-five, Sylvia Plath at thirty-one, Keats at twenty-six), while certain creative scientists live to a ripe old age (George Washington Carver lived to the age of seventy-nine, Einstein, seventy-six; and Werner Karl Heisenberg, seventy-five). Cassandro (1998) decided to investigate for possible explanations, and in the process (a funny thing happened on the way . . .) he discovered a major factor that appears to affect the mortality of creative geniuses: versatility. His findings (which have not yet been replicated or verified) show that nonversatile creative writers (for example, poets who achieve nothing but excellent poetry, like Plath and Keats) die, on average, ten years earlier than more versatile creative writers. Writers who are versatile in the field of writing (for example, both poetry and drama for Shakespeare, who died at fifty-two) live longer than nonversatile creative writers, while writers who are versatile both within and outside their field live even longer (for example, William Carlos Williams, a poet, novelist, and physician, who died at eighty).

Creative scientists exhibit the opposite trend. Nonversatile creative scientists live longer than creative scientists who are versatile in their field (Linus Pauling, the chemist, died at ninety-three; Galileo, a physicist, mathematician, and astronomer, at seventy-eight), and these creative scientists live even longer than those who are versatile both within and outside their field (Leonardo da Vinci, physicist, mathematician, architect, and painter, died at sixty-seven). On the average, Cassandro found that nonversatile creative writers die ten years earlier than their more versatile peers, while nonversatile creative scientists live five years beyond their more versatile peers. He associates each of these premature mortality groups with a tendency to mental illness. To a certain degree, singular devotion to a single creative writing outlet is less healthy than a more versatile lifestyle, and singular devotion to a single scientific endeavor is more healthy than a more versatile lifestyle.

Of course, exceptions abound. How would someone like Albert Schweitzer fit in? Here was a physician, musician, missionary, and writer who lived until he was ninety. Was he a versatile scientist or a versatile artist?

Application

Assess the level of balance in your life. To the extent that more focus can be beneficial to someone trying to achieve too much in too many different fields, simplify your life. To the extent that more diversity can relieve the stress that may accompany devotion to a single pursuit, balance your life with an additional pursuit.

TOPIC 11.10 Sex and Longevity

Based on a study of 918 men between the ages of forty-five and fifty-nine, research epidemiologists George Davey Smith of the University of Bristol and Stephen Frankel of Queen's University, Belfast, Northern Ireland, reported in the December 1997 *British Medical Journal* that there appears to be a rather strong relationship between rate of sexual orgasm and length of life. The men were followed up ten years later and analyzed on the basis of three groups: those who had two or more orgasms per week, fewer than one per month, or a number between these two extremes. The death rate for the least sexually active men was twice as high as that for the most active, while the death rate for the intermediate group was 1.6 times that of the most active group. While some have criticized the methodology of the study, following its implications could not be harmful in and of itself, certainly! On the other hand, we need to be alert for studies that confirm or challenge these findings, as well as for studies that include women.

Application

Rest assured that frequent orgasms do not appear to affect mortality adversely. However, if you have less frequent sexual activity and wish to hedge your bets longevity-wise, don't go looking for more mates or browbeat your partner into reluctantly increasing her or his frequency: simply take things in hand.

A Final Word on Aging Gracefully

In his book *Older and Wiser* (1997, pp. 228–244), Richard Restak lists "thirty steps you can take to enhance your brain in the mature years." I have reviewed his list, added to and subtracted from it, combined items, and modified them. Here's my revision of Restak's list:

1. Stop smoking.
2. Do weight-bearing exercises daily.
3. Don't rely on any particular food, drug, or chemical to promote longevity.

4. Maintain normal levels of blood pressure, blood sugar, and cholesterol.

5. Avoid a sedentary lifestyle; don't stop being active just because you are slower.

6. Prefer standing exercises to sitting exercises.

7. Walk at least four hours a week.

8. Practice balancing daily (for example, while in a line) by standing on one leg for as long as possible, then the other, and so on, alternating.

9. Reduce stress, or change (reframe) your attitude toward stressors.

10. Indulge your curiosity to the max.

11. Enjoy your coffee and other caffeine-drink energizers.

12. Nap.

13. Don't fret about the possibility of memory loss; work on developing and improving your memory with books (see Chapter Twenty-Six) and gadgets (such as palm-held computers).

14. Don't worry about becoming senile.

15. Keep working—gainfully or not—at something you enjoy for as long as possible.

16. Minimize spare time.

17. Avoid excessive use of alcohol.

18. Keep challenging your mental abilities, from doing crossword puzzles to learning new skills and knowledge.

19. Keep a diary in some form that you enjoy.

20. Avoid social isolation. Engage in many diverse kinds of activities with other people: if you get "retired" from your church choir, start a choir for seniors; if you live alone, get a pet.

21. Remain active on the Internet. Use it as a support group, information source, and means of communication with family and friends. Start and maintain a family web page.

22. Continue to stimulate your five senses with art, food, people, and nature in its abundance.

23. Accept the fact that your ability to concentrate will shorten (to about fifteen minutes), and take three- to five-minute breaks between fifteen-minute concentration periods.

24. Enjoy games as a way to nurture your ability to concentrate.

25. Accept being a slower organism and avoid activities that rely on speed of response: replace speed with wisdom.

26. Maintain—even increase—your sense of humor.

27. Maintain your friendships and develop new ones.

28. Prefer a diet with a moderate caloric intake, with a predominance of fresh fruits and vegetables.

29. Women after menopause should consult with their physician regarding the risks and advantages of taking estrogen supplements.

30. Take melatonin as a sleep aid.

31. Follow the research on dehydroepiandrosterone (DHEA), and begin taking it when the studies consistently point to its safety and effectiveness in promoting physical and mental vitality; if you're already in your seventies, you might consider taking it now. Ask your physician.

If thirty-one steps are too overwhelming, try these seven conclusions from the California Human Population Laboratory's study conducted in the 1970s (Hobson, 1994, p. 188). People who followed six out of the seven recommendations lived longer and in better health. The suggestions are listed in order of importance, with good sleep having the largest effect on health and longevity:

1. Sleep.

2. Exercise.

3. Eat breakfast.

4. Don't snack.

5. Watch your weight.

6. Do not smoke.

7. Use alcohol moderately.

SUGGESTED RESOURCES

Fossel, M. (1996). *Reversing Human Aging.* New York: Morrow.

Friedan, B. (1993). *The Fountain of Age.* New York: Simon & Schuster.

Keeton, K. (1992). *Longevity: The Science of Staying Young.* New York: Viking Penguin.

Medina, J. J. (1996). *The Clock of Ages.* Cambridge: Cambridge University Press.

Restak, R. M. (1997). *Older and Wiser.* New York: Simon & Schuster.

Ricklefs, R. E., and Finch, C. E. (1995). *Aging: A Natural History.* New York: Scientific American Library.

Schaie, K. W. (1994, April). "The Course of Adult Intellectual Development." *American Psychologist, 49*(4), 304–313.

Part Three

Sex,
Gender,
and
Relationships

The Birds and the Bees

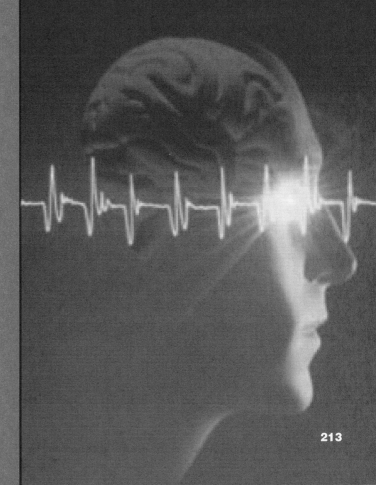

12

Sex and Gender

The Wiring Is Different

66 There is one phase of life that I have never heard discussed in any seminar

And that is that all women think men are funny and all men think that weminar. 99

—Ogden Nash

erhaps the facet of brain research of most general interest is that of the differences between males and females. Should we call these supposed differences gender- or sex-related? P. J. Caplan, M. Crawford, J. S. Hyde, and J.T.E. Richardson (1997) assert that *sex* is a noun that refers to biology while *gender* is a verb that refers to behavior. Put differently, males and females are bimodally distributed, with two large clusters at either end of the distribution and fewer in the middle area, and masculinity and femininity are normally distributed, with many members of the group in the middle area and fewer at the extremes. There are not only males and females, but also males with female-differentiated brains and females with male-differentiated brains, as well as people whose brain-body differentiation is somewhat ambiguous. People whose sex is ambiguous are far outnumbered by those whose gender role is ambiguous. Having a high amount of estrogen and being able to have babies relate to sex, while seeking a career in nursing and being able to do math usually relate to gender.

To the degree that a behavior is susceptible to environmental influences that are different for males than for females, it has a gender-related difference, not a sex difference. Sex differences should refer only to those that are attributable exclusively to biological factors. While this sounds simple and clear, it can become despairingly murky. Many differences have both biological and environmental influences. For example, we know that the menstrual cycle affects verbal and math performance in females; this suggests that differential performance on math and verbal scores between males and females is sex-related. But we also know that in countries where legislation has mandated the minimization of opportunity differences between males and females—particularly in the United States and Sweden—differences in math and verbal performance are diminishing significantly. Sandra Bem (1993) expresses these relationships well:

> No matter how many sex differences are someday shown to have a biological component, that knowledge will thus add little or nothing to our understanding of why women and men have universally played such different—and unequal—roles in virtually every society on earth. . . . So yes, women might turn out to be more biologically nurturant than men on the average, but that should make them psychiatrists, not secretaries. And yes, men might also turn out to have a higher aptitude for mathematics than women on the average, but that would not explain why so many more women have a high aptitude for mathematics than have careers requiring one.

This chapter summarizes the findings from cognitive science research on sex and gender differences that have some practical applications. I will endeavor to use the terms *sex* and *gender* properly, reserving *sex differences* to refer only to differences that are resistant to environmental influence. I confess in advance, however, that following this distinction is very difficult indeed. See Appendix B for a listing of some of these reported differences.

A word of warning: Whenever I refer to differences between the sexes, keep in mind that these differences are *averages* unless otherwise specified. This means, for example, that although males have a higher average score on math tests, some males score lower than females and some females score higher than males. In addition, only time will tell which of these reported differences are free of cultural influences.

To the degree that a man exhibits characteristics that are typically more female (language, emotion, nurture), he is said to have a *female-differentiated brain.* Conversely, to the degree that a woman exhibits characteristics that are typically more male (math proficiency, spatial ability, aggression), she is said to have a *male-differentiated brain.* To avoid having to constantly repeat the mouthfuls "male-differentiated brain" and "female-differentiated brain," I will use the terms *male, male brain, female,* and *female brain;* they all are intended to refer to the fuller term. I will also occasionally use the full term as a reminder. When I intend to refer to men and women and not just to their brains, I will use the terms *men* and *women.*

TOPIC 12.1   In the Womb

Several biological differences delineate where the brains of men and women begin. The male-differentiated brain has a thicker right cerebral cortex, a corpus callosum (which connects the hemispheres) that is thinner relative to brain weight, denser neurons, nuclei up to eight times larger than those of the female brain, and a hypothalamus that works on the principle of negative feedback to maintain constancy. The female-differentiated brain has a thicker left cerebral cortex, a corpus callosum that is thicker relative to brain weight, neurons that are less dense, smaller nuclei, and a hypothalamus that works on the principle of positive feedback to increase fluctuation in the system—that is, highs get higher and lows get lower, resulting in more emotionality.

The result is that the two brains are hard-wired differently: the male for doing and the female for talking. The male Doer tends to become more proficient in math, spatial reasoning, and what Moir and Jessel (1991) call the five characteristics of the male-differentiated brain: aggression, competition, self-assertion, self-confidence, and self-reliance. All of these characteristics are highly correlated with testosterone levels, whether in males or females. The very highest levels of testosterone, however, do not produce the highest math scores; slightly lower levels do.

Females who excel in math usually also exhibit the five male traits, and females who exhibit the five male traits tend to score higher in math and visual-spatial skills. The female Talker tends to become more proficient in language, sensory awareness, memory, social awareness, and relationships. Much of this is apparently due to the relatively thicker corpus callosum in the female-differentiated brain, which allows freer communication between the two hemispheres. In an effort to describe how this differentiation looks as pictured by various measures of brain activity, Moir and Jessel (1991) provide a summary, shown in Table 12.1.

The more concentrated activity for language production in females that is shown in the table may account for their verbal superiority as measured by various tests, and the more concentrated

Table 12.1. Location of Brain Function by Gender.

Function	Location
Language mechanics	Men: Left hemisphere front and back Women: Left hemisphere front[a]
Vocabulary	Men: Left hemisphere front and back[a] Women: Left and right hemispheres front and back
Visual-spatial perception	Men: Right hemisphere[a] Women: Right and left hemispheres
Emotion	Men: Right hemisphere Women: Right and left hemispheres

Source: From *Brain Sex: The Real Difference Between Men and Women* by Anne Moir and David Jessel, 1991, New York: Carol Publishing Group/Lyle Stuart. © 1989, 1991 by Anne Moir and David Jessel. Reprinted by permission of Carol Publishing Group.
[a]Denser, more specific, and highly localized concentrations of neural activity, which are associated with superior performance.

activity for visual-spatial perception in males may account for their visual-spatial superiority. Apparently, the advantage of the denser concentration is that fewer possibilities exist for interrupting or interfering with neural activity. Male-differentiated brains, in fact, find it easier to handle multitasking, such as talking while building something. Talking, which uses the left hemisphere, doesn't interfere in a major way with building, which is visual-spatial and uses the right hemisphere. Because the female-differentiated brain handles visual-spatial tasks in both hemispheres, building and talking, which both use the left hemisphere, interfere with each other.

One major structure that affects this pattern of specialization is the corpus callosum, which connects the two hemispheres. It is up to 23 percent thicker in the female-differentiated brain relative to brain size, providing the female brain with appreciably more connections, or synapses, between the two hemispheres. This degree of connection between the two hemispheres has been shown to be related to articulateness and fluency in language. The male's separation of language specialization in the left hemisphere and emotional specialization in the right helps to explain his traditional ineptness at talking about feelings; the neural basis of his feelings has far fewer connections with his language production via his thinner corpus callosum. The female, with her emotions seated in both hemispheres and with a thicker corpus callosum, has greater access to both her own feelings and the feelings of others as she produces her language. The male, with vocabulary-making powers seated only in the left hemisphere, is more proficient at developing vocabulary (hence the incredible mountains of male-created jargon and technical terminology), yet the female is more proficient at using the vocabulary that she does have.

Apparently the key to differentiation lies in our mothers' hormone levels during pregnancy. The effects are easier to experiment with in animals. If a pregnant rhesus monkey is injected with testosterone, a female offspring will exhibit one or more male traits, such as aggressive play or mounting. The female chaffinch can't sing; it doesn't have the synapses for singing that are present in the male. If male hormones are injected into the female chaffinch, the appropriate synapses develop, along with the accompanying ability to sing. When the ovaries of newborn female rats are removed, a check after they've reached adulthood reveals thicker right hemispheres, with an accompanying increase in spatial ability—a male trait. And when the testes of newborn male rats are removed, a similar check reveals thicker left hemispheres—a female trait.

Studies are revealing that men who behave as if they have female-differentiated brains in fact possess lower levels of testosterone, and women who behave as if they have male-differentiated brains possess higher levels of testosterone. In a fascinating line of research, Doreen Kimura, a clinical neuropsychology professor and professor emeritus at the University of Western Ontario in London, Ontario, Canada, has identified a relationship between body asymmetry and gender-related behavior. Namely, men and women with larger right testicles or breasts tend to exhibit more typically masculine behavior (aggression, spatial ability, math proficiency), while men and women with larger left testicles or breasts tend to exhibit more typically feminine behavior (nurturance, verbal ability). Variations in androgens (male sex hormones) and estrogens (female sex hormones) can affect both body asymmetry and the degree and direction of gender differentiation in the brain in the following ways:

Excess androgen in female embryo	Male-differentiated brain with male appearance and behavior
Excess estrogen (no androgen) in female embryo	Excessively female appearance and behavior (Turner's syndrome)
Excess androgen in male embryo	"Super" male (aggressive, hairy, and so on)
Excess estrogen in male embryo	Female-differentiated brain with male appearance and behavior

Events during pregnancy that can affect the hormone level of the unborn child include the following:

- Mutations within the chromosomal matter

- Major or sustained stress, such as war, rape, or bereavement, which suppresses testosterone

- Renal dysfunction, such as congenital adrenal hyperplasia, which produces too much testosterone

- Injections, as when mothers take estrogen for diabetes

- Barbiturates (taken by 25 percent of pregnant women from the 1950s through the 1980s)

- An extra chromosome (XXY in a boy yields low testosterone)

- Vigorous exercise (spurt exercise, such as tennis, increases testosterone; sustained exercise, such as a long run, lowers it)

Although the brain is wired in the womb, the differences are most noticeable after puberty, when the brain becomes fully activated as a result of being bathed in hormones.

Applications

1 Do not take any medication during pregnancy until you've carefully weighed the possible consequences. If you are in doubt, consult a neuropharmacologist (a specialist in pharmaceuticals for the nervous system). Be especially cautious during the first four months, when neurons are migrating.

2 Be accepting of your level of performance in various areas. Work to improve, always, but accentuate your strengths. If you sense that you are stronger at spatial skills than verbal skills, don't blame fate or your parents or your boss for not having done more to develop your verbal skills. The chances are that the discrepancy in skill level is hard-wired and permanent. Work to improve a skill to its next level, but don't begrudge how far you have to go to be perfect. Have a sense of humor about your natural gifts. There is so much to learn and so little time to learn it; don't moan about what seems impossible to learn. Instead, be attracted to what seems natural. As the Delphic Oracle said, "Know thyself."

3 Value typical females for cooperation and relationship building, among much else. Value typical males for competition and achievement, among much else. Know that achievement and relationship building are both important for success in today's business environment. Look at them as complementary assets in terms of meeting customers' needs and competing in a continual improvement business environment.

TOPIC 12.2 Sexual Identity

Whether we see ourselves as male or female is primarily determined by our genetic makeup. Brown University developmental geneticist Anne Fausto-Sterling (1993) proposes that sexual identity is really a continuum that ranges from female to male. Bimodal, to be sure, it is nonetheless a distribution, with points in between. While the medical literature uses the term *intersexual* to describe people who are in between (for example, someone with a penis who menstruates; see her story about Levi Suydam), Fausto-Sterling proposes three intermediate points: "herms" (hermaphrodites, with one testis and one ovary), "merms" (male pseudohermaphrodites with testes, no ovaries, and some form of female genitalia), and "ferms" (female pseudohermaphrodites with ovaries, no testes, and some form of male genitalia). Estimates have placed these intersexual categories at a level somewhere between 2 and 4 percent of births. Other writers question Fausto-Sterling's three intersexual categories, preferring to refer to them as a single complex of configurations known as the "transgender" category.

In spite of the difficulty of nomenclature, there appears to be agreement that the traditional medical practice of performing "clarifying surgery" at an early age serves the community more than the person who is born intersexual. What little evidence is available suggests that the problems accompanying "corrective" surgery (loss of erotic sensitivity and depression over lost body parts, for example) are more detrimental to the intersexual than problems associated with socialization (taking showers in gym class and showing secondary sexual features, for example). Fausto-Sterling and others (see the letters to the editor in *The Sciences,* July–August 1993, pp. 3–4, in response to her March–April article) propose that society should support intersexuals while they learn to accept their sexual identity as something that is more interesting and complex than being simply male or female.

A Dutch research team led by Dick Swaab at the Netherlands Institute for Brain Research in Amsterdam has identified a brain structure common to transsexuals—people with the primary and secondary characteristics of one sex who feel they belong to the opposite sex—that is more common among men. A section of the hypothalamus called the BSTc is 50 percent larger among males than among women, regardless of their sexual orientation (that is, whether they are homosexual or heterosexual). Among transsexual men (men who feel that they are really women trapped in the body of a man), the BSTc is not only smaller on the average than other men's; it is also smaller than women's. Most of these men report feelings of liberation after a sex-change operation.

Applications

1 If you are a parent or a surgeon faced with the decision to surgically clarify the sexuality of a newborn or older infant, seek further information from an emerging literature and support service network on transgender and intersexuality issues. Fausto-Sterling concludes that in her ideal world, transgender people should have a say in any medical interventions. Read Fausto-Sterling, *Myths of Gender* (1992), and Fausto-Sterling and Rose, *Love, Power, and Knowledge* (1994). Also see the story of John/Joan by Milton Diamond and Keith Sigmundson, of the University of Hawaii at Manoa's Pacific Center for Sex and Society, in the March 1997 *Archives of Pediatric and Adolescent Medicine.*

2 Sexual identity consists of more than gonads and other organs. Behavioral patterns and preferences (hairstyle, clothing fashions, mannerisms, and nurture versus aggression, among others) also must be allowed a full range of expression. If an intersexual is comfortable with a variety of gender-related fashions as well as a variety of organs, others should not force such an individual into the Procrustean clarity of a Rhett Butler male or a Melanie Wilkes female.

3 Contact and/or join the support network of the Intersex Society of North America; P.O. Box 31791; San Francisco, California 94131.

TOPIC 12.3 Sexual Orientation

The emerging evidence points in the direction of a strong genetic basis for sexual orientation, whether we are attracted to members of the same or a different sex. Richard Pillard of Boston University School of Medicine summarizes the research evidence in the June 1992 *Harvard Health Letter:*

- Homosexuality runs in families.

- Homosexuality appears randomly in birth order.

- Homosexuals exhibit early childhood gender nonconformity.

- Monozygotic (identical) twins have the highest concordance rate; if one is homosexual, there is a 50 percent probability that the other will be too.

In addition, a recent finding suggests a major biological difference: the third interstitial nucleus of the anterior hypothalamus is of equal size in women and homosexual men but is twice as large in heterosexual men. The meaning of this discovery is unclear; it is hoped that further research will clarify it.

Several other studies have emerged in support of Pillard's conclusions. Michael Bailey reported in the March 1993 *Archives of General Psychiatry* on a study of seventy-one sets of identical female twins, thirty-seven sets of fraternal female twins, and thirty-five sets of adoptive sisters. In each set, at least one was lesbian. For the identical twins, 48 percent of those identifying themselves as lesbian or bisexual also had a sister who was lesbian. For the fraternal twins, this was true of only 16 percent, and for the adoptive sisters, it was true of only 6 percent. In another study, Doreen Kimura reported in the December 1994 issue of *Behavioral Neuroscience* that in a study of the fingerprint patterns of 182 heterosexual men and 66 homosexual men, twice as many homosexuals (30 percent) as heterosexuals (16 percent) showed more ridges on the left hand than on the right (most men show more ridges on the right hand). These print patterns are completely formed within four months of conception. Women and gay men have a greater incidence of higher left-hand ridge counts.

This finding is related to earlier findings that gays and lesbians have a higher incidence of left-handedness and that a significant number of gay men hear equally well in both ears (most people hear better through the right ear). The latter finding supports earlier findings that homosexual men have larger connections between the two hemispheres. Kimura and Carson (1995) report that both men and women with higher left-hand ridge counts excel at typically feminine tasks such as those involving nurture and verbal skills, and that both men and women with higher right-hand ridge counts excel at typically masculine tasks such as those involving aggression, math, and spatial skills.

Two other recent discoveries add to the argument: Dean Hamer, of the National Cancer Institute, has demonstrated that many gay brothers share a strip of DNA passed down from their mothers. And Dennis McFadden, a University of Texas at Austin neuroscientist, has found that the inner ears of lesbians respond to sounds in a manner that resembles a male's response more than a female's.

Laura Allen and Roger Gorski of UCLA reported the results of a study they made of the brain tissue of thirty-four homosexual men, seventy-five presumed heterosexual men, and eighty-four presumed heterosexual women (*Proceedings of the National Academy of Sciences,* August 1992). The anterior commissures (a communication link between the two brain hemispheres) of the homosexual men were 34 percent larger than those of heterosexual men and 8 percent larger than those of the women, while the anterior commissures of the women were 13 percent larger than those of the heterosexual men. This finding appeared to be confirmed in a later report by Sandra Witelson, a psychiatry professor at McMaster University in Hamilton, Ontario, Canada. Her study was based on a sample of twenty-one men.

Even stronger support for the genetic basis of gender orientation has recently come from the laboratories at the University of Texas Southwestern Medical Center at Dallas, Stanford University, Brandeis University, and Oregon State University. These four collaborators reported that the male fruit fly (drosophila) possesses a powerful high-level gene that governs his sexual behavior (*Cell,* December 13, 1996). One mutation of the gene leads to indiscriminate, or bisexual, behavior; another mutation removes the desire to mate; and yet another mutation removes the ability to perform the "courtship buzz." Yet fruit flies with all three mutations are perfectly healthy otherwise. In the first mutation mentioned, indiscriminate males who are confined together without females all engage in the behaviors of courting and being courted by each other.

Apparently sex hormones are not an important determining factor. Although there is a small difference in testosterone levels between heterosexual and homosexual groups, a greater difference exists within groups. In one comparative study, the highest testosterone level belonged to a homosexual male subject.

Lest we see the evidence as all one-way, here is a clear reminder that parts of the animal kingdom present strong evidence for environmental influence. Russell Fernald, a neuroscience professor at Stanford University, has found that male cichlids who reach the top of their (fish) dominance hierarchy undergo biological changes: their colors appear, the hypothalamus enlarges, and they become sexually potent. On the other hand, if they fall (or sink) from the top of the hierarchy, they turn brown, their hypothalamus shrinks, and they become impotent. All determined by their environment? Or an environmental trigger for genetically determined programming?

And in a more human vein, Daryl Bem, a Cornell University psychologist, argues for an interactionist interpretation of sexual orientation (D. J. Bem, 1996). Although Bem accepts an inborn biological influence on sexual orientation, he also sees a strong cultural, or environmental, influence. More specifically, Bem says that we grow up seeing ourselves as more similar to one gender or the other, and the gender we view as different from us is the gender that we view as more "exotic." As our hormones urge sexual arousal, this "exotic" attitude is transformed into an "erotic" attitude. More research is required to support this aspect of Bem's theory. His view is certainly more cautious than a purely genetic or purely environmental explanation of sexual orientation. However, sexual orientation, like other life choices (business, religious, dietary, exercise, and academic choices, for example), is built on a biological foundation. Environmental add-ons do not eradicate that foundation, nor does the foundation prevent add-ons.

In support of Bem's argument for cultural influence, at the American Psychological Association's 1998 Annual Conference, Marc Breedlove, a professor of psychology at the University of California, Berkeley, reported new evidence that sexual orientation is subject to environmental manipulation (summarized in the *APA Monitor*, October 1998, p. 25). In male rodents, the medial amygdala is crucial for sexual arousal around female rodents. If the medial amygdala, which detects pheromones, is excised or reduced in size, then arousal doesn't occur. The size of this part of the brain can be controlled by externally manipulating the flow of androgens, with a flood of testosterone restoring the medial amygdala to normal size and, as a consequence, restoring the rodent to full arousal capability. Breedlove concludes that by extension, it is likely that environmental influences on human androgen levels also affect arousal capability. However, he has not performed the human research, and several questions are unanswered. For example, although the male rodent's medial amygdala is larger than the female's, Breedlove does not report whether the male rodent, in addition to losing interest in females, becomes aroused around other males when his medial amygdala is shrunk to the size of a female's.

Conservatives such as the Family Research Council think tank are advocating "conversion therapy" for changing homosexuals to heterosexuals. The American Psychological Association and the American Psychiatric Association have both issued policy statements opposing conversion therapy. Their opposition is based on their stand that homosexuality is not a mental illness and, hence, is not in need of treatment.

Application

Homosexuality appears to have a strong genetic component. To the degree that it is not a choice, it is also not a moral issue. Apparently, homosexuality and heterosexuality are as natural as blond or brown hair. Accept homosexuals and heterosexuals as equals, and don't try to change a person's preference or make fun of something that cannot be changed.

TOPIC 12.4 Gender Medicine

Traditionally, medicine has treated the male and female body as equivalent, except for baby-making capabilities. As JoAnn Manson, co-director of the Boston's Nurses' Health Study, puts it: "Medical literature and practice have been based on the 70-kilogram man" (*Boston Globe Magazine,* April 27, 1997, p. 13). Recent research, however, has uncovered the need for a more gender-specific approach to medicine. In the forefront of this gender-specific research is the National Institutes of Health, where the $628 million, fifteen-year Women's Health Initiative is housed. Among its findings is the discovery that women differ from men in a substantial number of medically significant ways. For example:

- Their immune systems function differently: women have higher immunoglobulin levels for fighting viruses.

- They metabolize drugs differently, including Valium and benzodiazepine, alcohol, acetaminophen, lidocaine, and aspirin.

- They have a higher prevalence of migraine headaches.

- They have a higher occurrence of depression.

- Most autoimmune diseases, including multiple sclerosis, lupus, and rheumatoid arthritis, are more common among women.

- Women come around more quickly after anesthesia.

- A woman's heart is two-thirds smaller than a man's and beats faster.

- A woman's risk of heart disease increases fourfold at menopause.

- Same-gender organ transplants are more successful.

- Tobacco exposure has more impact on a woman's lungs.

- Men produce estrogen throughout their lives at higher levels than women do after menopause.

- A woman's bone mass decreases at maturity relative to a man's.

- Women live on average seven years longer than men (this gap is widening; it was two to three years at the turn of the century).

- Aspirin reduces a man's risk of stroke, but not a woman's.

- Women are more likely to die after use of some heart medications, such as antiarrhythmia drugs.

Note also the brain differences between men and women cited earlier in this chapter.

Premenopausal women suffer heart disease less often than men, probably due to the palliative effect of abundant estrogen and progesterone, their natural beta-blockers. This, in combination with traditional physicians' tendency to see women's somatic complaints as hysterical, has contributed to women's heart disease symptoms being taken less seriously, As a result, women are more likely to die from their first heart attack than are men, and women are more likely to have a second heart attack within a year of their first.

All of this has led to a revolution in women's medicine from reproductive medicine to gender medicine. In the forefront of this movement, Columbia University's College of Physicians and Surgeons in New York has instituted the Partnership for Women's Health. The director, Marianne J. Legato, is leading the development of a database that includes sex-based findings about biological differences. Its purpose is primarily educational.

Applications

1 When you consult your physician about a specific condition or treatment, ask him or her if there are any sex-specific features that should be taken into consideration.

2 Ensure that your physician is familiar with the Partnership for Women's Health gender medicine database.

TOPIC 12.5 The Math-Verbal Controversy

In addition to documenting the hard-wired differences in brain structure and their possible impact on math and verbal performance, research continues to explore a very close relationship between hormone levels and individual performance. A higher testosterone level results in more sexual activity, more aggression, and higher math and spatial performance (as well as maze performance in rats). In females, performance is related to the menstrual cycle. From day 1 (the first day of menstruation) through ovulation, estrogen starts low and rises. From ovulation through the end of the cycle, progesterone is high and, for the most part, estrogen is high. This relationship is portrayed in Figure 12.1.

Regardless of hormone levels, females on the average test higher on verbal performance than on fine-motor coordination, and higher on fine-motor coordination than on math and spatial skills. When their hormone levels are higher, they

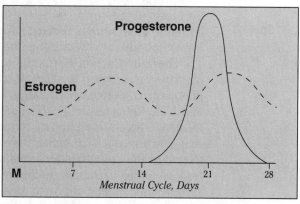

Figure 12.1. Female Hormone Levels Throughout the Monthly Cycle.
Source: From *Brain Sex: The Real Difference Between Men and Women* by Anne Moir and David Jessel, 1991, New York: Carol Publishing Group/ Lyle Stuart. © 1989, 1991 by Anne Moir and David Jessel. Reprinted by permission of Carol Publishing Group. *Note:* M = menstruation.

have higher average scores on verbal skills and fine-motor coordination, but even lower scores on math and spatial skills. In fact, during menstruation (when their estrogen and progesterone levels are at their lowest), women score 50 to 100 percent higher on mental rotation tests. Regardless of their hormone levels, females perform on average higher on verbal skills and fine-motor coordination than males and lower on math and spatial skills than the male average (Kimura and Hampson, 1990). Figure 12.2 illustrates this pattern.

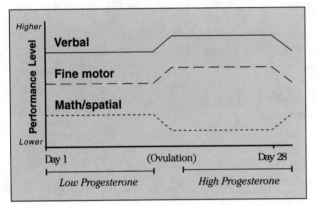

Figure 12.2. Female Hormone Levels and Their Relation to Performance.

If the same relationship of hormones to performance holds true for males, then males should do their best in math and spatial skills in the morning (testosterone levels are highest around 8:00 A.M.) and their best in verbal and fine-motor skills (although not at levels as high as those of the average female) from midafternoon through early evening (testosterone levels are lowest around 8:00 P.M.). This is purely my hypothesis; as far as I know, no research exists to support or reject it. Kimura and Hampson (1990) have found that males score higher on mental rotation tests in the spring (when testosterone is lowest) than in the fall (when testosterone is highest). Apparently the relationship is curvilinear: too much testosterone interferes with spatial performance.

These findings of hormonal influence on cognitive performance must be understood in relation to the findings of environmental influence on the same performance. P. J. Caplan, M. Crawford, J. S. Hyde, and J.T.E. Richardson (1997) point out that all of these cognitive performance levels are subject to improvement by learning and practice. The appropriate stance, because the final word is unavailable, is to regard the cognitive performance of females and males as a function of many variables, including hormones, biological structure, stereotypes, career opportunities, peer group models, role expectations, and verbal and nonverbal communication of expectations—in other words, as the interaction of environment and inheritance.

Zanna and Pack (1975) conducted a fascinatingly complex experiment that highlights the difficulty of interpreting differential cognitive performance for the sexes. (To aid in following this description, consult Figure 12.3.) A group of women were assessed on their self-reported gender roles. The women were identified as having traditional or nontraditional views (for example, they believed either that mothers should raise the children or that both the mother and the father should share equally in raising them). At a later point in time,

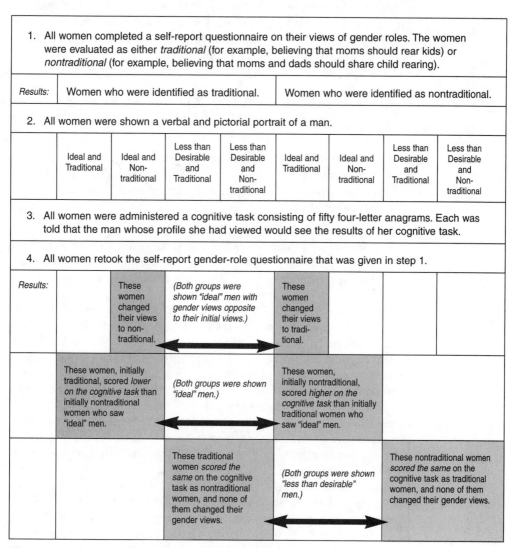

Figure 12.3. Zanna and Pack's Experiment on Gender Roles.

each of the women was given a verbal and pictorial profile of one man. Half of the men were "ideal" males (rich, handsome), while the other half were "less than desirable." Within each of these two groups, half of the men espoused traditional gender roles and half espoused nontraditional roles. All the women were then administered a cognitive task (fifty four-letter anagrams) as well as another gender-role questionnaire (remember, they had taken a similar test in the beginning). Each woman was informed that the man whose profile she'd viewed (ideal or less than ideal, traditional or nontraditional) would be shown the woman's score.

The results:

- If they were shown the ideal male picture, women changed their gender-role preference in the second testing to match that of the profiled ideal male!

- Women who initially expressed nontraditional views and who were shown pictures of an ideal male scored higher on the anagram test than did the traditional women who were shown the ideal male pictures.

- Both the traditional and nontraditional women who were shown pictures of less than desirable men performed equally well on the test, regardless of their gender-role views, and they did not change their gender-role preferences to match the male's.

In a similar study, Morier and Seroy (1994) used males as the subjects; these males also adjusted their views on gender roles, like the women above, to match the roles of the more desirable women.

In support of Zanna and Pack's findings, Claude Steele (1997) finds that women underperform in math achievement, based on their predicted scores, when they are told that the test produces differential results by sex. When they are told that women tend to score lower than men, they do. But they do not underperform when they are given the identical math questions and are told that they produce gender-free results. Steele refers to this as "stereotype threat" (p. 614; see also Topic 24.16).

Another interesting finding relative to math performance is that the female-differentiated brain tends to solve math problems by talking through them (hence, the female Talker), while the male-differentiated brain solves math problems nonverbally. Females manipulate math concepts with verbal labels, while males manipulate the concepts in abstract mental space without conscious use of language. (My wife cannot talk while studying a map in the car; I can.) One consequence of this difference is that the female-differentiated brain typically takes longer to solve a math problem.

Recent studies show that the gap in spatial ability between the sexes remains constant but that the math gap was cut in half between 1982 and 1989. To the degree that the gap is cultural in origin, societies that reduce experiential differences between boys and girls should see these differences diminish. In Charlotte, North Carolina, during the 1997–98 school year, a total of 267 females enrolled for calculus, compared to 292 males (provided by Sue Henry of the Charlotte-Mecklenburg Schools' Educational Services Department). This represents a dramatic increase from the 1950s, when female enrollment was minimal. On the other hand, Larry Hedges and Amy Nowell of the University of Chicago examined six major national surveys of U.S. teenagers' mental performance (Hedges and Nowell, 1995). They found that the gaps between boys and girls in math, spatial skills, and reading showed essentially no change from 1960 to 1992. In addition, they found that boys' scores showed greater variability, with disproportionately more boys scoring in the extremely high and low ranges, except in reading comprehension and writing, in which a disproportionately large number of boys scored in the low range (but not in the high range, as they did in math).

I have not seen math scores broken down by subtests; perhaps the differences are related to differences between computational skills, which would appear to be more left-brain-oriented and basically syntactic, and word-problem skills, which appear to be right-brain-oriented, since they are three-dimensional and spatial. Computational ability is more similar between the sexes and word-problem ability is more discrepant.

Evolutionary theorists Irwin Silverman and Marion Eals of York University in Toronto have considered subtests for spatial skills. They theorize that evolutionary necessity accounts for two distinct kinds of spatial skill: mental rotation and spatial memory. Man the hunter was selected for his ability to navigate and find his way home, while woman the gatherer was selected for her ability to remember where the good edible plants were to be found. Several lines of recent research tend to confirm this theory. Along with Krista Phillips, also of York, they found that people with higher estrogen (both men and women) perform worse on mental rotation tests: women worse than men, and men with higher estrogen levels worse than men with lower levels. Also, women score highest on mental rotation tests during menstruation, when estrogen is lowest.

In a new protocol in which subjects are asked to peruse a room for a couple of minutes, women remember objects and their relative location better than men—unless they are told to remember, in which case performance is more similar; women excel at "incidental memory." In still another confirming vein, women find their way better when using landmarks and concepts (such as "left turn"), while men find their way better when using distances and directions (such as north and south). Further support for this line comes from Heinrich Stumpf and Douglas Jackson (1994), who factor-analyzed cognitive ability for 90,142 female and 96,968 male German medical school applicants. Two of the resulting factors, reasoning and memory, showed clear gender advantages for men and women, respectively.

A brief note: the University of Michigan's Barbara Fredrickson reported that women's concern with their looks lowers their math scores (Fredrickson and others, 1998). She and her research team had men and women, separately, change into swimsuits, then fill out self-image questionnaires and take a math test. The women who felt bad about their body image as they took the tests while wearing a swimsuit scored lower than the women who didn't care. The men didn't feel bad; they felt either OK or silly, but not bad, so there was no interference with their math performance.

Applications

1 If you have a female-differentiated brain and you must take a math test like an actuarial exam or a financial audit, attempt to schedule it during the first two weeks of the menstrual cycle, between the first day of your period and ovulation. It is likely that your scores will be higher during this time. If you must take a verbal test, like a graduate oral or written exam, or make a major sales presentation, attempt to schedule it during the second two weeks of the menstrual cycle, between ovulation and the beginning of your period. If you must take a test that has both verbal and math components, such as the SAT, GRE, GMAT, or LSAT, schedule it according to which part of the test is your greater priority, math (first half of the cycle) or verbal (second half of the cycle).

2 If you administer tests—for example, as a human resources selection specialist or a teacher—then be flexible in scheduling the tests, whether with males or females. When possible, permit people to select the time of day and day of the week that best suits them.

3 The typical school curriculum from kindergarten through adult education is biased toward the female learner, with a predominance of oral and verbal methods and a minimum of visual and hands-on methods. In this environment, the female Talker finds it easier to excel over the male Doer. If you are a teacher or a student, examine your curriculum for its sexual fairness and recommend changes.

4 Do not administer a timed math test to women (or, actually, to anyone) unless speed at computation is a bona fide occupational qualification. See Sternberg's definition of intelligence in Topic 22.3. He makes a strong case against timed intelligence tests in *The Triarchic Mind* (1988).

5 If possible, females should put off written reports until the second half of their menstrual cycle, when their verbal ability is higher. *(Contributed by Jane Howard)*

6 Schedule meetings with men early in the morning when you want challenging alertness and problem-solving ability, and late in the afternoon when you want their agreement (males are less aggressive then). *(Contributed by Jane Howard)*

7 Males should schedule math and spatial tasks early in the day, verbal tasks such as writing and conversation later in the day. *(Contributed by Jane Howard)*

8 Work to get beyond negative feelings about your appearance. Understand that how you feel about your appearance affects your mental performance. Find a reasonable mode of appearance, accept it, and then don't worry about it. For example, I think I look OK in khaki pants, so I have a bunch of them and always wear khaki, never fretting about the appearance of other kinds of pants.

TOPIC 12.6 Hormones and Emotions

During the several days preceding the onset of the monthly menstrual period, the woman's body experiences a dramatic drop in progesterone and estrogen production. This is an example of *positive feedback,* in which changes tend to increase in their initial direction of change, as opposed to *negative feedback,* in which changes tend to return to the original state. The result of this positive-feedback phenomenon is an emotional volatility commonly referred to as *premenstrual tension* (PMT) or *premenstrual syndrome* (PMS). It affects an estimated 5 to 10 percent of all women. Approximately 50 percent of females' psychiatric and medical emergency hospital admissions and 50 percent of females' criminal acts occur at this time; most assignments of females to solitary confinement in prison take place during the premenstrual period. In September 1991, the U.S. Department of Agriculture reported that elevated (1,300-milligram) daily doses of calcium relieve some of these symptoms; American women average about 600 milligrams of calcium per day. It is not clear how the calcium works. An elevated level may result in optimum calpain production for cleaning out synapses so that the body's endorphins can work more effectively, or it may result in clogged synapses that dull a pain message. I suspect the former.

The equivalent of a woman's hormone depletion in a man is an excess of testosterone. The normal peaks in male testosterone levels are: early in the morning (they are 25 percent lower in evening hours), during rapid-eye-movement (REM, or dream) sleep, and in early autumn (they are lowest in spring). Males experience six or seven peaks in their testosterone level each day, with accompanying variations in the five male characteristics of behavior (competition, aggression, self-reliance, self-assertion, and self-confidence; see Topic 12.1). Excessively high testosterone takes these characteristics to a grotesque extreme: the cocksure (extreme self-confidence) loner (extreme self-reliance) driven (extreme self-assertion) to dominate (extreme aggression) whatever the cost (extreme competitiveness). Testosterone production soars in the teenage years; as a result, the highest crime rates are among boys thirteen to seventeen years old. Moir and Jessel (1991) talk of the two equivalent mood disorders as PMT (premenstrual tension) and VMT (violent male testosterone). Heino Meyer-Bahlburg of the New York State Psychiatric

Institute, however, finds that castration has little effect on male violence in general, only on sexual violence. This points to the contribution of other factors, such as low serotonin and GABA levels, in combination with testosterone.

Pioneering work by British researcher Katharina Dalton (1987) has yielded two significant findings relative to PMT: (1) administration of progesterone calms the rage center of the brain and (2) a drop in blood sugar results in a rise in adrenaline and a drop in progesterone. Holly Anderson has opened a PMT clinic based on this research: the PMS Treatment Center in Arcadia, California.

Applications

1 A simple, self-administered remedy for women with troublesome mood swings is to try snacking every two to three hours in order to sustain blood sugar levels throughout the day. Women who have a tendency toward violent moods that won't go away should consult an endocrinologist for both pharmaceutical and nonpharmaceutical treatment.

2 Women who have a tendency toward violent mood swings need to understand this reality. They also should mention this tendency to others and deal with the mood swings with appropriate humor after the fact. Men (and other women) need to avoid taking a woman's premenstrual mood swings personally; it helps if they can find appropriate ways to respond (such as "Wow! You're furious!" or "You have a right to be mad" or "You're right; good point") and then get on with things.

3 Men who have a tendency to "take no prisoners" need to understand this reality. They should follow up such episodes with humorous or self-deprecating comments (such as "Boy! I just couldn't let go of my position, could I? I was a real bastard"). To minimize the possibility of exhibiting killer behavior when an important high-risk situation is coming up, they should try preceding the situation with long, strenuous exercise—for example, a forty-five-minute run or lap swim or a sixty-minute brisk walk.

4 It is important for both males and females to pick up the pieces after their hormone-driven outbursts. At a minimum, they should say

"I'm sorry" or its equivalent (such as giving flowers or some other token). At another level, decisions made during outbursts should be reconsidered.

5 Women might try consuming more calcium products, such as milk or yogurt, before their periods.

6 For current information on PMS/PMT, call PMS Access, a national organization for PMS information in Madison, Wisconsin, at 800-222-2767.

TOPIC 12.7 Vision

Research has shown that male-differentiated brains have better visual discrimination in the blue end of the spectrum, and female-differentiated brains have better visual discrimination in the red end. Males have better visual discrimination in bright light (day vision), while females have better discrimination in subdued light (night vision).

Applications

1 Where extremely fine color discrimination is necessary, allow for the fatigue, error, and slowdown that might accompany an attempt to concentrate on an end of the spectrum that is not your "natural" end.

2 When testing employees for color discrimination, be aware that you will rarely find employees who are equally strong at both ends of the spectrum.

3 Females may be safer drivers at night, although I have not seen any hard data to support this.

4 Be aware in workplace design that brightly lit areas are more fatiguing for females and dimly lit areas are more fatiguing for males. Allow variations in brightness throughout the facility as much as possible. Vary lighting in break areas to give individuals a choice.

5 In a romantic setting, don't assume that the male is unromantic because he wants more light or that the female is romantic because she is comfortable with less light. Females can see better with less light than males.

TOPIC 12.8　Space

Research has shown that females are more comfortable being in close physical proximity to other females than males are being close to other males. (See also Topic 34.11.) As a general rule, males require more work space than females. However, this is not a reason for discriminating with regard to space. Understand that accepting a smaller space should not necessarily be taken as a sign of low ambition; some people, especially those with female-differentiated brains, are very comfortable with less space. Conversely, wanting a larger space should not necessarily be taken as a power play; some people, especially those with male-differentiated brains, become uncomfortable, or even stressed-out, in a smaller space. It is possible that this difference was genetically favored when women were primarily cave dwellers during the day and men roamed the fields as hunters.

Applications

1 Allow males to create a sufficiently comfortable space between themselves and other males.

2 Trust people to tell you how much space they need in order to be comfortable.

3 When overnight accommodations are necessary, if possible, let people choose single or double rooms. Females will generally feel more comfortable sharing a room than males. *(Contributed by Jane Howard)*

TOPIC 12.9 The Effect of Odors on Females

Females are more sensitive to odors than males. It takes a stronger odor to get a typical man's attention than a woman's. This is likely a genetic artifact of natural selection for mothers, who must be alert to olfactory indicators of their infants' distress. This gender difference has been definitely established (remembering, of course, that exceptions are common), but its cause is speculative. Researchers believe that it is related to higher levels of estrogen.

A long-suspected phenomenon among women—menstrual synchrony—has been confirmed by researchers at the University of Chicago (*Nature,* March 12, 1998). The senior researcher, Martha McClintock, finds that pheromones—odorless and colorless scents found among animals and humans—from one female affect the timing of menstruation of other females. Taking cotton swabs from the underarms of women at different times during menstruation, researchers found that pheromones from specific phases affect other women differently. For example, extracts from the follicular phase (early in the cycle) shortened others' cycles, while extracts from the ovarian phase (midcycle) lengthened others' cycles and those from the luteal phase (after ovulation) had no effect on others' cycles. This finding is likely to be the signal for an intense new line of human pheromone research with implications for mate selection, xenophobia, nepotism, dominance struggles, and friendships. (See the related discussion on histocompatibility complexes in Topic 13.1.)

Applications

1 Be sensitive to the fact that women regard certain odors as offensive. They do so because the female-differentiated brain has more alert smell receptors than the male-differentiated brain. Women are not being stereotypically prissy any more than men are being stereotypically macho when they are aggressive—this behavior is a result of their different hormonal makeups.

2 There are many tasks that require an acute sense of smell: cooking; chemical analysis; safety inspections, such as those for gas leaks; quality inspections, including perfume testing; even lie detection, which measures perspiration. Consider that females as a group have more sensitivity in olfactory detection.

3   Be aware that it is normal for women who are living in close proximity (roommates, office mates) to experience a convergence in the timing of menstruation. Research is under way to find possible applications in the areas of infertility and birth control.

TOPIC 12.10   Gender Differences in Taste

Female-differentiated brains are more sensitive to sweet tastes and male-differentiated brains are more sensitive to salty tastes. Hence, the typical female requires more salt to satisfy her and the typical male needs more sugar. A classic example is my wife's tendency to oversalt food when she cooks and my tendency to oversweeten hot chocolate when I make it from scratch. Notice how, generally, women tend to shake salt on their meals for a longer period than men, while men tend to add more sugar to their coffee or tea (if they sweeten it at all).

Applications

1   In food preparation, female chefs should try not to oversalt their dishes and male chefs should not oversweeten theirs. Folks can always add salt or sugar to suit their taste.

2   Don't be offended if you're female and a male adds sugar to your prepared dish; don't be offended if you're male and a female adds salt to your prepared dish!

TOPIC 12.11   Automatization

Males and females who are injected with extra testosterone show an ability to persevere at automatized behaviors. These are behaviors that do not demand excessive mental or physical exertion once they have been learned, but that are subject to fatigue effects over time (Moir and Jessel, 1991). Examples include solving basic arithmetic problems, walking, talking, maintaining balance (for example, standing guard), maintaining observation (for example, being a military sniper or a quality inspector), and writing. Injected groups show a lower decline in skills as the day wears on. Those who are not injected get tired and make more mistakes. The "automatizers," with extra testosterone, tend to be more focused and single-minded and are more often associated with upward mobility and success. Estrogen is known to suppress automatized behavior, especially just after puberty, when girls' academic performance tends to decline. Boys begin to exhibit automatized behaviors during puberty, when their system ratchets to a new level of testosterone.

Applications

1 Females who are engaging in automatized behaviors will require more frequent breaks to maintain a given skill level.

2 Females can be more consistently productive in nonautomatized areas—for example, sales, research and development, supervision, training and development, planning, analysis, and creative activities.

3 Promotional policies should not be based exclusively on performance at automatized skills. Management tasks do not consist of automatized behavior, so promoting those who are good at it incurs the risk of creating managers who convert their success at these behaviors into inappropriate management behaviors, such as supervising too closely and pushing, pulling, or riding employees without letup. Nonautomatizers are more likely to develop effective coaching, counseling, and listening skills.

A Final Word on Sex and Gender

The final word has not been written on the causes and changeability of sex and gender differences. Keep in mind that all of this research deals with averages, and that individuals do not obey the law of averages. Only groups do. So when we think of sex and gender differences, we should not automatically think that individual "X" can be described by those differences. It is likely that she or he can, but not a given. Just because men, on average, are not as nurturing as women, this does not mean that I am less nurturing than most women. In fact, I love babies and can't resist the opportunity to hold them and go "goo-goo." This does not make me a woman, but it does suggest that I have a "feminine" dimension to my personality.

In an extremely well written article using rigorous standards, Amy Eagly (1995) of Purdue University wrote in the *American Psychologist* that eight gender differences in behavior pass her test for significance: (1) mental rotation, (2) facial expressiveness, (3) frequency of filled pauses in speech, (4) incidence of masturbation, (5) attitudes toward casual sexual intercourse, (6) tender-mindedness, (7) nurturant tendencies, and (8) the velocity, distance, and accurateness of throwing a ball. All other gender differences, she finds, are too small to affect our notion of what we view as purely feminine or masculine. While these differences form the basis of a stereotype, they are not consistently present in only one sex. So even though most women exhibit more expressive faces, there will always be someone like Robin Williams. And although most men have more casual attitudes toward sexual intercourse, there will always be someone like Erica Jong.

SUGGESTED RESOURCES

Bem, S. L. (1993). *The Lenses of Gender: Transforming the Debate on Sexual Inequality.* New Haven: Yale University Press.

Caplan, P. J., Crawford, M., Hyde, J. S., and Richardson, J.T.E. (1997). *Gender Differences in Human Cognition.* New York: Oxford University Press.

Crawford, M. (1995). *Talking Difference: On Gender and Language.* Thousand Oaks, Calif.: Sage.

Moir, A., and Jessel, D. (1991). *Brain Sex: The Real Difference Between Men and Women.* New York: Carol.

13

Love and Relationships

The Wiring Is the Name of the Game

> **There are two kinds of sex— for babies, and fore play.**
>
> —*P. J. Howard*

Yes, cognitive science has something to say about how we form and maintain relationships. Our sexual identity (see Topics 12.2 and 12.3) and relationship preferences begin to form in the womb. A wide range of current research is establishing not only the value of being in a relationship, but also the way to maintain it. In a delightful word from avian research, for example, Tony Tremontin, of the University of Washington's zoology department, tells us that a male sparrow housed with a female sparrow experiences a 15 to 20 percent growth in his forebrain area. Tremontin suspects that if this growth in the forebrain area is also true for human male-female couples, it will have a corresponding effect on language development. This chapter will explore a variety of such issues, including the formation of relationships, love styles, affairs, sexual performance, and relationship maintenance.

TOPIC 13.1 Factors Influencing Partner Selection

Love! What is it? First, it is practically universal. William Jankowiak, of the University of Nevada–Las Vegas, and Edward Fischer, of Tulane University, studied 166 cultures and concluded that at least 147 of them showed evidence of the existence of romantic love. Although it is prevalent around the world, romantic love is not limited to marriage, and marriage is not limited to romantic love; many cultures permit and even encourage arranged marriages.

Several factors appear to influence the initial attraction. First, as Swiss researchers reported, females have clear preferences for certain male body odors (*Proceedings of the Royal Society of London*, 1995). Namely, they prefer the smell emitted by men with the major histocompatibility complexes (MHCs) that are most different from their own. A complicating factor is that women on the birth control pill prefer men with similar MHCs; so what happens when a woman who is on the pill falls in love, marries, goes off the pill, and wonders how she got attached to the smelly partner beside her.

A second factor was identified by Galdino Pranzarone, a psychologist at Roanoke College in Salem, Virginia, who found that people have established an image of their ideal lover and ideal love behavior patterns by the age of ten (see the discussion of schemas in Topics 23.4, 25.4, and 35.1). Helen Fisher, a research associate at the American Museum of Natural History, describes the physiological changes that accompany the recognition of the ideal partner as involving a rush of phenylethylamine (PEA), dopamine, and norepinephrine, all natural amphetamines. The feeling of euphoria associated with this neurochemical flooding can last up to three years, then weakens. Divorces and separations multiply around the end of the fourth year of love relationships. Having a second child can prolong the physiological state for another four years. If childbearing ends after the second child, the stage is set for the possibility of the "seven-year itch" made famous by Marilyn Monroe. Couples who are able to find satisfaction with each other after the euphoria dissipates apparently do so by generating increased amounts of endorphins (more similar to morphine than to amphetamines), which are associated with a sense of calm and security (the so-called "runner's high"). In addition, long-term couples benefit from oxytocin (called the "cuddle chemical" because it is produced during nursing and intercourse), which is manufactured by the pituitary gland during lovemaking, leading to feelings of satisfaction.

Fisher calls these phases *imprinting* (MHCs), *attraction* (PEA, dopamine, and norepinephrine), and *attachment* (endorphins and oxytocin). Anthony Walsh (1996), a psychobiologist at Boise State University in Idaho, observes that the natural amphetamines associated with attraction and its attendant euphoria act pretty much like pharmaceutical amphetamines: people build up a tolerance over time and need an increasingly large dose to be satisfied. At around the third year of the cycle, the body can't produce enough PEA to maintain the attraction.

> "Husband," said the woman, "have you caught nothing today?"
>
> "No," said the man, "I did catch a flounder who said he was an enchanted prince, so I let him go again."
>
> "Did you not wish for anything first?"
>
> "No," said the man, "what should I wish for?"
>
> "Ah!" said the wife.
>
> —"The Fisherman and His Wife,"
> *Grimm's Fairy Tales*

Applications

1 If you are a woman taking the birth control pill, before you become irrevocably attracted to someone, spend some time with that person while you're off the pill to ensure histocompatibility.

2 If you desire a long-term relationship, ensure that you find substantial features about your mate that you respect and admire, so that when the attraction phase wears down after several years, you will still derive your daily dose of endorphins for the long term.

TOPIC 13.2 Love Styles

Phillip Shaver, a psychologist at the University of California, Davis, has conducted extensive research on love, or attachment, styles (see Mallandain and Davies, 1994). Using two different models and studying twins in the California Twin Registry, Shaver has concluded that love style is determined primarily by environmental influences.

One model he has used was developed by Mary Ainsworth and John Bowlby, who found that in their first year, infants grow into one of three ways of relating—*secure, anxious,* or *avoidant*—based on how their parents or caregivers treat them. The secure child sees the mother as supportive and feels free to explore the world, the anxious child views the mother as an unpredictable caregiver and commits his or her life to earning the mother's love, and the avoidant child sees the mother as rejecting and consequently discounts his or her own needs. Although Shaver finds that these three styles appear to persist into adulthood, he has elaborated on them by using the six-part model developed by sociologist John Lee of the University of Toronto. Lee gives Greek names to the six attachment styles:

Agape: Selfless, spiritual, giving

Eros: Passionate, confident, self-disclosing; enjoys intimacy

Pragma: Requires the partner and relationship to satisfy certain preexisting conditions

Storge: Companionable, friendship-oriented, reliable

Ludus: Fun, exciting, non-self-disclosing; prefers multiple partners

Mania: Dependent, jealous, conflicted; yearns for love but experiences disappointment

People with the first four styles tend to prefer mates with the same style: for example, Eros mates with Eros. The last two styles, however, are a bit more tricky. While people with the first four styles exemplify the adage "Birds of a feather flock together . . . ," Ludus and Mania tend to mate with other styles. This makes sense. If both partners avoid intimacy and long-term relationships, as in the case of Ludus, there is less chance of the couple staying together than there would be if at least one member of the pair were less avoidant, and if both partners are jealous and dependent, as in the case of Mania, they are less likely to stay together than if one partner is more secure.

These six styles appear to be heavily influenced by one's up-bringing and to be an elaboration of the secure, anxious, and avoidant styles. To understand this elaboration, it is helpful to see the relationship between these six styles and the Five Factor Model of personality (see Topic 4.4 and Chapter Twenty-One for more explanation):

Agape:	Related to high Agreeableness
Eros:	Related to high Extraversion
Pragma:	Related to high Conscientiousness
Storge:	Related to high Extraversion and Conscientiousness
Ludus:	Related to high Extraversion and Openness, low Agreeableness and Conscientiousness
Mania:	Related to high Negative Emotionality and low Agreeableness

Applications

❶ Know your attachment style and consider the attachment styles of people with whom you find yourself becoming serious. The likelihood of long-term satisfaction is increased when your styles are compatible, as outlined above. Imagine Storge partnering with Pragma only to find after four years when the "amphetamines" wear off (see Topic 13.1) that the companion is no longer available and Storge must look elsewhere for friendship while Pragma pursues his or her own agenda.

❷ Consider conflicts in relationships, when they occur, as more likely to be caused by stylistic incompatibilities in values and expectations than to be caused by the other person in an intentional and hurtful way. Rather than saying, "You don't love me anymore," consider saying, "Your style of loving is different from mine."

TOPIC 13.3 The Ideal Mate

David Buss (1994), with a group of international collaborators, polled over ten thousand men and women from the United States to Indonesia in an effort to determine what people want in the ideal mate. Buss, who was schooled in the evolutionary biology tradition that sees contemporary behavior as the result of natural selection, found that after intelligence and kindness (which both sexes ranked as the top feature of the ideal mate), men preferred women who were physically beautiful and youthful over those with high earning potential, while women preferred good earning capacity and ambition over physical attractiveness.

In a related study, William Tooke of the State University of New York at Plattsburgh found that during courtship, men tend to exaggerate their earning potential and ambition and women tend to exaggerate their youthfulness and beauty, each relaxing into their more natural levels of ambition and appearance after attachment has been secured.

Applications

1 If ambition or appearance is important to you in a mate, be aware of the possibility that your intended is deceiving you in order to win your attachment. Look to the past for her or his natural behavior by interviewing friends and perusing yearbooks.

2 Talk with your intended in order to confirm whether his or her levels of ambition or appearance are authentic or a soon to be abandoned enticement.

3 If you are liberated from these classic needs of your animal and primitive ancestors, then smile at the antics of your anachronistic cousins and get on with your life.

TOPIC 13.4 Maintaining Relationships

Males are wired to do, and females are wired to talk (Moir and Jessel, 1991; see the earlier discussion in Topic 12.1). Expecting a male to talk and only talk can be highly uncomfortable for the male and rather unproductive as well. Expecting a female to engage in an activity without talking can be equally uncomfortable and unproductive for the female. In order to keep communication between males and females at the maximum, both should attempt to initiate serious conversation when the male is engaged in some form of physical activity, such as walking, trimming his fingernails, or gardening. In a scene from the movie *City of Angels,* the doctor friend of Meg Ryan, advancing his case for a proposal of marriage, recommends that they "get away" for a while. She says, "Why not right now? Let's just spend the next five minutes together, with nothing else on our minds." He says, "Five minutes? Doing what?" As a typical male, he just doesn't get it. She wants to chat intimately with him, but the very thought makes him uncomfortable. He wants to be "doing" something.

On another front, the University of Washington's John Gottman studied 130 newlyweds for six years for the purpose of finding ways to predict marital success and failure. A commonsensical finding emerged: men who accepted the influence of their wives and wives who presented requests, complaints, or suggestions in a warm, even humorous, manner were most likely to be in happy marriages for the long term. The gist of this report (*Journal of Marriage and the Family,* February 1998) is consistent with the behavior common to the midrange of the Agreeableness dimension of the Five Factor Model of personality (see Topic 4.4 and Chapter Twenty-One). In a related finding, Gottman reported that the use of interpersonal listening and communication techniques such as "active listening" were not predictive of marital success. Perhaps this is because therapists teach troubled partners such techniques too late in their downward spiral.

Applications

1 In most male-female relationships, conflict arises when the female wants to talk and the male wants to act; the classic example is the female preference in lovemaking for greater foreplay and the male preference for immediate release. The solution to this type of conflict is to allow the other person's style to be expressed: the male agrees to talk if he is allowed to continue working in the yard, and the female agrees to work in the yard with him if he will talk with her. Males need to be willing to listen and respond while doing, and females need to be willing to "do" as a stage for talking. For example, a male and female who go to a ball game or museum may discuss family matters during appropriate lulls. Or they may just go for a drive together, with the male driving (doing) while they are talking. An alternative is to set aside exclusive times to talk without doing and vice versa.

2 Any negotiating team should include females; they provide a willingness to talk and work on relationships that balances the males' desire for a quick fix.

3 Human resource functions in organizations should include females in decision-making or advisory roles.

4 One way to get males to talk more is to make something of a game or contest out of it. A traditional male is more likely to engage in talk when he can see communication skills as a set of tools to master. That way he is not just "talking"; he is practicing a skill set.

5 Neither a doormat nor a deaf ear be. For optimum satisfaction in a long-term relationship, make sure that neither of you gets your way to the exclusion of the other party. Harold Kelley (Kelley and Thibaut, 1978) describes this ideal relationship as "interdependent." Interdependence exists when neither person experiences costs (pain, labor, drudgery) that exceed rewards (life's pleasures).

TOPIC 13.5 Affairs

David Buss (1994) reports that women, 25 percent of whom have extramarital affairs, tend to explain their affairs as resulting from dissatisfaction with the marital relationship: they're looking for a replacement. On the other hand, men who have affairs are as likely to feel good about their primary relationship as they are to be unhappy with it. Another sex difference has to do with jealousy. Buss points out that the human female is the only species whose ovulation cannot be observed. Hence, her mate never knows visually when she is fertile. As a result, a man tends to be especially jealous when his woman simply has intercourse with another man, regardless of the seriousness or length of the attachment; if she becomes pregnant, he has no way of knowing if the child is his, and he risks spending resources on another man's child. (Perhaps in the era of DNA testing, this evolutionary vestige will disappear.) On the other hand, the woman generally cares less if her man has a one-night stand; she is more threatened by a competing serious attachment that could result in her loss of resources. This is all understandable from an evolutionary point of view (D. M. Buss, 1994; H. E. Fisher, 1982, 1995): in the past, the woman needed to keep an extra relationship offstage in case a saber-toothed tiger eliminated her man, yet she fought against her man's keeping up such a relationship for fear that she'd lose her resource provider. The man needed to ensure the survivability of his kind by planting his seed abundantly, but he fought against his woman's doing the same, not wanting to rear another man's child. Hence, the proverbial double standard.

Applications

1 If you are a woman, you should understand that typically, a man's jealousy is not triggered by a long-term serious relationship on your part, but by the single sex act itself. Consider that your need for an affair may be attributable to dissatisfaction with your marriage. This should be a signal to work on the marriage. Get help.

2 If you are a man, you should understand that typically, a woman's jealousy is not triggered by a one-night stand, but rather by an ongoing relationship on your part. If you require such a long-term outside relationship, this is a signal that the marriage is in trouble. Get help.

3 In the case of both men and women, attachment style (see Topic 13.2) also plays a part in the need for an intimate relationship with one's partner. For example, if you are a Ludus married to an Eros, you need to give Eros permission to find a deeper relationship elsewhere.

TOPIC 13.6   Appreciating Attachment Needs for the Long Term

Donald Kiesler (1996) has provided us with a definitive review of the literature on relationships. He identifies two crucial principles for the long-term viability of relationships, marital or otherwise: the *interpersonal reflex* (p. 6) and the *behavior concordance model* (p. 49). The interpersonal reflex principle states that "any interpersonal act is designed to elicit from a respondent reactions that confirm, reinforce, or validate the actor's self-presentation and that make it more likely that the actor will continue to emit similar interpersonal acts" (p. 6). When Neil Diamond laments, "You don't give me flowers anymore," he is revealing that either (1) he is no longer behaving in a way that encourages the woman to continue giving him flowers or (2) she has given up on him as a mate and is focusing elsewhere. In either case, things need fixing.

The behavior concordance model has established that "individuals will feel pleasant affect when they behave consistently with their traits" (p. 49) and unpleasant affect when they behave inconsistently with their traits. Have you ever heard of people who were "not happy unless they were unhappy"? Pity the worrier who has nothing about which to worry, the gregarious talker who has no ears around, the ambitious worker who has no goal. They are unhappy campers. The relevance to relationships is this: to maximize the chances of your happiness and the happiness of your mate, ensure that you validate the core behaviors (traits, values, interests, attitudes, and skills) of your mate and that they validate yours. More importantly, during the initial phase of the relationship, learn what these core behaviors are and decide early on whether you feel good about validating them for a lifetime.

Applications

1   Be careful that you don't validate someone's behavior unintentionally; you may dig yourself into such a deep hole that you can't get out. A friend faked orgasm with her mate for years. The consequence? He didn't develop as a lover, and she grew resentful.

2   On the other hand, be careful that you don't invalidate someone's behavior that you wish to maintain. Be careful with "You shouldn't have done that" responses, because the other person is likely to, in fact, stop doing that. Or if you wonder why a friend hasn't asked you back for dinner, look for the possibility that you neglected to confirm your enjoyment of the last dinner (by returning the favor, taking a house gift, writing a note, mentioning it favorably at a later date, and so on).

3   If you are in the beginning phases of a relationship, romantic, work, or otherwise, and you know that you want the relationship to be long-term, learn all you can about the other person's core values and behaviors and share as much of your core values and behaviors as you can. This might not seem important during the honeymoon or "amphetamine" phase, but it makes all the difference in the world when, after the initial euphoria wears off, you are a Willie Nelson groupie left to live life with a Mozart maniac or a Sierra Club enthusiast tied to an unrecycler who drives a gas-guzzler.

TOPIC 13.7 Sexual Fantasies

University of Vermont psychologists Harold Leitenberg and Kris Henning reported in the *Psychological Bulletin* (May 1995) that 95 percent of adults have sexual fantasies and, Freud's views to the contrary notwithstanding, people with more active sex lives have more fantasies, not the other way around. The median number of daily sexual fantasies for males is seven; five are prompted by events (for example, an attractive woman appears on the scene), while two arise spontaneously from within. For women, the median number is five daily, three from external cues and two from within. Men are more likely to fantasize about having multiple sexual partners, with an average of 1.96 partners per fantasy; women have an average of 1.08 partners per fantasy.

Application

Accept sexual fantasies as normal and unavoidable.

TOPIC 13.8   Personality Traits and Sexual Behavior

The two most widely researched dimensions of personality are Extraversion (aka Positive Emotions) and Negative Emotionality (aka Neuroticism or Emotional Stability). (See Chapter Twenty-One for a more extensive discussion of these dimensions.) G. D. Wilson, in his essay "Personality and Social Behavior" (in Eysenck, 1981), summarized a wide variety of behavioral correlates of personality dimensions. Several of these correlates relate specifically to sexual behaviors. They are listed in Table 13.1.

Remember that these associations are not absolutes. Not all highly extraverted people, for example, demonstrate all the associated behaviors. These are trends, not inevitabilities. It is useful, however, to get a sense of the degree to which one's behavior is typical of that of other people with a similar personality. Many factors can explain exceptions to the trends provided in such tables, including mores, opportunities, incentives, exposure to diverse lifestyles, parenting styles, and limitations resulting from social circumstances.

Application

If your partner's behavior is something other than what you prefer, realize that there is a strong likelihood that this difference in sexual behavior is attributable to the way your partner's personality is built and is not a reaction to, or judgment of, you. In other words, don't

Table 13.1. Sexual Behaviors Correlated with the Personality Dimensions Extraversion and Negative Emotionality.

Low Negative Emotionality ("Resilient")	High Negative Emotionality ("Reactive")
Males report fewer sexual urges	Males report more sexual urges, more frequent erections, more masturbation
Females report more orgasms during intercourse	Females report fewer orgasms during intercourse
Less sexual pathology and dissatisfaction reported	More sexual pathology and dissatisfaction reported
Less nervous about sex	More nervous about sex
Less easily excited sexually	More easily excited sexually
Less sexual hostility	More sexual hostility
Less guilty concerning sex	More guilty concerning sex
More petting	Less petting
More acts of sexual intercourse	Fewer acts of sexual intercourse
More oral-genital sex	Less oral-genital sex

Low Extraversion ("Introvert")	High Extraversion ("Extravert")
Report somewhat less satisfaction with sex	Report more satisfaction with sex
Less engagement in fellatio and cunnilingus	More engagement in fellatio and cunnilingus
Engage in less sexual foreplay	Engage in more sexual foreplay
Average fewer than three sexual positions	Average more than three sexual positions
Fewer sexual partners over time	More sexual partners over time
Larger proportion are virgins	Smaller proportion are virgins
Less comfortable with physical closeness and touching	More comfortable with physical closeness and touching
Relatively less pursuit of interpersonal intimacy	Maximizing of interpersonal intimacy

take differences in sexual preferences personally, as a kind of rejection. To the degree that sexual behavior is very important to you, realize the importance of partnering with someone whose personality is similar to yours. If you're more introverted, don't date an extravert and then be perturbed because she or he acts consistently with an extravert's "nature."

TOPIC 13.9 Inbreeding

Although mating with a cousin is only slightly less risky than mating with a nonrelative (cousins have a 90 percent chance of producing a healthy offspring; nonrelatives, a 94 percent chance), inbreeding on a large scale has a significant downside (Jones, 1994). In areas where one founder or a relatively small number of founders established a community that has remained resistant to mingling with the outside world, deadly diseases or undesirable deformities have emerged. Some examples: porphyria among Afrikaners, blindness among the inhabitants of Tristan da Cunha, an enzyme defect among Kurdistan Jews, and a stunted, six-fingered hand among the Pennsylvania Amish. The most dramatic instance of the negative effects of inbreeding is that of the Lake Maracaibo Venezuelans, where four thousand out of ten thousand people either have Huntington's disease or are at risk of contracting it.

Application

Celebrate mating between people of diverse backgrounds, through which undesirable genes can become extinguished. In diversity is strength.

SUGGESTED RESOURCES

Buss, D. M. (1994). *The Evolution of Desire.* New York: Basic Books.

Diamond, J. (1997b). *Why Is Sex Fun? The Evolution of Human Sexuality.* New York: Basic Books.

Fausto-Sterling, A., and Rose, H. (1994). *Love, Power, and Knowledge.* Bloomington: Indiana University Press.

Fisher, H. E. (1982). *The Sex Contract.* New York: Morrow.

Fisher, H. E. (1995). *Anatomy of Love: A Natural History of Mating, Marriage, and Why We Stray.* New York: Fawcett.

Hatfield, E., and Rapson, R. L. (1993). *Love, Sex, and Intimacy: Their Psychology, Biology, and History.* Reading, Mass.: Addison-Wesley.

Kelley, H. H., and Thibaut, J. W. (1978). *Interpersonal Relations: A Theory of Interdependence.* New York: Wiley.

Kiesler, D. J. (1996). *Contemporary Interpersonal Theory and Research: Personality, Psychopathology, and Psychotherapy.* New York: Wiley.

LeVay, S. (1996). *Queer Science: The Use and Abuse of Research into Homosexuality.* Cambridge, Mass.: MIT Press.

Walsh, A. (1996). *The Science of Love: Understanding Love and Its Effects on Mind and Body.* Amherst, N.Y.: Prometheus.

Part Four

*What
We Know
About
Brain
Repair*

Illness
and Injury

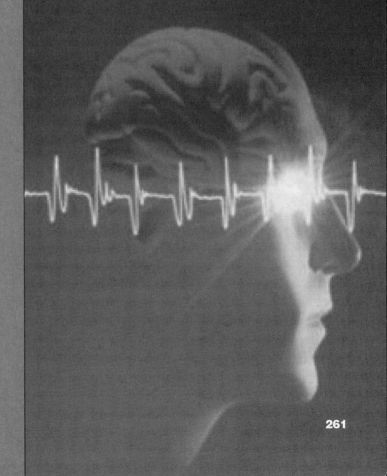

14

Brain-Related Disorders and Their Treatment

Background Information

*L*ittle Jimmy was five years old and had never spoken a word. His parents had tried every known resource—from speech pathologists to faith healers—to help Jimmy talk. One Saturday morning at breakfast, little Jimmy whined, "My damn eggs are cold!"

His parents exclaimed, "Jimmy, we're certainly glad to hear you finally talk! But why've you waited so long, and only to curse like a little sailor?"

Jimmy replied, "Everything's been all right up 'til now!"

> **" *A journey of a thousand miles must begin with a single step.* "**
>
> —Lao-tzu,
> The Way of Lao-tzu

In general, our brains appear to function within acceptable limits. We may be more sleepy than we like, or more nervous than we like, but we're able to hold a job, to advance in our careers, to enjoy long-term relationships, and to entertain ourselves. But sometimes the brain goes awry: that is, it begins to function outside these acceptable limits in a way that makes it hard, and sometimes impossible, to hold a job or manage a relationship.

This chapter provides some background on therapeutic approaches to brain disorders, while the next four chapters address specific categories of disorders. This chapter also includes a discussion of psychoneuroimmunology (PNI). PNI is not a mental disorder; rather, it is the study of the nervous system, endocrine system, and immune system considered as if they were a single system. To the degree that we embrace the principles of PNI, we establish the best possible psychophysical environment for staying physically and psychologically well.

Neurobehavioral Disorders

It should become clear after reading the next several chapters that neurobehavioral disorders are not simply "in one's head." For many years, mental disorders from depression to dyslexia were believed to be solely attributable to childhood mistreatment, lack of discipline or will, or some such nonbiological source. Only something as blatantly palpable as a brain tumor was sufficiently "physical" in nature so that people were willing to 'fess up to it in public. One could say "My son has a brain tumor" without adversely reflecting on oneself, whereas saying "My son has a depressive disorder" seemed to acknowledge a kind of personal failure or inadequacy. We now know better. Sure, environment can play a role, but we have learned that the so-called mental disorders are in fact physical.

Ivan Goldberg, a New York City psychiatrist, proposes in an Internet posting that the phrase *neurobehavioral disorder* be substituted for *mental disorder* or *mental disease*. When his patients ask what it means, he says something like this: "It is an illness in which thoughts, feelings, images, and behavior are largely the result of a neurochemical disturbance in the brain." This emphasizes the fact that "there is but one self, not a neurobiological self and a psychological self."

In a thoughtful discussion of mental illness in the January 26, 1998, *Newsweek* ("Is Everybody Crazy?"), Sharon Begley describes what psychiatrists and neurologists are calling a continuum of diagnosis. For example, if a dozen or so gene markers are involved in dopamine regulation, then the behavior of people with one or two genetic markers will be less extreme than the behavior of people with all twelve markers. This would be like the difference between someone who is moderately impulsive (with only two or three markers) and someone who constantly flirts with disaster.

Treatment Alternatives

Generally, treatment for brain-related illnesses will fall under one or more of five categories: psychotherapy, pharmacotherapy, mechanotherapy, complementary therapy, and autotherapy. Or, more familiarly, talk therapy, drug therapy, electronic therapy, nontraditional therapy, and self-help.

Psychotherapy

Traditional wisdom has maintained that psychotherapy is not effective. However, in a major study of the effectiveness of psychotherapy, *Consumer Reports* ("Mental Health," 1995) challenged this stance based on the results of a survey of its readership. Seligman (1996) summarized the report in a special issue of the *American Psychologist,* "Outcome Assessment of Psychotherapy." The key to understanding the *Consumer Reports* findings hinges on an important distinction: academic research versus field research. In the traditional academic research paradigm, a single treatment is evaluated over a relatively brief time span, and the therapist's personality is eliminated through random assignment and control groups. In field research, as typified by the *Consumer Reports* study, the therapist-patient relationship is evaluated over the entire length of their association, whether it lasts two weeks or two years, a day or a lifetime. In academic research, the treatment is the subject of the study, while in field research, the therapist-patient relationship is the subject of the study.

Thus, academic research demonstrated that specific therapies—gestalt, transactional analysis, cognitive, behavioral, and other therapies—showed few positive effects. However, when the subject of the study changed to the patient-therapist relationship, dramatic improvements were reported. The difference is this: in the field, therapists don't use just one treatment method, such as gestalt therapy, for a defined period of time and quit. Rather, they tend to try a treatment method and, if it doesn't appear to work, they'll switch to another one. Under these more realistic field conditions, patients report highly satisfactory results for psychotherapy. In fact, Seligman (in Horgan, 1996) maintains that only two drugs are superior to talk therapy: lithium for manic depression and tranquilizers for schizophrenia.

Psychotherapy can be divided into two formats: individual talk therapy and group therapy. The former ranges from the so-called brief therapies of one or two sessions to psychoanalysis, which can extend for years. The latter ranges from informal support groups, in which people with a similar concern (for example, long-term caregivers) get together and talk with the aid of a therapist, to traditional group therapy, in which people with a variety of conditions (for example, control freaks, nonassertives, and such) confront their problems with the aid of the therapists and each other.

Pharmacotherapy

In its ideal form, this type of therapy is practiced by a therapist who is committed to an ongoing relationship with a patient and who prescribes medication as an enhancement of the ongoing individual or group therapy. The drugs may be prescription (Prozac) or non-prescription (St. John's Wort, melatonin). As a general rule, pharmaceuticals are less effective when they are unaccompanied by psychotherapy. All too often, a primary care physician will prescribe a medication such as Ritalin or Prozac, both of which have become fashionable, under one of two conditions: either (1) the patient does not have the disorder and the drug provides only cosmetic relief or (2) the patient does have the disorder and the drug provides some relief, but the relief is less dramatic and less long-lasting than would be the case if the patient had a continuing relationship with a psychotherapist.

Increasingly, a new descriptor is popping up in the pharmaceutical landscape—that of "rational" drugs. Traditional pharmaceutical research and development could be defined as pre-genome. In other words, before the Human Genome Project began in the early 1990s to slowly identify the relationship between specific genes and specific disorders, a hit-or-miss, "shotgun" quality typified much pharmaceutical research. The more recent line of rational drugs has built on the known chemical relationships between one or more genes and a specific disorder. The term *rational* applies to this more deductive form of development—hence, rational drugs. Typically, these drugs are more precise in their aim; as a consequence, they have fewer adverse side effects. It is as though researchers now have a kind of blueprint for building new drugs.

In contrast to therapy with rational drugs, which treat diseases that are genetic in origin, *gene therapy* uses genes as a distribution system. This remarkable process begins with a benign virus, introduces into its DNA a new gene that will produce the desired chemical, then injects the virus into the desired area of the brain, thus bypassing the blood-brain barrier. The benign virus then multiplies, becoming a regional drug factory that deposits increasing and permanent supplies of the desired chemical. As an example, the adeno-associated virus (AAV) is modified with the human gene for the enzyme tyrosine hydroxylase (TH). Once it has been implanted, TH is released, which in turn converts the amino acid tyrosine into L-dopa, the precursor molecule for dopamine.

Mechanotherapy

This category includes any electrical (brain wave machines, biofeedback, vibrators), surgical, mechanical (acupuncture, massage implements), physical (hand massage, Rolfing, various touch techniques), or other devices or procedures, not including talk or drugs. One approach currently enjoying wide and diverse exploration is the electrode implant with impulse generator, in which an electrode is surgically placed in a specific part of the brain. When it is active, the electrode stimulates neurons that relate to a specific response, such as tremor, a mood change, stiffness, appetite, or pain. Medtronics Inc. manufactures these devices. The Food and Drug Administration approved them for general use in August 1997. A typical procedure costs around $25,000 and is normally covered by insurance.

Complementary Therapy

Candace Pert (1997) has documented the beneficial effects of a wide variety of alternative (she prefers the term "complementary") therapies that are not traditionally accepted by mainstream therapist providers or insurance companies. These include, but are not limited to, massage; Rolfing; body psychotherapy; biofeedback; hypnotherapy; music, art, dance, and humor therapy; acupuncture; Ayurveda; naturopathy; macrobiotics; body work; acupressure; bioenergetics;

Feldenkrais; Hellerwork; Alexander technique; myotheraphy; reflexology; chiropractic; transcendental meditation; yoga—the list goes on. Pert sees these "mindbody" therapies as assisting in promoting the free flow of peptides and other "molecules of emotion" that is essential to general health and well-being. She provides an extensive list of resources, by category, in Appendix B of her book *Molecules of Emotion* (1997).

Autotherapy

Power to the people. Never before in history have such informational resources been available to the average individual. From lending libraries to the Internet, we can look up our ailments, attempt diagnosis, and, when confident, treat them. In roughly two-thirds of the cases, this can't hurt, as two-thirds of all ailments are self-limiting: they will go away with time and respect for the ailment (for example, with rest). Self-help therapy is consistent with many of the findings from the growing field of psychoneuroimmunology (for more information, see Topic 14.2).

In fact, if you would like information on a topic that is not found in this book, try your local reference librarian or search on the World Wide Web. Just doing a keyword search in Yahoo or some other search engine, such as Lycos or Infoseek, can yield a multitude of resources (chat rooms, document repositories, support groups, current information summaries, article and book references, and addresses of researchers and scholars, for example) about a multitude of medical topics. Norman Cousins (1979, 1989) has ably demonstrated that taking an active part in your own treatment improves your chances of recovery.

The ideal treatment is probably a combination of elements of all four modes of treatment. One clinic that manages to put it all together in a comprehensive therapeutic environment is the Biscayne Institutes in North Miami Beach, Florida, Marie DiCowden, executive director. The clinic's holistic approach to patient care is described in the April 1997 *APA Monitor* (p. 38). Imagine getting a massage before engaging in an hour of psychotherapy!

A Note on Placebos

The word *placebo* comes from the Latin for "I shall please." The placebo effect, therefore, is what happens when the "very act of undergoing treatment—seeing a medical expert, for instance, or taking a pill—helps the patient to recover" (W. A. Brown, 1998, p. 90). Walter Brown, a psychiatrist at the Brown University School of Medicine, recommends the cautious and appropriate use of placebos in treating disorders that research has shown to be positively affected by placebo treatment. These disorders include asthma, angina pectoris, the common cold, high blood pressure, depression, anxiety, and general aches and pains. Placebos are any medically originated interventions that are believed by the physician to be inert—that is, to have no research-documented curative effect. The placebo can be a "sugar" pill, an injection of water, something nonprescriptive to ingest (such as an herb tea, chicken soup with rice, or a spoonful of honey), an exercise, acupuncture, something externally applied (such as an ice pack, mud pack, "brain wave" machine, or hot bath), a regimen (a twenty-minute nap after lunch, a thirty-minute walk before dinner, and a warm cup of milk before bed every day), or the experience of the trappings of the medical art itself (using the stethoscope, the reflex hammer, the tongue depressor, or the otoscope). Anne Harrington, a science historian at Harvard, calls placebos "lies that heal" (*New York Times,* October 13, 1998, p. F1).

Because the research on the effectiveness of placebos is so convincing (in one study, 40 percent of a group of depressed patients improved after taking placebos), Brown believes that physicians should seriously consider prescribing them in place of drugs that may have undesirable costs and side effects. If they don't work, then they can try medications. The success of these interventions is explained by expectancy theory. According to expectancy theory, we are trained by classical conditioning to associate certain consequences with specific actions. Take a pill; feel better. Hence, if it looks like a pill and we are told it's a pill by an authority figure, we expect it to act like a pill, and our bodies typically anticipate that action. Brown is appropriately cautious concerning the ethics of such interventions. He writes (1998):

> A doctor could explain the situation to a patient in the following manner: "You have several options. One is to take a diuretic. It will probably bring your blood pressure down, but it does have some side effects. There are also other treatments that are less expensive and less likely to cause side effects and that help many people with your condition. Some find that herbal tea twice a day is helpful; others find that taking these pills twice a day is helpful.

These pills do not contain any drug. We do not know how the herbal tea or these pills work. They may trigger or stimulate your body's own healing processes. We do know that about 20 percent of the people with your type of high blood pressure get their blood pressure into the normal range using this approach. If you decide to try one of these treatments, I will check your progress every two weeks. If after six weeks your blood pressure is still high, we should consider the diuretic."

Mark Ardis, a retired Veterans Administration psychiatrist, psychiatric administrator, and university professor, has strong reservations concerning the use of placebos (personal communication). He points out that the health of the relationship between the patient and the therapist is crucial to the successful outcome of treatment. In many cases, if the patient even suspects that the physician is using placebos, that relationship is likely to deteriorate.

TOPIC 14.1 Genetics and Disease

Figure 14.1 illustrates the relationship between environmental nurture and genetic predisposition for genetically based diseases. Generally, the relationship is interactive—the better the nurture and the lower the genetic predisposition, the better the chances are of not contracting a genetically based disease. The poorer the nurture and the higher the predisposition, the better the chances are of contracting the disease. High nurture combined with a high predisposition and low nurture combined with a low predisposition are each more of a toss-up: high nurture will not guarantee suppression and low nurture will not guarantee expression of a genetically predisposed disease.

Only 3 percent of all human diseases are caused by a single

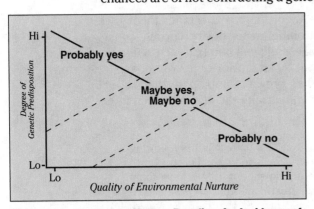

Figure 14.1. The Nature-Nurture Paradigm for Incidence of Genetically Based Diseases.

defective gene, and these diseases are not major killers like cancer. John Rennie points out that more complex diseases "involve a host of genes that merely nudge a person's predisposition to develop an illness" (*Scientific American,* June 1994, p. 90). The notion that single genes cause specific diseases has led to the phrase "myth of genetic determinism," with the accompanying notion that one's genotype equates to one's fate. Because of the complex interaction between multiple genes and multiple environmental effects (diet, drugs, behavior, climate, stress, exercise—the list goes on), Rennie concludes that "genetic tests for [specific] illnesses can never by themselves predict an individual's future with perfect clarity."

Applications

1 The best nurture can only minimize the chances of getting a disease toward which you are genetically predisposed. When you contract a disease following good nurture, assume a genetic predisposition; don't feel as if the nurture was somehow inadequate. Continued good nurture will facilitate recovery. (See Topic 14.2 for a related discussion of psychoneuroimmunology.)

2 Conversely, don't assume that avoiding a disease is the result of excellent nurture; you may simply be genetically resistant.

TOPIC 14.2 The Immune System and Psychoneuroimmunology

Descartes's mind-body dualism has traditionally dominated medical thinking: adjust the body to fix a bodily problem and adjust the mind to fix a mental problem. However, recent research suggests that a single system exists in which mental symptoms (for example, depression) can have either a mental cause (for example, job loss, divorce, death of a close friend) or a physical cause (for example, poor internal regulation of melatonin). This field, called psychoneuroimmunology (PNI), is the study of the feedback loop, traced by Karen Bulloch of the University of California, San Diego, between the brain and the immune system—the lymphocytes (white blood cells residing in lymph), thymus, spleen, and marrow. In this system, lymphocytes attack and neutralize invaders, and natural killer cells (NKs) fight viruses and tumors.

The loop works like this: the brain can emit chemicals under stress that depress the immune function, so that stress leads to disease, or the immune system can produce chemicals such as lymphokines in the thymus that can cause depression; in this case, disease leads to stress. Edwin Blalock, a physiology professor at the University of Alabama in Birmingham, discovered that the cells of the immune system can produce the same hormones as the brain and that immune-system cells have the same receptors as brain cells. He says that immune cells act like a classic sensory organ, sending messages to the brain the way the eyes and ears do.

The original discovery of the mind's control over immune-cell levels was made by psychologist Robert Ader and immunologist Nicholas Cohen at the University of Rochester in the mid 1970s. They gave a saccharine solution to rats, followed by an injection of cyclophosphamide, which induces nausea and reduces the immune function. Rats who continued drinking the saccharine solution without the cyclophosphamide injections showed a continuing drop in immune function. Ader gave the field its name: psychoneuroimmunology.

Increasing evidence suggests that people's emotional states affect their immune levels. Sandra Levy of the Pittsburgh Cancer Institute found joy level to be the second-best predictor of survival time for patients with recurrent breast cancer. (The best predictor was the length of disease-free intervals.) She found that more than half of the fluctuation in the NK level could be attributed to psychological factors, including the patient's perceived social support and how she coped with stress. Other studies by Levy; Lydia Temoshok of the University of California, San Francisco; and Carrie Millon of the University of Miami School of Medicine point to the high relationship between a patient's level of assertiveness and fighting spirit and his or her immune level. Temoshok studied men with AIDS and found that more assertive men had higher immune levels. Millon found that men infected with the AIDS virus had higher immune levels if they were narcissistic and strong-willed.

The Healing Brain (Ornstein and Sobel, 1987) is a highly readable treatment of this subject. The authors relate amazing stories of the power of the mind's control over the body, including one experiment in which a placebo treatment had the same pain-reducing ability as 8 milligrams of morphine. They also say that the brain is more of a pharmacy than a computer. Another interesting treatment is found in Norman Cousins's *Anatomy of an Illness* (1979, pp. 67–69), where he tells of the witch doctor in Albert Schweitzer's village. The two doctors had an arrangement to provide three levels of service to the villagers: bend, mend, and send. The witch doctor provided two levels: one for those with vague complaints such as stomach pains, which he treated by the traditional methods (for example, "bending" the patient's spirits with incantations), and one for those with simple specific complaints such as cuts and bruises, which he and his assistants treated with modern first aid (for example, "mending" with iodine). For the third level—complex specific complaints such as a broken leg—the villager was referred ("sent") to Albert Schweitzer.

The late Franz Ingelfinger, editor of the *New England Journal of Medicine,* wrote in his last article (Ingelfinger, 1980) that he judged 85 percent of all human illnesses to be addressed by the immune system. Ever since Seneca, who wrote, "It is part of the cure to wish to be cured," people have debated the effect of the mind on the healing process. In fact, in many ways, this debate is at the core of cognitive science. Herbert Benson, of the Mind/Body Clinic of New England Deaconess Hospital in Boston, uses the relaxation response—the body's reaction to activities such as meditation and aerobic exercise—on patients with hypertension; he reports that 80 percent are able to reduce either blood pressure or drug dosage. Psychologist Gregg Jacobs of Harvard University's Mind/Body Medical Institute (founded by Benson) reports that it takes only five minutes of the relaxation technique to detect dramatic brain wave changes. Jacobs has used the techniques to cure insomniacs.

David C. McClelland of Boston University (McClelland, 1986; McClelland and Kirshnit, 1988) has found salivary immunoglobulin type A to be

- Low among people with a high need for power when they are stressed and out of control

- High among people who are experiencing love

- High among people who are temporarily experiencing positive emotions (as in watching a film of Mother Teresa)

- High among those with a stronger sense of humor

Cousins (1989) is careful to explain that people should not abandon medical assistance in favor of exclusively concentrating on positive emotions to cure disease. He urges patients to accept medical diagnosis and treatment but to augment it by taking an active role in the healing process. He says that patients who don't deny the diagnosis but defy the verdict seem to do better than others (p. 45). This sense of "defying the verdict" is what Cousins means by "hardiness," discussed in Topic 20.2.

Applications

1 To ensure maximum functioning of your immune system during both sickness and health, maintain your sense of humor, have positive expectations (hope and trust in medical processes), play an active role in the healing process, and stay relaxed by removing or minimizing your stressors and dissipating stress when it occurs.

2 Several books about PNI are available for both caregivers and seriously ill patients. Start with Cousins (1989), LeShan (1989), Siegel (1987), and Simonton, Simonton, and Creighton (1980). A must-read is the recent *Molecules of Emotion* (1997) by Candace Pert, discoverer of the endorphin receptor.

3 Seek out doctors with a more holistic approach. *(Contributed by Rick Bradley)*

4 Make a commitment for yourself and your close friends, family, and associates to be supportive of one another, spread good humor, and show appropriate optimism.

5 When you are faced with higher than expected levels of sickness at home or at work, look to stress as a possible cause. Identify the stressors and eliminate them as much as possible.

6 Encourage yourself to increase the level of humor in your life, both humor that you initiate (tell jokes, be witty, go to comedic plays and movies, be around funny people, read humorous books) and humor that you react to (let yourself belly-laugh, don't always hold back). Norman Cousins calls a good belly laugh "internal jogging."

7 Develop a sense that you are in control of your life and a fighting spirit that stays on the lookout for ways to improve your situation. Remember the Alcoholics Anonymous version of the Serenity Prayer: "God, grant me the serenity to accept the things I cannot change today, the courage to change the things I can today, and the wisdom to know the difference." To accept too much negativity in your life is to be personally responsible for lowering your own immune level. (See more on motivation in Chapter Twenty.)

8 If you have a sick family member or friend, look for funny get-well cards instead of sad, depressing ones. When my mother had cancer, I sent her lots of funny cards. After recovery, she decided they were good "medicine" and began sending this type of card instead of the serious, somber versions. *(Contributed by Jane Howard)*

9 Kiecolt-Glaser and Glaser (1992) identify eight specific behavioral strategies for improving immune function: aerobic exercise, relaxation, social support, learned control such as biofeedback, classical conditioning, cognitive training, therapy, and self-disclosure (talking or writing about one's problems).

10 For pain management, try repeating positive words or phrases privately while ignoring thoughts that try to intrude on your awareness. Let the words or phrases fully occupy your conscious awareness.

11 If you are a prospective medical student, ensure that your medical school offers course work in nontraditional healing. According to a 1996 survey by the Association of American Medical Colleges, 92 of 125 medical schools offer such programs.

12 Demand that your managed care provider include benefits for nontraditional healing methods. In a 1997 survey of eighty HMOs conducted by Landmark Healthcare, 58 percent indicated that they either currently offered alternative therapies or planned to offer them within one to two years.

13 Subscribe to these resources:

Mental Medicine Book/Tape Catalog; phone: 800-222-4745.

Mental Medicine Update, a mind-body health newsletter edited by David Sobel and Robert Ornstein; Center for Health Sciences; Los Altos, California; phone: 800-222-4745.

Mind-Body Health News, a quarterly resource for mind-body study groups; Mind-Body Health Study Group Network; Washington, D.C.; phone: 202-393-2210.

TOPIC 14.3 Treatments for Pain

The Nature of Pain

The sources of pain vary from pressure (being hit) to puncture (being stuck), but all pain is communicated through synaptic structures called nociceptors. These receptors, which are committed to relaying pain messages, follow two pathways:

1. From the source of potential pain (for example, a fingertip) to the spinal cord and back to the source, resulting in a reflex action (jerking the finger off a hot stove). This is a warning path.

2. From the source of actual pain (for example, the burned area of the finger) to the brain and back, resulting in the sensation of pain. The inflamed area produces prostaglandins, which act on the nociceptors to transmit pain messages. How much pain we feel depends on the threshold for activating our nociceptors. This threshold is a function of genetics, physical condition, attitude, and attentional focus (for example, boxers don't really feel the pain of being hit until they stop focusing on the fight itself). The following Applications offer some treatments for pain.

Applications

CURRENT TREATMENTS

1 Narcotic analgesics such as morphine and codeine actually block the pain message at the nociceptor. However, the body develops a tolerance for these drugs, so this is only a short-term solution.

2 More powerful than morphine and lacking the side effects is Abbott Laboratories' new painkiller, ABT-594, which is derived from the poison contained in the skin of the Ecuadorean frog *Epibpedobates tricolor.* ABT-594 (now being referred to as epibatidine) appears to be emerging as the drug of choice for treating severe and unrelenting pain, especially because it lacks the addictive quality of morphine.

3 Roughly two-thirds of those who suffer chronic pain experience relief with either cognitive-behavioral psychotherapy or nonaddictive drugs. Because of the social toll of untreated chronic pain, doctors are beginning to prescribe narcotics for the other third (*APA Monitor,* December 1996, p. 22).

4 The PNI literature contains a vast number of suggestions for self-managing pain as well as illness in general (see Topic 14.2).

5 Anesthetics such as novocaine and ether block all sensation, not just pain.

6 Neurontin (gabapentin), a drug currently on the market for epilepsy, also is effective as a pain reliever.

7 SNX-111, made from the venom of poisonous snails, is under development and appears to ease pain by blocking calcium receptors.

8 NMDA-receptor blockers, already approved for epilepsy, are in the clinical-trial stage as a possible pain reliever.

9 Hot and cold applications such as heat lamps and ice activate other nerve endings that compete with the nociceptors for attention.

10 Electrical stimulation such as transcutaneous electrical nerve stimulation works the same way as heat and cold.

11 To soothe pain in infants, nursing them, holding them, and feeding them sucrose, alone or in combination, have been shown to be calming (*APA Monitor,* December 1996, p. 21).

12 Stress-reduction techniques appear to be effective against pain (see Topic 20.4).

13 Patient-controlled analgesia, an intravenous administration, is used for pain.

14 Biofeedback uses visual feedback to promote mental self-control of pain.

15 Deep relaxation (self-hypnosis) induces a generally numb feeling; for example, fewer pregnant women require epidurals during delivery when they use deep-relaxation techniques (*Journal of Women's Health,* Winter 1993). For a list of hypnotherapists in your area, send a stamped, self-addressed envelope to the American Society of Clinical Hypnosis, 2200 East Devon Avenue, Suite 291; Des Plaines, Illinois 60018-4534.

16 Mild, over-the-counter analgesics such as aspirin work at the site of the pain to reduce inflammation and block production of prostaglandins. Four classes of over-the-counter analgesics are currently available. Their pros and cons are listed in Table 14.1.

17 Tips for over-the-counter analgesics:

• Heat and moisture can affect their quality, so store them away from the bathroom in a cool, dry area.

• Avoid "extra-strength" pain relievers; they are more expensive per milligram than normal doses and they make it harder to control precise dosage.

Table 14.1. Pros and Cons of Over-the-Counter Analgesics.

Class	Trade Names	Advantages	Disadvantages
Aspirin	Bayer, Anacin, Ecotrin, Bufferin	Cheapest; reduces fever, swelling, stiffness; reduces chance of heart attack, stroke, and digestive tract cancer	Hard on stomach, Reye's syndrome when given to young child with flu or chicken pox
Acetaminophen	Tylenol, Aspirin-free Anacin	Reduces fever, easier on stomach, fewest side effects	No effect on swelling and stiffness; liver damage when taken with three alcoholic drinks per day
Ibuprofen	Advil, Nuprin, Motrin-IB	Lasts longer than aspirin and acetaminophen; better on stronger pains; reduces fever, swelling, stiffness	Aggravates stomach upset when taken with three alcoholic drinks per day; boosts blood pressure; liver, kidney, stomach disease
Naproxen	Aleve	Lasts longest; best with strongest pain; helps swelling, fever, stiffness	Most expensive; same disadvantages as ibuprofen

- Avoid products with caffeine mixed with analgesics. Consumers Union questions their effects in the combined form. If you want caffeine with your single-ingredient pain reliever, ingest it as coffee or another product of your choice.

- To ease the effect on your tummy, take analgesics on a full stomach with a full glass of water and avoid lying down for a half hour.

- If you take medicine for high blood pressure, avoid all analgesics but aspirin, as they can elevate blood pressure. Consult your physician if you are unsure.

FUTURE POSSIBILITIES

❶ For more (and free) information, write The Neurological Institute; P.O. Box 5801; Bethesda, Maryland 20824.

2 Follow the work of scientists such as Mich Hein of the Scripps Research Institute, La Jolla, California; Charles Arntzen of Texas A&M University; and Richard Curtis III of Washington University in St. Louis. They are using recombinant DNA technology to develop plants that deliver medication, as in potatoes that prevent gastroenteritis (Arntzen) and alfalfa sprouts that carry a cholera vaccine.

TOPIC 14.4 Caring for Caregivers

Those who fall into the role of providing long-term care (for example, for Alzheimer's patients) develop health problems of their own. The emotional and physical pressures associated with around-the-clock caregiving often lead to the kinds of diseases normally associated with prolonged stress. The Canadian Study of Health and Aging has presented evidence that Alzheimer's caregivers have more health problems than other people of the same age, as well as more health problems than people caring for a loved one at home with a disease other than Alzheimer's. Periodic temporary relief that allows the caregiver to get away for a couple of hours at a time appears to minimize such health complications.

Applications

1 Two interventions have been found to be effective in helping caregivers maintain their immune level: teaching them relaxation and other stress-reduction methods and providing them with respite when they feel they need it, so they can go to a movie, go shopping, or just walk.

2 If you are a caregiver, or if you know one, find a support group of people you can call on for short-term relief. Most cities have a clearinghouse that will put you in touch with providers of respite care. Don't be a martyr; it's not healthy.

3 To keep current on caregiving, get on the mailing list for the Family Survival Project for Brain-Impaired Adults; 425 Bush Street, Suite 500; San Francisco, California 94108; phone: 415-434-3388.

SUGGESTED RESOURCES

Brown, W. A. (1998, January). "The Placebo Effect." *Scientific American,* pp. 90–95.

Cousins, N. (1979). *Anatomy of an Illness.* New York: Norton.

Cousins, N. (1989). *Head First: The Biology of Hope.* New York: NAL/Dutton.

Hafen, B. Q., Karren, K. J., Frandsen, K. J., and Smith, N. L. (1996). *Mind/Body Health: The Effects of Attitudes, Emotions, and Relationships.* Needham Heights, Mass.: Allyn & Bacon.

Horgan, J. (1996, December). "Why Freud Isn't Dead." *Scientific American,* pp. 106–111.

"Mental Health: Does Therapy Help?" (1995, November). *Consumer Reports,* pp. 734–739.

Seligman, M.E.P. (1994). *What You Can Change and What You Can't.* New York: Knopf.

Seligman, M.E.P. (1996, October). "Science as an Ally of Practice." *American Psychologist, 51*(10), 1072–1079. [Special issue: "Outcome Assessment of Psychotherapy"].

Web Sites

Charles A. Dana Foundation home page:
www.dana.org

U.S. Office of Disease Prevention and Health Promotion:
www.healthfinder.gov

15

Structural Disorders

Bats in Your Belfry

66 Art thou not, fatal vision, sensible

To feeling as to sight? or art thou but

A dagger of the mind, a false creation,

Proceeding from the heat-oppressed brain? 99

—William Shakespeare,
Macbeth

A combination of genetic and environmental contributions can render the brain structurally—that is, biologically and chemically—out of sorts. The result of structural damage or alteration can slow down or speed up function and can range from the dulling of function in retardation to the massive electrical storms of epilepsy. This chapter explores the state of causal associations and therapeutic possibilities for six structural disorders: attention deficit hyperactivity disorder, dyslexia, epilepsy, retardation, schizophrenia, and tumors.

TOPIC 15.1 **Attention Deficit Hyperactivity Disorder (ADHD)**

Nature of the Disorder

Roughly 5 percent of children have attention deficit hyperactivity disorder (ADHD), with boys holding the edge over girls (Biederman and Faraone, 1996). It accounts for about half of the referrals to children's psychiatric clinics. No more than one in five of these cases carries over into adulthood. ADHD involves poor regulation of the catecholamine family of neurotransmitters, specifically dopamine and norepinephrine, among the synapses in the frontal area of the brain, particularly the right area, and the basal ganglia (*Archives of General Psychiatry,* July 1996). These two areas, which are associated with focusing attention, blocking distractions, and inhibiting behavior, are up to 10 percent smaller in ADHD children. In essence, their brains fail to fire inhibitory processes, thus leading to uncontrollable motoric behavior. ADHD occurs in families, pointing to a genetic basis, and is associated with poor environmental conditions. Although 49 percent of ADHD cases involve no other mental disturbance, 51 percent are associated with other disorders: depression (11 percent), anxiety disorders (11 percent), conduct disorders (7 percent), or some combination of the three. A combination of ADHD and conduct disorders predicts later antisocial disorders and alcohol or drug dependence, ADHD and depression predicts later manic depression, and ADHD and anxiety predicts later anxiety disorders.

Symptoms

The symptoms of ADHD are inattentiveness, impulsivity, and motoric overactivity, starting during the early grades and interfering with social and academic performance. The *Diagnostic and Statistical Manual of Mental Disorders (DSM-IV)* lists a total of nineteen specific symptoms. Symptoms must occur in at least two different settings, such as home and school. Doctors typically diagnose ADHD into one of three categories: predominantly inattentive (usually called just "ADD"), predominantly hyperactive, or combined.

In the Charlotte-Mecklenburg (North Carolina) schools, teachers look for the following fourteen behaviors as indicators; they must be severe, must have lasted for six months, and must have started before age seven (*Charlotte Observer,* December 5, 1993):

1. Often fidgets or squirms in seat
2. Has difficulty remaining seated
3. Is easily distracted
4. Has difficulty awaiting turn in groups
5. Often blurts out answers to questions
6. Has difficulty following directions
7. Has difficulty sustaining attention to tasks
8. Shifts from one uncompleted activity to another
9. Has difficulty playing quietly
10. Often talks excessively
11. Often interrupts or intrudes on others
12. Often does not seem to listen
13. Often loses things necessary for tasks
14. Often engages in dangerous activity without considering the consequences

Martin Teicher of Harvard Medical School's McLean Hospital reported the results of a new protocol to assess for ADHD that is 90 percent accurate (*Journal of the American Academy of Child and Adolescent Psychiatry,* March 1996). In this procedure, a child performs a high-vigilance task with a television screen. The child watches the screen for fifteen minutes, only occasionally being asked to respond. This boring procedure intentionally (and unfortunately!) resembles traditional expectations for classroom behavior. Throughout the procedure, an infrared motion-analysis device monitors movements fifty times per second.

Applications

CURRENT TREATMENTS

Ritalin (methylphenidate, an amphetamine) is the treatment drug of choice, with upward of two million prescriptions in the United States, about 90 percent of them for children. Normal doses range from 5 to 20 milligrams daily. Ritalin works by stimulating the production of neurotransmitters, including dopamine and norepinephrine. In general, ADHD sufferers have low neurotransmitter production, which leads to poor impulse control. Ritalin attempts to normalize this production. Possible side effects include loss of appetite (which typically vanishes after one month of use), as well as crankiness, headaches, or drowsiness as the drug's effects wear off.

Joe Stegman, a pediatrician in Concord, North Carolina, cautions that taking Ritalin can only calm the brain. It should be accompanied by family counseling so that the family's lifestyle does not foster ADHD any more than necessary. For example, Stegman cautions that ADHD children should avoid violent television programs, candy-coated cereal, long bus rides to school, and other situations that can aggravate the condition.

Although not all ADHD children take Ritalin, many children who are merely restless take it unnecessarily. Just as Prozac is often prescribed wrongly to help adults take the rough edges off their personality, Ritalin is often prescribed for children's rough edges that do not reflect ADHD. As the ability to maintain reasonably healthy relationships at home and work is a test for genuine depression, so the ability to maintain healthy school and social performance is a test for genuine ADHD.

FUTURE POSSIBILITIES

1 Jay Giedd and a team at the National Institute of Mental Health used magnetic resonance imaging to identify brain asymmetries in ADHD boys. Non-ADHD boys have an anterior frontal area, caudate, and globus pallidus that are 4 to 6 percent larger in the right hemisphere than they are in ADHD boys. Further research must determine if this asymmetry is a cause of ADHD or a result of treatment. It should be noted that hyperactivity can also occur among people who have a genetic defect associated with a thyroid disorder.

2 An innovative approach being used with some ADHD cases that meet certain requirements is electroencephalographic neurofeedback. For specific information on this technology, as well as a position paper on its use with ADHD, check out the Allied Products web site: www.biof.com/neuroarticles.html.

3 For the most current information, try the Attention Deficit Disorder Association hot line: 800-540-2791.

TOPIC 15.2 Dyslexia

Nature of the Disorder

Once thought to be mostly caused by stress (we now point to a gene on chromosome 6), dyslexia (difficulty in reading) has been estimated to afflict up to 15 percent of the population. It appears to be related to the poor synchronization of two neural systems in the brain. Dyslexic patients have magnocellular layers ("large" cells in the visual pathway) that are 27 percent smaller and less well organized than comparable areas in the brains of nondyslexic people. On the other hand, dyslexic and nondyslexic individuals have parvocellular layers ("small" cells in the visual pathway) of comparable size and organization. In processing perceptual information, such as letters on the printed page, magnocellular cells transmit more slowly than parvocellular ones. As a result, visual information (printed words) and auditory information (spoken words) don't work together. Auditory content is processed at normal speeds, but visual content is not. Appropriate treatments for dyslexia equalize the speeds of these two perceptual systems. Paula Tallal, co-director of the Center for Molecular and Behavioral Neuroscience at Rutgers University, and Michael Merzenich of the Keck Center for Integrative Neuroscience at the University of California, San Francisco, have developed a computer-based therapy that varies the duration and amplitude of sounds in a video-game format.

Sally Shaywitz (1996) has identified five myths about dyslexia:

1. Dyslexics engage in mirror writing. (Not necessarily. Mirror writing is a common developmental phenomenon among

dyslexics and nondyslexics. Dyslexics have phonological problems, not writing problems.)

2. Dyslexia should be treated with eye training. (There is no evidence to support this.)

3. Boys are more often dyslexic than girls. (No. This is a bias of traditional research methods. Current data show the distribution to be pretty much identical for boys and girls.)

4. One can outgrow dyslexia. (No. For many, it continues into adulthood. They can read, but slowly.)

5. Dyslexics can't be smart. (No. The two are independent. William Butler Yeats, Albert Einstein, and George Patton were dyslexic.)

Symptoms

The classic symptom of dyslexia is a discrepancy between intelligence (or ability) and achievement (or performance). The symptoms differ widely, from spelling problems to hesitant oral reading production; different symptoms call for different treatments. The later a child is diagnosed as reading-disabled, the harder it is to teach that child to read and the more likely it is that the disability will leave psychological scars. Louisa Moats, project director of the National Institute of Child Health and Human Development Early Intervention Project in Washington, D.C., has identified indicators appearing as early as thirty months of age, including a slowed-down ability to name numbers, colors, or objects, that point to later reading disabilities.

Applications

CURRENT TREATMENTS

1 To treat dyslexia, consult your neurologist for the latest information on how to pharmaceutically or behaviorally equalize the transmission of magno and parvo cells.

2 If you grew up thinking that dyslexia was primarily a reaction to stress, understand that current research believes that most cases of dyslexia have a physical basis. Until they have been treated, be sympathetic with dyslexics' need to take their time processing perceptual information. For them, proceeding slowly is not a sign of less intelligence.

3 Because of their phonological deficits, dyslexics respond better to the whole-word method of reading instruction than to the phonics approach. Dyslexics often need surrounding context cues in order to identify a specific word. Therefore, multiple-choice tests, which provide virtually no context, particularly penalize them.

4 Paula Tallal and Michael Merzenich have founded a company, Scientific Learning Principles, based in San Francisco, that will develop a CD product employing their video learning program and market it as an interactive CD-ROM. They have a web site at http://www.scilearn.com.

FUTURE POSSIBILITIES

1 Perform a keyword search on the World Wide Web using "dyslexia." You will find a wide variety of support groups and informational sources for both children and adults. One such resource is the National Institute of Neural Disorders and Stroke at www.ninds.nih.gov/healinfo/disorder/dyslexia/. Once you have found a site that you particularly like, check it with some frequency as a way of keeping abreast of newly developing information.

2 Because dyslexia is considered a genetic defect, cures are not realistically expected, but treatments certainly are. One line of research (as yet unproductive) is the development of a drug that equalizes the tempos of the magno and parvo cells.

3 David Pauls of Yale University is part of a research team that has identified two genetic markers for dyslexia, one on human chromosome 15 that is associated with single-word reading and another on chromosome 6 that is associated with phonetic ability. It is hoped that this line of research will lead to increasingly effective treatments for dyslexia.

4 Try getting on the mailing list for the Orton Dyslexia Society; Chester Building; 8600 LaSalle Road, Suite 382; Baltimore, Maryland 21204-6020; phone: 410-296-0232.

5 For information on the broader subject of learning disabilities, visit the web site focused on children's learning disabilities at www.ldonline.org.

TOPIC 15.3 Epilepsy

Nature of the Disorder

About 1 percent of the U.S. population have a brain condition for which no single cause is known. Genes are suspected in half of the cases, but the other half point to an array of causes, including lead poisoning, prenatal problems, disease, tumor, head injury, stroke, infection, and drug or alcohol abuse. Epilepsy describes a pattern of electrical storms called seizures, which are set off by a brief period of electrical firing at a rate up to four times above normal.

Applications

CURRENT TREATMENTS

1 About two-thirds of epileptics improve by taking anticonvulsant drugs such as Tegretol (carbamazepine), while still more can improve with surgical procedures. However, thousands remain whose epilepsy is impervious to all known treatments.

2 A new treatment, just approved in 1997, is an implant that stimulates the vagus nerve (reported in the *Chicago Tribune,* January 5, 1998, p. 1). Manufactured by Cyberonics, Inc., in Texas, and dubbed the "NeuroCybernetic Prosthesis System," the device consists of a set of coils placed around the vagus nerve and connected to a generator the size of a stopwatch that is surgically implanted under the skin of the chest. The generator sends a thirty-second burst of electricity followed by a five-minute lull, continuing in alternation. Apparently, these bursts disrupt seizure patterns, amounting to what some have called a pacemaker for the brain.

FUTURE POSSIBILITIES

1 In an effort to increase participation in genetic studies, the Epilepsy Foundation of America has set up a web site for the purpose of putting people who think they have inherited epilepsy in touch with researchers. You may visit this site at www.efa.org/index/htm. By participating, you can help in isolating the particular genes that are associated with the dozen or more specific types of epilepsy. At present, researchers have found only a few genes that are associated with three or four types of epilepsy. More volunteers are necessary. Drugs in use for epilepsy before 1994 were not based on genetic research, whereas the new "rational" drugs such as Gabitril (tiagabine hydrochloride) address specific properties defined by newly identified genes associated with epilepsy (C. A. Walsh, 1997). With the identification of more genes comes the possibility of more and better rational drugs that will close the treatment gap.

2 Physicians at Boston's Beth Israel Deaconess Medical Center have transplanted 400,000 pig fetal cells into the brain of a middle-aged man with severe epilepsy. Researchers will watch to determine if the animal cells survive and affect the patient's condition. Beth Israel plans additional "xenotransplants" over the next several years.

TOPIC 15.4 **Retardation**

Nature of the Disorder

A developmental disorder that afflicts between 1 and 3 percent of the population, retardation is defined as a failure of the individual to perform age-appropriate motor, language, intellectual, or self-help behaviors. Its onset, severity, and causation cover a wide range. Onset can be before birth (prenatal), during birth (perinatal), or up to age eighteen (postnatal). Roughly 75 percent of cases of retardation have prenatal causes, 10 percent are perinatal, and another 10 percent are postnatal; 5 percent are simply hard to understand and classify. The severity of retardation can range from borderline to severe.

The most common prenatal cause is Down's syndrome, with congenital rubella and fetal alcohol syndrome also causing many cases. Perinatal causes include prematurity and infections, with birth trauma actually accounting for only a small portion. Postnatal causes include trauma and tumors. Causation is extremely complex, with upward of forty different causes, some of which are related to trauma, some to disease, some to genetics, and still others to diet, poisons, and environment. Only an estimated 25 percent of cases have a clear-cut causation identified, with the remainder in a huge "unexplained" category.

Applications

CURRENT TREATMENTS

Prenatal family genetic screening and counseling can prevent the occurrence of retardation caused by genetic factors. Prenatal counseling also can educate parents to avoid dietary, drug, and other causative factors, such as malnutrition and alcohol or lead poisoning. Counseling can also identify diseases that could harm the fetus to which the mother may be prone—she can be taught how to avoid contracting such diseases. Current treatments are aimed at helping retarded individuals to learn behaviors at the most advanced possible level. Many are able to live independently, while others must live in a specially structured environment.

FUTURE POSSIBILITIES

1   Current research is focused on a variety of techniques, including the use of gene therapy, neuronal cell growth factors, and "rational" drug development. Evan Snyder, for example, of Children's Hospital (Boston) and Harvard Medical School, has reported his work on mucopolysaccharidosis (MPS) (*Nature,* March 23, 1995). In MPS, an enzyme is deficient in the brain, and Snyder and his team are experimenting with a process learned from rat research in which good enzyme-producing cells are transplanted into the target area.

2   For current information, try visiting the many web sites dedicated to mental retardation. A good one to start with is www.healthanswers.com/database/ami/converted/001523.html.

TOPIC 15.5 Schizophrenia

Nature of the Disorder

Schizophrenia typically begins during the teenage or early adult years in upward of 1 percent of the population. U.S. rates are similar to those in both developed and undeveloped countries. The criteria used to diagnose schizophrenia in the *DSM-IV* include

- Speech and thought disorders
- Hallucinations and delusions
- Psychomotor disturbance (immobile or restless)
- Inappropriate emotional responses
- Bizarre behavior
- Lessened intellectual and self-help ability

Schizophrenia is a chronic condition; symptoms must endure for at least six months to earn the diagnosis. Early on, it can be confused with several other disorders, including depression, mania, and substance abuse, and can range from slightly to totally disabling. Based on the different symptom sets, the diagnosis may be for any one of five different subtypes: catatonic, disorganized, undifferentiated, residual, or paranoid. Some cases last for only one or several episodes with a return to normal or near normal, while others slowly improve or slowly worsen. Sex differences in responses to antipsychotic drugs and in age of onset suggest that sex hormones influence the course of the disease. In addition, socioeconomic status appears to influence the course of the disease, with three factors playing a significant role:

1. Lower income and status
2. An urban environment
3. The demands for socialization placed on adolescents and young adults

EEG, PET, MRI, and CT evaluations all reveal abnormalities in the brains of schizophrenics, and recent studies indicate that the abnormal brain patterns are present before the onset of symptoms. This suggests that schizophrenia is the result of developmental problems in the brain and nervous system. While some forms of the disease may be associated with one specific gene, the greater likelihood is that several genes are implicated, suggesting a tangle of causes (genetic and environmental) for each of the subtypes. To date, linkage studies have identified regions on chromosomes 6, 15, and 22 as being possible addresses for schizophrenia-related genes (Wyatt and Henter, 1997).

Applications

CURRENT TREATMENTS

Treatment is directed at relieving symptoms. Traditional medications have aimed at blocking dopamine receptors, as well as targeting specific symptoms such as low affect. More recent medications have been more of a "cocktail" in which multiple ligands are addressed in addition to dopamine. These include clozapine, olanzapine, risperidone, and sertindole. These newer medications have a record of fewer relapses and fewer, and milder, side effects. Pharmacotherapy must be accompanied by psychotherapy, and researchers are improving their knowledge of environmental scenarios that trigger episodes in specific patients. Gerard Hogarty, the lead researcher of a psychiatric team at the University of Pittsburgh's School of Medicine, reported in the November 1998 issue of the *American Journal of Psychiatry* that a three-year psychotherapy regimen called "personal therapy" resulted in improved adjustment and fewer relapses (in comparison to pharmacotherapy alone). In contrast to psychoanalysis, personal therapy concentrates on the present-day life of the patient. Patients are educated to the idea that their brains are unusually sensitive to stress and are trained in ways to recognize stress and cope with it.

FUTURE POSSIBILITIES

(1) In addition to the well-established dopamine connection to schizophrenia, researchers have recently discovered that phencyclidine (PCP), when abused as a street drug, can initiate schizophrenia-like behavior. PCP's special action blocks the receptors for glutamate, a critical neurotransmitter involved in intercellular communication. Glutamate's role in the drama is currently under investigation.

2 In addition, researchers are exploring the possible ramifications of the fact that schizophrenics are the heaviest smokers of all those with mental disorders. Apparently, nicotine gives some relief, and that connection is under investigation.

3 As with other disorders of the mind-brain, researchers are using all available imaging devices to localize the active areas of the brain that are unique to specific symptoms. As the areas are mapped, interventions can be designed to address them based on the characteristics of these parts of the brain.

4 One current area of research has identified that there appears to be an optimal time to aggressively begin administering antipsychotic medications, which is earlier than the traditional practice. Patients whose drug therapy was begun earlier in the history of the disease appear to exhibit greater improvement in the long term.

5 Increasing evidence points to maternal influences before and during pregnancy that are associated with later onset of schizophrenia in the child. These include deficiencies in nutrition of the mother, immunological incompatibilities between the mother and the fetus, and the effect of influenza contracted by the mother during the second trimester of pregnancy. As more evidence accumulates, legislation can assist in reducing sources that are associated with schizophrenia's onset.

6 For current information on schizophrenia, call the National Alliance for Research on Schizophrenia and Depression at 516-829-0091. Also visit the web site of the same group at http://www.mhsource.com/narsad.html.

TOPIC 15.6 Tumors

Nature of the Disorder

Tumors (also called neoplasia; the field is called neuro-oncology) form as the direct result of bad genes (Louis, 1995). Two kinds of genes, *oncogenes,* which promote cell growth, and *suppressor genes,* which retard cell growth, normally act in balanced concert. Tumors form when either the oncogenes are overactive or the suppressor genes are underactive. Tumors can occur in glial cells (gliomas), meningeal cells (meningiomas), Schwann cells (schwannomas), and immune-system cells (lymphomas), but only rarely in normal neurons, because they do not divide after birth. In the United States, around seventeen thousand brain tumors are newly diagnosed annually, over two-thirds of them gliomas. They are the second most frequent kind of cancer in children, behind leukemia. More commonly, tumors occur in older people because of the complex mixture of influences—inherited, external environmental (for example, gases), and internal environmental (for example, disease)—that interact to start the process.

Applications

CURRENT TREATMENTS

Most gliomas and lymphomas resist therapy and lead to death within several years. Meningiomas and schwannomas are typically benign and capable of surgical removal. The key issue with tumors, however, is "location, location, location." Remote areas of the brain can harbor tumors whose removal would be extremely risky.

One complication of surgical removal is the inevitable destruction of neurons, either from having been crushed by the tumor or from the surgical invasion. At present, it is thought that these lost cells will not regenerate. However, loss of function as a result of neuronal damage can sometimes be recovered using the property of plasticity in neighboring cells. Plasticity is the capacity of cells to take on new functions. Rehabilitation processes are designed according to the nature of the tumor and the outcome of the surgery.

FUTURE POSSIBILITIES

1 A promising new gene therapy technique is under study at the University of Pennsylvania. Researchers have inserted a gene into benign viruses that later commands the viral cells to manufacture the enzyme thymidine kinase. Once the enzyme has been injected into the tumor, it attacks both cancerous and noncancerous cells. The doctor then administers the drug ganciclovir, which the thymidine kinase converts into a powerful toxin that prevents tumor cells from making further DNA, hence arresting further cell division.

❷ An excellent way to keep current, as well as to find support, is to join the Massachusetts Institute of Technology's discussion group on the Internet. To subscribe, send an E-mail message to listserv@mitvma.mit.edu and leave the subject line blank. In the body of the message, type:

subscribe BRAINTMR {your first name} {your last name}

❸ For excellent current information, visit Al Musella's web site at http://www.lanminds.com/local/brain/trial.html. Al got hooked on the discussion group when his sister-in-law was diagnosed with a brain tumor. From there, he began posting to his web site information on every brain tumor clinical trial going on in the United States.

❹ Two other excellent neuro-oncology information sites on the web are www.aneuroa.org/nlinkst97.html and http://weber.u. washington.edu/~chudler/disorders.html. On both sites, look for the section called "Neuro-oncology."

❺ Call the American Brain Tumor Association at 847-827-9910 or visit their web site at neurosurgery.mgh.harvard.edu/abta/.

SUGGESTED RESOURCES

Biederman, J., and Faraone, S. (1996, Winter). "Attention Deficit Hyper-activity Disorder." *On the Brain* (Harvard Mahoney Neuroscience Institute Letter), pp. 4–7.

Livingstone, M. S., Rosen, G. D., Drislane, F. W., and Galaburda, A. M. (1991). "Physiological and Anatomical Evidence for a Magnocellular Defect in Developmental Dyslexia." *Proceedings of the National Academy of Science, 88,* 7943–7947.

Pennington, B. F. (1991). *Diagnosing Learning Disorders: A Neuropsychological Framework.* New York: Guilford Press.

Shaywitz, S. E. (1996, November). "Dyslexia." *Scientific American,* pp. 98–104.

Shaywitz, S. E., and others. (1992). "Evidence That Dyslexia May Represent the Lower Tail of a Normal Distribution of Reading Ability." *New England Journal of Medicine, 326*(3), 145–150.

Walsh, C. A. (1997, Winter). "Epilepsy: Genes May Build the Road to Treatment." *On the Brain* (Harvard Mahoney Neuroscience Institute Letter), pp. 1–3.

Wyatt, R. J., and Henter, I. D. (1997, May–June). "Schizophrenia: An Introduction." *BrainWork: The Neuroscience Newsletter* (Charles A. Dana Foundation), 7(3), 1–3, 8.

16

Insults and Injuries

A Blow-by-Blow Account

66 An injury is much sooner forgotten than an insult. 99

—Philip Dormer Stanhope,
Earl of Chesterfield

Perhaps the Earl of Chesterfield was not thinking of insults and injuries to the brain when he penned his pearl, but a parallel exists. In fact, insults in the form of early childhood abuse appear to have a disturbingly long, and often permanent, life. This chapter explores brain disorders that can be attributed to injury: abused child syndrome, cerebral palsy, concussion, headaches, spinal cord injury, and stroke.

TOPIC 16.1 Abused Child Syndrome

Nature and Causes of the Disorder

Intense stress from severe physical or sexual abuse floods the brain with hormones, including adrenaline, noradrenaline, cortisol, and opiates; this results in the eventual shrinkage of the hippocampus. The left hippocampus typically shrinks more than the right, with the former reportedly shrinking up to 26 percent and the latter up to 22 percent of their normal size (Mukerjee, 1995).

Daniel Alkon committed his career to discovering the secret of how to reverse the effects of early abuse, only to become convinced of its impossibility. He reported on his findings in his book *Memory's Voice* (1992). According to Alkon, a kind of neural commitment occurs (pp. 162–164):

> [The result of this lifework] was not what I expected to find when I set out, energized by a sense of mission to wrestle with trauma's grip on the human psyche.... I didn't understand then, as I do now, that the actual biology of experience's influence on our brains is not the same in most of adulthood as it is in early childhood.... The adult brain's networks are to a significant degree hard-wired.... These are not styles that can be trained. They are ingrained, built into a permanent template. When we wish to counsel change in others or consider it for ourselves, it seems essential, therefore, to know the basic terrain of the behavioral landscape. New training and radically different experience may be able to modify familiar behavior, but the networks will not change with learning in adulthood as they can when we are growing up. The chemistry of personality has already been determined.... These thoughts do recommend an attitude of humility toward the possibilities of change for people.

The most disturbing part of this hard-wiring process, Alkon points out, is that "the emotional importance of what has been learned in critical periods determines its permanence. If only the brain changes of adult learning were more like those of childhood. Perhaps then we could be more ambitious. As it is, for now, these differences limit our freedom and, to a degree, seal our fate" (p. 164). A person traumatized by abuse, Alkon learned, cannot dissolve the hard-wired networks of increasingly thick myelination built up over months and years of emotional trauma. As an adult, such a person must search for a partner who shares these attitudes shaped by abuse, or who does not pose a challenge to the maintenance of these attitudes. Neither surgical, pharmaceutical, nor other therapeutic methods, according to Alkon, have succeeded in overcoming these abuse-built neural networks, glazed with the chemicals of fear, anger, and depression and fired in the kiln of these intense emotions.

One phenomenon that compounds the problem of early abuse is that of early neuronal commitment. A kind of commitment of neurons appears to be made in humans sometime between eight and twelve months of age. Once they are committed, the neurons ignore unfamiliar stimuli. Janet Werker, of the University of British Columbia in Vancouver, finds that babies who are exposed only to English from birth can recognize consonants that do not occur in English from the language of the Thompson tribe (located in the Thompson and Fraser valleys of southwest British Columbia) up until eight months of age, but at twelve months they cannot discriminate between the Thompson consonants. Stephen Pinker (1994) reports that with less drastic subtleties in phonetic differences, one can learn to speak a nonnative language like a native speaker up through age seven. Apparently, then, different levels of neuronal commitment are operating.

Symptoms

Up to 20 percent of survivors of abuse suffer from either dissociation or post-traumatic stress disorder (PTSD). In dissociation, often used by children who are unable to escape the abuse, the victims separate their experience from conscious awareness, in essence feeling detached from the experience in such a way that it doesn't appear to happen at all. On the other hand, in PTSD, the victims relive the abusive and/or severely stressful memory and try to avoid situations that remind them of it.

Sexually abused girls suffer a dramatically altered developmental pattern. Although there is some variation among them, these girls can be found to mature physically earlier, have different hormonal reactions, and have impaired immune functions (DeAngelis, 1995). They tend to suffer generally higher levels of arousal, as evidenced by sustained higher levels of catecholimines. This hyperarousal is associated with sleep disorders, nervousness, depression, and anxiety. Ongoing collaborative research into abuse victims is being conducted by Penelope Tricket of the University of Southern California and Frank Putnam of the National Institute of Mental Health's Laboratory of Clinical Psychology.

Applications

CURRENT TREATMENTS

1 A variety of treatments are being tried, from eye-movement therapy to the "counting method." For an excellent summary of available resources, visit the abuse and trauma pages of the OurPlace Support Forum's web site: ourworld.compuserve.com/homepages/Arael_Et_Al/TRMA-RX.htm.

2 For a book that summarizes current prevention and treatment issues, get Wolfe, McMahon, and Peters, *Child Abuse: New Directions in Prevention and Treatment Across the Lifespan* (1997).

3 If you know a child who appears to be experiencing abuse, know that the longer it goes on the harder its effects will be to reverse. Act now!

FUTURE POSSIBILITIES

For breaking news in the treatment of abuse victims, get on the mailing list for the National Crime Victim's Research and Treatment Center; Medical University of South Carolina; Charleston, South Carolina 29425.

TOPIC 16.2 Cerebral Palsy

Nature of the Disorder

About two to four out of every thousand births result in irreversible damage to brain cells that govern voluntary muscle movements, sensations, and mental faculties. About one out of every twenty babies who weigh less than three pounds suffers this damage. These very low birth weight babies account for roughly 28 percent of all cases of cerebral palsy (CP). The damage may also be caused by bleeding in the brain or by a dying off of white matter that leaves holes in the midst of various nerve connections. In other cases, the damage occurs in early infancy because of some accident or trauma.

Symptoms

Symptoms typically appear anywhere from three months of age to as late as age two. The symptoms are nonprogressive and can include one or more of a long list, including spasticity (the most common symptom), paralysis, perceptual abnormalities, speech defects, and seizures. Life expectancy is normal, except for very low birth weight infants with CP, whose average life expectancy is twenty years. The intellectual ability of people with CP can range from severely retarded to extremely bright.

Applications

CURRENT TREATMENTS

Because there is no cure for CP, the goal is to create the greatest possible independence. This may include use of physical therapy, braces, hearing and seeing aids, drugs, special schooling, and, for extreme cases, institutionalization. Prescriptions could include muscle relaxants and anticonvulsants. Some cases require surgery to correct joint, muscle, and feeding problems.

FUTURE POSSIBILITIES

1 In the December 11, 1996, issue of the *Journal of the American Medical Association* (reported in the *New York Times,* December 11, 1996, p. 13C), Diana Schendel and colleagues from the Centers for Disease Control and Prevention in Atlanta reported a significant finding in the prevention of CP, and possibly also mental retardation, among premature infants. Based on a clue from rat studies, they tracked all women in the Atlanta area from 1986 to 1988 who gave birth to infants weighing less than three pounds. Their findings: infants whose mothers were given intravenous magnesium sulfate (a drug commonly used to prevent premature delivery or given to women with high blood pressure to prevent convulsions) were 90 percent less likely to have CP and 70 percent less likely to be mentally retarded than those whose mothers had no drugs or some other drug during premature labor. Although controlled studies must be completed before outright recommendation of this procedure, doctors associated with the study are concerned about the ethics of denying women this option, considering the results to date. More recently, Karen Nelson at the National Institutes of Health has confirmed the association of higher magnesium levels with a lower incidence of developing CP. However, as of mid-1998, the way magnesium relates to CP was unclear.

2 Keep current with information from these two web sites: www.familyinternet.com and the National Institute of Neural Disorders and Stroke's web site at www.ninds.nih.gov/healinfo/disorder.

TOPIC 16.3 Concussion

Nature of the Disorder

A concussion occurs when the head sustains a strong blow that results in loss of consciousness, however brief. After the blow, the brain then hits the skull in a "counterblow." In more severe cases, often as the result of twisting the neck during the blow, pressure is put on the brain stem, where basic involuntary life functions are controlled. Bleeding or other damage may occur. Often, people who sustain a concussion cannot remember the events surrounding the blow.

Symptoms

Symptoms include vomiting, pupils that are different sizes, confusion, seizures, coma, muscle weakness, or unusual walking patterns.

Applications

CURRENT TREATMENTS

The American Academy of Neurology has established guidelines for three levels of concussion (note that the examples are drawn from the sports world, which has the highest incidence of concussion):

Grade 1: No perceptible loss of consciousness; mild confusion and loss of coordination; symptoms are gone in fifteen minutes. (Check every five minutes for symptoms; if they have cleared after fifteen minutes, the individual may resume normal activity. If a player in a sport suffers multiple grade-1 concussions, she or he may return to play only after a neurological assessment and one symptom-free week.)

Grade 2: No perceptible loss of consciousness; mild confusion and loss of coordination; symptoms last more than fifteen minutes. (Remove a player from the game; examine him or her frequently; conduct a neurological assessment. The player may return after one week with no symptoms after rest or exertion. If a player suffers multiple grade-2 concussions, he or she may return only after being symptom-free for two weeks.)

Grade 3: Loss of consciousness, either for seconds or minutes. (Take the patient by ambulance for an emergency neurological examination. With brief unconsciousness, a player may return to a game after one symptom-free week; with longer periods of unconsciousness, the player may return after two symptom-free weeks.) These last two guidelines are for adults. The guidelines differ for young people.

If a young person in an athletic situation has a concussion, typically she or he should not resume athletics for three months. Immediately after the concussion, the person should be still and quiet. Brain injury rates are higher for those who have sustained prior concussions with unconsciousness. Repeated concussions have a cumulative effect on one or more mental functions. With uncomplicated concussions, full recovery is typical.

For a complete copy of the American Academy of Neurology guidelines, call 612-623-8115.

FUTURE POSSIBILITIES

Stay current with information on concussions by visiting the National Institute of Neural Disorders' web site at www.ninds.nih.gov/healinfo/disorder. Information is also available from the Brain Injury Association at 202-296-6443.

TOPIC 16.4   Headaches

Nature of the Disorder

Most headaches are associated with vasoconstriction (tightening of the blood vessels). Vasoconstriction can be offset or prevented by limiting consumption of foodstuffs with tyramine, an amino acid believed to be associated with vasoconstriction. (See Table 16.1 for a list of tyramine-containing, migraine-precipitating foods.) Menstrual migraines can be eliminated by finding the precipitating foods from the list in Table 16.1 and avoiding them, starting several days before the onset of menses and continuing until it's over. One friend has successfully eliminated her menstrual migraines by cutting out sugar two to three days before the expected onset of menses, another friend by eliminating alcohol consumption two to three days before menses. For nonmenstrual migraines, an individual would simply eliminate a suspected food until a migraine occurred, then assume that the food hadn't been the cause of the headache and eliminate another food.

Gallagher (1990) concludes that most headaches can be limited or eliminated by pharmaceutical methods or by nonpharmaceutical methods such as diet or biofeedback. Once a headache begins, however, dietary methods are ineffective: it's time for drugs.

Table 16.1. Migraine-Precipitating Foods.

Meat and Fish	Fruits	Beverages
Pickled herring	Canned figs	Alcoholic
Chicken livers	Raisins	Caffeine
Sausage	Papaya	(limit to 2 cups
Salami	Passion fruit	per day)
Pepperoni	Avocado	Chocolate milk
Bologna	Bananas	Buttermilk
Hot dogs	Red plums	
Marinated meats	Citrus fruit	
Aged, canned, or cured meats	(limit to ½ cup per day)	

Vegetables	Dairy	Other
Fava beans	Aged and processed	Soy sauce
Lima beans	cheese	MSG
Navy beans	Yogurt (limit to ½ cup	Meat tenderizer
Pea pods	per day)	Seasoning salt
Sauerkraut	Sour cream	Canned soups
Onions		TV dinners
		Garlic
		Yeast extracts

Baked Goods	Desserts	Nuts
Fresh-baked breads	Chocolate	
Sourdough		

Source: From *Drug Therapy for Headache,* edited by R. Michael Gallagher, 1990, New York: Marcel Dekker. © 1991 by Marcel Dekker, Inc. Extracted from the National Headache Foundation Diet, Chicago, Illinois. Reprinted by permission.

Applications

CURRENT TREATMENTS

❶ Experiment: Systematically eliminate different foods from the list in Table 16.1 before expected headaches. If a headache happens, resume that food and next time try eliminating another. Or try eliminating combinations of foods.

2 Consult with your physician for pharmaceutical assistance. If this produces no results, read Gallagher (1990) and discuss some of his recommendations with your physician.

3 For further information, call the National Headache Foundation at 800-843-2256.

4 Significant relief is available for menstrual migraines through a new dopamine-related drug called bromocriptine. Also, for migraine, large daily doses (400 milligrams) of Vitamin B-2 (riboflavin) have been shown to have preventive value: migraine sufferers who took B-2 had 37 percent fewer reported migraines than those who did not take the vitamin (*Neurology,* February 1998). And when the B-2 takers did have a migraine, the attack was shorter than for a placebo group.

5 Two recently approved treatments are zolmitriptan (a designer drug acting on serotonin receptors; it provides relief within two hours for two-thirds of recipients) and sumatriptan nasal spray (which could begin pain reduction as early as fifteen minutes after administration; it helps two-thirds of recipients).

FUTURE POSSIBILITIES

1 The March 1998 issue of *Archives of Neurology* reported that 59 percent of migraine sufferers who took a combination of three nonprescription drugs—acetaminophen, aspirin, and caffeine—within two hours of migraine onset found that their pain subsided or disappeared.

2 Martin A. Samuels, chair of the Department of Neurology at Boston's Brigham and Women's Hospital, argues that because migraine sufferers' stomachs do not empty well, oral pills are less effective. He finds that the inexpensive suppository Indocin works almost as well as expensive injections. He recommends that if suppositories don't appeal, a stomach relaxer should be tried along with oral pills to help improve absorption of the active ingredients.

TOPIC 16.5 | Spinal Cord Injury

Nature of the Disorder

Upward of ten thousand incidents of spinal cord injury (SCI) occur in the United States annually, the majority of them in metropolitan and industrial areas. About 80 percent of the injuries happen to people between the ages of sixteen and thirty, with males accounting for 82 percent overall. Vehicular accidents cause 40 percent, with sports, assaults, and falls contributing to most of the remainder. Injuries are classified as consisting of either partial or completely severed spinal cords. Completely severed cords cannot be rejoined at present, nor can feeling or movement be regained in body parts below the break.

Applications

CURRENT TREATMENTS

Although recent studies have shown that megadoses of methyl-prednisolone aid in restoring some degree of neurological function, treatments will vary depending on the point and degree of the separation. A variety of pharmaceutical and orthopedic options are available. For a good summary of the state of knowledge about spinal injury as of April 1997, see the special issue of *BrainWork: The Neuroscience Newsletter* ("Spinal Cord Injury," 1997). Full text copies of the newsletter are available on the Internet at www.dana.org/dana/brainwrk.html.

FUTURE POSSIBILITIES

Lars Olson, Henrich Cheng, and Yihai Cao of the Karolinska Institute in Sweden reported a major step in spinal cord reconstruction: the ability to successfully grow nerve cells across gaps in the severed spinal cords of adult rats (*Science*, July 26, 1996). Researchers took nerve cells from the rats' chests, formed them into filaments called "bridges," and fitted them into a ⅕-inch gap in their spinal cords. After several months, their once-motionless, dragging hind legs began to show voluntary movement. Within a year, the rats could partially support their weight and walk to some degree. An unusual feature of this technique that may account for the researchers' dramatic success is that they connected one end of each "bridge" to gray matter (the inner core of the cord) and the other end to white matter (the outer cover). Needless to say, intense efforts are under way to refine the technique and to ultimately experiment with humans.

For a web site with a listing of organizations that provide information and support, try http://neurosurgery.mgh.harvard.edu/paral-r.htm. For the larger subject of traumatic brain injury, try www.tbidoc.com.

TOPIC 16.6 Stroke

Nature of the Disorder

Strokes (also called brain attacks or ischemia) hit 700,000 people in the United States every year, making stroke the third most fatal disease, following heart attack and cancer. The attack on the brain is initiated by the circulatory system, which blocks the path of oxygen and other nutrients to the brain because of a disease within the circulatory system itself.

Symptoms

Symptoms that an attack has begun may include any or all of the following: headache, dizziness, confusion, visual disturbance, loss of speech, slurred speech, difficulty swallowing, and weakness or paralysis on one side of the body.

The effects of stroke include paralysis, loss of speech, and mood disorders, depending on just where the damage occurs. Recent research indicates that damage to the left hemisphere results in more depressive moods (activity in the left hemisphere is associated with positive moods), while damage to the right hemisphere (associated with more negative moods) results in more manic and hallucinatory moods. Roughly one-third of strokes are fatal, another one-third result in some degree of handicap, and the remainder result in complete (or close to complete) recovery.

Applications

CURRENT TREATMENTS

The best prevention for stroke is to take maximum care of one's circulatory system. After that, many doctors recommend that at a certain point in your life (my doctor recommended that I start at age fifty-five), you take one coated aspirin each morning as a preventive; aspirin eases blood flow through its thinning, anticoagulant properties. In addition, Matthew Gillman of the Harvard Community Health Plan reports that stroke risk declines 22 percent for every three servings of fruits and vegetables eaten daily, where one serving equals ½ cup (*Journal of the American Medical Association,* April 12, 1995).

The treatment for a brain attack depends on the nature of the attacking force. One must first determine the kind of circulatory problem that caused the attack. The initial cell death that occurs within ninety minutes of the attack sets off a program of systematic follow-on destruction that can last for days. If appropriate action can be taken before that ninety minutes are up, the chances of minimizing damage and maximizing recovery are improved. A new drug that dissolves blood clots, a "tissue plasminogen activator (TPA)," will improve the outcome of stroke if it is administered within two hours of onset. However, Stuart Lipman of Brigham and Women's Hospital reported in the February 1998 issue of *Nature Genetics* that TPA damages nerve cells in addition to breaking up clots.

FUTURE POSSIBILITIES

A variety of research efforts are under way, including studies of how such players as glutamates, neurotrophins, free radicals, nitric oxide, and calcium act before, during, and after a brain attack. Another hotly debated topic is the role of fat consumption in stroke. A controversial article in the *Journal of the American Medical Association* (December 24, 1997) reported a positive relationship between *all* kinds of fat that are consumed—saturated, unsaturated, and polyunsaturated—and the absence of stroke: the more fat consumed, the less likely an individual is to have a stroke. This research, based on the Framingham Heart Study, was reported by Matthew Gillman, the same person who reported (see above) that every three servings of fruits and veggies reduced stroke chances by 22 percent! We must await clarification. Researchers commonly point to studies conducted in Crete, a region where both heart disease and stroke are low and low levels of saturated fat are coupled with low levels of overweight among the population. Interestingly, the Cretans have a high fat content in their diet, but it is monounsaturated fat, as in olive oil.

A University of Alabama at Birmingham team has reported excellent results in arm and leg rehabilitation (Pidikiti and others, 1996). The technique involves immobilizing the good arm or leg and forcing use of the damaged one.

For an excellent web site on the subject of stroke, try visiting the University of Alabama in Birmingham's "Comprehensive Stroke Center" at www.uab.edu/neurol/stroke.htm. You will be especially interested in the "StrokeLinks" option, which puts at your fingertips major Internet resources on the subject of stroke.

SUGGESTED RESOURCES

Alkon, D. L. (1992). *Memory's Voice: Deciphering the Brain-Mind Code.* New York: HarperCollins.

DeAngelis, T. (1995, April). "New Threat Associated with Child Abuse." *APA Monitor, 26*(4), 1, 38.

Mukerjee, M. (1995, October). "Hidden Scars." *Scientific American,* pp. 14, 20.

Wolfe, D. A., McMahon, R. J., and Peters, R. D. (1997). *Child Abuse: New Directions in Prevention and Treatment Across the Lifespan.* Thousand Oaks, Calif.: Sage.

17

Degenerative Conditions

Slowly Falling Apart

*I*n a sense, the degenerative conditions discussed in this chapter are like accelerated aging. But even normal aging does not require us to experience the terrifying loss of memory, coordination, and clarity that these conditions can entail. This chapter discusses five degenerative diseases: Alzheimer's disease, Huntington's disease, Lou Gehrig's disease, multiple sclerosis, and Parkinson's disease.

> **" *Forgive,
> O Lord, my little
> jokes on Thee*
>
> *And I'll forgive
> Thy great big
> one on me.* "**
>
> —*Robert Frost*

For the most part, cures for these degenerative conditions are dependent on the ability to find ways to replace damaged and deceased neurons. In the spring of 1992, Samuel Weiss and Brent Reynolds of the University of Calgary (Canada) Faculty of Medicine discovered reserves of immature brain cells in adult mice that could be coaxed into dividing into new cells. This phenomenon had been thought possible only in embryos. The implications for humans are now being studied. (To underscore the rapidity of research developments, it is now eight months since I wrote the last several sentences, and Fred Gage, along with a team of Swedish scientists, has just announced the successful detection of regenerated brain cells.) However, the successful regeneration of human or animal brain cells, although it is a major breakthrough, is just the first step in a long research-and-development process.

TOPIC 17.1 Alzheimer's Disease

Nature and Causes of the Disorder

At the 1996 meeting of the Society for Neuroscience, attendees could choose from among over five hundred presentations on Alzheimer's disease (AD). AD afflicts four million senior Americans (and almost half of those aged eighty-five and over) and is sure to increase with the aging baby-boom cohort. Apparently, a concatenation of bad genes, poor education, head injury, and normal aging processes works diabolically to produce beta-amyloid and neurofibrillary tangles. Beta-amyloid is a protein composed of forty-two amino acids that form toxic deposits, or "plaque," on the brain's neurons. The neural tangles result from an abnormal protein, tau protein, within the cell that constricts and distorts fibers. These processes appear to be controlled by at least three genes (*Neuron,* November 15, 1997): APP, which, when it is flawed, produces amyloid-precursor protein, the raw material for plaque; Presenilin 1, which affects cell repair and cell death; and APO-E4, which affects the speed at which plaque is deposited. Apparently, the mutated APP alone is associated with late onset of AD, while the presence of the other two are associated with earlier onset (Presenilin 1) and rate of onset (APO-E4). Huntington

Potter, of Harvard Medical School's Department of Neurobiology, reports that these genes apparently do not perform inside neurons but rather work inside the cells of neighboring microglial cells and astrocytes, which in turn release the free radicals that kill off the nerve cells (*Cell,* October 1997). Others, including Davis Parker, Jr., of the University of Virginia, believe that the process starts in the neuron's mitochondria, where, because of a genetic defect, energy production goes awry and produces free radicals rather than energy. In either case, the brain essentially oxidizes, or slowly burns itself up, leaving plaque and tangled fibers as evidence of what once was.

The effect of this toxic process is a progressive, neurodegenerative disease that typically begins in one's seventies or eighties. A variation, called early-onset Alzheimer's, can begin during middle age. The first symptoms of this buildup of plaque (from beta-amyloid protein) and tangled nerve fibers (from tau protein) are memory problems; then, over a period of years, problems develop with personality, cognition, and general physical functioning.

Huntington Potter discovered an early diagnosis for AD, using analogical reasoning. While looking for Down's syndrome features that it might be reasonable to expect in AD because they share the same chromosome, Potter found that AD-destined individuals show a hypersensitivity to tropicamide (the synthetic version of atropine), used by eye doctors to dilate pupils in order to have a good look at the retina. AD subjects, both before and after onset of the disease, need only 1/100th of the normal amount of tropicamide for satisfactory pupil dilation. So we now have a rather effective diagnostic procedure (*On the Brain,* Winter 1995).

Richard Mayeux, leader of a study at Columbia University's College of Physicians and Surgeons, and coauthor Ann Saunders, of Duke University, report in the *New England Journal of Medicine* (February 19, 1998) that a simple blood test for the presence of the APO-E4 gene, coupled with the presence of dementia, can reduce the AD misdiagnosis rate from the 1997 rate of 45 percent to a significantly lower rate of 16 percent.

For a brief yet insightful story of the progression of AD, read Lawrence Altman's feature story on Ronald Reagan in the *New York Times* (October 5, 1997, pp. 1, 34).

Applications

CURRENT TREATMENTS

❶ Donepezil (Aricept) was approved by the Food and Drug Administration in November 1996. It functions in one of two ways: either it improves memory or it slows down the progress of AD by preventing the breakdown of acetylcholine, which is deficient in AD patients. This represents an improvement over Cognex (tacrine), which has a similar purpose but more side effects. Europeans have been treating AD patients with ginkgo biloba extract, which improves blood flow to the brain, although in doing so, it decreases the blood's clotting ability.

❷ Yaskov Stern and his colleagues at Columbia University studied 593 New Yorkers at risk for AD. They found that people who either had fewer than eight years of schooling or lower-skilled jobs were twice as likely to end up with AD, while those with both of these two conditions were three times as likely to develop dementia as those who were more highly educated and more highly skilled. Pursuing higher education and higher skills is something that all of us can do with minimal fear of undesirable side effects!

❸ The amount of exercise engaged in regularly between the ages of twenty and fifty-nine is directly related to the risk of AD. In a study of 373 people, both those with AD and healthy individuals, neurologists Arthur Smith and Robert Friedland, of Case Western Reserve University School of Medicine, compiled an exercise score based on the number of hours of exercise per month multiplied by an intensity factor. The higher the score, the less likely one's chance of developing AD.

FUTURE POSSIBILITIES

Many lines of research are under way, including the following:

❶ Pills are being studied that can offset the effect of mutated genes that are relevant to AD.

❷ Estrogen therapy has been shown to improve memory among Alzheimer's patients; the Women's Health Initiative, which follows eight thousand women, is specifically looking at the effect of estrogen on the onset of AD. Barbara Sherwin of McGill University has demonstrated that administering estrogen to women has clear effects in preventing, delaying, and reversing dementia and AD. Her results apply only to verbal memory; visual and spatial memory appear to be unaffected by estrogen levels. University of Southern California neurologist Victor Henderson suspects that these beneficial effects may also be true for men (*BrainWork: The Neuroscience Newsletter,* January–February 1998).

❸ Researchers at Johns Hopkins University and the National Institute on Aging have identified a significant reduction in the risk of getting AD among those who take nonsteroidal anti-inflammatory drugs (NSAIDs), such as aspirin, ibuprofen, and naproxen, for periods of two years. The doses for the different drugs, however, are unknown, and the side effects of inappropriate use could cause people to wind up with a disease or condition, such as kidney failure, other than the one they were perhaps unnecessarily trying to prevent.

❹ Still another line of research has yielded a slowing-down effect after the onset of AD with ginkgo extract (specifically, Egb 761), but doses are unclear and it can interact with other treatments such as NSAIDs, which could cause both excessive blood thinning and anticoagulation.

❺ One treatment that is close to availability is a new class of drugs—ampakines—being developed by Gary Lynch of the University of California at Irvine. Ampakines intensify the level of AMPA-glutamates, a chemical necessary for interneuronal communication, and have been shown to improve memory. Clinical trials are under way.

❻ William Klunk of Western Psychiatric Institute in Pittsburgh is working with a tissue dye called Chrysamine G, which appears to have the property of preventing beta-amyloid from expressing its toxic effect on brain neurons—a kind of shield, as it were.

❼ Some suspect that beta-amyloids, or possibly the immune system itself, increase free radicals; they are exploring treatment with antioxidants.

8 Rachel Neve at McLean Hospital in Belmont, Massachusetts, is pursuing a variation of the beta-amyloid molecule joined with molecules associated with the APP gene. This combination (called "C-100") has been shown to be more toxic than beta-amyloid in its normal state.

9 A team headed by Jeffrey Gray at Maudesley Hospital's Institute of Psychiatry in London has developed a technique that manufactures brain cells from rat embryos, injects them into diseased rat brains, and then frees them to migrate to the diseased area and repair or replace the damaged cells. Rats so treated have recovered from severe ischemic attacks and have subsequently learned complex tasks. The researchers have started a company, ReNeuron, dedicated to researching, developing, and eventually selling the product.

10 Mark Mattson, a University of Kentucky neurobiologist, leads a team at the university's Sanders-Brown Center on Aging in the investigation of calorie intake's relation to the onset of AD. In research with rats, Mattson's team reported that rats with a restricted calorie intake were successful in resisting injected toxins that mimic Alzheimer's, Parkinson's, and Huntington's diseases (*Annals of Neurology,* January 1999). Rats that ate all they pleased showed significantly less resistance to the AD-like agent. In human terms, this would suggest an optimum daily intake of 1,800 to 2,000 calories. The mechanism perhaps involves the fact that stress results from reduced intake, followed by the activation of genes that protect the body during low intake. No mention is made of the long-term effects of such a pattern.

11 The July 1998 issue of *Nature Medicine* presented three articles with apparent breakthrough news: the related reports confirm that beta-amyloid is the prime nerve cell killer and that a peptide has been developed that arrests and corrects the progress of cell death. This new peptide binds to the good amyloid gone bad; it both prevents it from twisting further and straightens out the hardened twists to their formerly benign condition. These animal studies will result in human trials by early 2000. Researchers are confident that both prevention and cure are around the corner.

12 If you have an interest in AD, you should keep informed about all these lines of research. One way is through frequently visiting the Alzheimer's disease web site at www.alzheimers.com.

TOPIC 17.2 Huntington's Disease

Nature of the Disorder

Huntington's is the result of one single dominant gene; each child of an affected parent has a 50 percent chance of getting the disease. Huntington's typically begins by killing off cells in the caudate nucleus sometime during one's forties. The result is a gradual loss of control of the person's intellect, emotions, balance, and speech. Typically, a pattern of involuntary movements, referred to as Huntington's chorea, accompanies the other symptoms. Approximately fifty thousand people have the disease in the United States; the normal progression of the disease leads to death within fifteen to twenty years of the initial symptoms.

The Huntington's gene, discovered in 1993, produces a protein referred to as "huntingtin." The normal form of huntingtin typically contains between 10 and 35 glutamine molecules, whereas the mutant version contains a minimum of 38 molecules and up to as many as 100. This repeated sequence has been described as a kind of chemical "stuttering" (*Los Angeles Times,* August 8, 1997, p. A1). The normal version of huntingtin is necessary to sustain life, and apparently 38 molecules is the threshold at which huntingtin transmogrifies and becomes lethal. In 1995, researchers at Johns Hopkins University announced the discovery of a protein that binds to huntingtin and dubbed it "Huntington's Associated Protein–1," or HAP-1 (*Nature,* November 23, 1995).

Applications

CURRENT TREATMENTS

There are no known treatments.

FUTURE POSSIBILITIES

Current research is aimed at preventing HAP-1 from binding to huntingtin in mice. Researchers are attempting to find a pharmaceutical that will somehow interact with the HAP-1 protein and the glutamine 38+ chain to prevent the clustering and buildup that eventually kills off brain cells.

Keep current by visiting the Huntington's disease web site at www.interlog.com/~rlaycock/what.html.

TOPIC 17.3 Lou Gehrig's Disease

Nature and Causes of the Disorder

In the United States, Lou Gehrig's disease (amyotrophic lateral sclerosis, or ALS) is at about twenty-five thousand cases with about five thousand new cases each year. It was named after the New York Yankees star who died from it in 1941. ALS attacks the motor neurons of the brain and spinal cord that control the muscles. This progressive condition affects strength, speech, swallowing, and breathing, but it does not affect intellect, vision, hearing, taste, touch, or smell and typically it does not affect sexual, bowel, or bladder functions.

Researchers continue to investigate the cause of ALS. Only 10 percent of the cases run in families and, of that 10 percent, only one in five has a known genetic origin. How are the other 98 percent of the cases explained? The best explanation at present is that ALS results from a combination of some kind of genetic predisposition and some kind of environmental assault (such as the inhalation of strong petrochemicals). Some researchers think that ALS is actually a combination of several different diseases.

Applications

CURRENT TREATMENTS

1 There is no known cure. Two current treatments aimed at slowing the disease's progress involve an injection and an implant. The implant is a genetically engineered capsule of about 100,000 cells of ciliary neurotrophic factor (CNTF) that releases CNTF at a normal rate. It is manufactured by CytoTherapeutics Inc. in Providence, Rhode Island. The injection uses the drug myotrophin, a genetically engineered form of human insulin-like growth factor (IGF-1). It appears to slow the progress of ALS by a factor of about 25 percent.

2 For information and support, visit the web site of Doug Jacobson (he has ALS) at www.phoenix.net/~jacobson/beatals.html.

FUTURE POSSIBILITIES

In the fall of 1998, an international study began human tests for a hockey-puck-sized pump that delivers brain-derived neurotrophic factor (BDNF) at a steady rate. BDNF, a synthetic protein similar to one that naturally occurs in the brain, has had only minimal effectiveness when administered by injection.

TOPIC 17.4 | Multiple Sclerosis

Nature of the Disorder

Multiple sclerosis (MS) is the second most common neural disease among young adults, after head injury. MS affects about 300,000 people in the United States and typically begins somewhere between the ages of twenty and forty. An autoimmune dysfunction, MS occurs when the immune system mistakenly identifies brain and spinal cord tissues, and particularly the myelin sheath that covers axons, as foreign invaders and attempts to get rid of them. The result is an eating away of myelin in a region called a "plaque" that can cover a length from several millimeters to over a centimeter. In some cases, this attack succeeds in destroying the axon itself. After some time, the process of inflammatory demyelination is halted by suppressor cells and, depending on the severity of the attack, the processes of remyelination and recovery of function may occur, only to be subjected to another attack months or years later.

Major symptoms can include weakness, paralysis, tingling, numbness, disturbed vision, balance and coordination problems, slurred speech, lack of control of the bladder and bowel, chronic pain, and severe fatigue. Sensations will spontaneously stop, then renew at a different location. Episodes vary in length from days to months. Because diagnosis is based on multiple sites of inflammation separated in time, early diagnosis is difficult, but new MRI techniques are making early diagnosis a possibility.

About one-fourth of the cases of MS are relatively mild, and about one-third are severe. Half of the people with MS are disabled after ten years, and more than one-third cannot walk after thirty years (Riskind, 1996). Twice as many women as men contract MS, and Caucasians are more likely to suffer MS than other ethnic groups. Eight or more genes appear to be associated with the disease, with particular focus on a region of chromosome 6 that is associated with the immune system. The concordance rate is rather low between identical twins, however, suggesting that an unknown environmental agent triggers MS.

Applications

CURRENT TREATMENTS

A cure is unavailable at present. Some relief from the fatigue of MS is available to about half of the MS population through amantadine, a dopamine enhancer. For severe flare-ups, an adrenal steroid hormone called methylprednisolone can shorten the episode but does not appear to retard the overall progress of the disease. These drugs treat symptoms, whereas beta-interferon (Betaseron, Avonex), a natural immune agent, provides more long-term benefits for some MS patients. Given in the early stages, a new drug—copolymer 1 (Copaxone)—can reduce both the rate of flare-ups and the overall progress of the disease for patients with milder MS.

FUTURE POSSIBILITIES

1 Current research is exploring a variety of possible environmental triggers in three different areas: immune cells from mutant genes, viruses, and pregnancy (particularly prolactin production). The British biotechnology group Plc is currently at work on a new drug based on a major discovery. Steven Jacobson, principal investigator for the Viral Immunology Section of the National Institute of Neurological Disorders and Stroke (NINDS), strongly suspects that a version of the human herpesvirus may be the trigger that initiates MS in many cases (*BrainWork: The Neuroscience Newsletter,* January–February 1998).

2 To keep current, visit the web site of the International Federation for Multiple Sclerosis at www.ifmss.org.uk/.

TOPIC 17.5 Parkinson's Disease

Nature of the Disorder

Around 1.5 million people in the United States suffer from Parkinson's disease (PD), most of them over forty. While the initiating cause of PD is unknown, onset is associated with the death of cells in the substantia nigra and the striatum. We start off life with about one million so-called dopamine cells; through normal aging we lose about half of them. In PD, one's portion of dopamine cells drops dangerously low, to somewhere between 50,000 and 100,000. As a consequence, the level of dopamine, which is crucial for coordinated muscle movements, may be 80 percent less than normal. Because of this dopamine drop-off, the balance between acetylcholine and dopamine becomes out of kilter. Apparently, this balance is also crucial for coordination of movement. Interaction with other neurotransmitters such as serotonin, norepinephrine, and GABA, as well as deficiencies in these neurotransmitters, may also be involved.

The symptoms that signal PD include stiffness, tremor, slowness, reduced movement, and problems with balance and walking. The disease is progressive, and survival after onset is typically ten to fifteen years.

Parkinson-like symptoms have recently resulted from the illegal use by several young people of a drug called MPTP, which was found to directly damage cells in the pyramidal tract of motor neurons. Some think that PD may in fact produce a chemical similar to MPTP, and that hunch forms one line of current research in better understanding the disease.

Applications

CURRENT TREATMENTS

1 Because there is no definite cure, treatment is aimed at reducing the symptoms. The most common treatment for PD is levodopa, or L-dopa, which the body transforms into dopamine. Others are amantadine (believed to release dopamine), carbidopa (which prevents the breakdown of dopamine by the enzyme MAO-B), bromocriptine (which stimulates the three different dopamine receptors), and pramipexole or Mirapex (which controls tremor).

2 Three different surgical procedures are currently hot topics in the PD community, but as they are still experimental, they are listed below as future possibilities. They are in fact available if you can get on the waiting list and travel to the sites that are trying them.

FUTURE POSSIBILITIES

1 An exciting line of research is resulting from the young people who took MPTP and developed PD-like symptoms. Researchers injected MPTP into monkeys and induced PD symptoms, then looked for an agent that would reverse the symptoms. They have apparently found it in "glial-cell-line-derived neurotrophic factor" (GDNF; see *Nature,* April 1996). GDNF appears not only to prevent MPTP from destroying substantia nigra cells, but also to resuscitate the useless dopamine-producing cells to some degree; however, the effects only last for a month in monkeys, so repeated injections are necessary. Clinical trials with humans are now under way. GDNF will not pass the blood-brain barrier, but gene therapy appears to be an effective way to introduce GDNF into the target neurons.

2 In 1988, the first implants of six- to eight-week-old human fetal tissue were placed in the brains of PD patients. Over time, these young cells started producing dopamine to various degrees. Curt Freed, director of the University of Colorado's National Parkinson Foundation Center of Excellence, has completed a few dozen of these procedures. A third were unsuccessful, a third were moderately successful (patients still needed about 70 percent of their original drug dosages), and the final third were extremely successful: patients regained normal movement with minimal or, in one case, no use of drugs. Legal and ethical concerns currently hamper development of this process.

3 Another (and legal) course of trial implants involves the use of pig dopamine cells. Beginning in 1995 and continuing through 1997, twelve PD patients at Harvard University Medical School were implanted with pig cells (six patients with Huntington's disease have also been implanted). Preliminary results are exciting, but researchers estimate that release for mainstream use is probably a decade away.

4 Another procedure being developed is the pallidotomy, which involves partial destruction of the cells in the globus pallidus. Low dopamine levels cause that area to become overactive, and the pallidotomy brings the levels under control, according to the lead researcher, Mahlon DeLong of Emory University. Other sites currently doing pallidotomies include the Loma Linda University Medical Center, Massachusetts General Hospital, Boston University, Deaconess Hospital in Boston, New York University, the University of Arkansas Center for Medical Sciences, and Mt. Sinai School of Medicine in New York City. Pallidotomies were popular before the availability of L-dopa in the 1960s, when the procedure was all but abandoned. Swedish neurosurgeon Lauri Laitinen caused a revival of the pallidotomy with a published research report in 1992 (*Boston Globe,* June 19, 1995, p. 29). The revival of pallidotomies is based on the availability of improved imaging methods that better pinpoint the lesions. However, pallidotomies are at best, and at present, only a temporary relief of symptoms and not a cure. Refinements of the procedure may improve its results and reduce its side effects.

5 Among other experimental approaches is the implantation of electrodes in various areas. The Movement Disorders Program at Allegheny General Hospital in Pittsburgh, for example, is treating Parkinson tremors by implanting an electrode in the thalamus through a dime-sized hole drilled in the skull. A lead wire runs under the skin's surface to an impulse generator located in the vicinity of the collarbone (*Pittsburgh Post-Gazette,* September 2, 1997, p. C1). Called a thalamic stimulator, this device is similar in look and concept to the heart pacemaker. It is made by Medtronics Inc. and is intended not just for Parkinson's tremors but for non-Parkinson's tremors as well. The technique was pioneered by Richard Trosch, a neurologist at the Detroit Medical Center (*Detroit News,* August 25, 1997, p. D1).

6 At least one version of PD—referred to as "familial Parkinson's"—is thought to be inherited, and research is under way to identify the gene and its nature. A team headed by Roger Duvoisin of Robert Wood Johnson Medical School, New Brunswick, New Jersey, and Mihael Polymeropoulos of the National Institutes of Health has reported that the gene is located in a small region of chromosome 4 (*Science,* November 15, 1996). Once the gene's specific address is isolated, research can begin on possible ways to prevent and/or treat familial PD.

7 To keep current, browse the various web sites listed at www.santel.lu/SANTEL/diseases/parkins.html. This site contains links to twenty or more other web sites, each of which stresses a different aspect of PD. The best of these sites for general information is Harvard's web site: "The Parkinson's Web." You can also call the American Parkinson's Disease Association at 800-223-2732.

SUGGESTED RESOURCES

Riskind, P. (1996, Fall). "Multiple Sclerosis: The Immune System's Terrible Mistake." *On the Brain* (Harvard Mahoney Neuroscience Institute Letter), pp. 1–4.

Web Sites

ALS site (Doug Jacobson's site):
      www.phoenix.net/~jacobson/beatals.html
Alzheimer's disease:
      www.alzheimers.com
Huntington's disease:
      www.interlog.com/~rlaycock/what.html
Parkinson's disease:
      www.santel.lu/SANTEL/diseases/parkins.html

18

Mood Disorders and Addictions

Chemicals Gone Haywire

66 *As crude a weapon as the cave man's club, the chemical barrage has been hurled against the fabric of life.* 99

—Rachel Louise Carson,
The Sea Around Us

Depression, anxiety, addiction, and bulimia all have at least one thing in common: they result from chemical peculiarities and can be treated chemically. Whether the peculiarity stems from environmental pollution, weather conditions, genetic pranks, an unbalanced diet, or insufficient or inappropriate exercise, these disorders, which were once thought to be "in one's head" and evidence of a failure of will, all stem from excesses or deficiencies of some naturally occurring chemical. We will look at six disorders: addictions, anxiety, depression, manic-depressive illness, seasonal affective disorder, and eating disorders.

TOPIC 18.1 Addictions

Nature of the Disorder

In the vicinity of thirty million Americans are addicted to some substance, whether it's alcohol, cocaine, or a related substance. Addiction is defined as a compulsive craving for a substance in spite of destructive consequences for oneself and others. George Koob, director of psychopharmacology at Scripps Research Center, adds to this definition by stipulating that true withdrawal from addiction involves a negative affect during the absence of the preferred stimulus. Recent research has revealed that no matter which substance is involved, nicotine or alcohol, heroin or amphetamines (or chocolates and sex!), all abused substances activate the same circuit for pleasure. Originally identified through PET scans of cocaine-addicted patients, this circuit runs from the amygdala and anterior cingulum to the outer reaches of the two temporal lobes. The circuit is called the median forebrain bundle or, more popularly, the hedonic highway. The one kind of cell that is common among sites along this circuit is the D2 dopamine receptor. Three to four weeks after the addict's last cocaine dose, for example, this pleasure circuit shows unusually low activity on a PET scan. Cocaine, amphetamines, Ritalin, nicotine, and marijuana all inhibit reuptake of dopamine. (Addiction to caffeine does not follow this pathway; caffeine gets its effect by blocking the sedative adenosine.)

Apparently, the repeated episodes of unnaturally intense baths of dopamine provided by the cocaine or other addictive substance damage the effectiveness of the dopamine delivery system. This could be the result of reduced dopamine supply, deadened receptors, and/or shrunken cells that contain D2 dopamine receptor sites. In fact, Eric Nestler, of Yale University School of Medicine's Laboratory of Molecular Psychiatry, has found that the dopamine cells along this pathway in rats shrink by 25 percent (Goleman, 1996). Often addicts take their drugs not to feel high, but just to feel normal, to stop the craving caused by decreased dopamine function. The craving typically subsides after 1 to 1½ years, but many researchers believe that the pleasure circuit never really returns to normal.

George Koob refers to this increased threshold as "allostasis" (*Science,* October 1997). The new set point established by addiction requires increased volumes of the preferred stimulus. During withdrawal, or absence of the stimulus, levels of dopamine, opioids, serotonin, and GABA all decrease, while cortisol—the stress hormone—increases. All of this activity leads to pain, anxiety, dysphoria, and panic attacks.

Applications

CURRENT TREATMENTS

The craving apparently cannot go away; it can only be displaced through some combination of autotherapy (as in twelve-step self-help groups), psychotherapy, and/or pharmacotherapy. Because each addictive drug follows a slightly different path along the median forebrain bundle (also called the mesolimbic dopamine system), no single drug can work to restore dopamine balance. The real challenge is getting the addict to stay off the substance for at least a year and preferably for eighteen months. Any program must provide the support necessary to get through that withdrawal period. Two school-based programs get positive reviews in the literature (*APA Monitor,* September 1997, p. 30): Life Skills Training (LST) and the Midwestern Prevention Project (Project STAR). LST was developed by Gilbert Botvin of the Cornell University Medical College Project. STAR was developed by psychologists at the University of Southern California and has been fully implemented in the Indianapolis schools. Both use secondary school teachers to train students in specific coping skills and have yielded good results in stopping smoking, alcohol, and drug abuse. Both programs also build on the practice of encouraging extracurricular organizations to sponsor activities such as drug-free sports events, smoke-outs, and parent involvement. Another highly touted program, Drug Abuse Resistance Education (DARE), apparently fails to do more than reduce cigarette smoking (*Health Education and Behavior,* April 1997, pp. 165–176).

FUTURE POSSIBILITIES

1   Alan Leshner, director of the National Institute on Drug Abuse, believes that there will never be a "silver bullet"—one drug that addresses all addictions (Goleman, 1996). Rather, he feels that eventually a kind of "neurochemical cocktail" will be available for restoring balance to the dopamine system for each of the different addicting substances.

2   Researchers at the Brookhaven National Laboratory in Upton, New York, report encouraging results with a new drug—GVG—that in rodents and primates appears able to block both the high of cocaine and the craving for it. Human trials began in 1998. As of February 1999, GVG had not been released. Watch for the results on www.pet.bnl.gov, Brookhaven Lab's web site. GVG is an epilepsy drug that controls dopamine levels. Higher dopamine levels are associated with the cocaine high, and GVG appears to prevent these elevated levels. In a similar vein, naltrexone blocks the effects of alcohol on the opioid system. Alcohol enhances GABA (an inhibitor) and activates endorphins and dopamine. Naltrexone stands guard, preventing these chemical reactions.

TOPIC 18.2 Anxiety: A Family of Disorders

Nature of the Disorder

Fear: of being in death's hands (panic disorder), of being covered with germs and obligated to continually wash oneself clean of them (obsessive-compulsive disorder), of being in an airplane (phobia). These fears belong to a family of anxiety disorders that appears to be traceable to a common gene. Klaus-Peter Lesch and Armin Heils, of the University of Wurzburg, reported in *Science* (January 1997) that one variant of this "worry gene" leads to more serotonin production, while another variant leads to less. Discovery of this anxiety gene should expedite and clarify decisions regarding the nature of specific anxiety disorders and treatments for them.

About 25 percent of all Americans experience an anxiety disorder at least once in their lifetime, with women experiencing anxiety disorders at three times the rate of men. Annually, twenty-five million people in the United States suffer from anxiety disorders. Because of the stigma attached to overt acknowledgment and treatment of mental disorders, many people who suffer from anxiety disorders attempt to "self-medicate" with alcohol, tobacco, and nonprescription drugs. This contributes to an estimated $250 billion in lost wages and productivity for American employers.

Symptoms

Anxiety disorders have the following symptoms:

Obsessive-compulsive disorder: Worry caused by repeated thoughts that intrude through the day. They are typically accompanied by a repetitive series of behaviors. There are over five million cases of obsessive-compulsive disorder in the United States. Some are apparently caused by bacterial infections. For information, visit www.ocdresource.com or call 800-NEWS-4-OCD.

Phobias: The experience of crippling worry and tension in the presence of specific settings (such as snakes, airplanes, heights, or tests), often accompanied by trembling, stomach problems, headache, and muscle tension. Around eight million people in the United States have phobias. For information, contact Phobics Anonymous at 619-322-2673.

Panic disorder: A paralyzing sense of terror that strikes without warning, often accompanied by dizziness, racing heart, hyperventilation, and chest pain. Researchers suspect that panic disorder is closely related to disturbances, probably genetic, in the vestibular system of the brain, which controls our sense of balance. Panic attacks may be set off by a hypersensitive "suffocation alarm" in the body. Around six million people in the United States suffer from panic disorder. For information, call the National Institute of Mental Health hot line at 800-647-2642.

Generalized anxiety disorder (GAD): A tendency to expect the worst without clear evidence, with particular worries about finances, health, job, and family. Individuals often can't relax, sleep, or concentrate on the task at hand. This disorder affects the quality of work and home life, unlike pure stress. The approximately seven million

Americans with GAD know that their worry is excessive but can't do anything about it. For information, call 888-ANXIETY.

Applications

CURRENT TREATMENTS

Most anxiety disorders can be treated effectively with a combination of psychotherapy (especially cognitive and behavioral therapy) and pharmacotherapy (especially benzodiazepines and antianxiety agents such as Xanax and Valium and antidepressants such as Zoloft, Prozac, Paxil, and Luvox). Some anxiety disorders can be treated successfully with psychotherapy alone. Check with a therapist for specific treatment recommendations. Or take a look at Edward Hallowell's *Worry: Controlling It and Using It Wisely* (1997).

FUTURE POSSIBILITIES

Clearly more than one gene is involved in setting the stage for the various anxiety disorders. Each gene makes its own protein, and ultimately pharmaceuticals will be available to address specific gene activity.

To keep current on anxiety-related disorders, get on the mailing list of the Anxiety Disorders Association of America; 6000 Executive Boulevard, No. 513; Rockville, Maryland 20852; phone: 301-231-9350.

In addition, the National Institute of Mental Health maintains the following web site with breaking information on anxiety disorders: www.nimh.nih.gov/anxiety.

TOPIC 18.3 Depression

Nature of the Disorder

Depression is thought to be a malfunction of the monoamine neurotransmitters, including norepinephrine, serotonin, and dopamine. About seventeen million people experience one or more episodes of depression annually. One person in six will experience at least one depressive episode in a lifetime; the incidence within a depressive's family is even higher. Depression attacks all ages. Out of every six people whose depression is serious enough for hospitalization, one dies from suicide. Risk factors for depression include heart disease, Parkinson's disease, stroke, immune dysfunction, previous depressive episodes, and substance abuse. Factors that adversely affect an individual's chances for recovery include continual stress, coexisting medical and psychological problems, alcohol and substance abuse, and adverse socioeconomic circumstances.

The longer that symptoms go without diagnosis and treatment, the more resistant they become to treatment. About two-thirds of depressives seek help, yet about 90 percent of those seeking help are undertreated (for example, with a single visit and prescription from a primary care physician). One difficulty in treating depression is that the results of therapy are not immediate. Typically, improvement is not noticed for three to four weeks, and, with the expense of treatment, many depressives abandon therapy. Researchers at the Dean Foundation in Madison, Wisconsin, have estimated the average daily cost of treating depression to be about $12.25 per patient per day, but this cost is offset by a cost of $13.28 in unnecessary medical services for depressives who are not being treated for depression (reported in Veggeberg, 1997). Moreover, employers lose about $23 billion annually because of lost production and absenteeism associated with depression.

In a related series of findings, researchers have found that men with low cholesterol are three times as likely to experience depression and high stress and to die a violent death, including suicide (*British Medical Journal,* September 14, 1996, pp. 637 ff.). Both men with naturally low cholesterol (below 160) and men who have reduced their cholesterol by diet and/or medication show this tendency. Traditionally, we have thought that the lower the cholesterol, the better. But recent research suggests that the optimal level is between 160 and 199. Less is apparently not better. This phenomenon is attributed to its association with low serotonin, which is a metabolite of animal fat, along with cholesterol. Can't win for losing! (I am not aware of a similar study done with women. However, the same principle should work. Low cholesterol is associated with lower serotonin levels, and increasing serotonin is a treatment for depression.)

While we're on the subject of men and depression, men suffer depression at half the rate that women do, but they more often fail to get treatment. Depression is seen by many as "unmanly." Recent open discussions of male depression by such public figures as Dick Cavett, Mike Wallace, and William Styron have paved the way for a higher proportion of afflicted men to seek help. A good book on the subject of male depression is Terrence Real's *I Don't Want to Talk About It: Overcoming the Secret Legacy of Male Depression* (1997). Dick Cavett (1992) wrote about his recovery from depression through psychopharmacology combined with talking therapy.

One mitigating factor that accounts for the lower incidence of depression among men was discovered in 1998 by researchers at McGill University in Montreal. Using positron emission tomography, they found that men produce serotonin at a rate 52 percent higher than women. They speculated that in the past, warring and hunting men were subject to more stressors, so an abundance of serotonin became an adaptive trait with high survival value.

Symptoms

The symptoms of depression, according to Jerrold F. Rosenbaum (*On the Brain* [Harvard Mahoney Neuroscience Institute Letter], Spring 1996), include two or more weeks of

- Depressed mood
- Loss of interest or pleasure
- Excessive guilt
- Impaired concentration
- Fatigue and loss of energy
- Appetite and sleep changes
- Agitated or retarded motor behavior
- State of being suicidal

Scott Veggeberg, in *BrainWork: The Neuroscience Newsletter* (September–October 1997), adds these symptoms to the list:

- Unexplained aches and pains
- Unexplained crying spells
- Indifference toward former interests

- Social withdrawal

- Indecisiveness

- Feelings of worthlessness

- Overall negative affect, including anger, worry, agitation, anxiety, irritability, and pessimism

Four or five of these symptoms experienced daily over a two-week period should alert an individual to the possibility of being in a depressed state. Dysthymia, a milder form of depression, is characterized by the same symptoms but in less severe form; these less severe symptoms can last for more than two years.

Apparently, although some genetic causes have been acknowledged, depression is largely environmental in origin, as evidenced by the large variation in incidence rates across cultures. Myrna Weissman, a professor in the School of Public Health at Columbia University, headed up a ten-nation survey of depression (*Scientific American,* November 1996, pp. 24–25), using the same methods for all of the countries. (Note that the list doesn't distinguish between rural and urban areas. It would be interesting to know if rural areas have a lower incidence than urban areas.) The research revealed that the percentage of the population in each locale that would experience at least one depressive episode lasting one year or more was as follows:

Country	Percentage
Taiwan	1.5
Korea	2.9
Puerto Rico	4.3
United States	5.2
Germany	9.2
Canada (Edmonton, Alberta)	9.6
New Zealand (Christchurch)	11.6
Italy (Florence)	12.4
France (Paris)	16.4
Lebanon (Beirut)	19.0

This wide range of occurrence for depression certainly argues for strong cultural influences. On the other hand, Weissman (E-mail: mmw3@columbia.edu) found several patterns that held true for all ten countries:

1. Each country's rate was highly correlated with its divorce and separation rates, except for Lebanon, which has suffered war for the last fifteen years.

2. Women were twice as likely as men to suffer depression.

3. Separated or divorced men were more likely to suffer depression than separated or divorced women.

4. The average age of first depression fell into a fairly narrow range, from thirty-four in Italy down to twenty-four in Canada.

5. Manic depression (bipolar disorder) showed much less magnitude and variability across the ten countries, ranging from 0.3 percent in Taiwan to 1.5 percent in New Zealand. This confirms other studies that have posited a stronger genetic component for bipolar depression than for unipolar depression.

Applications

CURRENT TREATMENTS

❶ In a review in *Professional Psychology: Research and Practice* (December 1996), David Antonuccio and William Danton, both of the University of Nevada School of Medicine, and Garland DeNelsky, of the Cleveland Clinic Foundation, reported that psychotherapy, particularly cognitive-behavioral therapy or interpersonal psychotherapy, should be the treatment of choice for unipolar depression because of its superior long-term outcome and lower medical risk than either drugs alone or drugs combined with psychotherapy. Psychotherapy, then, is at least as effective as pharmacotherapy, even for severe depression. Furthermore, they assert, there is no evidence that drug treatment can improve the results of psychotherapy for depression, although psychotherapy can improve the results of drug treatment. Considering that the relapse rate for treating depression with drugs alone is upward of 60 percent, psychotherapy should always accompany pharmacotherapy. Antonuccio, Danton, and DeNelsky argue that medication should not be used to treat depressive children or adolescents and should be prescribed with caution for adults.

② Three classes of drugs are associated with the treatment of depression: tricyclic antidepressants (TCAs), monoamine oxydase (MAO) inhibitors, and selective serotonin reuptake inhibitors (SSRIs). The older tricyclics (Elavil, Pamelor) and lithium had unpleasant side effects and have been replaced by the SSRI drugs—Prozac, Zoloft, and Paxil (fluoxetine, sertraline, and paroxetine)—and MAO inhibitors (including the increasingly popular herb, St. John's Wort). Monoamine oxydase gobbles up extra neurotransmitters (including serotonin) in the synapse, and MAO inhibitors prevent such a feast, thus making more serotonin (among other neurotransmitters) available in the synapse. SSRI drugs supposedly work by preventing serotonin in the synapse that has not been absorbed by postsynaptic receptors from being reabsorbed by presynaptic receptors, thus keeping it available in the synapse for immediate and future absorption. Thus, if one has a low supply of serotonin, the proportion available for use is maximized. It is sort of like taking a bottle of water out of the refrigerator, taking a swig, and keeping it with you in case you want more, rather than putting it back in the fridge.

However, the monoamine system is complex, and its workings are not apparent. There are at least fourteen different subtypes of monoamine receptors, and it is terribly easy, and tempting, to over-simplify what happens: "Raise serotonin levels and you'll be happy." Yeah, right! It's not that simple. In fact, Ivan Goldberg of Columbia University, in an Internet posting (E-mail: ikgl@columbia.edu), writes, "It is very clear that SSRIs do not work as antidepressants by inhibit-ing the reuptake of serotonin. It is clearly established that 1 mg/day of fluoxetine is all that is needed to fully block the reuptake of serotonin. If blocking the reuptake of serotonin were both necessary and suffi-cient, patients would not need higher doses to get over their depres-sions. I know no patient who has had an optimal response to such a low dose."

Normally, patients take one 20-milligram capsule of SSRI (the actual range of doses is from 5 to 300 milligrams daily) for no more than one year, although some take it for longer periods. The possible side effects include the following:

- Weight loss (in fact, SSRIs have been found successful in treating some cases of bulimia)
- Delay in achieving orgasm (SSRIs have been prescribed to help some men with premature ejaculation problems) and/or failure to reach orgasm, although many accept this side effect because they are glad to feel good enough to have sex in the first place!
- Akathisia, or outbursts of temper and/or violence
- Gastrointestinal problems, fatigue, and nervousness

Many experts feel that SSRIs are overprescribed. More than 60 percent of SSRI prescriptions are written by primary care physicians or obstetrician-gynecologists who do not follow up with ongoing talk therapy and evaluation. Of the more than fifteen million SSRI prescriptions written annually, many are not written for depression but are given by sympathetic physicians to patients who are unsatisfied with the rough edges on their personality. Thus, SSRI drugs have become something of a cult phenomenon, a kind of plastic surgery for the persona, for people who want a quick fix to achieve social and career success.

Julian Whitaker, in his newsletter *Health and Healing* (January 1998), points out that over time, SSRIs can reduce the overall supply of serotonin. He prescribes instead tryptophan (an amino acid), which is the precursor of 5-HTP (5-hydroxytryptophan), and/or 5-HTP, the precursor of serotonin. Whitaker comments that supplying these raw materials to increase the production of serotonin has only a few mild side effects, the worst being occasional diarrhea. He says that daily doses of 50 to 100 milligrams of 5-HTP on an empty stomach are helpful for most people; some take 100 milligrams three times a day and others may take up to 900 milligrams daily. He recommends that patients start the prescription in the evenings, because 5-HTP can cause drowsiness.

In a study of 536 adult depressives, a research team led by Gregory Simon of the Center for Health Studies in Seattle compared three treatment groups, two using tricyclics (desipramine or imipramine) and one using an SSRI, fluoxetine (reported in the *Journal of the American Medical Association,* June 26, 1996). Their findings after six months of treatment were as follows:

- There was no difference among the three groups in the overall effectiveness of the drugs.
- There was no difference in the length of time it took the drugs to become effective.
- There was no difference in total cost.
- There was no difference in remission rates.
- Tricyclic users reported more side effects.
- Twenty-seven percent of tricyclic users discontinued medication early, compared with 9 percent of fluoxetine users.
- Forty percent of tricyclic users switched to another medication, compared to 20 percent of fluoxetine users.

Their conclusion: the patient and physician may choose whichever drug they prefer. Note that Paxil (paroxetine) appears to be the antidepressant of choice for patients suffering depression as a direct result of a heart attack (*Journal of the American Medical Association,* January 28, 1998).

3 Robert Hirschfeld, a psychiatrist with the University of Texas Medical Branch in Galveston, insists that the family of a depressive must become involved with the treatment. He believes that treatment for depressives whose families have not bought into the process is prone to failure (reported in Veggeberg, 1997).

4 Apparently women respond better to drugs that affect serotonin only, while men respond better to drugs that address both noradrenaline and serotonin. This is part of a growing body of research, such as that of Susan Kornstein of the Medical College of Virginia, on how the sexes and their respective hormonal profiles respond differently to drugs.

5 Many depressives self-medicate by resorting to nicotine (see Topic 6.6). Others self-medicate by abusing alcohol or drugs. Summarizing recent findings on the co-occurrence of substance abuse and mood disorders, Brenda Patoine (*BrainWork: The Neuroscience Newsletter,* May–June 1998) recommends the following for people suffering from both disorders:

- Stop drinking alcohol, even moderately; it interferes with depression medication.
- Get treatment from someone with expertise in both areas.
- Don't assume that treating one disorder will also treat the other one.

6 Leslie Taylor, of the Dean Foundation in Madison, Wisconsin, is confident that 80 percent of depressives can be satisfactorily treated but says that 35 percent of those who are treated abandon treatment within the first month. Taylor recommends intense follow-up and monitoring, such as scheduling visits in advance and having the therapist phone the patient from his or her office. In one study (reported in Veggeberg, 1997), Taylor found that twenty patients all completed a six-month treatment program that included such intense follow-up and monitoring of compliance.

FUTURE POSSIBILITIES

1 In addition to close monitoring and follow-up, another promising approach is what Martin Seligman of the University of Pennsylvania has dubbed a depression "vaccine" (*APA Monitor,* October 1994; see Chapter Twenty for more information on his work). He proposes that we train young people in optimism or, more precisely, in a positive explanatory style (see Topic 20.1). Seligman's research has shown that a negative explanatory style is associated with depression and that his model for a positive explanatory style is both (1) learnable and (2) effective in reversing and preventing depression. In experiments with ten- and eleven-year-olds and also with college freshmen, two years after learning the optimism model the younger subjects showed a 50 to 100 percent reduction in their depression rate compared to controls, while the eighteen-year-olds showed just a slight to moderate reduction. He is convinced that teaching a positive explanatory style at an early age, in effect, "immunizes" children against depression and possibly against other mental problems. With childhood depression rates roughly ten times greater now than two generations back, we should regard this finding as something of a mandate. In fact, the California legislature has mandated training in self-esteem as a weapon to crack the welfare cycle, but Seligman says that self-esteem training misses the mark. His explanatory style model doesn't.

2 On the pharmaceutical front, England has approved reboxetine (Edronax), which has been more effective than Prozac in treating severe depression. This new drug does not address serotonin; rather, it enhances the presence of norepinephrine. Also, for many centuries, Europeans have been using the herb hypericum (St. John's Wort). It has few, mild side effects and enhances serotonin, norepinephrine, and dopamine. At the time of this writing, Duke University psychiatrists were beginning a multisite, double-blind study in order to evaluate St. John's Wort as compared to Zoloft and a placebo; 336 depressed patients were to receive one of the three treatments, with the St. John's Wort dosage set at 900 milligrams per day.

3 One new line of research comes from Wayne Drevets of the University of Pittsburgh, who led a team that has discovered that the brains of depressive patients, compared to nondepressives' brains, are missing 40 to 90 percent of their glial cells in the anterior cingulum of the prefrontal cortex (a part of the "hedonic highway"— see Topic 18.1). On the other hand, these same depressive patients' regular neurons were all intact; just the glial cells were depleted. Glial cells provide structural support for neurons, as well as growth nutrients that provide the "fuel" that drives neurotransmitter production (*Newsday,* October 21, 1997, p. A8).

4 New York Medical College researchers report that approximately 25 percent of people who are hospitalized for depression or suicide appear to carry the gene for Wolfram syndrome (a form of diabetes that entails deterioration of eyesight) (*Molecular Psychiatry,* January 1998, pp. 86–91). Research is under way to determine how this knowledge can help in the treatment of depression.

5 Merck & Co. researchers reported in the September 11, 1998, issue of *Science* that a new drug code-named MK-869 appears to be a robust treatment for depression, targeting a heretofore mysterious chemical in the brain called substance P. Substance P is abundant in the area of the brain associated with the negative emotions, and the new drug appears to block substance P with far fewer side effects than Paxil or Prozac.

6 On the dietary front, researchers at the National Institutes of Health report a strong relationship between low levels of omega-3 fatty acids and depression, as well as other mental disorders. Omega-3 polyunsaturated fatty acids are found primarily in fish. A few fish high in omega-3 fatty acids are listed here:

Fish	Grams of Omega-3 Fatty Acids per 100 Grams of Fish
Raw mackerel	5
Raw salmon	4
Marinated salmon	4
Smoked salmon	3
Fillet of herring	3
Tuna in oil	2

In Asia, where fish consumption is high, depression levels are low. In several recent studies, fatty acid supplements led to a decrease in depressive symptoms and a decrease in schizophrenic hallucinations.

7 For the most current information on depression, get on the mailing list of the National Foundation for Depressive Illnesses; P.O. Box 2257; New York, New York 10116; phone: 800-248-4344.

TOPIC 18.4 Manic-Depressive Illness

Nature and Causes of the Disorder

Affecting about 1 percent of the population, manic-depressive illness (MDI, or bipolar disorder) is a more uncommon form of depression (see Topic 18.3) in which an exhilarating period of heightened physical and mental energy, which can last from days to weeks, spins out of control into a delusional state, which then typically crashes into a major depressive episode. The process is cyclical, with manic and depressive phases interspersed with normal periods. The composer

Robert Schumann suffered from it, and achieved with it, until his suicide by starvation in 1856. At present, the only known cause of the manic phase of MDI is the excessive presence of inositol, an enzyme that participates in the communication process between neurons.

Symptoms

The depressive phase of manic depression involves the same symptoms reported for depression (see Topic 18.3). Symptoms of the manic phase include "exaggerated optimism . . . , decreased need for sleep without feeling fatigue, grandiose delusions . . . , excessive irritability, aggressive behavior, increased physical and mental activity, racing speech, flight of ideas, impulsiveness, poor judgment, easily distracted [and] reckless behavior, i.e., spending sprees, rash business decisions, erratic driving, flagrant affairs" (Veggeberg, 1997, p. 2).

Applications

CURRENT TREATMENTS

Lithium is used to bind inositol in order to make it unusable, thus calming the communication process. Anticonvulsives are also prescribed for the manic phase. Antidepressants are sometimes used for the depressive phase, but drugs such as Prozac and Zoloft can trigger a manic episode.

FUTURE POSSIBILITIES

About fifteen groups around the world are attempting to isolate the genes associated with manic depression. Studies of twins lend support to the hunt; most believe that one gene is located on chromosome 18, while some are looking at chromosome 21.

For current information, contact the National Depressive and Manic-Depressive Association (DMDA) at 800-826-3632.

TOPIC 18.5 **Seasonal Affective Disorder**

Nature and Causes of the Disorder

Also called "winter depression," seasonal affective disorder (SAD) apparently results from the inefficiency of the body's system that produces melatonin (see more information on melatonin in Topic 7.9). Normally, the pineal gland produces melatonin in the absence of sunlight (even for blind people). This flooding of melatonin is apparently critical for sleep. In the morning, with sunrise, the presence of natural light (you can do the same thing with a good lamp) signals the pineal gland to shut down production of melatonin. This leads to alert wakefulness. In SAD, apparently, the pineal gland, fooled in some people by winter's darkness, continues to produce melatonin into the day, with a resulting inability to shake off the night's slumber.

Symptoms

Symptoms of SAD include inactivity, negative affect, weight gain, craving for carbohydrates, increased sleep time, decreased libido, and daytime sleepiness (Thayer, 1996). This disorder affects about 5 percent of the population, females more than males. It tends to let up in spring and summer, although a summer variant has been noted.

Applications

CURRENT TREATMENTS

Upon waking, the person with SAD is exposed to a bank of bright lights of about 2,500 lux (roughly equal to a window open to normal sunlight) for about two hours, looking directly at the light source from time to time. The individual, apparently "starved" for light, should experience a resetting of the body clock and an attendant return of a normal mood.

TOPIC 18.6 Eating Disorders

Nature and Causes of the Disorder

Statistics on eating disorders are difficult to assess, with some estimating that upward of one-third of all Americans suffer from one of the eating disorders to some degree. Anorexia nervosa (starving oneself), bulimia nervosa (dieting, binging, and purging), binge eating disorder (compulsive eating), anorexia athletica (compulsive exercising), night-eating syndrome (consuming over one-half of one's daily food after 7:00 P.M.), and nocturnal sleep-related eating disorder each have a complex set of causes, including biological, social, family, and psychological sources. While anorexia and bulimia primarily afflict females between ten and thirty-five years old (somewhere between 5 and 10 percent of anorexia and bulimia patients are males), cases have been reported from as young as six years of age to as old as seventy-six. The lower incidence among males is attributed to societal approval of the strong, muscular, more bulky image for males. In fact, many believe that the primary cause of eating disorders is the ideal image that daily forces itself upon readers, listeners, and viewers of the popular media. In South Korea, as recently as the 1970s, the ideal image for a female was full-figured. These women were thought to be more sexy, more beautiful, and more able to bear healthy children. But decontrol of broadcasting has unleashed a flood of Western body image material throughout the culture, so that today the diet industry in Korea is flourishing, with entrepreneurs hawking everything from diet pills to liposuction. The statistics for South Korea now roughly parallel those of the United States (*Los Angeles Times* release, October 26, 1997).

Symptoms

Symptoms for each of the disorders are complex and are best not summarized. They include such diverse behaviors as skipping meals, experiencing relationship problems, and talking excessively about food. Excellent profiles of the symptoms for each disorder are available at the web site for Anorexia Nervosa and Related Eating Disorders, Inc.: www.anred.com.

Applications

CURRENT TREATMENTS

Without treatment, one out of five people with eating disorders will die prematurely. Treatment reduces that rate to one out of thirty to fifty. About 60 percent of those who are treated recover, but not all make a full recovery. Current treatment could include one or more of the following: hospitalization, medication, dental work, individual counseling, group counseling, family counseling, nutritional counseling, and support groups. Consult a physician or mental health professional for specific recommendations.

FUTURE POSSIBILITIES

Although little research evaluation is available at the present, a promising new approach has been taken by Peggy Claude-Pierre. She has labeled eating disorders the "confirmed negativity condition" and has established a therapeutic environment that consists of twenty-four-hour unconditional love and support. The Montreux Counseling Centre in Victoria, British Columbia, is her residential treatment site. The treatment is expensive, has a high staff-to-patient ratio, and is based on a five-step process. Read about it in her book *The Secret Language of Eating Disorders* (1999); an abridged version is available on audiocassette from Random House (order at www.randomhouse.com).

Expect major discoveries in the next ten years. This field is relatively new. For a summary of current research on the physiology of appetite, see Topic 5.3. Follow new developments with these two web sites: www.eating-disorder.com and www.anred.com.

Also, contact Eating Disorders Awareness and Prevention, Inc., at 206-382-3587, and the National Association of Anorexia Nervosa and Associated Disorders at 847-831-3438.

SUGGESTED RESOURCES

Claude-Pierre, P. (1999). *The Secret Language of Eating Disorders: The Revolutionary New Approach to Understanding and Curing Anorexia and Bulimia.* New York: Vintage Books.

Foreman, J. (1996, December 17). "Anxiety: It's Not Just a State of Mind." *Boston Globe,* p. C1.

Goleman, D. (1996, August 13). "Brain Images of Addiction in Action Show Its Neural Basis." *New York Times,* p. C1.

Hallowell, E. M. (1997). *Worry: Controlling It and Using It Wisely.* New York: Pantheon Books.

Nemeroff, C. B. (1998, June). "The Neurobiology of Depression." *Scientific American,* pp. 42–49.

Real, T. (1997). *I Don't Want to Talk About It: Overcoming the Secret Legacy of Male Depression.* New York: Scribner.

Seligman, M.E.P. (1991). *Learned Optimism.* New York: Knopf.

Veggeberg, S. K. (1997, September–October). "The Big Story in Depression: What Isn't Happening." *BrainWork: The Neuroscience Newsletter* (Charles A. Dana Foundation), 7(4), 1–3.

Whybrow, P. C. (1997). *A Mood Apart: Depression, Mania, and Other Afflictions of Self.* New York: Basic Books.

Web Sites

National Institute of Mental Health site on anxiety disorders:
www.nimh.nih.gov/anxiety

Obsessive-compulsive disorder site:
www.ocdresource.com

Part Five

Emotions,
Motivation,
Stress,
and Burnout

Being in Control

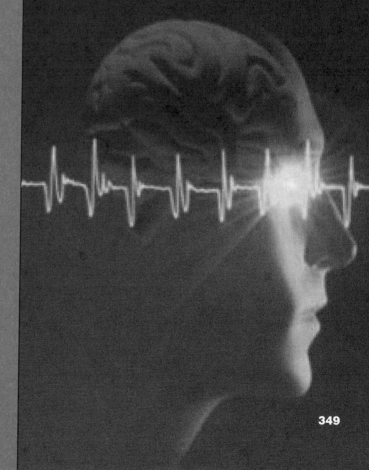

19

EQ, Call Home

Getting Savvy About Your Emotional Side

> **66 Anger raiseth invention, but it overheateth the oven. 99**
> —George Savile, Marquess of Halifax

*T*he word *emotion* comes from the Latin *emovēre* (*e* = away, *movere* = to move), which means to move out of or agitate. The etymology of the word is closely related to that of *motivation*. Both suggest action, in the sense of a state that is the opposite of standing still or being calm and laid-back. This action is related to an individual's goals: motivation is action in pursuit of a goal, while emotion is action resulting from situations that enhance

> "Emotion turning
> back on itself,
> and not leading on
> to thought or action,
> is the element
> of madness."
> —John Sterling

or threaten a goal. Hence, to the degree that I'm motivated, I'm pursuing a goal. To the degree that I'm emotional, I'm perceiving either a threat to my goal (negative emotion) or significant progress toward my goal (positive emotion).

Emotions weren't the subject of serious study by cognitive scientists until recently. This field of study is still young, and several theories are competing for followers. I have included in this chapter the material that appears to be most compatible with the overall direction of cognitive research.

TOPIC 19.1 A Model for Emotions

A review of several major recent works on the theory of emotions (Lazarus, 1991a; Plutchik and Kellerman, 1989; J. G. Thompson, 1988) suggests a five-step model to describe what might happen to someone during an emotional situation:

1. *The event:* Something happens (for example, a remark, a gesture, an accident) that potentially relates to one of the person's goals as either a threat or an enhancer.

2. *Perception of the event:* The individual becomes fully aware of the event (for example, through seeing, hearing, or reading).

3. *Appraisal of the perceived event:* The person determines whether or not the event relates to a goal. The value of the goal will directly affect the strength of the emotion.

4. *Filtering of the appraisal:* The status of the person's body (sleepy, alert, and so on) influences the intensity of her or his appraisal (for instance, very threatening or only mildly threatening). This filter can include past events with a strong emotional association. For example, the first funeral I attended was also my first introduction to the fragrance of gardenias. The nearness of gardenias still filters an event with a melancholy element. Joseph LeDoux (1996) writes extensively of this memory-emotion relationship.

5. *Reaction to the appraisal:* The person channels his or her appraisal into some form of coping (from the Middle French

couper, to strike or cut). The strength of the reaction is a direct function of the value of the goal concerned and the degree of certainty that the event will thwart or enhance attainment of that goal.

Applications

1 Know that the reaction to the appraisal (step 5) can be either cognitive or emotional. Normally, when goals appear to be thwarted or enhanced by an event, emotions precede cognitions. These emotions can last for less than a second or for a lifetime, partly depending on whether we decide to will the cognitive part of the reaction to ultimately subdue the emotional part. See Seligman's ABCDE technique (Topic 20.1) for ways to cognitively short-circuit a disturbing emotional event.

2 Analyze events and filters, and look past situations for patterns. *(Contributed by Rick Bradley)*

3 Put up these mottoes:

"We are disturbed not by things, but by the views we take of things."

—**Epictetus,** *The Encheiridion*

"There is nothing either good or bad, but thinking makes it so."

—**William Shakespeare,** *Hamlet*

TOPIC 19.2 **The Appraisal Filter: What Triggers Emotions**

The notion that the mind serves as a kind of gatekeeper for emotional behavior is at the core of the cognitive theory of emotions. The opposing theory, developed earlier in this century, is that a person reacts automatically, without mental intervention, whenever certain emotion-evoking stimuli appear. Today, a consensus is emerging that embraces the notion that events with the potential to elicit emotional responses must first pass the appraisal activity of the mind. This appraisal activity is typically rapid. It may have several components and may be sequential or simultaneous, but researchers agree that it takes place between stimulus and response. When we receive "news" from our environment, it is neither good nor bad until our appraisal process has passed judgment.

Antonio Damasio (1994) has written an entire book that explores the appraisal process. The thrust of his book is startlingly unexpected: he says that rational decision making and planning cannot occur without access to the emotions. In dozens of ways, Damasio illustrates the point that emotions are necessary for reasoning to occur. Studying patients with brain damage that had severed the frontal reasoning area from the amygdala's emotional resources, he found that these patients performed normally on traditional intelligence tests but were unable to plan and make rational decisions. They appeared to be locked into the present and past. Damasio explains it this way. People form "dispositional representations" (such as traits, values, opinions, and schemas) over time; these representations are linked to "somatic markers" that register pain or pleasure when the representations are activated. His brain-damaged patients who were unable to experience their somatic markers couldn't make decisions. They were stymied, with no gut-level pointers to favor one alternative over another. They were unable to anticipate future pain or pleasure in connection with specific alternatives. With their decline in emotion came a concomitant decline in reasoning. Or, as Damasio put it, "The powers of reason and the experience of emotion decline together" (p. 77). Far from being an "unwelcome intrusion" or a "supernumerary mental faculty" (p. 75), the emotions are inextricably linked to rationality as the critical link in evaluating our perception of everyday events.

> **"Reason generates the list of possibilities. Emotion chooses from that list."**
>
> —Richard Wrangham and Dale Peterson, *Demonic Males*

Lazarus (1991b, p. 827) has identified six ingredients that comprise the act of appraisal:

1. *Goal relevance:* Does this news relate to one of my goals or values?

2. *Goal congruence or incongruence:* Does this news serve to enhance or thwart my goal or value?

3. *Goal content:* How is my ego involved? (The answer helps to tap the relevant emotional response—for example, anger versus guilt).

4. *Source of blame or credit:* Where does the responsibility lie, with me or thee?

5. *Coping potential:* Can I handle the consequences of this news or event?

6. *Future expectations:* Will things get better or worse?

Lazarus calls the first three elements *primary appraisal* and the last three *secondary appraisal.* Lazarus's secondary-appraisal elements resemble Seligman's three elements of learned optimism: personalization, pervasiveness, and permanence (see Topic 20.1).

These six mental-appraisal interventions control the gate that determines whether or not a perceived event leads to an emotional response. In reading the manuscript of this book, Rick Bradley commented that no one could use this process without a personal commitment to truth.

Applications

1 Commit your goals to writing. Document situations that promote or thwart goal attainment. Analyze for patterns. *(Contributed by Rick Bradley)*

2 Make a personal commitment to truth. *(Contributed by Rick Bradley)*

3 Make a list of your personal hot buttons—the words, phrases, actions, or situations that cause you to become angry or emotional. Determine in advance what you will do to alter your normal response the next time one of your hot buttons is pushed.

TOPIC 19.3 Emotions' Home: The Body as Catalyst

J. G. Thompson (1988) identifies four ways in which biological mechanisms can influence emotion-related neurotransmitter levels. These mechanisms can influence the degree to which an emotion gets expressed, depending, of course, on the prior or simultaneous appraisal process. It's as though these four mechanisms serve as a kind of catalyst, influencing the *degree* but probably not the *kind* of emotional response. They are

1. *Genetic vulnerability:* This is a very complex issue. See Chapter One for a discussion of this topic.

2. *Diet:* Many of the chemicals that block or facilitate the development and transmission of emotion-related neurotransmitters can, at this point, only be manufactured within the body. See Kolata (1976, 1979) for a more complete treatment.

3. *Hormone level:* In the complex interaction of hormones with neurotransmitters, hormone levels that are too high or too low can sometimes have a dramatic impact on the intensity of an emotional response. Research seems to be stuck at the chicken-and-egg stage here: do hormones control neurotransmitter levels or vice versa? Although it is not clear how the causal relationship works, it is clear that hormone levels are related to emotional response. As an example, we know that estrogen levels are directly related to left-brain activity (Kimura and Hampson, 1990).

4. *Circadian rhythm:* The degree to which we are able to satisfy the sleep-wake cycle and live with the twenty-five-hour day can affect our hormone and neurotransmitter levels, intensifying our emotional response. That is why we may be more testy, tearful, or giggly during sleep deprivation or jet lag.

Applications

1 The single most effective way to keep emotional responses comfortable is to stay in good physical condition, using the right diet (see Chapter Five), aerobic exercise plan (see Chapter Eight), sleep habits (see Chapter Seven), and stress management program (see Topic 20.5).

2 If Application 1 doesn't work satisfactorily, consult appropriate cognitive scientists, such as neurosurgeons, psychiatrists, or neuropharmacologists.

3 See the discussion of personality arousal systems in Topic 21.4.

TOPIC 19.4   The Origins of Violence

Wrangham and Peterson (1996) write that among the primates, the capacity for violent aggression (including battering, rape, and infanticide) has been common to all, but its actual expression is a function of vulnerability. Vulnerability itself is a function of one's degree of social protection. Apes who live in smaller groups, such as orangutans and chimpanzees (the latter live in groups of two to nine), experience more violence, because the individual apes have fewer resources for forming protective alliances. Those who live in larger groups, such as bonobos, or pygmy chimpanzees (with an average of seventeen), and gorillas, benefit from the social protection available from the implicit alliances in the larger group. Safety is found in numbers (p. 143).

The forces that cause a species to evolve into larger groups have to do with the "costs" associated with grouping. These costs include the availability of snack food from the jungle floor. Groups are easier to form when abundant snack food is available. Bonobos developed into peaceable, nonaggressive colonies because of the topography of their homeland south of the Zaire River, where tree fruits and floor plants abound. Lots of snacks, lots of cohorts, lots of alliances and friendships, and lots of peace. Chimps, on the other hand, evolved north of the Zaire River, where the dearth of floor plants forced them to split up in order to forage. No snacks, competition for scarcer foods, few alliances to prevent aggression. Humans evolved three million years ago in a savanna near the chimps. Our need to forage makes us more like the chimps and less like the peaceable bonobos.

This pattern is an excellent example of the interaction of nature and nurture. Although aggression is common to all apes (nature), some had social protection and some didn't (nurture), resulting in the more peaceable bonobo and the more aggressive chimps and humans. Wrangham and Peterson (1996) point out that specific acts of aggression are caused by pride in one's status. If this status (for example, the status of the alpha male or the All-American running back) is never challenged, then there is no need for violence. One's nature doesn't express itself. But dominant primates, especially males, do not like to grovel. So when their dominance, or position in the hierarchy, is challenged, a quick mental calculation ensues, something like this:

1. The status quo is disturbed by a perceived threat.
2. The dominant member evaluates the threat and asks: "Can I win or not?"
3. If the dominant member feels confident of winning, then aggression takes place.
4. If the dominant member feels unsure of winning, then she or he avoids immediate engagement, delaying until an effective coalition can be formed.

In a related area of research, serotonin levels have been shown to be highly subject to nature-nurture interaction (*APA Monitor,* April 1997). Stress combined with severe living conditions or a harsh upbringing can lower levels of serotonin. Low levels of serotonin are associated with poor impulse control and have been shown to accompany alcoholism, aggression, depression, and suicide. In addition to low serotonin levels, researchers have identified another neurotransmitter that increases aggression and sexual violence—nitric oxide (NO). Rats low in NO are missing the gene that encodes for the enzyme nitric oxide synthase, from which NO emerges. The enzyme monoamine oxidase A (MAO-A) is known to break down chemicals associated with overreactivity to stress; it is lower in more violent men. The gene encoded for MAO-A, which is sex-linked, has been identified by researchers at Massachusetts General Hospital (*Science,* October 22, 1993).

Applications

1 Understand that the most effective way to deal with aggression is by forming alliances. When you are vulnerable to the aggressive advances of someone else, form friendships and alliances that are publicly visible to your aggressor. There is safety in numbers. Consider the aggressor-boss in the movie *9 to 5* and the effective coalition formed by the three secretaries! Remember that once an alliance has been formed, whether to aid or thwart aggression, the members need ongoing grooming for long-term stability and dependability. "Grooming" among primates typically involves picking nits; among humans, this would translate into subservient behavior, such as offering to help with some unpleasant chore—covering the phones, washing dishes, and the like.

2 Find a way to boost the serotonin levels of significant people in your life who are prone to aggression: dietary fats, aerobic exercise, serotonin reuptake inhibitors, and success experiences are several options.

TOPIC 19.5   Coping Mechanisms

Once we have appraised a situation as threatening or enhancing our well-being, we tend to follow one of four coping styles (J. G. Thompson, 1988):

1. *Verbal:* This left-hemisphere response suggests, for example, an individual who responds with vindictive thoughts but without any accompanying physiological arousal.

2. *Nonverbal:* This right-hemisphere response suggests, for example, an individual who feels upset but doesn't know why; that is, he or she doesn't relate the upset to an event or emotion but instead may think it's the flu.

3. *Both verbal and nonverbal:* This style is characterized by a high cognitive response (left hemisphere) and a high somatic response (right hemisphere), as when someone thinks, "I'm really letting my anger get me down."

4. *Neither verbal nor nonverbal:* With this style, a person chooses to see the event as neutral (neither threatening nor enhancing) with respect to her or his goals and values; therefore, no cognitive (mental) or somatic (physical) coping is required. This coping style is similar to the one in Seligman's ABCDE technique (see Topic 20.1). With respect to this style, I like to recall Graham Greene's comment that hatred is a failure of the imagination.

Applications

1 Understand that positive emotions are responses to events that are perceived as enhancing attainment of one or more of our goals. Positive emotions are healthy; they promote a feeling of satisfaction with life. We can increase the experience of positive emotions by changing our goals if not enough enhancing events happen, changing our environment (see Sternberg's three problem-solving strategies in Topic 22.3), or changing our interpretation of events (we may be seeing events as threats when, in fact, they are enhancers, even if they are only weak enhancers).

2 The emotion of angry hostility places us in a double bind: both holding it in and venting it are bad for the heart (Ironson and others, 1992) and the immune system. The secret to dealing with anger is to express it without getting angry. Get it out, deal with it, and get over it.

3 Daniel Goleman (1995) presents a multitude of methods for considering alternative responses that could follow an appraisal of an event as threatening or enhancing. One example is "Red Light, Yellow Light, Green Light," developed by Yale University psychologists as a part of the Social Competence Program for Troup Middle School, New Haven, Connecticut:

Red light: Stop and reflect when the emotion is first recognized.

Yellow light: Consider alternative interpretations and actions.

Green light: Pick the most satisfying ones and implement them.

4 Seligman's ABCDE model is an excellent approach to reconsidering how an event is appraised. See Topic 20.1.

5 Bruce Arnow, an assistant professor in the Stanford University School of Medicine's Psychiatry and Behavioral Sciences Department, points out (1996) that many people with weight problems tend to eat as a way of assuaging emotions. Table 19.1 lists more constructive strategies for managing one's emotions.

TOPIC 19.6 The Behavioral Approach to Emotions

Most of the research on emotions has occurred at the molar, or behavioral, level. Many efforts have been directed toward listing the primary emotions. Various studies have worked with anywhere from five hundred to several thousand words that describe emotions. Most of these studies have tended to accept two primary dimensions of emotion: *evaluation* or *valence* (pleasant versus unpleasant) and *level of arousal* (alertness versus sleepiness). Lazarus (1991a) points out that pleasure and pain, rather than being emotions, are some of emotions' raw materials. The "circumplex" model (see Figure 19.1) locates each of the emotions on an *x-y* coordinate system based on these two dimensions. Anger, for example, would be located in the area suggesting unpleasant evaluation and high arousal. Sadness would be located in the area of unpleasant evaluation and low

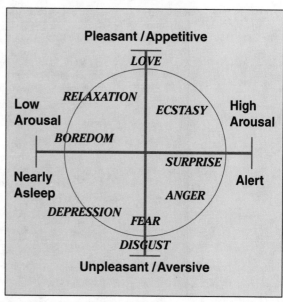

Figure 19.1. The Circumplex Model of Emotion.
Note: Only a sampling of emotions has been placed on the circumplex.

Table 19.1. Strategies for Emotional Management.

Emotion	Anger	Frustration	Anxiety	Sadness	Boredom or Loneliness
The Task	Eliminate the cause of anger or release the anger itself.	Overcome a sense of failure or disappointment.	Relieve or get away from your worries.	Restore your enthusiasm and positive mood.	Find companionship.
Suggestions	Perform a productive physical task. Talk or act it out with a pet. Do aerobic exercise (walk or run around the block). Act it out with loud music, dance, shout. Play a physical game such as darts, have a pillow fight, use a punching bag. Meditate in your own way.	Write out your accomplishments. Make a prioritized list and begin knocking off items in order. Put together a modest party. Read Jack Canfield and Mark Hanson's *Chicken Soup for the Soul.* Read Seligman's *Learned Optimism* (1991). Read friends' comments in your old school annuals. Do a favor for someone.	Practice Benson's "relaxation response" (Benson with Klipper, 1990). Call an old friend. Engage in a repetitive activity like crafts or weeding. Read a favorite writer. Meditate. Reminisce through old picture albums. Enjoy a good TV or video comedy. Write to someone or in your journal.	Exercise. Act on the source of the sadness (visit it, write about it, or commemorate it). Plant or arrange some flowers. Immerse yourself in nature. Play music that touches your soul. Enjoy watching a romantic comedy like *Sleepless in Seattle.* Compare yourself to others with a greater loss.	Rent some movies and watch with a friend. Join a club with your interests in mind. Take a class or workshop. Visit others who are lonely (in hospitals, nursing homes). Get active on a committee for your children's school, your alma mater, or your office. Be a volunteer (a Big Brother or Sister, for example).

Source: Based on "Cognitive-Behavioral Therapy for Bulimia Nervosa" by Bruce Arnow, in J. Werne (Ed.), *Treating Eating Disorders,* 1996, San Francisco: Jossey-Bass.

arousal, excitement would be located in the area of pleasant evaluation and high arousal, and so on. A good current discussion of the circumplex method of listing and differentiating emotions is available in Plutchik and Kellerman (1989).

A currently popular taxonomy of emotion (Baker, Zevon, and Rounds, 1994) maintains that positive emotions do not differ in quality, only in degree, and that negative emotions differ in kind as well as degree. Accordingly, love, surprise, delight, and ecstasy would all be similar in kind but different in degree, from less intense to more intense. Some have maintained that there are only three pure emotions—ecstasy, terror, and despair—with all other emotions simply combinations of those three (see Schlosberg, 1954); however, most researchers seem to list somewhere between six and eight primary emotions. A popular model, for example, is the hexagon (see Rozin, 1997), which includes around the six points of the hexagon, in order, happiness, surprise, fear, sadness, disgust, and anger. The clearest listing of the emotions that I have found is that of Plutchik and Kellerman (1989). In Table 19.2, I have italicized the column labeled "Subjective State," which contains the terms we commonly refer to as the emotions. But from glancing through the other columns, you can readily see that there are many ways of describing emotional activity.

Applications

❶ Use Table 19.1 to become aware of your emotional patterns. If you find a pattern that is dysfunctional for you, make up your mind to deal with it either through learning a self-control skill on your own (such as Seligman's ABCDE model, described in Topic 20.1) or through engaging in a therapeutic relationship with a counselor.

❷ For serious emotional disorders that leave someone unable to hold a job or a relationship, consult with a neurosurgeon, psychiatrist, or psychopharmacologist.

Table 19.2. Emotional States and Parallels.

Biological Regulatory Process	Behavioral Expression	Adaptive Function	Subjective State	Personality Trait Expression
Avoid	Withdraw	Protection	*Fear*	Timid
Approach	Attack	Destruction	*Anger*	Quarrelsome
Fuse	Mate	Reproduction	*Joy*	Affectionate
Separate	Distress signal	Reintegration	*Sadness*	Gloomy
Ingest	Eat	Incorporation	*Acceptance*	Trusting
Eject	Vomit	Rejection	*Disgust*	Hostile
Start	Examine	Exploration	*Expectation*	Demanding
Stop	Freeze	Orientation	*Surprise*	Indecisive

Source: From *The Measurement of Emotions*, Vol. 4 of *Emotion: Theory, Research, and Experience,* edited by R. Plutchik and H. Kellerman, 1989, Orlando: Academic Press. © 1989 by Academic Press, Inc., Orlando, Florida 32887. Reprinted

TOPIC 19.7 The Biological Approach to Emotions

Compared to other aspects of brain research, the emotions have suffered from relative inattention. Much of the research on emotion has been conducted at the behavioral, or molar, level and has been centered on the researchers' play toy of choice—factor analysis. Factor analysis begins with a large amount of measurement data and attempts to find patterns (factors, clusters) within those data.

As the Decade of the Brain draws to a close, a current project is attempting to map the various emotions onto specific brain regions. One of the tests that is used to determine how many distinct emotions exist is isolation by brain area. Two emotions had been so located by the time of this writing: fear, involved in a pathway terminating in the amygdala (see LeDoux, 1996), and disgust, whose primary activity is in the basal ganglia (see Rozin, 1997). It is of interest to note that obsessive-compulsive disorder, which is associated with excessive reactions to conditions that cause disgust, also involves a disturbance in the basal ganglia.

Diagnostic Extreme	Ego-Defense Regulatory Process	Coping Style	Social Control Institution
Anxious	Repression	Avoidance	Religion
Aggressive	Displacement	Substitution	Police, war, sports
Manic	Reaction	Reversal	Marriage and family
Depressed	Compensation	Replacement	Religion
Hysterical	Denial	Minimization	Psychiatry, shamanism
Paranoid	Projection	Blame	Medicine
Obsessive-compulsive	Intellectualization	Mapping	Science
Borderline	Regression	Help-seeking	Games, entertainment

by permission of the author and publisher.

At the time of this writing, very few molecular, or microscopic, findings are etched in stone. For example, the region of the brain called the amygdala has been strongly positioned as the "rage" center; however, the actual research findings have been inconsistent. Although surgical removal of the amygdala can eliminate rage, bizarre eating patterns and sexual behaviors sometimes follow. The inconsistency of the results is attributed to two factors: (1) the redundancy principle, which suggests that because of duplication of function it is impossible to pin any one function to a single location in the brain, and (2) the difficulty of absolute surgical precision, which makes it impossible to perform a procedure precisely the same way on two successive occasions—that is, without invading a neighboring area that was previously left intact or leaving an area untouched if it was removed in a previous, similar operation. Nonetheless, some general principles are emerging (see Borod, 1999):

- A pleasure center seems to exist called the median forebrain bundle, which runs parallel to the pain center.

- A pain center seems to exist called the periventricular system, which runs from the hindbrain or medulla to the forebrain, parallel to both the median forebrain bundle and the RAS (see Chapter Two).

- Frontal structures are associated with emotional expression and right-hemisphere posterior cerebral structures are associated with emotional perception.

- Stimulation of the posterior hypothalamus excites the sympathetic nervous system (the fight-or-flight response).

- Stimulation of the anterior hypothalamus excites the para-sympathetic nervous system (the relaxation response).

- Damage to the parietal, temporal, or occipital lobes results in no appreciable change in emotional activity.

- Damage to the frontal lobe can result in major increases or decreases in emotionality.

- The left frontal lobe houses positive and negative emotional processes; the right frontal lobe houses only negative processes.

- If the same site in one human's brain is stimulated at different times, different emotions can be produced.

- Hormone levels influence the intensity of an emotional response.

- Levels of specific neurotransmitters affect one's propensity toward specific emotions; for example, high melatonin leads to depression, low melatonin to high sexual appetite, high epinephrine to elation, high prolactin to anxiety. For more on this topic, see Kolata (1976, 1979).

- Each emotion seems to have unique physiological responses; for example, anxiety leads to greater phasic increases in systolic blood pressure, anger leads to greater phasic increases in diastolic blood pressure, fear leads to vasoconstriction or narrowing of the blood vessels (which makes the skin pale), and anger leads to vasodilation or widening of the blood vessels (which makes the skin flush). Progress is slow in describing these unique responses because of the difficulty of eliciting one single emotion and measuring its accompanying processes (J. G. Thompson, 1988).

- The physiological responses to emotion (cardiovascular, musculoskeletal, thermoregulatory, respiratory, gastrointestinal, urinary, and reproductive) can result in related disorders, such as headache, stomach pain, blushing, sweating, Raynaud's disease (vasoconstriction in the digits of the hands and feet), muscular tightness, and diarrhea.

- These physiological disorders seem to be mutually exclusive: people who sweat don't blush and people who blush don't have chronic headaches.

- One emotion elicits different physical symptoms in different individuals: anger can elicit headache in one person, sweat in another.

- Physiological disorders are only partially connected to conscious awareness of one's emotional state.

Application

Develop an appreciation for the fact that emotional responses, whether weak or strong, have complex origins. They may be attributed to brain structure, body chemistry, stress, habit, or personal cognitive intention. Do not assume that you know the cause of someone's emotionality. If knowing the cause is important, consult with a variety of specialists, such as neurosurgeons, neuropharmacologists, or psychiatrists. Never forget that although many emotions can be controlled by personal will, some people's emotions are held captive by aberrant biochemical forces.

TOPIC 19.8 EQ Versus IQ

Daniel Goleman legitimized research on emotions in one fell swoop with the publication of *Emotional Intelligence* in 1995. Again looms that word *intelligence*. Sternberg (see Topic 22.3) calls intelligence "mental self-management." Extending that definition, then, emotional intelligence (EI) is a specific aspect of intelligence, namely, "emotional self-management." Research clearly shows that emotional and mental intelligence are all part of the same bundle. Sternberg's definition of mental self-management, then, should include emotional components.

In fact, we can find all of the elements of Goleman's five-part model of EI (1995, pp. 43 ff.) covered in some aspect of Chapter Twenty-One (on personality) or Chapter Twenty-Two (on intelligence) of this book. The five-part model of EI was actually developed by Yale University psychologist Peter Salovey (Salovey and Mayer, 1990). The five elements are presented in Table 19.3.

The five elements of EI are closely related to the anatomy of emotions presented in the first four topics of this chapter. The five-

---

Table 19.3. The Salovey-Goleman Five-Part Model of Emotional Intelligence, with Its Analogues in the Big-Five Personality Theory and in Sternberg's and Gardner's Theories of Intelligence.

Element	Explanation	Analogue in the Big Five	Analogue in Sternberg	Analogue in Gardner
Self-awareness	Ability to monitor one's own feelings	O3: Feelings (*high*)	A part of contextual intelligence	Intrapersonal talent
Self-management	Ability to handle one's own feelings in such a way that they do not disrupt one's life	N: Negative Emotionality (*low*)	A part of contextual intelligence	Intrapersonal talent
Self-motivation	Ability to remain in Csikszentmihalyi's "flow" state	C: Conscientious-ness (*high*)	A part of componential intelligence	None
Other-awareness	Awareness of emotions in others and an attendant empathy for them	O3: Feelings (*high*) A2: Straightfor-wardness (*mid*) A3: Altruism (*high*) A6: Tender-minded-ness (*high*)	A part of contextual intelligence	Interpersonal talent
Relationship management	Social compe-tence that enables one to interact smoothly with others	Negative Emotionality (*low*) Extraversion (*high*) Agreeableness (*high*)	A part of contextual intelligence	Interpersonal talent

Source: Adapted from *Emotional Intelligence* by D. Goleman, 1995, New York: Bantam Books.

step model of emotion presented in Topic 19.1, for example, can be plugged into the Salovey-Goleman model in several ways. Self-awareness relates to step 3, which is the point at which an individual consciously or unconsciously appraises the significance of an event. Self-management relates to step 5, which involves consciously planning how to cope. Self-motivation refers to the way in which an individual uses step 5—coping—to manipulate the events of step 1. By manipulating environmental demands and challenges with respect to his or her personal resources, a person can influence the degree to which he or she stays in the "flow" channel (see Topic 30.3). Other-awareness relates to step 2 of the five-step model and how the individual perceives the behavior of others. Relationship management relates to phase 5, coping strategies.

Personally, I prefer the five-step model presented in Topic 19.1 because it presents emotion as a process that moves from an event through appraisal to coping. Whatever model is used, education in emotional self-management should be a high priority. In a study released in the November 1993 issue of the *Journal of the American Academy of Child and Adolescent Psychiatry,* researchers concluded that from 1976 to 1989, children aged seven to sixteen showed a significant worsening in 45 out of 118 specific emotion-related problems, with improvement coming in only one area. Whatever model we choose, it is clearly time to address the issue.

Applications

1 A new area of school curriculum development has sprung up around EI called SEL, for Social and Emotional Learning. For information on specific course material, write: The Collaborative for the Advancement of Social and Emotional Learning (CASEL); Yale Child Study Center; P.O. Box 207900; 230 South Frontage Road; New Haven, Connecticut 06520-7900.

2 Get hold of *How to Raise a Child with a High EQ,* by Lawrence Shapiro (1997), or *Playwise: 365 Fun-Filled Activities for Building Character, Conscience, and Emotional Intelligence in Children,* by Denise Chapman Weston and Mark S. Weston (1996).

3 Try identifying hot lines and web sites that provide good advice. Two examples: call Beverly Mills's Child Life hot line at 800-827-1092 or E-mail her at bevmills@aol.com.

④ Review Reuven Bar-On's 133-item Bar-On Emotional Quotient Inventory (EQ-i), published by Multi-Health Systems Inc. (Bar-On, 1996). Visit their web site at www.mhs.com.

⑤ Review the 33-item EI inventory developed by Nicola Schutte and her associates at Nova Southeastern University, Fort Lauderdale, Florida (Schutte and others, 1998).

⑥ Another EI instrument is the Executive EQ, authored by R. Cooper and A. Sawaf (1997).

⑦ Peter Salovey and J. D. Mayer have developed a CD-based EI instrument. Find out more at www.virtent.com/ei.

TOPIC 19.9 Emotions Versus Moods

Robert Thayer (1996, p. 5) points out that emotions are caused by events, whereas a mood is a "background feeling that persists over time." Moods do not have a causal factor the way emotions do (see Topic 19.1). Rather, moods reflect the state of one's body on two dimensions: relaxation and energy level. An individual's energy level is closely related to the time of day (the circadian rhythm, as described in Topic 7.2), with the highest energy typically in late morning and early evening (see Figure 19.2). During the low-energy periods—morning, midafternoon, and late evening—people are most susceptible to increased tension. More introverted people exhibit high energy earlier in the day, while more extraverted people exhibit high energy later. So move the curve in the figure somewhat to the left for Introverts, somewhat to the right for Extraverts.

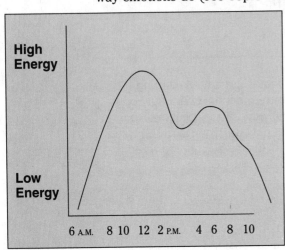

Figure 19.2. Natural Highs and Lows in Energy During Normal Waking Hours.
Source: Adapted from *The Origin of Everyday Moods: Managing Energy, Tension, and Stress* by Robert E. Thayer, 1996, New York: Oxford University Press.

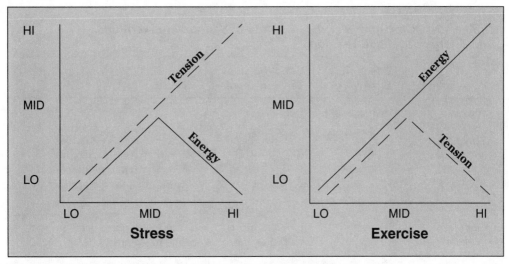

Figure 19.3. The Effect of Stress and Exercise on Energy and Tension.

Thayer finds that positive moods are associated with high energy levels, negative moods with tension. The most positive are high-energy, low-tension moods; the most negative are high-tension, low-energy moods. Depression is an example, according to Thayer, of an intense bad mood, with low energy and high tension. Mood is highly susceptible to personal control: we can alter our mood. Stress and exercise have the most profound effect on mood, as illustrated by Figure 19.3. The various methods traditionally used to alter mood are presented in Table 19.4. Note that most methods can potentially affect both tension and energy.

The final word is that events don't cause moods. Moods are the result of your body state, which is determined by the interaction of biorhythm, diet, exercise, atmosphere, sleep, stress level, and drugs. Moods affect how we interpret events. Hence, they are an important part of the filter that affects the appraisal of events described in Topics 19.1 and 19.2.

Applications

The Applications for this topic appear in Table 19.4.

Table 19.4. Changing Mood: The Effect of Various Interventions on Energy Level and Tension.

Intervention	Effect on Energy Level	Effect on Tension Level	Notes
Yoga	Increase	Decrease	
Ten-minute brisk walk	Increase	May decrease	Energy level is enhanced for thirty to ninety minutes afterward; fatigue disappears within one to two minutes of beginning walk.
Aerobic workout	Increase	More vigorous workouts more likely to reduce	Energy increase occurs about one hour later.
Sugar snacks	Immediate increase	Increase	Energy level falls below pre-snack level one hour later.
Good night's sleep (seven to eight hours)	Increase	Decrease	Loss of sleep decreases energy and increases tension.
Nicotine	Increase	Decrease	Lasts for only a few minutes.
Alcohol	Increase	Lessens inhibitions, but doesn't really decrease tension	Effect is temporary and only at the beginning of the episode.
Caffeine	Increase	Increase	
Benzodiazepine (Valium)	Increase	Decrease	
Increase in negative ions (cleaner air)	Increase	Decrease	

TOPIC 19.10 **A Note on Deception**

In two recent major works on the problem of deception (Ekman, 1985; R. Rogers, 1997), the results are clear: we cannot reliably determine whether another person is lying. To quote Paul Ekman (1985, p. 97): "No clue to deceit is reliable for all human beings, but singly and in combination they can help the lie catcher in judging most people."

The most common technique for detecting lies is to observe whether or not a person exhibits stressful symptoms while answering questions about which she or he has or could have "guilty knowledge"; this might be done with a polygraph, interviews, film analysis, or other methods. So, for example, if I answer "No!" when I'm asked if I ate the last piece of cake and then my skin turns pale, I develop a nervous twitch in my shoulder, and I look away, normally you would suspect that I'm lying.

Ekman has identified two common exceptions to this rule. He calls one the Brokaw hazard, which consists of judging a person's responses without baseline data; it is named for NBC's Tom Brokaw, who interpreted circumlocution in an interview as a sign of lying, not allowing for the fact that many people both tell the truth and use circumlocution. If I *always* respond with a paling of the skin, a twitch, and a glance out the window, that pattern of behavior does not indicate any more stress than usual; hence it is no clue to deceit.

Ekman calls the second exception the Othello error. In Shakespeare's *Othello,* Desdemona was afraid that Othello wouldn't believe her. Her concern led to stress symptoms during her encounter with him, and, as a result, he didn't believe her. Her stress came not from lying, but from worrying about being thought to be lying: "Why I should fear I know not, Since guiltiness I know not; but yet I feel I fear" (V, ii, 38–39). This reflects the fact that some people can lie without exhibiting stress, and some can exhibit stress symptoms without lying. A low voice can lie and a high voice can tell the truth. My stress symptoms could appear as a result of my fear of not being believed, rather than of getting caught.

The bottom line is that stress symptoms reveal only one thing—stress. Stress is not deceit. The polygraph is not a lie detector; it is a stress detector and should be called that. For a good discussion of the severe limitations of the polygraph as a lie detector, see Ekman

(1985) or R. Rogers (1997), or obtain the definitive evaluation of the polygraph published by the Office of Technology Assessment (OTA) in Washington, D.C. The OTA concluded that the claims for the polygraph's validity (published for the most part by polygraph vendors) were not supported by scientifically acceptable research findings. Daniel Greenberg, editor of *Science and Government Report,* a Washington newsletter, sums it up as follows: "The survival of the polygraph is a monument to the yearning of wishfully thinking scientific illiterates for certainty where none exists."

In a new line of research, but one not yet admissible into U.S. courts, Lawrence A. Farwell of Human Brain Research Laboratory, Inc., in Burke, Virginia, uses sensors to establish brain wave patterns in suspects. The device builds on the fact that a specific memory network established in the brain is measurably activated when recalled. Each subject gives off regular brain wave patterns when perceiving meaningless objects. When the subject perceives a familiar object, the memory network associated with it is instantly activated, appearing as a kind of "murmur" on the screen. Referred to as Farwell Brain Fingerprinting, this new technique depends on the skill of the operator in presenting visual stimuli that only a guilty person would know.

Applications

1 Don't rely on a polygraph as an absolutely reliable employment screening device.

2 Ekman (1985) provides an appendix that lists thirty-eight questions to use in assessing the probability that a person is lying. If you must frequently render judgments on whether people are lying, use Ekman's list as a guide.

3 Follow the development of Farwell Brain Fingerprinting as an aid in ascertaining guilty knowledge.

SUGGESTED RESOURCES

Damasio, A. R. (1994). *Descartes' Error: Emotion, Reason and the Human Brain.* New York: Grosset & Dunlap.

Ekman, P. (1985). *Telling Lies.* New York: Norton.

Goleman, D. (1995). *Emotional Intelligence.* New York: Bantam Books.

Goleman, D. (1998). *Working with Emotional Intelligence.* New York: Bantam Books.

Lazarus, R. S. (1991a). *Emotion and Adaptation.* New York: Oxford University Press.

LeDoux, J. (1996). *The Emotional Brain: The Mysterious Underpinnings of Emotional Life.* New York: Simon & Schuster.

Plutchik, R., and Kellerman, H. (Eds.). (1989). *The Measurement of Emotions.* Vol. 4 of *Emotion: Theory, Research, and Experience.* Orlando: Academic Press.

Rogers, R. (Ed.). (1997). *Clinical Assessment of Malingering and Deception* (2nd ed.). New York: Guilford Press.

Thayer, R. E. (1996). *The Origin of Everyday Moods: Managing Energy, Tension, and Stress.* New York: Oxford University Press.

Thompson, J. G. (1988). *The Psychobiology of Emotions.* New York: Plenum.

Motivation, Stress, and Burnout

Taking Charge of Your Life

> **Action may not always bring happiness; but there is no happiness without action.**
> —Benjamin Disraeli

What is motivation and how can we increase it? The word *motivation* derives from the Latin *motivus,* a form of *movēre,* which means "to move." The difference between being motivated and unmotivated, then, is whether or not the subject in question is moving. A classic example of an unmotivated person is the so-called couch potato, who sits or lies unmoving while watching seemingly endless hours of television. The remote-control zapper is the only thing that moves.

Generally, motivation is described as goal-oriented behavior. The vast literature on the subject of motivation revolves around two aspects of goals: how an individual rates his or her chances of attaining a goal successfully and how he or she rates the value of the goal itself. The problem with motivation comes when individuals who have a good chance of success choose not to pursue a goal that they value highly.

For most of us, when life is going well, whatever that means to us individually, we are motivated. When adversity knocks us down, those of us who are motivated get back up and get on with life. The less motivated tend to become resigned to their fate and to accept what life hands them. You've heard the expression, "When the going gets tough, the tough get going." I think that statement refers to motivation. In this chapter, we will take a careful look at the difference between those of us who find it easier to bounce back and those who find it harder, and we will explore ways to compensate for that difference. We also will look at stress. If motivation is behavior in pursuit of a goal, then stress is how we feel when our pursuit of a goal is thwarted.

We have been talking about motivation at the molar, or environmental, level. Research is pointing to mounting evidence of a molecular, or biological, basis for goal-oriented behavior. It is important to remember that in all probability, 50 percent of the variance in motivation can be accounted for by our genetic inheritance. Therefore, our levels of testosterone, cortisol, guanosine monophosphate, and other "molecules of emotion" (Pert, 1997); the constitution of our endorphin gene; the distribution of the various kinds of immune cells in our system; and our hemispheric dominance—all of which affect our motivation, or level of action—are essentially set from conception. The research indicates that we primarily influence these levels downward. This means, for example, that the pursuit of hardiness allows us to fully utilize our genetic endowment of natural killer cells but probably does not increase our normal level. On the other hand, allowing stress, pessimism, and negative feelings to dominate our minds can actually lower our motivational resources.

At the risk of oversimplifying, the physiological processes that accompany a motivated state can be summarized as follows:

- Optimal functioning of the immune system (see Topic 14.2)

- Optimal functioning of the cerebral cortex (cortical alertness; see Chapter Two)

- Moderate activation of the limbic system (moderate stress; see Chapter Two)

- Optimal diet and exercise (see Chapters Five and Eight, respectively)

- Effective functioning of the "pleasure center" of the brain (see Topic 19.7)

The degree to which we see ourselves or others as more or less motivated can be accounted for by either attitude or physical makeup. We can't change our physical makeup without resorting to pharmaceuticals, surgery, or genetic engineering. In a serious case, we might wish to consult a team consisting of a neurosurgeon, a psychiatrist, a neuropsychologist, and a genetic engineer to explore the possibilities of getting fixed. Otherwise, we must explore more molar, or environmental, approaches. If we choose not to tamper with nature, we can at least maximize what we've got by ensuring that our nurture is as good as it can be.

As we scan the current writing on motivation, two closely related approaches rise to the surface: Seligman's work on optimism and Cousins's work on hardiness.

TOPIC 20.1   Seligman: Optimism Versus Helplessness

Martin Seligman, in his book *Learned Optimism* (1991), describes how rats and humans learn to be helpless. When either rats or humans experimentally learn that they have no control over their environment, they give up trying to exert control. Whether the bothersome stimuli are electroshocks or noise, unsuccessful attempts to stop them are followed by defeatist despair. Seligman has found three ingredients of this learned helplessness among humans, which he contrasts to learned optimism. The three ingredients are *personalization, permanence,* and *pervasiveness.* Depending on how we typically respond to success or adversity along these three dimensions, we are described as optimistic or pessimistic. In Table 20.1, I have summarized the healthy, more motivated explanatory style and the less healthy, unmotivated explanatory style.

> "I had rather have a fool to make me merry than experience to make me sad."
>
> —William Shakespeare, *As You Like It*

Table 20.1. Seligman's Explanatory Styles.

Explanation of Adversity

Optimist	Pessimist
It's someone else's fault (external personalization).	It's my fault (internal personalization).
It's only temporary (not permanent).	It's gonna last forever (permanent).
It won't affect other areas of my life (limited pervasiveness).	It'll affect every area of my life (universal pervasiveness).

Explanation of Success

Optimist	Pessimist
I made it happen (internal personalization).	Someone else made it happen (external personalization).
This is one in a line of many successes (permanent).	It'll never happen again (not permanent).
The effect will ripple throughout my life (universal pervasiveness).	It won't help me in any other areas of my life (limited pervasiveness).

Seligman concludes from his research that the optimistic explanatory style is associated with high motivation, success, achievement, and physical and mental health, whereas the pessimistic explanatory style is associated with the opposite traits. In addition, he finds that certain pessimistic people who constantly ruminate about their misfortune in life and brood about the pessimistic aspects of personalization, permanence, and pervasiveness are at high risk for depression.

Notice that the preferred explanatory styles are opposite in their response to success or adversity: the more healthy (optimistic) explanatory style for success (internal, permanent, and pervasive) is in fact unhealthy (pessimistic) as a way to explain adversity. Conversely, the more unhealthy (pessimistic) way to explain success (external, temporary, and limited) is the healthy (optimistic) way to explain adversity. Figure 20.1 illustrates this model as a flowchart.

Benjamin Libet, a neurophysiologist at the University of California, San Francisco, has demonstrated that brain activity precedes consciousness. Hence, he concludes, intentions are spontaneous and actions are intentional. We choose our actions based on a spontaneous set of alternatives, so there is a point in time before an emotional reaction during which we can select a more optimistic response, as opposed to a more pessimistic one. See Restak (1991).

A word of warning. The goal of understanding the explanatory style is not to create a world of Pollyannaish optimists. Too much optimism, like too much pessimism, is typically counterproductive. On the other hand, psychologists Katri Raikkonen and Karen Matthews, of the University of Pittsburgh School of Medicine, report that people with more pessimistic outlooks have an average blood pressure that is about five points higher (both systolic and diastolic) than that of optimists. In addition, among people who have suffered one heart attack, pessimism predicts a second, more lethal heart attack more accurately than physical condition. And a University of Michigan research team headed by Christopher Peterson has reported that people (especially males) who "catastrophize" events, seeing them as part of a worldwide pattern of evil and pain, tend to

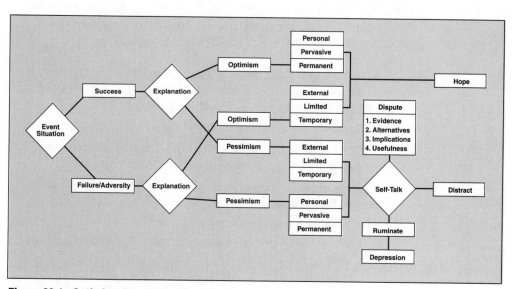

Figure 20.1. Optimism-Pessimism Flowchart.
Source: Designed by the Center for Applied Cognitive Studies, based on the work of Martin E. P. Seligman in *Learned Optimism*, 1991, New York: Knopf.

die before age sixty-five. Moreover, they are more likely to die by suicide or accident (*Psychological Science,* March 1998).

Applications

❶ Get a copy of Seligman's *Learned Optimism.* It is an easy read, intended for the layperson. He provides both an adult's and a child's version of his Explanatory Style Questionnaire, from which you can obtain a sense of how you compare to the rest of the population with respect to optimism and pessimism. The questionnaire also includes much research on the ability of the explanatory style to predict job or sports success, and it has a fascinating section on psychohistory—the ability of the explanatory style to predict the future (specifically, presidential elections). A computer-scored version of the Explanatory Style Questionnaire is available from Martin Seligman at 215-898-2748 in Philadelphia.

❷ Learn to use Seligman's ABCDE model. Seligman has found success in teaching a form of learned optimism to people with a pessimistic explanatory style, using the ABCDE approach. "ABC" refers to how we react negatively to success or adversity, while "DE" refers to how we can rethink the pessimistic reaction into an optimistic one. The letters are defined as follows:

> *A (Adversity).* Recognize when adversity hits. For die-hard pessimists, successes are a form of adversity; they say, "It won't last," "I was just lucky," or "Too little, too late."
>
> *B (Beliefs).* Be aware of what you believe about the adversity.
>
> *C (Consequences).* Be aware of the emotional and other consequences of your belief about that adversity.
>
> *D (Disputation).* Question whether your beliefs are the only explanation. For example, ask:
>
> - What is the evidence for my beliefs?
> - What are other possible explanations for what happened?
> - What are the implications of my believing this way, and do they make it worth holding on to my beliefs?
> - How useful are my beliefs? Do I or others get any benefits from holding on to them, or would we benefit more if we held other beliefs?

E (Energization). Be aware of the new consequences (feelings, behaviors, actions) that do or could follow from a different, more optimistic explanation or set of beliefs.

Here is an example of the ABCDE model as I applied it to a specific situation. My train of thought went like this:

1. I didn't finish this chapter by the end of the Thanksgiving holiday as I promised my wife and myself I would do. *(Adversity)*

2. I'm an incurable procrastinator who'll never meet my goals. *(Beliefs: a personal, pervasive, and permanent explanation, which is therefore pessimistic)*

3. I might as well abandon this project and settle for a life of less ambitious projects. That way, my wife won't be disappointed with me when I miss deadlines. *(Consequence)*

4. Wait a minute! Lots of writers set unrealistic deadlines. Besides, my wife and I did several things together and with her parents that had a very positive impact on our relationship. And if sticking to my schedule were so all-fired important to her, she could have insisted on doing some of those things without me. *(Disputation)*

5. I'll talk about my schedule with her and get her input on whether the remainder of the schedule is important to her. If not, I'll push my deadlines back. If so, I'll ask her assistance and cooperation in finding ways to make more time for writing. I really don't want to give up this project. It's exciting, even if it is a little off-schedule. *(Energization)*

❸ If you or someone you know would like assistance in developing a more optimistic style, select a psychotherapist who practices cognitive therapy, a directive therapy aimed at changing the way a client perceives her or his environment, which is closely allied with Seligman's research.

❹ If you are a ruminator (someone who talks silently and continually to himself or herself in a negative vein, as in "I'm going to fail. I'm no good . . ."), then you need to learn more than just a more optimistic explanatory style. You need to learn how to jerk away from the hold that pessimistic thoughts have on you. Seligman suggests several distracting techniques in his book, including wearing a rubber band on your wrist (snap it when you start ruminating) and creating physical distractions (such as slapping the wall or doing isometric exercises), as ways to pop the pessimistic preoccupation out of your mind.

5 For some people, visualization techniques are effective both for removing pessimistic thoughts and for encouraging optimistic ones (see Gawain, 1978). Here is an example. First, get a clear picture of the unpleasant thought in your mind, with your eyes closed. Then, as though you were turning a television control knob, make the image lighter and lighter until all you see is white light. Slowly bring it back into view, continuing to make it darker until all you see is blackness. When the unpleasant image reappears, take control of it and reduce it to whiteness or blackness, whichever you prefer. You can do the same with sounds in your head that are unpleasant and stressful, such as parental scripts: try turning up the imaginary volume knob until they are so loud that they sound like static; then gradually turn them down until they are inaudible.

6 Seligman has developed a technique with which you can assess the attributional style of a public figure, such as your mayor or coach, by studiously watching television clips and reading newspaper and magazine accounts. If you send $3.00 (as of this writing), Seligman will send you the necessary instructions to conduct a CAVE (content analysis of verbatim explanations). Mail to: Dr. Martin Seligman (or Peter Schulma); Department of Psychology; University of Pennsylvania; 3815 Walnut Street; Philadelphia, Pennsylvania 19104-6196.

7 Michael Lewis of the Robert Wood Johnson Medical School (formerly Rutgers University Medical School) in Piscataway, New Jersey, reports that most girls grow up with a pessimistic explanatory style. Parents and teachers tend to lavish more praise on boys. Be aware of this tendency and be sure to encourage young girls to attribute their successes to their ability and their failures to bad luck.

8 Seligman has conducted extensive research on the benefits of teaching young children how to be in control of their explanatory style. The results of this research, along with practical applications and exercises for young children, are presented in *The Optimistic Child* (Seligman, Reivich, Jaycox, and Gillham, 1995).

TOPIC 20.2 Cousins: The Four Ingredients of Hardiness

Norman Cousins (1989), who himself recovered from three life-threatening illnesses, became a primary popularizer for the new field of psychoneuroimmunology (see Topic 14.2). Cousins summarizes a large body of research and experience with a quote from Seneca: "It is part of the cure to wish to be cured." This attitude—wanting to play an active role in curing oneself—is the essence of the moti-

> **"A light heart lives long."**
>
> —William Shakespeare,
> *Love's Labour's Lost*

vated person. Cousins calls it "hardiness" and says that it is composed of four ingredients. I have summarized them as follows:

1. *Positive expectations (versus negative expectations):* Expecting successful outcomes for oneself and others

2. *Relaxation (versus stress):* Dissipating stress through appropriate methods

3. *Positive emotions (versus negative emotions):* Maintaining a sense of humor and joyfulness

4. *Active role (versus passive role):* Being a doer, not just being done unto

Applications

1 Rosenthal and Jacobson (1968) lit the torch on the power of the self-fulfilling prophecy, or the Pygmalion effect. Their lesson is simple: expect bad things and bad things tend to happen; expect good things and good things tend to happen. See also Topic 32.3.

2 Topic 20.4 provides abundant information and suggested Applications for ways to dissipate stress.

3 Give yourself permission to be humorous and to enjoy the humor of others. Explore the various ramifications of humor in Chapter Nine.

4 Focus on positive emotions. See fewer horror films, more inspirational films; listen to music in a major key. In one study, students who were randomly assigned to watch films of Mother Teresa had higher levels of salivary immunoglobulin A, a measure of the level of immune-system functioning, after viewing than did students assigned to watch films of Nazis.

5 The Society for the Preservation of Barbershop Quartet Singing in America has documented the positive effect of singing on health. Call 800-876-SING for more information. *(Contributed by Jack Wilson)*

6 Give a damn! Robert Sternberg (see Topic 22.3) says that three basic strategies are available to affect the world around us: change me, change thee, and change the situation. Use them. Don't stick with a strategy type that's not working. If you do what you've always done, you'll always get what you've always gotten!

7 The Eastern concept of Chi is defined as the force we feel when our life is in balance. A study of Eastern philosophy, science, and literature will lead us in the direction of self-control, which is the essence of optimism and hardiness.

TOPIC 20.3   Selye and Trait Dissonance

Hans Selye once wrote of the rabbit and the turtle. Some of us approach life more like a rabbit, running from place to place, nibbling when we can, shooting off in all directions. Others approach life more like a turtle, proceeding methodically from point to point with careful attention to detail, taking things one at a time. Both extremes are healthy. What is unhealthy, or stressful, is trying to be different from our nature. For example, the rabbit says to her or his turtle spouse, "You never want to go anywhere or do anything." The turtle, feeling guilty, decides to become a rabbit for the night and go bar-hopping with the rabbit spouse. That, Selye says, is what causes stress—being untrue to our nature.

It is stressful to attempt to be someone different from who we are, to try to be solitary when our nature is to be gregarious. Being true to our nature is, in some ways, the ultimate goal (as in "to thine own self be true . . ."). Attempting to be something different is an obstacle to that goal. Along with Selye's work, a growing body of literature points to the fact that congruence between people's nature and the nature of their activities (whether at work, at play, or in their home life) is a crucial prerequisite for contentment with their pursuit of the goal. In order for them to be fully motivated, their personality traits, talents, special abilities, values, and beliefs should be compatible with their life tasks. Don't expect a recluse to be motivated to sell, a creative thinker to be motivated to be a good proofreader day in and day out, or a sow's ear to be happy in the role of a silk purse. (See the discussion of the behavior concordance model in Topic 13.6.)

Applications

1 To what degree do you expect others to be like you—to use your vocabulary, to walk at your speed, to talk as fast or slowly as you do? Do you feel that people are inferior to you if they talk more slowly than you do? (This is a classic source of misunderstanding between a New Englander and a Southerner.) Be aware of these judgments, and don't let such surface behaviors be mistaken for indicators of ability. (Rick Bradley recalls a former manager whose perception of a co-worker was that he was "slow" because he had an unhurried gait.)

2 When you feel pressured to change your personality to meet with a spouse's, friend's, or boss's approval, it's time to sit down with that person and talk it through. If you are unsuccessful, you may need to bring in a third party (counselor, consultant, friend) to help establish the necessity of maintaining your differences in personality and behavior. Don't ignore the conflict; that will only lead to resentment and may rupture the relationship.

TOPIC 20.4 What Is Stress and How Can We Relieve It?

If motivation is action, then the study of motivation is the study of why some people act while others don't. Biologically, the definition of inaction is death. People who are continually thwarted from goal attainment enter into a kind of living inaction, or living death. The term "burnout" has come upon the scene to describe those who are alive but not active (see Topic 20.7). What is burnout? Most simply, it is the result of unrelieved stress; it can be reached through one of two routes: more intense, shorter-term stress or less intense, longer-term stress (Golembiewski, 1988).

What exactly is stress? Jeffrey Gray (1971) defines stress, along with fear and anxiety, as one of the emotions. (See Chapter Nineteen for a discussion of emotions.) An emotion is a reaction to an actual, expected, missing, or removed reinforcing event (a reward or a punisher). Fear is a form of emotion associated with the desire to terminate, escape from, or avoid a dangerous event, which might be internal or external. Anxiety differs from fear in that fear deals with actual or threatened dangers, whereas anxiety deals with imagined or unreal dangers (R. J. Campbell, 1989). Because it includes both fear and anxiety, stress may be defined as the emotion that results from the desire to terminate, escape from, or avoid a real or imagined, current or imminent, negatively reinforcing event. This negatively reinforcing event is usually referred to as a *stressor*. More simply, stress occurs when something interferes with a person's goal attainment. Or, put another way, stress occurs when the body's normal homeostasis has been disturbed (Sapolsky, 1994). The "something" that interferes is the stressor. Stressors can be anything from fear-arousing enemies to anxiety-arousing fantasies.

> "He who has health, has hope; and he who has hope, has everything."
>
> —Arabian proverb

One's *perception* of an event or situation as goal-deterring is crucial in determining its actual effect as a stressor. Woody Allen has said, "Eighty percent of success is showing up." Accordingly, 80 percent of the effect of a stressor is our perception of it as deterring us from a goal. Or, put another way, if I do not perceive an event as keeping me from pursuing and attaining my goals, I do not perceive it as stressful. Stress, then, is in the eye of the beholder. The critical test for a situation's having achieved stressor status is whether the individual feels out of control. Stress is the point at which an event or circumstance makes the individual say, "I have lost control of my destiny." Or, as Chinua Achebe borrows from Yeats in the title of his novel, *Things Fall Apart.* More fully:

> *Turning and turning in the widening gyre*
> *The falcon cannot hear the falconer;*
> *Things fall apart; the center cannot hold;*
> *Mere anarchy is loosed upon the world.*
>
> **—William Butler Yeats, "The Second Coming"**

Just as the falconer feels the falcon slipping out of reach, so the stressed individual feels life's goals falling below the horizon, out of sight. There is no light at the end of the tunnel. There is no balm in Gilead. Things are out of control.

Stressors are not only negative and hostile, as when we are evicted from a home; they may also be positive and friendly, as when we move into a new home. In both cases, prolonged stress can be harmful, causing us to feel the need to get away from the stressor.

When stress occurs, our bodies mobilize for one of the three F's: freeze, fight, or flee (the fight-or-flight syndrome). This mobilization includes the following changes:

- Dilation of the pupils, for maximum visual perception even in darkness

- Constriction of the arteries, for maximum pressure to pump blood to the heart and other muscles (the heart goes from one to five gallons pumped per minute)

- Activation of the adrenal gland to pump cortisol, which maintains pupil dilation and artery constriction by stimulating the formation of epinephrine and norepinephrine, sensitizing adrenergic receptors, and inhibiting the breakdown of epinephrine and norepinephrine

- Enlargement of the vessels to the heart to facilitate the return flow of blood

- Metabolism of fat (from fatty cells) and glucose (from the liver) for energy

- Constriction of vessels to the skin, kidneys, and digestive tract, shutting down digestion and maximizing readiness for the fight-or-flight syndrome

Control of this process lies in the hypothalamus, which acts as a control console. Stimulation of the front part of the hypothalamus calms the emotions (the parasympathetic nervous system response), while stimulation of the back section activates the mobilization processes (the sympathetic nervous system response). This is known as the general adaptation syndrome (GAS). The term *general adaptation syndrome* originated with Hans Selye (1952); a complete and more technical, but highly readable, description of it can be found in R. Williams (1989).

Normally, stress comes and goes, like the tides. Fears and anxieties, for most of us, subside shortly after their onset. Ira Black (1991) reports that a sympathetic nervous system stimulation of thirty to ninety minutes can result in a 200 to 300 percent increase in enzyme and impulse activity for twelve hours to three days and, in some cases, for up to two weeks. But what happens when fears and anxieties don't subside? What happens when stressors don't go away and the feelings of fear and anxiety persist over time? In a word, the high levels of cortisol become toxic. During this sustained period of GAS, when the posterior hypothalamus is active, the performance of the immune system (see Topic 14.2) is seriously impaired. Minor results of this stress-related impairment include colds, flu, backaches, tight chest, migraine headaches, tension headaches, allergy outbreaks, and skin ailments. More chronic and life-threatening results can include hypertension, ulcers, accident-proneness, addictions, asthma, infertility, colon or bowel disorders, diabetes, kidney disease, rheumatoid arthritis, and mental illness. Killers that can result include heart disease, stroke, cancer, and suicide. In addition, chronic stress can result in energy depletion, depression, insecurity, impotence or frigidity, apathy, emotional withdrawal, confusion, insomnia, chronic fatigue, helplessness or hopelessness, anxiety, lack of concentration, and poor memory.

Thomas Kamarck, of the University of Pittsburgh, and his team of researchers report that in a study of 901 Finnish men, those exhibiting the highest mental stress also showed blood vessel blockages similar to those associated with smoking and elevated cholesterol (*Circulation,* December 2, 1997, pp. 3842–3848). Further research is under way to determine the degree to which prolonged stress causes plaque buildup in the arteries, leading to higher risk for stroke and atherosclerosis. Sonya Lupien, of Montreal's McGill University, has found that prolonged high levels of cortisol shrink the hippocampus, with resulting memory impairment (*Nature Neuroscience,* May 1998). Meanwhile, a new study led by Elizabeth Gould, of Princeton University, and Bruce McEwan, of New York's Rockefeller University, has found that marmoset monkeys manufacture thousands of new neurons in the hippocampus every day. Surely, they avow, humans do also. (In October 1998, Fred Gage and a group of Swedish associates announced the first observed regeneration of brain neurons.) What this suggests is the following process:

1. Prolonged stress produces sustained high levels of cortisol.

2. The hippocampus shrinks as a result.

3. The production of new neurons is significantly reduced.

4. Memory, mood, and other mental functions are affected.

In a separate review of the literature on stress, McEwan and Schmeck (1996) summarize by identifying five clear markers for stress-related physical damage: blood pressure, blood sugar, cholesterol, cortisol, and abdominal fat. If one or more of these five have not been affected, then we may conclude that for the individual in question, stress-related damage has not been sustained.

How do we prevent stressors from occurring or stop them once they begin? The simplest answer lies in the word *control.* If we resign ourselves to the inevitability of long-term stress, it will continue to ravage our bodies. However, if we decide that we have some degree of control and can limit or prevent stressors, the effects of stress can be minimized or even eliminated.

Applications

❶ If any of the disorders listed above affect you or those close to you, confirm with your physician the possibility that they are stress-related. Then identify and list the stressors that cause a continued feeling of tightness in the chest, rapid heartbeat, acid stomach, and so on. Consider specific ways you can control each stressor, using the techniques in the following Applications. You might also seek the assistance of a psychotherapist who is trained in stress-reduction strategies.

❷ *Relax:* Meditation, hypnosis, deep breathing, napping, saunas, and just resting quietly—all these and other methods are equally effective. Research says that meditation techniques are no more effective than other relaxation techniques (see Druckman and Bjork, 1991). Popular magazines and other media commonly advertise or otherwise feature commercial "relaxation techniques" that consist of some mechanical, sensory, or meditative technique. As a general rule, unless you really want to spend money to learn to relax, just go to the library and read Herbert Benson's classic, *The Relaxation Response* (1990). The "Joy Touch," which can only be learned in workshops—

at a charge, of course—is an example of a commercial approach with no data to suggest that it is any more effective than Benson's relaxation response. I'm reminded of a favorite saying of mine: "Meditation is not what you think."

The state of mind during hypnosis is no different from that of the normal, awake, alert mind. Hypnosis is a guided form of conscious selective attention and dissociation characterized by suggestibility. Even the best subjects do nothing under hypnosis that they wouldn't do otherwise. See an excellent summary of research on hypnosis in the *Harvard Health Letter,* April 1991, pp. 1–4.

3 *Escape:* Do anything that "takes your mind off" the stressors, such as reading, watching television, listening to music, pursuing hobbies and crafts, or cooking. When our minds are filled with such activities, limbic arousal shuts down and cortical arousal takes over. As we take part in a totally absorbing pursuit, any activity in the posterior hypothalamus moves to its forward area and to subsequent parasympathetic arousal.

4 *Exercise:* Although any exercise is helpful in relieving stress, aerobic exercise is best. The simplest definition of aerobic exercise is any physical activity that keeps the heart pumping at elevated levels continuously for twelve to thirty minutes. Jogging, swimming, and brisk walking are aerobic, for example, while tennis, golf, and basketball are not (unless they are played nonstop; see Appendix C for more examples). For further discussion, see Covert Bailey's excellent book, *The New Fit or Fat* (1991). See Chapter Eight for more discussion on this topic.

5 *Don't rely on sex:* Sexual orgasm releases the sympathetic nervous system's grip and leads to a parasympathetic response. But because sex drive and stress levels are inversely related, a person under extreme stress probably would not find sexual activity the release that others might. Instead, those who are experiencing extreme stress should probably try some other strategy, such as those in Applications 2–4 and 6–15, before trying sex. When high stress levels have been reduced, sexual activity can arise more spontaneously.

6 *Eat and drink moderately:* Ingestion of moderate amounts of food or nonalcoholic beverages assists in dissipating stomach acids and returning stress levels to normal.

7 *Visualize:* Richard Restak (1991) relates an Eastern three-step technique for relieving "monkey mind," otherwise known as jumpiness or jitteriness. First, stare at an object, such as a plant. Then close your eyes and visualize that same object. Finally, open your eyes to confirm your visualization. This form of meditative observation, by focusing your attention, will calm you. (For more information on visualizing, see Topic 20.1, Application 5.)

8 *Laugh:* Cousins (1989) reports that ten minutes of belly laughs can provide two hours of pain-free sleep. (See the extended treatment of humor and laughter in Chapter Nine.) Edward O'Brien, of Marywood University in Scranton, Pennsylvania, found that college students who had to give impromptu speeches had heart rates of 100 beats per minute while they were speaking, but those who watched an episode of "Seinfeld" beforehand performed with heart rates of only 80 to 85 beats per minute.

9 *Seek relief:* Make the necessary arrangements for getting away from stressors. Have lists of babysitters, substitute caregivers, and temporary help. Use your creativity and the creativity of others to develop ways to relieve stress, such as neighborhood dinner co-ops and babysitting co-ops. Research says that simply knowing that relief is available is relaxing in and of itself. Air traffic controllers are more relaxed if they know they can call on relief when they need it. Usually, when flextime is initiated in organizations, few people use it; just knowing that it is an option is comfort enough. In one experiment, subjects taking a test were randomly assigned to one of two conditions: both groups had noise outside their room, but only the members of one group were told they could shut the door if the noise became bothersome. The group given permission didn't close the door, yet its members scored higher than the members of the group without permission.

10 *Reframe the stressor:* Find a new way to explain your stressor so that it becomes less stressful. See Seligman (1991) and Bandler and Grinder (1982).

11 *Consider medication:* For severe long-term stress, you might consult a physician for pharmaceutical relief when other measures prove to be ineffective. The goals of medication could include:

- Blocking alpha and beta receptors for adrenergic neuro-transmitters to prevent sympathetic arousal
- Shutting down cortisol production in the adrenal gland (for example, by using alprazolam and ketoconazole)
- Inhibiting the release of epinephrine and norepinephrine (the neurotransmitter GABA inhibits production of epinephrine and norepinephrine; Valium is one of the catalysts for GABA)
- Increasing cholinergic neurotransmitters (for example, acetylcholine) and sensitizing muscarinic receptors, resulting in the release of cyclic guanosine monophosphate, which stimulates a parasympathetic response (the heart slows, pupils contract, and digestion is stimulated)

Drugs can help to prevent or shut down a sympathetic response and bring on a parasympathetic response. One result of failure to shut down sympathetic arousal is Type A behavior. See Topic 20.6 for more information on this behavior.

12 *Get a pet:* Handling pets is a great stress reliever, which explains the popular practice of taking pets to rest home patients. *(Contributed by Rick Bradley)*

13 *Develop a corporate policy:* Listed below are several corporate policies or practices that have the effect of instilling in employees a sense of having some control over the quality of their work life:

- Pay for performance
- Flextime
- Cafeteria benefits
- Two-way performance appraisals
- Negotiated rather than imposed goals
- Employee involvement programs
- Explicit management responses to employee suggestions
- Career development with visible, active support
- No boss for consistent performers
- Self-directed work teams
- An effective ethics code that contains a whistle-blowing policy

- Dual career paths
- A focus on team results

14 In the vein of more is better, here is a list of eighteen "stress busters" by three researchers who suggest that extreme measures are not mandatory for stress reduction: look for smaller victories. Cardiologist Thomas Kottke of the Mayo Institute, cardiologist Robert S. Eliot of Scottsdale's Institute of Stress Medicine, and neuroscientist Robert Sapolsky of Stanford University suggest these modest measures:

- Every day, take thirty minutes to one hour to do something you really like to do, whether it's taking a bubble bath or playing with a child.

- Strengthen your ties with your family.

- Don't accept trouble in your marriage—do something about it.

- Recognize that people with some sort of religious belief experience less stress; consider giving religion an increased role in your life.

- Stress is often a matter of one's point of view. Consider alternative interpretations of your situation; see difficult situations as challenging rather than enraging.

- Exercise in whatever quantity is possible. Don't fail to exercise just because you can't get in thirty minutes; lesser quantities do have a positive effect on stress.

- Cut back at least a little on fats, sugars, smoking, and alcohol. Small changes will have some results, plus the satisfaction of knowing that you're headed in the right direction.

- Don't spend time looking for the nearest parking space. Drive up to a distant space and enjoy the walk.

- Give or receive a massage.

- Make sleeping well a priority. (See Chapter Seven.)

- If your job is a major irritant and you can't leave it, try getting more control over the parts of the job that cause the most fear, anger, depression, or uncertainty. There is no job that can't be improved to some degree.

- Change what you can, and don't waste time trying to change what you can't.
- Delegate, train the delegatees, and trust them, whether at work or at home.
- Don't try to be perfect at everything. Identify two or three top priorities and do them perfectly; accept imperfect performance in tasks with lower priorities.
- Avoid the FUD factor—fear, uncertainty, and doubt.
- Do whatever you can, at home, work, or play, to avoid the feeling that you're not in control.
- Be assertive: don't say yes when you mean no, no when you mean yes.
- Be clear on your goals; don't spend any time, energy, or resources on activities that don't matter to you.

Now don't go out and try to implement all of these stress busters! Consider them to be something like a cafeteria line and take what seems appropriate for you.

15 Rock! No, not the music! Nancy Watson, of the Rochester (New York) School of Nursing, found that nursing home patients who used rocking chairs from ½ to 2½ hours per day over six weeks reported less emotional distress, fewer requests for pain medication, and improved balance.

TOPIC 20.5   Stress and Arousal

Although there is evidence that many kinds of arousal exist, including both limbic and cortical arousal, research over the years has proceeded as though there were only one general type. One of the more popular examples of this research has come to be known as the Yerkes-Dodson law (Figure 20.2). It has two aspects:

1. There is an optimal level of arousal. Too low a state of arousal, as when you are sleepy, appears to result in errors of omission, while too high a state of arousal, as when you

are jittery from too much caffeine, results in errors of commission. In other words, when you are underaroused, you may leave things out, skip things, and be forgetful; when you are overaroused, you may hit the wrong key while typing, act impulsively, and lose proper restraint.

2. The optimal point of arousal for complex tasks is different from the optimal point for simple tasks. Higher arousal (for example, that extra cup of coffee) is more conducive to performing simpler tasks, while lower arousal is more conducive to performing more complex tasks (see Topic 6.3).

Redford Williams (1989) has identified a hierarchical relationship between three different forms of arousal. The kind of arousal described here as the Yerkes-Dodson law might be described as normal cortical arousal. Williams describes two other forms of arousal that can suppress cortical arousal, regardless of whether an individual is under- or overaroused cortically. The first is what he calls "focused attention and aggression," such as the arousal exhibited in athletic competition or military observation duty. Focused attention and aggression is accompanied by higher than normal levels of testosterone and is characterized by partially suppressed cortical arousal; therefore, both creativity and problem-solving ability are reduced. The other kind of arousal is what we have called the general adaptation syndrome (see Topic 20.4) or

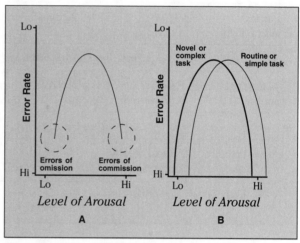

Figure 20.2. The Yerkes-Dodson Law.
Note: (A) Normal optimal level of arousal. (B) Simple, routine tasks require a somewhat higher level of arousal than complex, novel ones.

the fight-or-flight syndrome. During GAS, high cortisol levels are accompanied by virtually total suppression of cortical arousal. The three states, plus the sleep state, are shown in Table 20.2, based on concepts developed by Redford Williams (1989).

Table 20.2. The Four States of Arousal.

Sleep	Normal Arousal	Focused Attention and Aggression	Fight-or-Flight Syndrome
Typical Behaviors During This State			
Rest, dream	Solve problems and be creative	Productivity, routinized behavior	Automatic pilot survival mode
Active Neurotransmitters			
Melatonin	Acetylcholine, dopamine, serotonin	Testosterone	Epinephrine, norepinephrine, cortisol
Condition During Normal Arousal			
Partially suppressed	Active	Accessible	Accessible
Condition During Focused Attention			
Almost totally suppressed	Partially suppressed	Active	Accessible
Condition During Fight-or-Flight			
Almost totally suppressed	Almost totally suppressed	Almost totally suppressed	Active

Source: Based on ideas in *The Trusting Heart: Great News About Type A Behavior* by R. Williams, 1989, New York: Times Books.

Applications

1 If you happen to let yourself get overstimulated—for example, by drinking too much of a caffeinated beverage—switch to a task that is simpler and more repetitive than the task at hand (for example, switch from writing to cleaning up). You will make fewer errors and the increased energy level required will help to dissipate the high arousal. Otherwise, go exercise!

② If you must perform a particularly complex task, such as writing an involved report or reviewing a complex set of numbers, switch to a noncaffeinated beverage, limiting yourself to approximately one heavily caffeinated drink every six hours. (For me, one cup of strong, home-dripped coffee equals two to three cups of standard commercial brew, with respect to its caffeine effect.) See Topic 6.3 for additional information on caffeine.

③ If you are concerned that focused attention and aggression is or will be interfering with your mental self-management, try aerobic exercise to calm you down before the big presentation, meeting, or date. The exercise will lower your testosterone level and its accompanying aggression.

TOPIC 20.6 Williams: Type A Research

Redford Williams, in his book *The Trusting Heart: Great News About Type A Behavior* (1989), defines Type A behavior as a cyclical form of hostile behavior that originates with cynicism, progresses into anger, culminates in an outburst of aggression, and recycles whenever the original cause of the cynicism recurs. Williams defines the onset of Type A behavior as the fulfillment of negative expectations. He contrasts the cynicism of Type A with the trust of Type B: cynicism expects the worst and has a toxic effect on the body, while trust expects better and has a nontoxic effect. What makes the Type A and Type B responses different is that while both types can be cynical and hostile, the Type A person has a physiological defect that prevents restoration of the parasympathetic response following sympathetic arousal.

In his research at Duke University Medical School and elsewhere, Williams has learned that Type A personalities' brain wave patterns take longer to return to normal after sympathetic arousal because their parasympathetic response is sluggish. This is also known as *parasympathetic antagonism*. It is directly related to their lower production within the neurons of cyclic guanosine monophosphate, which directly triggers parasympathetic responses. Williams accounts for about 50 percent of Type A cases by postulating a low-endorphin gene that results in prolonged sympathetic arousal.

For the other 50 percent, Williams points to childhoods with low trust and low touch. Far less Type A behavior exists in Japan; Williams accounts for this by pointing to the reputation of the Japanese for unconditional love in child rearing. While American kids take an average of 17.5 seconds to resume crawling toward a toy after an "angry mother" comment, Japanese children average 49 seconds; they are less accustomed to angry comments and as a result the comments have a stronger impact.

Williams suggests that Type A personalities can use three kinds of strategies to gain control over their uncontrolled sympathetic response: religion, behavior modification, and medicine.

Applications

1 *Religion:* In Jerusalem's Hadassah Hospital, heart disease is four times higher among "secular" Jews. In Evans County, Georgia, churchgoers show lower blood pressure than nonchurchgoers. Williams suggests that religion typically urges individuals to be less concerned with love of self, more with love of others. Such behavior, followed consistently, would short-circuit the whole Type A response by breeding trust rather than cynicism. An exception was seen in a study of 2,850 North Carolinians led by Keith Meador of the psychiatry department at Vanderbilt University Medical Center in Nashville, Tennessee. He found that Pentecostal Christians (Church of God and Assembly of God) exhibit an incidence of depression three times higher than that of other religious groups.

2 *Behavior modification:* In addition to various communication skills available from books and workshops, such as assertiveness, conflict management, and negotiation skills, Williams suggests his twelve-step approach, which I summarize as follows:

1. Monitor your cynical thoughts.

2. Confess your hostility and seek support to change.

3. Stop cynical thoughts.

4. Reason with yourself.

5. Put yourself in the other person's shoes.

6. Laugh at yourself.

7. Practice the relaxation response.

8. Try trusting others.

9. Force yourself to listen more.

10. Substitute assertiveness for aggression.

11. Pretend that today is your last.

12. Practice forgiveness.

3 *Medicine:* See Topic 20.4, Application 11.

4 Williams and his wife, Virginia, wrote *Anger Kills* (1994) as a "how-to" approach to addressing the issues surrounding Type A behavior. It includes a self-assessment tool and seven chapters of specific applications.

TOPIC 20.7 Golembiewski: Burnout—The Ultimate State of Demotivation

Robert Golembiewski of the University of Georgia has developed a phase model for burnout (Golembiewski, 1988). The eight phases are defined by levels of depersonalization, sense of personal achievement, and emotional exhaustion (see Table 20.3). Phase 1 exhibits little or no depersonalization, a reasonable sense of success and job worth, and little or no emotional fatigue, whereas phase 8 exhibits high depersonalization (people are seen as objects without innate value), absence of a personal sense of accomplishment or worth, and emotional exhaustion (a sense of being unable to cope anymore).

In a sample of over ten thousand people, 43 percent scored in phases 1 to 3 (no burnout), 13 percent scored in phases 4 and 5 (borderline burnout), and 44 percent scored in phases 6 to 8 (from moderate to extreme burnout). Physical measures of cholesterol, uric acid, blood pressure, number of sick days used, weight, smoking, drinking, and so on appear to increase uniformly along this model. For example, phase 1 shows lower levels of cholesterol, with levels getting progressively higher through phase 8.

We defined burnout earlier as the result of prolonged stress. Golembiewski gets more specific by defining it as having a sense that we and others have no worth, with no energy to do anything about

Factors of Burnout	Phases							
	1	2	3	4	5	6	7	8
Depersonalization	Lo	Hi	Lo	Hi	Lo	Hi	Lo	Hi
Personal achievement[a]	Lo	Lo	Hi	Hi	Lo	Lo	Hi	Hi
Emotional exhaustion	Lo	Lo	Lo	Lo	Hi	Hi	Hi	Hi

Table 20.3. Golembiewski's Phase Model of Burnout.

Source: From *Phases of Burnout* by R. T. Golembiewski, 1988, New York: Praeger. Reprinted by permission of the author.
[a]Reversed: A low score equals a higher sense of personal achievement.

it. Notice the similarity of his definition of burnout to Seligman's definition of pessimism (personal, pervasive, and permanent helplessness) (Seligman, 1991). Seligman's research focuses on depression and Golembiewski's focuses on burnout, but the working mechanisms appear to be similar. Burnout appears to be the organizational form of depression.

Golembiewski's research had two findings that are particularly important in dealing with the results of burnout. First, he found that burnout did not occur randomly throughout organizations. Instead, it seemed to occur in clusters of workers with a common supervisor. His conclusion was that the quality of the supervisor is responsible for the lion's share of burnout in organizations. Second, he found that people appear to use two different styles to deal with their stress: active and passive. When they reach the stage of burnout, passives have to take extended vacations or personal leave in order to restore their emotional resources and sense of worth, while actives might benefit more from workshops, self-help materials, and wellness programs.

Applications

1 If you are a human resources administrator, you should use employee surveys, Golembiewski's survey, or good common sense (sick-leave patterns, for example) to determine where the actual or potential pockets of burnout are in your organization. Then determine whether you need to train or replace the supervisors in those pockets. Some organizations are experimenting with eliminating the role of supervisor by developing self-directed work teams. For Golembiewski's survey, write to: Dr. Robert Golembiewski; Department of Political Science; Baldwin Hall; University of Georgia; Athens, Georgia 30602; phone: 404-542-2970; E-mail: rtgolem@arches.uga.edu.

2 Provide seminars, self-help materials, wellness programs, and employee counseling resources to assist highly stressed employees in learning ways to cope more effectively.

3 For people with more passive styles of dealing with burnout, the strategies in Application 2 won't work. With passives, you may need to be prepared to offer extended leave followed by transfer to a new work unit upon return.

TOPIC 20.8 The Effect of Odors on Relaxation

Lavender-chamomile scents reportedly reduce stress; lemon, jasmine, and cypress scents induce a positive mood; and basil, peppermint, pine, eucalyptus, and clove are "refreshing . . . invigorating," according to Junichi Yagi of Shimizu Technology Center America. Gary Schwartz of the University of Arizona in Tucson finds that within one minute, spiced apple scent yields more relaxed brain waves and an average drop in blood pressure of 5 millimeters per person. Spiced apple scent has also been associated with the prevention of panic attacks (Ackerman, 1990).

William H. Redd, of the Memorial Sloan-Kettering Cancer Center in New York, has experimented with bursts of heliotropine to relax patients undergoing magnetic resonance imaging. These patients frequently suffer anxiety, panic, and claustrophobic attacks, which cause average delays of fifteen minutes. This results in the loss of approximately $62.5 million annually in the United States (Kallan, 1991). At the March 1991 meeting of the Society of Behavioral Medicine in Washington, D.C., Redd reported that among eighty-five patients, the heliotropine-receiving group exhibited 63 percent less anxiety than the controls.

Applications

❶ Chamomile, spiced apple, lemon, jasmine, eucalyptus, and peppermint are all available in tea-bag form. Consider offering them for breaks as a hot-drink alternative to decaffeinated coffee.

❷ In waiting rooms, entry halls, and other areas where you would like to put people at ease, consider naturally fragrant wood furniture (such as cedar or cypress), home-style fragrances (such as clove balls or potpourri), natural objects (such as pine needles or cones, a potted miniature pine tree, a bowl of apples), and oils (such as lavender) for a continuous source of relaxing fragrance. Hospitals in particular should work to rid waiting areas of that unique hospital smell; though I have no research data to back me up, I'm sure it is anxiety-producing.

❸ Use, where possible, tools that possess a natural texture and odor. There's too much plastic in the world. Picking up a ruler made of wood can add a bit of pleasurable fragrance to an otherwise cold and lackluster act. I've played on an aluminum harpsichord, and it just doesn't offer the same sense of pleasure as performing on a fragrant wooden instrument. I keep a plastic recorder for use on camping trips, but I never play it at home because it doesn't have the pleasing taste or smell of my rosewood version redolent of linseed oil.

❹ The odor of barbecue smoke makes a room feel smaller, while the odor of green apples makes the same room feel larger. Since we know that most women are more comfortable in smaller spaces and most men are more comfortable in larger spaces, try adjusting the perception of room size by freshening women's space with barbecue smoke, men's with green apple!

Some Final Thoughts on Motivation, Stress, and Burnout

What calls us to act? What motivates us? Put most simply, it is the perception that we are in charge of our lives. When we feel that we are out of control, it is usually because we perceive real or imagined deficiencies in our physical or mental makeup—we feel we are not

Table 20.4. Causes of Low Motivation and Possible Remedies.

Likely Causes	Possible Remedies
Physical	
Low testosterone	Take testosterone injections; participate in competitions at which you can win.
Parasympathetic antagonism	Take drugs that perform acetylcholine's function of sensitizing muscarinic receptors and the release of cyclic guanosine monophosphate (consult a neuropsychiatrist); follow Williams's twelve steps; take up religion.
Excess epinephrine, norepinephrine, or both	Participate in noncompetitive aerobic exercise.
Low epinephrine, norepinephrine, or both	Lower your blood sugar by exercise or fasting.
Left cerebral hemisphere underactive	Take drugs that increase blood flow and glucose metabolism in the left lobe (consult a neuropsychiatrist); use talking therapy; follow Seligman's ABCDE technique.
Low immune cell count	Remove stressors.
Mental	
Pessimistic explanatory style	Learn Seligman's ABCDE technique; seek out a good cognitive therapist.
Burnout	Take a long break or leave of absence with the assistance of a therapist; change jobs, or otherwise change the situation that is the source of the burnout; somehow find a new (and better) supervisor.
Stress (remember, the higher the stress, the lower the ambition; find your optimun level)	Find one or more strategies in Topic 20.4 that work for you; remove your stressors by changing yourself, changing others, or changing your situation.
Excessive reliance on external or extrinsic rewards	Explore ways to convert to internal or intrinsic rewards—take an active role in setting your goals and planning action strategies to reach them.
People don't pay sufficient attention to you	Try practicing neurolinguistic programming's matching and pacing.
Low expectation of self and others	Practice the Pygmalion effect; develop Cousins's sense of "hardiness" (see Topics 32.3 and 20.2).

strong enough, not fast enough, not insightful enough. These deficiencies can be addressed by specific strategies for improvement. At the risk of appearing to oversimplify the motivation problem, I have listed in Table 20.4 the state of research with respect to the likely causes of low motivation and possible remedies.

Above all, take charge! Cheerfully!

SUGGESTED RESOURCES

Benson, H., with Klipper, M. Z. (1990). *The Relaxation Response.* New York: Avon.

Caine, R. N., and Caine, G. (1991). *Making Connections: Teaching and the Human Brain.* Alexandria, Va.: Association for Supervision and Curriculum Development.

Cousins, N. (1979). *Anatomy of an Illness.* New York: Norton.

Cousins, N. (1989). *Head First: The Biology of Hope.* New York: NAL/Dutton.

Gazzaniga, M. S. (1985). *The Social Brain.* New York: Basic Books.

Golembiewski, R. T. (1988). *Phases of Burnout.* New York: Praeger.

Petri, H. L. (1991). *Motivation: Theory, Research, and Applications* (3rd ed.). Belmont, Calif.: Wadsworth.

Sapolsky, R. M. (1994). *Why Zebras Don't Get Ulcers: A Guide to Stress, Stress-Related Diseases, and Coping.* New York: Freeman.

Seligman, M.E.P. (1991). *Learned Optimism.* New York: Knopf.

Seligman, M.E.P., Reivich, K., Jaycox, L., and Gillham, J. (1995). *The Optimistic Child.* Boston: Houghton Mifflin.

Selye, H. (1952). *The Story of the Adaptation Syndrome.* Montreal: Acta.

Williams, R. (1989). *The Trusting Heart: Great News About Type A Behavior.* New York: Times Books.

Williams, R., and Williams, V. (1994). *Anger Kills.* New York: HarperPerennial.

Part Six

Appreciating
Our Many
Gifts

Individual Differences

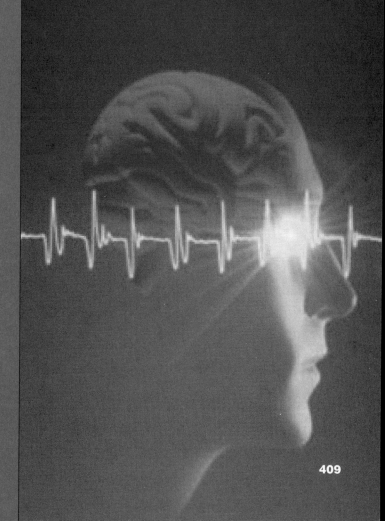

21

The Big Five

A Universal Language for Personality Traits

❝ *Should one tell you that a mountain had changed its place, you are at liberty to doubt it; but if anyone tells you that a man has changed his character, do not believe it.* ❞

—*Muhammad*

*T*he word *personality* stems from the Latin *persona,* which referred to the masks worn by actors in early drama. These masks provided clues to the enduring behaviors by which a specific actor could be recognized throughout the play. Recall the paired face masks—one frowning, one smiling—adorning theatrical facilities and publications. Today, the term *personality* refers to the sets of predictable behaviors by which

411

others recognize us as ourselves. These sets of behaviors go by the name of *traits.*

Do personality traits really exist? It is beyond the scope of this book to present the many points of view on this topic. I encourage you to begin with Walter Mischel's *Personality and Assessment* (1968) for a well-reasoned warning against the use of traits. Mischel's argument runs something like this: Say that procrastination is offered as a trait. Well, there are literally thousands of situations in which we may or may not procrastinate: mailing holiday gifts, depositing paychecks, cooking dinner, reading a professional book, scheduling a physical examination, writing a letter . . . The list could go on indefinitely. In addition, each item on the list could be subdivided: procrastinating at cooking dinner for unwanted guests, for our boss, for our lover, and so on. And even these could be subdivided: procrastinating at cooking dinner for our lover when we desire to break off the relationship, when we want to impress our lover with culinary flamboyance, when we want the chance to work closely together in the kitchen, when we hope that cooking will be abandoned in favor of dining out, or when we hope that if there is no food it will lead to quicker sex—with food following!

What Mischel means to say is that people act differently in different situations and never (well, hardly ever) exhibit a single behavior in every possible situation that could elicit it. Therefore, says Mischel, to label someone a procrastinator is not only irresponsible; it is impossible to prove. We would have to enumerate thousands of situations, with subdivisions, in order to say with confidence that a person is a procrastinator. Personality tests that attempt to measure the degree of a person's tendency toward a particular trait only ask a sample of ten to fifteen questions out of the universe of tens of thousands in order to make a statement like "Fran Doe is a procrastinator about 82 percent of the time." Says Mischel: "Poppycock!"

I and others who argue for the existence of personality traits, which are also called *temperaments* (see A. H. Buss, 1989, for an excellent summary), will grant that it is risky to use a dozen or so questionnaire items to form a conclusion about the degree of a particular temperament in a person (see a brief discussion of temperament in children in Topic 4.4). However, we can minimize that risk by careful selection, choosing only questions that all people can identify with in some way, such as "People tell me that they can depend on me to finish things when I say I will." In addition, by presenting two statements and asking which is more like the person most of the time (for example, "I prefer parties" and "I enjoy parties with lots of people"), we can ask the respondent to subjectively rewind the tape of his or her recent life and form a judgment as to which statement is a better fit. By using carefully selected items and question formats, we can obtain valid and reliable estimates concerning how a person will tend to respond across situations that invite behaviors related to a particular temperament. "If personality was primarily inconsistent," says Seymour Epstein (1997, p. 14), "then human behavior would be essentially unpredictable. One might as well select a spouse at random from a telephone book. The concept of responsibility would be meaningless, so one might as well imprison or release people at random. One could not write meaningful letters of recommendation, as it would be pointless to describe a person as conscientious, cooperative, aggressive, lacking in a sense of humor, and so forth, as none of these would have any predictive value."

> "If there be light, then there is darkness; if cold, then heat; if height, depth also; if solid, then fluid; hardness and softness; roughness and smoothness; calm and tempest; prosperity and adversity; life and death."
> —Pythagoras

The concept of the personality trait is widely accepted today. A trait is a dimension of personality that has the quality of a continuum. "Gregariousness" is a trait that describes a continuum of behavior on which people find themselves stretched out, ranging from a troglodyte like Ted Kaczynski to a rabble-rouser like Howard Stern, with people like you and me in between.

A popular, but receding, school of thought, as expressed in the literature surrounding the Myers-Briggs Type Indicator (MBTI) (Myers and McCaulley, 1985), has seen labels like "extravert" as bipolar; in other words, one either is or is not gregarious. I, and many of the researchers cited in this chapter, reject that dichotomization as simplistic and inadequate to describe the abundant diversity of our species. John Loehlin (1992, p. 119) explains:

An old issue in personality theory is whether human personality comes in distinct subvarieties—personality *types*—or is best conceptualized as varying continuously along dimensions—personality *traits*. Evolutionary biology has something to say on this point. For example, Tooby and Cosmides argue that the nature of human reproduction makes the emergence of genetically based personality types unlikely. That is because parental genes get reshuffled into new combinations in every generation, so that it becomes extremely unlikely that a system depending on a coherent set of genes could be transmitted as a unit from parent to child. What we should find, argue Tooby and Cosmides, is a general human nature, with variations on it provided by variation in individual genes that affect such things as thresholds of behavioral expression. About the only possibility of true emergent types would be on the basis of single genes that could act as switches between alternate courses of development.

A Warning About Using Labels

I think it is appropriate, when we talk about personality characteristics, to recall Paul Valéry's comment: "Seeing is forgetting the name of the thing one sees." Valéry is talking about the tendency to substitute labels for the thing itself. He urges us to beware of labels. Labels originate at the point where a careful observer has arrived at a single word or phrase to express a complex set of attributes that are under observation. Those who come upon the label at a later time must choose whether to reexamine the attributes before accepting the label or to simply accept the label on faith. If the stakes are high, it pays to reexamine the real thing, rather than automatically accepting the label. Here are two simple examples:

1. I label my feelings for my wife as love, but rather than simply repeating "I love you" to convey my feelings, I should reexamine my behavior from time to time to see if it is still saying what I mean by love. The Neil Diamond song "You Don't Send Me Flowers Anymore" is evidence of a label that has lost touch with its origins.

2. A death occurred in a major regional medical center because of excessive trust in labels. An inaccurately labeled drug container was sent from the pharmacy to the operating room, and because of assumptions by a pharmacist's technician and a surgeon that the label was correct, a patient died. Simply looking closely at the drug or smelling it would have prevented this unnecessary loss of life.

After presenting this warning, I must push on to insist that labels are a necessary shortcut. We simply do not have the time or energy to look freshly at everything; we must be selective. And the fact that our world is full of differences requires us to develop a language to talk about them. We could take pains to describe everyone we meet with the objective, descriptive detail of an anthropologist, but then we'd all have to be anthropologists. Indira Gandhi reportedly commented on the subject of diversity with the observation that an orchestra of one hundred violins does not hold our interest with anywhere near the power of the multi-instrument orchestra. Having acknowledged that we are different, let us proceed with learning a language to describe those differences.

But wait. Some, such as Mischel (1968), complain that we should avoid the use of labels, maintaining that there are simply not enough labels to go around to describe the billions of people on the Earth. Others, such as Hans Eysenck (Eysenck, 1967, 1970, 1981; Eysenck and Eysenck, 1985), have defended the use of personality labels. In the study of color, we find 340,000 discriminable points, each of which can be defined as a unique intersection of the three variables of hue, tint, and saturation. Likewise, if we were to propose ten personality variables, each with ten degrees of variation, that would be sufficient to describe ten billion unique individuals. This is more than enough to label everyone presently on this planet with no need for repetition. Our labels will be words like *extravert* and *agreeable*. Each label can vary in strength: just as we can have a 30 percent or 90 percent solution of hydrochloric acid, we also can have differing degrees of extraversion and agreeableness.

Labels are a kind of shorthand. The label "industrious" is like a computer macro that refers to a complex set of elements. We should never reify a label and give it a status equivalent to that of the behavior it refers to. But without the label, we would have no time to do many things. I simply cannot take the time to write a letter of reference for someone if I must specify the forty or fifty incidents that led me to describe that individual as industrious. I must use the shorthand of the label.

The Equalizer Model of Personality

I hereby propose the "equalizer" model of personality description. You know what an equalizer is—a series of knobs that go up and down to create different qualities and quantities of sound production. Imagine a huge equalizer designed to create multisensory experiences. The machine would have five channels—Sight, Sound,

Touch and Motion, Smell, and Taste—and each channel would have several component controls. Sight would have three components (hue, tint, and saturation); Sound four (pitch, rhythm, volume, and timbre); Touch and Motion six (shape, size, texture, temperature, direction, and speed); Smell seven (minty, floral, ethereal, musky, resinous, foul, and acrid); and Taste four (salty, sweet, sour, and bitter). See Ackerman (1990) for a readable and complete description of the senses.

Some of the components might be subdivided further; for example, shape could be divided into curve, length, and other subcomponents. By varying the control knobs, we could create a specific multisensory experience, such as "having wine and cheese in the late afternoon at an outdoor café on the Champs-Elysées." If we were to add another channel—Language—we could even have conversation in the background and foreground. Every multisensory experience can be described by determining the point on each scale that fits the experience. The illustration in Figure 21.1 tries to capture such an equalizer.

Now take the same idea and apply it to personality. The channels would be Intelligence—Domains, Intelligence—Components, Traits, Values, and Motivators. Each channel would have components: Intelligence—Domains would have eight (linguistic, musical, logical and mathematical, spatial, interpersonal, intrapersonal, kinesthetic, and natural observation); Intelligence—Components would have three (production, creativity, and problem solving); Traits would have five (Negative Emotions, Extraversion, Openness, Agreeableness, and

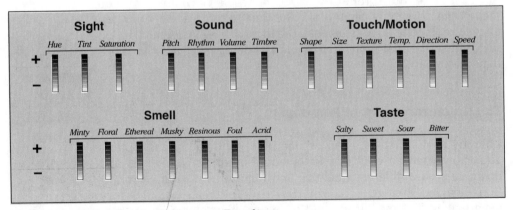

Figure 21.1. An Equalizer for Multisensory Experience.

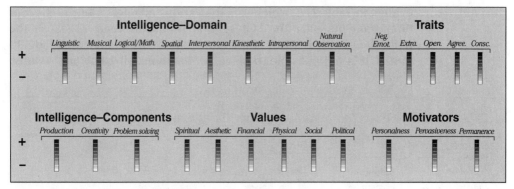

Figure 21.2. An Equalizer Model of Personality.

Conscientiousness), each with six different subcomponents; Values would have six (spiritual, aesthetic, financial, physical, social, and political); and Motivators would have three (personalness, pervasiveness, and permanence). Each person can be described by reference to points on each of the scales of the equalizer. The illustration in Figure 21.2 tries to capture this personality equalizer.

The difference in the two equalizers is crucial: whereas the multi-sensory-experience machine is hooked up to wires, microchips, lights, and amplifiers, the personality equalizer is hooked up to the central nervous system, the circulatory system, the endocrine system, and the musculoskeletal system, all of which, in turn, are hooked up to the external environment. This invites a logical question: to what degree are we free as individuals to modify the positions of our knobs? And as members of families, teachers, therapists, managers, and friends, to what degree can we modify the positions of the knobs of our children, spouse, patients, subordinates (and bosses!), students, and friends? Traditionally, personality has comprised four biologically based temperaments. We will discuss them next, then place them in the light of current genetic theory.

A History of Temperament Theory

Western civilization has operated under the paradigm of four personality temperaments since the early Greeks enumerated the four elements of air, fire, earth, and water, along with their associated personality traits (see Kuhn 1970, for a discussion of paradigms). The fixedness of this paradigm in the minds of Western thinkers is evident in Table 21.1, which lists the various manifestations of the four temperaments over the last several thousand years. Because the definitions of each set of four traits are not consistent from model to model, it is not possible to place, for example, all "sanguine"-related

Table 21.1. The Four Temperaments from Early Greece to the Present.

Source	Air	Fire	Earth	Water
Mythology	Apollo	Hermes	Zeus	Dionysus
Hippocrates	Phlegmatic	Melancholic	Sanguine	Choleric
The Elizabethans (Also Galen and Wundt)	Phlegmatic	Melancholic	Sanguine	Choleric
Native American	East/Eagle	West/Bear	South/Squirrel	North/Buffalo
Herrmann (1989)	Cerebral left	Cerebral right	Limbic left	Limbic right
Lefton, Buzzotta, and Sherberg (1985)	Q2, Submissive-Hostile	Q1, Dominant-Hostile	Q3, Submissive-Warm	Q4, Dominant-Warm
Hersey and Blanchard (1976)	S-1, Telling	S-4, Delegating	S-2, Selling	S-3, Participating
LIFO[a] (Atkins, 1978)	Conserving/Holding	Adapting/Dealing	Controlling/Taking	Supporting/Giving
AVA[b] (Clarke, 1956)	V3, Stability	V4, Structure	V1, Dominance	V2, Sociability
DISC[c] (Marston, 1987)	Dominance	Influence	Steadiness	Compliance
Keirsey and Bates (1978)	Troubleshooter	Visionary	Traditionalist	Catalyst
Social Styles (Merrill and Reid, 1981)	Analytic	Expressive	Driver	Amiable
Jung (1971)	Thinker	Intuitor	Sensor	Feeler
MBTI[d] (Myers and McCaulley, 1985)	Extravert/Introvert	Sensor/Intuitor	Thinker/Feeler	Judger/Perceiver
Kolbe (1990)	Follow through	Quick start	Implementor	Fact finder

[a]LIFO = life orientation.
[b]AVA = activity vector analysis.
[c]DISC = dominance, influence, steadiness, compliance.
[d]MBTI = Myers-Briggs Type Indicator.

traits in the same column. Don't attempt to find the commonality within each column; you'll get Excedrin headache number 4!

This four-factor model of temperament still persists. The most compelling argument to support it is made in Hans Eysenck's *The Structure of Human Personality* (1970). Eysenck presents the psychological dimensions of Extraversion and Neuroticism as the basis of his four-factor model (Figure 21.3). Each of the two dimensions forms an axis of a two-by-two grid, with the vectors that emerge from each of the four quadrants defining the four temperaments. But even Eysenck's work shows this four-factor model breaking down. In subsequent writings (Eysenck and Kamin, 1981; Eysenck and Eysenck, 1985), he portrays three dimensions (the third being Psychoticism) and their various combinations.

In the 1930s, Gordon Allport (Allport and Odbert, 1936) threw out a challenge to the psychological community: find the common synonym clusters in the roughly 4,500 words in Webster's unabridged dictionary that describe variations in normal human personality. Over the next forty years, many tried. The solution did not become apparent, however, until the availability of personal computers and of factor analysis programs designed to work on them. In the early 1980s, something approaching consensus emerged in the community of personality scholars: five, not four, factors best account for the broad categories of variability in human personality. As early as 1963, W. T. Norman defined these five factors, based on his careful factor analysis, as Emotional Stability, Extraversion, Culture, Agreeableness, and Conscientiousness (see Topic 21.2). An excellent summary of the research leading up to the definition of what we now know as the Big Five, or the Five-Factor Model, appears in John, Angleitner, and Ostendorf (1988). Digman and Inouye (1986, p. 116) summarize this trend in personality research as follows: "A series of research studies of personality traits has led to a finding consistent enough to approach the status of law. The finding is this: If a large number of rating scales is used and if the

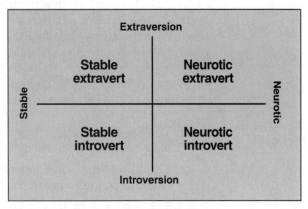

Figure 21.3. Eysenck's Four-Factor Model.

scope of the scales is very broad, the domain of personality descriptors is almost completely accounted for by five robust factors."

It is interesting to note an increasing convergence of Eastern and Western intellectual traditions. My introduction to this convergence came back in the 1960s when I read the works of F.S.C. Northrop— *The Logic of the Sciences and the Humanities* (1947) and *The Meeting of East and West* (1946)—and, more recently, when I read *The Tao of Physics,* by Fritjof Capra (1984). Now, while writing this chapter, I am reading *The Tao of Health, Sex, and Longevity,* by Daniel Reid (1989), in which Reid argues for the Eastern view of five elements (*wu-hsing*): wood, fire, earth, metal, and water. He proceeds to show how all of human existence, according to the Tao masters, is organized around these five elements, not the four of Western intellectual tradition. Can you sense the paradigm shifting underfoot?

The most important difference between the four-factor model as measured by the MBTI (Myers and McCaulley, 1985) and the Five-Factor Model is that the MBTI does not provide a direct measure of the first factor, Negative Emotionality (Norman's Emotional Stability, Costa and McCrae's Neuroticism). Yet, after Extraversion, it is the most extensively documented factor. McCrae and Costa (1989) have written an excellent article explaining the differences in the two models.

Six attributes of Big Five research help to explain the wide acceptance of the Five-Factor Model among personality researchers:

1. The same five factors emerge regardless of what factor analysis program is used.

2. The same five factors emerge regardless of the type of item used in testing: sentences, phrases, or words.

3. The same five factors emerge regardless of the people doing the ratings: professional psychologists, self-reports, spouse ratings, or peer ratings.

4. The same five factors emerge regardless of the language that is used.

5. The same five factors emerge regardless of the subjects tested (old or young, male or female, more educated or less educated).

6. An extremely high coefficient alpha (a measure of internal consistency) of .90 is associated with the five factors.

TOPIC 21.1 The Inherited Basis of Personality Traits

Neubauer and Neubauer (1990, pp. 38 ff.) write of the research on the genetic origins of personality traits (see the discussion in Chapter One). Among the traits for which strong evidence of an inherited basis exists are the following (see Topic 12.1 for information on the heritability of sexuality):

Aggressiveness	Excitability	Quickness to anger
Alcoholism (see Topic 6.1)	Imagination	Shyness
Autism	Language facility	Susceptibility to addiction
Depression	Leadership	Traditionalism
Empathy	Maturation rate	Vulnerability to stress
Engageability (aggressive pursuit of one's needs)	Obsessions	Weakness of will
	Person-versus-object orientation	

I must take pains to point out that one does not inherit the gene for a trait, or even the trait itself. The term *trait* is a shorthand way to refer to a correlated set of attributes—behaviors, attitudes, and values that tend to occur together in the same individual. These attributes are composed of specific behavioral responses, or habits, that are persistent over time, such as blushing. The specific behavioral responses are associated with the complex interaction of specific genes and environmental experiences. (See Figure 21.4.) For the relationship between genes and habits, see Figure 21.5. For an extended description of the relationship between genes, habits, and traits, see Zuckerman (1991).

Continuing research is aimed at determining both the makeup and the degree of heritability of personality factors: which factors seem to be especially influenced genetically and to what degree. Tesser and Crelia (1994), for example, have reported on the greater rigidity of attitudes that have high heritability components. R. Wright (1994, p. 81), on the other hand, argues that personality traits are more environmentally determined: "Genes that irrevocably committed our ancestors to one personality type should in theory have

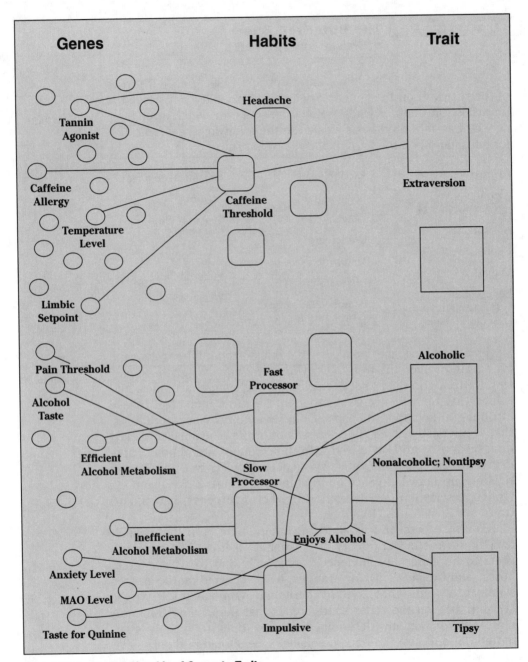

Figure 21.4. The Relationship of Genes to Traits.

lost out to genes that let the personality solidify gracefully." But their arguments are either-or. Traits, whether they are apparently more biologically based (such as sex drive) or apparently more environmentally based (such as sociability) are inevitably based on an interaction between one's genes and the environment. Both nature and nurture play a part. Among the environmental factors that Neubauer and Neubauer (1990) identify as tending to have the most impact on personality development are

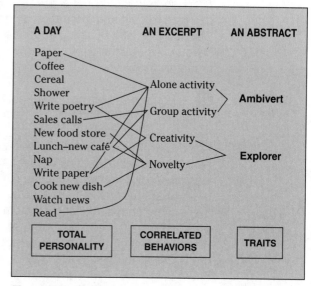

Figure 21.5. **The Relationship of Everyday Behaviors to Personality Traits.**

- The quality and quantity of language the child is exposed to

- The amount of play the child has

- Expressed affection

- The availability of toys

- The presence of parents

- The presence of other children

- The natural expression of emotion in the household

- Intellectual expectations (riddles, questions, problem solving, and so on)

- Control, limits, and discipline (deprivation and excess have a negative effect)

In summary, genetics would appear to be like a flower, with environment more like fertilizer, rain, or soil. Or, as Neubauer and Neubauer say, genes appear to set limits for the range of development. They are not a blueprint that fully defines the final product; instead, they establish the range of possible variation.

Applications

❶   As a parent, you can only do what your informed judgment suggests is appropriate. Realize that some traits will emerge in your offspring that you do not share. To deny the validity of these traits can lead to guilt and frustration on both your part and your child's. Develop the habit of taking your child's strengths and helping them develop. As Goethe wrote: "That which he has inherited has been made his own."

❷   If you are a therapist, manager, coach, or other "people developer," you will find that the people you deal with will exhibit some traits that relate well to a job they are trying to do and some that do not. It is reasonable to hold people accountable for their relevant strengths, but it is unreasonable to browbeat them for their weaknesses. For example, if you coach a boy's basketball team and a player shoots well but shies away from the responsibility of calling plays, work on his shooting. Don't make him play point guard and browbeat him for not being more of a playmaker. If you must make him play point guard, praise his shooting and be knowingly supportive of his efforts to make plays. Say, "I know that playing you at point guard is not using your strengths to your advantage, but for now you're the best person for the job. I won't expect you to perform as well as you do as a shooting guard, but I will support you in every way I can to make the best of the circumstances."

❸   In hiring or choosing someone to do a job, make the selection on the basis of the person's relevant strengths. Don't make the mistake of choosing employees because their credentials are generally impressive; hire them because their credentials are job-related. For example, a common mistake is to hire a creative, innovative person for a routine job. This will lead to a higher than necessary error rate and eventual turnover. If you must hire a creative person to do a routine job, make sure you both know that the routine job is only temporary and that a better job fit will come soon. Then manage the employee with understanding and support in the routine job. Say, "We both need to be aware that the time you spend as a bank teller will be boring much of the time, and as a result, you will be more error-prone than other tellers. Let's figure out what we can do to minimize error and keep you motivated during this rotation. When your next assignment comes along, your creativity will be more challenged. But for now, let's figure out a survival strategy."

4 As a general rule, don't try to change people. Learn to build on what they are and compensate for what they are not. I'll never love the chore of managing family finances, but I've made it bearable by figuring out a way to make it more interesting. I've done this by learning a computer program. I know people who have entered into marriage with the confidence that they would ultimately be able to change the less desirable traits of their future spouse. This typically leads to frustration and resentment as the change strategies prove to be ineffectual.

5 Don't confuse personality traits with learnable skills. There are many bodies of knowledge and specific skills that I could learn if I wanted to. In that respect, you could "change" me by teaching me a skill or a body of knowledge. But that learning doesn't mean that a personality trait will change as a result. I have an architect friend who hated to make presentations before groups. He is an introverted, idea-focused person. He knew he would never love presentations, but he decided that he would at least be good at it. He took Ty Boyd's seminar on public speaking and learned the skills involved in making effective presentations. Now he gets good marks for his presentations, even though he still doesn't like doing them and prefers being creative in the privacy of his office. But he is less anxious about his presentations because he knows the tricks of the trade.

6 With respect to adopted children, Eysenck and Kamin (1981, p. 51) write, "At no time do adopted children and foster parents correlate more than .10, and adopted children do not grow to resemble their adopting parents." I have friends who've taken it hard when their incorrigible adopted children haven't developed the kind of loving, nurturing, thoughtful behaviors the adopting parents have shown them. This should not be seen as a personal failure. The parents should continue to provide support and encourage skill and social development, but they need to help their adopted children to build on their strengths and limitations, rather than trying to force them into a path alien to their nature.

7 Nigel Nicholson (1998, p. 142) provides an excellent summary of the implications of evolutionary psychology for managers:

- Be aware that people always hear bad news loudest.
- Assign sensitive people, who can avoid communicating a sense of failure to people, to give performance appraisals.

- Remember that people resist change unless they are dissatisfied.
- Be aware that people usually think most creatively when they feel safe.
- People have a tendency to be overconfident, so check things out.
- Stereotyping strangers is natural, so build in opportunities to get beyond stereotypes.
- Rumors and gossip are natural. Don't eradicate them; just ensure that they are accurate.
- One-upmanship is natural. You can't get rid of it, but you don't have to take it seriously.
- Limit the size of the organizational entity with which a person identifies to 150 people.
- Remember that people prefer identifying with one group at work, not two or more.
- Hierarchy building is innate and ineradicable. Accept it, but realize that it doesn't need fuel as an accelerant.
- The drive to lead is inborn. Know that encouraging reluctant leaders has little likelihood of payoff.
- Don't blame people for failing to exert leadership in a crisis when they haven't demonstrated it before; accept that it's just not their nature.

8 How environment interacts with inheritance is an apparently mysterious process. But recent research (Loehlin, 1992) has identified four circumstances that can lead to the expression of a particular trait:

Passive: A predisposed individual is in an environment that supports the predisposed trait (a conscientious child attends a traditional school).

Active: A predisposed individual is recognized by someone else (or by herself or himself) and thereafter is encouraged in the predisposed trait (a teacher asks an extraverted child, or the child volunteers, to lead the class line to lunch).

Interactive: A moderately predisposed individual enters an environment supportive of the extreme form of the trait and then moves to the extreme (a moderately conscientious young adult enters the armed forces and excels).

Reactive: A predisposed individual is in an environment that is opposite to the trait (a teacher suggests that a selfish child enter the candy-striper program, or a shy child is reared by pushy, gregarious parents).

In the first three cases, the trait develops naturally; the fourth case leads to unnatural expressions.

⑨ Steven Pinker (1994) points out that a surprisingly large number of human behaviors are found universally among all documented human cultures. It is clarifying to view his list, which I have adapted somewhat and included in this book as Appendix D.

TOPIC 21.2 The Big Five

The most popular version of the Big Five (see the discussion in Topic 4.4) is the one developed by Costa and McCrae (1992). Their five dimensions are Negative Emotionality (or Neuroticism), Extraversion, Openness, Agreeableness, and Conscientiousness.

The Negative Emotionality Dimension

The Negative Emotionality dimension of the Five-Factor Model relates to one's threshold of response to stressful stimuli. At one extreme we have the Resilient, who tends to experience life on a more rational level than most people and who sometimes appears rather impervious to his or her surroundings. I think, for example, of my choir director, who didn't miss a beat during a dress rehearsal when the podium on which he was standing collapsed forward. He simply placed his feet at an angle like a snowplow and kept his baton moving. Of course, all the singers and instrumentalists broke out laughing at this classic example of nonreactivity. He's unflappable. This extreme is also the foundation for many valuable social roles— from air traffic controllers and airline pilots to military snipers, financial managers, and engineers.

At the other extreme, we have the Reactive, who experiences more negative emotions and reports less satisfaction with life than most people do. This is not meant to place a value judgment on Reactives, however; a susceptibility to negative emotions and discontent with life provide the basis for filling extremely important roles in our society, such as social scientists, academicians, and customer service professionals.

Along the continuum from Reactive to Resilient is the Responsive, who has a mixture of the qualities of both the Resilient and the Reactive. Responsives are more able to turn behaviors from both extremes on and off, according to what seems appropriate to the situation. Typically, however, a Responsive cannot maintain the calmness of a Resilient for as long a period of time or sustain the nervous edge of alertness of a Reactive (as, for example, would be typical of a stock trader during a session).

The Extraversion Dimension

The Extraversion dimension is about the degree of one's preference for being actively engaged with other people. On one hand, the Extravert tends to exert more leadership, to be more physically and verbally active, and to be more friendly and outgoing around others than most people. This extraverted profile is the foundation of many important social roles, such as salespeople, politicians, managers, and social scientists.

On the other hand, the Introvert tends to be more independent, reserved, steady, and comfortable being alone than are most people. This introverted profile is the basis of such varied and important social roles as production managers, physical and natural scientists, and computer programmers.

In between these two extremes is the Ambivert, who is able to move comfortably from outgoing social situations to the isolation of working alone. The stereotypical Ambivert is the player-coach, who moves easily from the leadership demands of a coach to the personal production demands of a player.

The Openness Dimension

The Openness dimension refers to the degree to which a person is curious about her or his inner and outer worlds. On one hand, the

Explorer has broader interests, is fascinated by novelty and innovation, would generally be perceived as liberal, and reports more introspection and reflection. Explorers are not unprincipled, but they tend to be open to considering new approaches. The Explorer profile forms the basis for such important social roles as entrepreneurs, architects, change agents, artists, and theoretical scientists.

The Preserver has narrower interests, is perceived as more conventional, and is more comfortable with the familiar. Preservers are thought of as being more conservative, but not necessarily more authoritarian. The Preserver profile is the basis for such important social roles as financial managers, performers, project managers, and applied scientists.

In the middle of the continuum lies the Moderate. Moderates can explore the novel with interest when necessary but consider too much novelty to be tiresome; on the other hand, they can focus on the familiar for extended periods of time but eventually develop a hunger for novelty.

This trait doesn't relate to intelligence; Preservers and Explorers both score well on traditional measures of intelligence. Instead, it helps to define creativity, since openness to new experience is an important ingredient of creativity.

The Agreeableness Dimension

The Agreeableness dimension is a measure of altruism versus egocentrism. At one end of the continuum, the Adapter tends to subordinate personal needs to the needs of the group and to accept the group's norms rather than insisting on his or her personal norms. Harmony is more important to the Adapter than, for example, broadcasting a personal notion of truth. Galileo, in recanting his Copernican views before the Inquisition, behaved like an Adapter. The Adapter profile is the core of such important social roles as teachers, social workers, and psychologists.

At the other end of the continuum, the Challenger is more focused on her or his personal norms and needs than on those of the group. The Challenger is more concerned with acquiring and exercising power. Challengers follow the beat of their own drum, rather than getting in step with the group. The Challenger profile is the foundation of such important social roles as advertising executives, managers, and military leaders.

In the middle of the continuum is the Negotiator, who is able to move from leading to following as the situation demands. Psychoanalyst and author Karen Horney (1945) described the two extremes of this trait as "moving toward people" (Adapter) and "moving against people" (Challenger). Tender-minded Adapters can become dependent personalities who have a minimal sense of self; tough-minded Challengers can become narcissistic, antisocial, authoritarian, or paranoid personalities who have a minimal sense of fellow feeling. This trait differentiates the dependence, or altruism, of the Adapter, the independence, or egocentrism, of the Challenger, and the interdependence, or situational response, of the Negotiator.

The Conscientiousness Dimension

The Conscientiousness dimension concerns self-control in the service of one's will to achieve. On one hand, the Focused person exhibits high self-control, resulting in a consistent focus on personal and occupational goals. In its normal state, this trait is characterized by academic and career achievement, but when it turns extreme, it results in workaholism. Focused people are difficult to distract. This profile is the basis for such important social roles as leaders, executives, and, in general, high achievers.

On the other hand, the Flexible person is more easily distracted, less focused on goals, more hedonistic, and generally more lax with respect to goals. Flexibles are easily seduced from the task at hand by a passing idea, activity, or person; that is, they have weak control over their impulses. They do not necessarily work less than Focused people, but less of their total work effort is goal-directed. Flexibility facilitates creativity, inasmuch as people remain open to possibilities longer without feeling driven to achieve closure and move on. This profile is the core of such important social roles as researchers, detectives, and consultants.

Toward the middle of this continuum is the Balanced person, who finds it easier to move from focus to laxity, from production to research. Balanced people would make ideal managers for either a group of Flexibles or a group of Focused people because they have some of both qualities. They can keep Flexibles reasonably on target without alienating them, and they can keep Focused people cautious enough to keep them from jumping to conclusions, relaxed enough to prevent them from suffering a coronary.

Summary

The five dimensions fit onto a bipolar continuum, which is a progression with graduated changes between two extreme and contrasting characteristics. For example, temperature is a bipolar continuum that is defined by the two extremes of hot and cold. I generally report a person's profile by placing the five scores in one of three zones in each bipolar continuum: high, medium, and low. A Big Five Feedback Form is included as Appendix E. Table 21.2 shows the Big Five traits with anchor words that describe extreme scorers. Midrange descriptors would consist of relatively equal anchors from each of the two extremes. For example, extreme Extraverts are usually talkative and sociable and extreme Introverts are usually quiet and private, while Ambiverts might see themselves as equally talkative and private.

Table 21.2. The Big Five Personality Dimensions with Anchors for Extreme Scorers.

Factor	Negative Emotionality	Extraversion	Openness	Agreeableness	Conscientiousness
High Score	*Reactive*	*Extravert*	*Explorer*	*Adapter*	*Focused*
High-Score Descriptors					
	Tense	Sociable	Curious	Accepting	Productive
	Alert	Optimistic	Liberal	Team player	Decisive
	Fast	Talker	Variety-seeking	Trusting	Organized
	Anxious	Happy	Dreamer	Agreeable	Dependable
Midscore	*Responsive*	*Ambivert*	*Moderate*	*Negotiator*	*Balanced*
Low-Score Descriptors					
	Content	Reserved	Efficient	Questioning	Spontaneous
	Controlled	Writing	Practical	Competitive	Chaotic
	Secure	Private	Conservative	Self-interested	Permissive
	Stress-free	Inhibited	Habits	Direct	Unfocused
Low Score	*Resilient*	*Introvert*	*Preserver*	*Challenger*	*Flexible*

The popularity of sociobiology (see E. O. Wilson, 1975) invites us to enjoy speculation about the evolutionary advantages of specific traits. The sociobiologist, or evolutionary psychologist, stipulates that in order to survive over the generations, a human personality trait (or animal trait, for that matter) must have clearly demonstrable survival value. Or, as D. M. Buss (1991) describes it, the survival values of the Big Five form a kind of "adaptive landscape." Consider: High Negative Emotionality is helpful in a fight, while low Negative Emotionality is helpful for patiently waiting through long periods of deprivation. High Extraversion is helpful in procuring mates, while low Extraversion is helpful in persevering in the solitary tasks of child rearing and being a hunter-gatherer. High Openness is helpful for innovating in the face of need, while low Openness is helpful for reaping the benefits of steady, repetitive production activities. High Agreeableness is helpful in nurturing relationships, while low Agreeableness is helpful in building empires. High Conscientiousness is helpful in achieving the discipline necessary for effective leadership; low Conscientiousness is helpful in providing the flexibility necessary to accomplish the needs of the moment.

And if possession of each of these extremes is adaptive, then certainly possession of both extremes is also adaptive. Hence, none of us is exclusively characterized by any one extreme. Even Extraverts have to go it alone. In fact, the current definition of a personality disorder is what happens when an individual loses the flexibility to use each of these opposing behaviors (for example, trusting and questioning) and rigidly (and maladaptively) persists in only one of the extremes. For example, a person who engages only in trusting and never questions anyone would have a dependent personality disorder.

Application

Two tests are commercially available for measuring the Big Five: the NEO Five Factor Inventory and the NEO PI-R (Costa and McCrae, 1992). The first is shorter (60 questions) and is self-scoring. The second test is longer (240 questions) and provides six "facet" scores for each of the five factors, for a total of thirty-five scores (five factors and thirty facets of these factors). The longer test has self-scoring and computer-scoring versions.

TOPIC 21.3   Facets of the Big Five

In developing a test to measure the Big Five, Costa and McCrae (1992) have found six facets that help in defining each of the five factors; they are listed in Table 21.3.

Table 21.3. The Facets of the Big Five Personality Traits.

Negative Emotionality	Extraversion	Openness	Agreeableness	Conscientiousness
Worry	Warmth	Fantasy	Trust	Competence
Anger	Gregariousness	Aesthetics	Straightforwardness	Order
Discouragement	Assertiveness	Feelings	Altruism	Dutifulness
Self-consciousness	Activity	Actions	Compliance	Achievement striving
Impulsiveness	Excitement seeking	Ideas	Modesty	Self-discipline
Vulnerability	Positive emotions	Values	Tender-mindedness	Deliberation

Source: From the *NEO PI-R Professional Manual* by P. T. Costa, Jr., and R. R. McCrae, 1992, Odessa, Florida: Psychological Assessment Resources. © 1978, 1985, 1989, 1992 by PAR, Inc. Adapted and reprinted by permission of Psychological Assessment Resources, Inc., Odessa, Florida 33556. Further reproduction is prohibited without permission of PAR, Inc.

Complete definitions of the thirty facets are available in Costa and McCrae (1992). Here are brief definitions:

Negative Emotionality Facets

N1   *Worry:* The level of worry and fear about how things will turn out.

N2   *Anger:* How quickly one comes to feel anger and bitterness.

N3   *Discouragement:* One's capacity for feeling sad and hopeless.

N4   *Self-consciousness:* Embarrassment or shame at awkward public situations.

N5   *Impulsiveness:* The tendency to yield to temptation.

N6   *Vulnerability:* The tendency to panic in emergency or stressful situations.

Extraversion Facets

E1   *Warmth:* One's capacity for affection, friendliness, and cordiality.

E2   *Gregariousness:* A preference for being around other people.

E3   *Assertiveness:* The tendency to express oneself forcefully and without reluctance.

E4   *Activity:* Level of energy; the tendency toward a fast-paced lifestyle.

E5   *Excitement seeking:* An appetite for the thrills of bright colors and noisy settings.

E6   *Positive emotions:* One's capacity for laughter, joy, and love; optimism; happiness.

Openness Facets

O1   *Fantasy:* The ability to create an interesting inner world through imagination and fantasy.

O2   *Aesthetics:* A wide and deep appreciation for art and beauty; sensitivity.

O3   *Feelings:* The ability to value and experience a wide range of positive and negative emotions.

O4   *Actions:* A preference for novelty and variety over the routine and familiar.

O5   *Ideas:* Intellectual curiosity; openness to new and unconventional ideas.

O6   *Values:* The willingness to examine social, political, and religious values; lack of dogmatism.

Agreeableness Facets

A1   *Trust:* The tendency to regard others as honest and well intentioned; lack of skepticism.

A2   *Straightforwardness:* Proneness to candor and frankness; tendency not to be deceptive or manipulative.

A3   *Altruism:* Generosity; consideration; the willingness to help others.

A4 *Compliance:* Proneness to submit to the will of others; cooperativeness as opposed to competitiveness; inhibition of aggressive feelings.

A5 *Modesty:* Humility; lack of arrogance or narcissism.

A6 *Tender-mindedness:* The ability to feel concern, pity, and sympathy for others.

Conscientiousness Facets

C1 *Competence:* The tendency to feel prepared and capable; high self-esteem; an internal locus.

C2 *Order:* A tendency to feel well organized and methodical; neatness; a tendency toward compulsiveness.

C3 *Dutifulness:* Strict adherence to one's conscience; reliability.

C4 *Achievement striving:* The ability to set high goals and focus on them; a tendency toward workaholism.

C5 *Self-discipline:* The capacity to motivate oneself to get the job done and resist distractions.

C6 *Deliberation:* The ability to think something through before acting on it.

McCrae and Costa reported in the *American Psychologist* in May 1997 that research samples had validated their thirty-facet structure in at least eight language and cultural groups that represented a good mix of cultural features: Chinese, English, German, Hebrew, Japanese, Korean, Portuguese, and Spanish.

Applications

❶ Remember that pure personality traits do not exist. For example, although Extraverts usually exhibit dominance, sometimes they don't and sometimes Introverts do. The five families of traits are merely an attempt to capture the more frequently occurring combinations of sub-traits. This sort of classification is helpful in understanding trends and probabilities, but we must always look freshly at individuals to see where they differ from the norm.

② In using personality traits as an aid for team building and group development, it is important to understand that there is no one right way to be. The task is to understand how best to use what you have learned about personalities to help you get work done more effectively. Most groups need to be cautioned about teasing one another when they first encounter differing personality traits.

TOPIC 21.4 The Physical Basis of Personality

Ongoing research is aimed at describing the biological, physiological, genetic, chemical, and—to sum it up in one word—physical basis of personality traits. I like to approach this subject by describing each of the Big Five dimensions as having its own "arousal system": a complex of physical factors that work together to determine the threshold at which an individual switches off a preference for behaviors at one end of the dimension and begins to prefer the opposite. For example, the threshold for Extraversion-Introversion would be associated with the point at which an individual has had enough of big, noisy, smelly crowds and begins craving quiet and solitude.

The arousal system for Negative Emotionality is based on the autonomic nervous system; its threshold is the point at which stressors take one out of a state of calm, known as parasympathetic arousal and associated with activity in the cerebral cortex, and into the general adaptation syndrome, or sympathetic arousal, associated with activity in the limbic system (see Chapter Two). In fact, researchers in the United States and Germany, led by Klaus-Peter Lesch of the University of Würzburg, have announced the discovery of a genetic marker for the negative emotions (*Science,* November 29, 1997). The gene in question comes in two forms, short and long, and is involved in the efficiency of serotonin transportation. Those in their sample of 505 people with one or two copies of the short form scored higher on self-report measures of anxiety, angry hostility, depression, harm avoidance, pessimism, fear of uncertainty, and fatigability. Having two copies of the short version does not appear to affect the level of negative emotions; people with two copies scored roughly the same as those with one copy. In addition to serotonin levels, the negative emotions are associated with high levels of monoamine oxydase (MAO), cortisol, and adenosine GMP (guanine monophosphate). All three influence levels of central nervous system arousal.

The arousal system for Extraversion is associated with the peripheral nervous system (Heller, 1993), and its threshold is associated with the point at which a person has experienced so much stimulation that he or she retreats into isolation. Caffeine, dopamine, endorphins, and the general efficiency of transmissions within the afferent and efferent peripheral nervous system are all associated with determining one's threshold for sensory stimulation. In addition, studies show that Extraversion is associated with increased activity in the right hemisphere and an accompanying tendency toward optimism and enhanced performance in the left visual field (Heller, 1993). Introversion, on the other hand, is associated with increased activity in the left hemisphere and an accompanying tendency toward pessimism and enhanced performance in the right visual field.

Moreover, Extraverts (who are also low in Negative Emotionality) show greater hypnotic susceptibility, which is related to the Extravert's faster path in habituating to physical stimuli. Introverts (who are higher in Negative Emotionality) show less hypnotic susceptibility and are slower to habituate. The speed of habituation is associated with the threshold of the peripheral nervous system. Because the Extravert has a higher threshold for sensory stimulation ("Sock it to me, baby"), it makes sense that Extraverts would habituate, or get used to, increased levels and sources of sensation more quickly than Introverts. Interestingly, Extraverts can be visually identified by observing the tendency for their eyes to make quick, darting movements to the left, an indication of enhanced performance in the left visual field (and the right hemisphere). The opposite is true for Introverts; check out their quick, darting eye movements to the right.

The arousal system for Openness is associated with novelty seeking and activation of the associative area of the cerebral cortex; its threshold is the point at which a person has experienced a surfeit of novelty, rejecting the new and craving the familiar. The threshold is determined by, among other things, levels of acetylcholine, dopamine, and noradrenalin and the condition of the myelin sheath.

The arousal system for Agreeableness is associated with the sex hormones, whose effects result in a person's opposing cravings for dominance and nurture, for challenge and submission. The threshold is defined as the point at which the individual will submit to a challenge from someone else; it is associated with the sex hormones as well as with serotonin, MAO, and oxytocin.

The arousal system for Conscientiousness is associated with the attentional focus system, with the threshold defined as the point at which an individual is distracted from the task at hand and engages in off-task behaviors. This threshold appears to be associated with levels of testosterone in both men and women, with higher levels associated with greater perseverance and ease in spending time automatizing new skills and behaviors (see Topic 12.11 for information on automatization).

Application

Remember that each of us has a real threshold that influences how much of a behavior we can productively and effectively engage in. I am an Ambivert and, on a recent week-long writing retreat in the North Carolina mountains, I "hit the wall" after five straight days of writing, an introverted activity. My body wanted no more; I'd reached my threshold for isolation and was craving stimulation. Such moments can be addressed by experiences that refresh and restore us, such as walking in the fresh air. On this particular day, I'd had both enough isolation and enough high Openness, so I restored myself (along with my wife) by taking a two-mile walk and then watching the semifinals of the men's NCAA basketball tournament with red wine, French bread, and smoked trout with all the trimmings.

When your body seems to be saying "Enough!" (enough stimulation, enough stress, enough isolation, enough focused attention, enough submission, and so on), give it a break and engage in an opposite activity for a while.

TOPIC 21.5 Personality Changes over Time

McCrae and Costa (1990), in their work with the Baltimore Longitudinal Study of Aging, have looked for changes in temperament over time. They found that up through the early twenties, the tendency is to score lower on Agreeableness and Conscientiousness than on the other three factors. They attribute this to the preoccupation of young people with identity formation (people who are low on Agreeableness are called Challengers) and to their low career commitment (those who are low on Conscientiousness are called Flexibles). By age thirty this difference has lessened as a result of increased Agreeableness and Conscientiousness and lessened Negative Emotionality, Extraversion, and Openness. Another way of saying this is that as we enter adulthood and the world of work, we become more emotionally stable, somewhat less sociable, a little more conservative, a little easier to get along with, and a little more goal-oriented (see Figure 21.6).

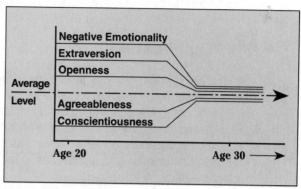

Figure 21.6. Development of Stability in the Adult Personality.

Applications

1 Be reasonably accepting of selfishness and impulsivity among youth, knowing that with understanding parents and societal nudging, people in their twenties tend to move toward a more cooperative and goal-focused adulthood.

2 Also be reasonably accepting of the higher emotionality, minimal time with self, and complaints of boredom of young people, for this too will change some over time.

TOPIC 21.6 Sex Differences in the Big Five

Virtually no differences exist between men and women on the Extraversion, Openness, Agreeableness, and Conscientiousness dimensions. Costa and McCrae (1992) report some small differences on specific facets within these dimensions. Women do tend to score a bit higher on the Negative Emotionality dimension. On only one of the Negative Emotionality facets—angry hostility—do women score the same as men. We do not know whether this difference on the Negative Emotionality dimension is the result of real differences in emotional control or whether women are simply more forthcoming in reporting their feelings. More research is needed.

Application

As a group, females tend to be more reactive—that is, they tend to make more overt responses to "good news, bad news" situations. This is not to say that males, who are less reactive, do not have internal reactions; they simply tend to show them less. Remember that this control can be either an asset (as in maintaining composure in stressful situations) or a liability (as in failing to show the intensity of a reaction to one's partner).

TOPIC 21.7   Relationships Versus Self-Development

McCrae and Costa (1990) identify the second and fourth factors (Extraversion and Agreeableness) as two traits that are particularly important in developing relationships. The Extraversion dimension reflects the quantity of relationships; the Agreeableness dimension reflects their quality. The other three factors—Negative Emotionality, Openness, and Conscientiousness—refer more to the development of the self, regardless of the relationship context.

Application

Understand that in building a relationship, it is important to continually communicate with one another, particularly on issues related to Extraversion and Agreeableness. See Costa and McCrae (1992) and McCrae and Costa (1990) for further discussion and examples.

TOPIC 21.8 Can You Change Your Personality?

For the most part, people are comfortable with the person they've become. Introverts like being introverted, Explorers like exploring, Balanced folk like being well-rounded, and Challengers like challenges. However, situations may exist in which people find that their personality conflicts with their job, their co-workers, their spouse, their child, or other significant people. The reality is that one's personality as an adult is unlikely to change. Daniel Alkon writes movingly of this in *Memory's Voice* (1992), a testament to his lifelong search to find a cure for the effects of childhood abuse. He recommends "an attitude of humility toward the possibilities of change for people" (p. 163) and says that "the adult brain's networks . . . are to a significant degree hard-wired" (p. 162). For more from Alkon, see Topic 16.1.

What can be done when we find our trait in conflict with our life situation? How can an Introvert improve, if not personally change, a relationship with an Extravert? Three kinds of strategies are available, identified as Applications below. Each kind of strategy is supported by a list of specific suggestions in corresponding appendixes.

Applications

1 *Development strategy:* Attempt to learn some behaviors that offset the effect of your extreme trait. For example, extreme Extraverts could establish the habit of one hour of private reflection every day (through reading, writing, or some other solitary activity). See other suggestions in Appendix F.

2 *Compensatory strategy:* Find a crutch, a "work-around," that relieves you of having to exercise a trait that is unnatural for you. For example, extreme Introverts who have responsibility for leading meetings could delegate the facilitation to a more extraverted colleague or team member. See other suggestions in Appendix G.

3 *Influence strategy:* Learn how people with opposite traits naturally act; then use that behavior selectively when influencing them is particularly important. For example, if you are an extraverted salesperson who must establish rapport with an introverted purchasing agent, instead of dropping by and inviting the agent to lunch (both are extraverted strategies), send some written materials and make an appointment in advance (both are introverted strategies). See other suggestions in Appendix H.

SUGGESTED RESOURCES

Alkon, D. L. (1992). *Memory's Voice: Deciphering the Brain-Mind Code.* New York: HarperCollins.

Costa, P. T., Jr., and McCrae, R. R. (1992). *NEO PI-R Professional Manual.* Odessa, Fla.: Psychological Assessment Resources.

Howard, P. J., and Howard, J. M. (1993). *The Big Five Workbook: A Roadmap for Individual and Team Interpretation for Scores on the Five-Factor Model of Personality.* Charlotte, N.C.: Center for Applied Cognitive Studies.

McCrae, R. M., and Costa, P. T. (1990). *Personality in Adulthood.* New York: Guilford Press.

Web Sites

Center for Applied Cognitive Studies web site with Big Five information: www.centacs.com

22

Getting Smart About IQ

The Many Ways to Be Intelligent

> 66 *Can there be any doubt that walking on the street involves intelligence?* 99
>
> —Robert J. Sternberg,
> The Triarchic Mind

When people speak of IQ (intelligence quotient, or mental age divided by chronological age times 100), they typically are referring to a score on some test of verbal, spatial, and numerical reasoning. Those scoring above 100 are seen as having an above-average IQ; those scoring under 100, a below-average IQ. It is this IQ score that the popular and academic media refer to when they speak of a person's IQ being high or low.

For example, the media write of the so-called "Flynn effect," named after the psychologist who has observed that across a dozen or so nations, IQ scores are increasing at a rate of three to seven points per decade (Flynn, 1999). The problem is that these test scores are not really based on any generally accepted theory of intelligence, nor do they help in predicting success in life (Epstein and Meier, 1989). In fact, the entire range of academic prediction tests (the SAT, GRE, ACT, LSAT, GMAT, MAT, and others) has been shown to predict only the first year of undergraduate or graduate school grades, when rote learning dominates the curriculum. These tests do not predict success in the later years of school, when more creative synthesis is required, nor do they predict work success (Sternberg, 1997b, pp. 71 ff.). In fact, Sternberg (1997b, p. 79) points out that traditional IQ (or ability) tests explain less than 10 percent of what society calls success. IQ tests originated in France as an academic screening device, and today, for the most part, they continue to be primarily an academic screening device.

At the beginning of *The Triarchic Mind,* Robert Sternberg (1988) provides a stimulating history of IQ measurement. He has suggested several problems with current IQ measures, including the following:

- Inappropriate use of the stopwatch

- Cultural bias

- Academic bias

- The assumption of a fixed quantity of IQ

- The lack of a generally accepted theory of intelligence

- The narrowness of verbal, spatial, and numerical reasoning as indicators of intelligence

- The assumption that verbally intelligent people read everything for detail

In this chapter, we will discuss three different kinds of definitions of intelligence: process, content, and structure. A summary of these three aspects of intelligence is presented in Table 22.1. The *process* definition is that of Robert Sternberg (1988), who describes the various processes at work during intellectual activity. The *content* definition is that of Howard Gardner (1983), who maintains that different kinds of intelligence exist within an individual, and that an individual has differing degrees of ability in each kind of intelligence. These two definitions complement each other: Gardner identifies several different unique domains, or playing fields, whereas Sternberg identifies the basic self-managing processes that operate regardless of domain. Consider the "resort" as an analogy. Gardner's domains are rather like different kinds of resorts, such as golf or tennis resorts, theme parks, tropical paradises, beaches, arts centers, cruise ships, campgrounds, luxury hotels, and sports camps. Continuing with this analogy, Sternberg's processes are rather like the management principles that apply to all resorts regardless of content, such as those involved in information systems, sales and marketing, people management, long-range planning, financial systems, and research and development.

Table 22.1. Three Approaches to Intelligence.

Approaches: Common Name	Approaches: Technical Name	Primary Names	Definition	Societal Relevance
Field (facts)	Domain	Gardner	Ones' ability to acquire and retain information in a given field of knowledge (talent)	Appropriate career choices Necessary for expert or professional status Cues for appropriate parenting and schooling
Mastery (use of facts)	Components	Sternberg	One's capacity for mental self-management	Appropriate role within a career The difference between managers and doers The difference between achievers and average performers
Engine (housing)	Biology and chemistry	Eysenck Zuckerman Brody	The combined effect of hereditary and environmental contributions to one's body and its component systems	The dependence of the speed, accuracy, and scope of one's intellectual efforts on the quality of one's physical body and the condition in which it is maintained

The third definition—*structure*—belongs to no one researcher but has been developed by such scientists as Hans Eysenck and Nathan Brody. Continuing with the resort management analogy, the structural definition of intelligence is much like the physical facility itself—its buildings, grounds, staff, equipment, supplies, and infra-structure—and the people who take care of it: construction workers, maintenance crews, inspectors, groundskeeping crews, food service workers, and sanitation workers. This description of the biological structure of intelligence applies regardless of content or process. It is molecular, whereas Gardner's and Sternberg's descriptions are molar. Figure 22.1 shows the relation of the three definitions to each other. The domains of intelligence (Gardner) are represented by the tennis court, golf course, and swimming pool, three separate and distinct areas of expertise; the structure of intelligence (Eysenck and others) is represented by the underground pipes and the structures with which they communicate; and the process of intelligence (Sternberg) is represented by the administration building at the top left.

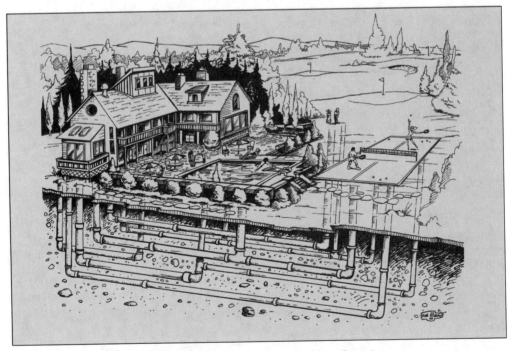

Figure 22.1. The Three Aspects of Intelligence as Illustrated by a Resort.

TOPIC 22.1 The Heritability of Intelligence

John DeFries, lead researcher for the Colorado Adoption Project, reports two strong findings concerning the heritability of intelligence (*APA Monitor,* May 1997). First, adopted children's cognitive ability correlates with the ability of their birth parents, and second, this correlation increases dramatically from age three to age sixteen. Second, the IQs of sixteen-year-old adopted children show no correlation with the IQs of their adoptive parents. These two findings point strongly to the significant contribution of inheritance to intelligence. In a recent meta-analysis of 212 studies, Bernie Devlin, a psychiatry professor at the University of Pittsburgh School of Medicine, reports that genes account for approximately 48 percent of differences in IQ scores, with prenatal care (about 20 percent), environmental effects, and chance accounting for the remainder (*Nature,* March 1998). Specific ways in which prenatal and postnatal care influence IQ are discussed in Chapter Four.

In related work, researchers have identified over a thousand genetic causes of mental retardation in its many forms. It is hoped that the fruits of this research will result in effective strategies for prevention and/or treatment.

Application

The brainpower of a child appears to be essentially set in her or his genetic endowment. Parents should provide a rich environment of love, toys, conversation, discipline, challenges, exercise, and nutrition to increase the likelihood that their children will use their potential to the fullest.

TOPIC 22.2 How Environment Shapes Intelligence

In 1994, Charles Murray and the late Richard Herrnstein caused a furor with the publication of their book, *The Bell Curve: Intelligence and Class Structure in American Life* (Herrnstein and Murray, 1994). They presented research to support the conclusion that about a fifteen-point difference in measured, traditional IQ (math, verbal, and spatial reasoning) exists between the predominantly African American lower class and the predominantly Caucasian upper class. Most researchers will agree with that conclusion. However, Herrnstein and Murray then claimed that the fifteen-point edge for Caucasians is accounted for by genetics, and that no environmental interventions can reduce the gap. In fact, they claimed, the gap is widening, with a dysgenic effect caused by the disproportionately higher birth rate among poorer African Americans. With that conclusion, a loud chorus rose in disagreement.

Robert Ornstein, in *The Roots of the Self: Unraveling the Mystery of Who We Are* (1993), recaps the dramatic impact that appropriate interventions have on the intelligence of lower-class children:

Vitamin and mineral deficiencies: A three-month dose of 200 percent of the recommended daily allowance for vitamins and minerals increases traditional IQ scores by an average of *four* points.

Birth weight: The average white infant weighs 3,286 grams at birth, while the average black infant weighs 3,069 grams. This is the result of cultural influences. Eradicating the difference in birth weight that results from inadequate prenatal care increases the average black IQ score by *five* points.

Ascorbic acid levels: Providing supplements for undernourished children who are deficient in ascorbic acid (vitamin C) increases their average IQ score by *three* points.

Head growth: Malnutrition retards brain and head growth in children, for an average effect of *five* to *six* points.

The mother's talking patterns: If IQ were exclusively genetic, then it shouldn't matter from which parent a child gets its genes. In studies of interracial couples, children with white mothers and black fathers scored an average of *six* to *seven* points higher than children of black mothers and white fathers. This effect is attributed to the observation that white mothers talk more with their children than black mothers do.

These five interventions alone could account for twenty-three to twenty-five points on a traditional measure of IQ.

In addition to Ornstein's summary of environmental factors, Sternberg (1997b) reports several additional significant factors:

- The degree of the primary caregiver's involvement with the child

- Avoidance of arbitrary punishment

- Organization of the child's schedule and environment

- Availability of play materials

- Variety in the child's daily opportunities

Citing the research of Bradley and Caldwell (1984), Sternberg states that these factors are better predictors of intelligence than is socioeconomic status.

Wendy Williams and Stephen Ceci (1997) address the issue of race and ability differences directly. After reviewing relevant trends over the last thirty years, they have formed three conclusions:

1. The gap between white and black students in ability and achievement has narrowed by between one-third and one-half. This is the result of increases in the test scores of black students.

2. The gap in intelligence scores between upper-class and lower-class families has decreased by about one-fourth.

3. The standard deviation of the Preliminary Scholastic Aptitude Test has remained stable, thereby mitigating the claims by dysgenic doomsayers that the gaps are widening.

In a review of Herrnstein and Murray's book in *Scientific American* (February 1995, pp. 99–103), Leon Kamin concludes that "the book has nothing to do with science."

Application

Do your part in leveling the playing field of life by lobbying in your part of the world for legislative guarantees of proper prenatal nutrition and postnatal child care with ample adult-child interaction (see Topic 28.1, "How Language Grows Up").

TOPIC 22.3 Sternberg's Process Definition of Intelligence

Sternberg defines intelligence as the capacity for mental self-management. I suppose this is the sort of thing Jean Piaget had in mind when he defined intelligence as "what you use when you don't know what to do" (quoted in Calvin, 1996, p. 1). These definitions obviously include more than the traditional word, number, and space problems of current IQ tests. Sternberg sees three large, inclusive domains in which self-management is necessary: the *componential* (or academic), *experiential* (or creative), and *contextual* (or "street-smart") domains. Figure 22.2 illustrates the relationship between these three domains. They take the form of six steps: (1) goal formation, (2) research, (3) strategizing, (4) tactics, (5) creativity, and (6) implementation.

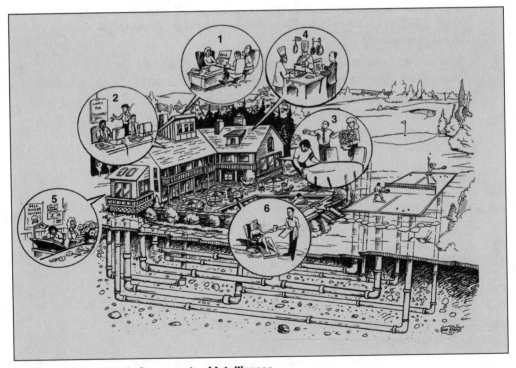

Figure 22.2. Sternberg's Components of Intelligence.
Note: (*1*) goal formation, (*2*) research, (*3*) strategizing, (*4*) tactics, (*5*) creativity, (*6*) implementation.

I like to call the componential domain of intellect the production function: it researches, plans, and executes a mental effort. Two typical examples of the componential function at work are the college research paper and the corporate annual report. Pointing to the same kind of process, Gazzaniga (1985) describes the "Interpreter" as seated in the left hemisphere of the brain. Sternberg's componential and contextual functions would appear to be a more detailed analysis of the function of Gazzaniga's Interpreter.

Another name for the experiential domain might be the "creativity" function. This function engages in the quest for originality—novelty, uniqueness, innovation, insight, and so on. (See Chapters Twenty-Nine and Thirty for further elaboration.) Sternberg identifies two aspects of dealing with novelty: how comfortable we are in dealing with new, unfamiliar experiences and how readily we understand these experiences and are able to make them a part of our normal routine, or *routinize* them.

The contextual domain is the problem solver, or, as Sternberg says, the street-smart function. Whereas the componential function deals with the efficiency of the mental effort and the experiential function deals with the originality of the effort, the contextual function deals with the rigidity of the effort. To the degree that a person always chooses the same strategy to solve problems, he or she is less intelligent than the person who calls upon different strategies that are appropriate to different occasions. The three main problem-solving strategy types are

1. *Altering yourself:* Maybe what I'm doing is causing the problem. Hence, if I change my behavior, I can solve the problem.

2. *Altering others:* Maybe what others (my spouse, boss, co-workers, friends) are doing is causing the problem. Hence, if I can change them, I can solve the problem.

3. *Altering the situation:* Maybe some features of the environment surrounding the problem (the workplace, home, organizational chart) are causing the problem. Hence, if I can change them, I can solve the problem.

To illustrate the three contextual problem-solving strategies, let's say that you experience a problem in your marriage. You could try changing your behavior (altering yourself), changing your spouse's behavior (altering others), or divorcing (altering the situation). The more intelligent (more mentally flexible) person will vary these three strategy types as problems arise. The less intelligent (more mentally rigid) person will tend to persist with the same strategy type. Rigid persisters become known as martyrs or doormats (always altering themselves), control freaks (always altering others), or quitters (always altering the situation). People with skill in this area maintain their flexibility by staying attuned to subtle verbal and nonverbal cues from their environment. Street-smart people are good at reading body language, for example. Figure 22.3 attempts to visualize how the mind manages itself according to Sternberg.

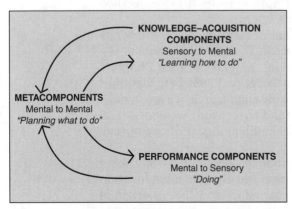

Figure 22.3. How Sternberg's Three Componential Elements Relate to Each Other.

KNOWLEDGE–ACQUISITION COMPONENTS
Sensory to Mental
"Learning how to do"

METACOMPONENTS
Mental to Mental
"Planning what to do"

PERFORMANCE COMPONENTS
Mental to Sensory
"Doing"

In a report to the 1997 meeting of the American Psychological Association in Chicago, Regina Colonia-Willner shared research on expert managers and how they reflected Sternberg's emphasis on situational flexibility. She tested 200 bank managers, 43 of whom were considered expert, with the rest simply ordinary. Sternberg's measure of contextual or situational flexibility (street smarts), which she referred to as "successful intelligence" to match the title of a book by Sternberg (1997b), was significantly better at identifying the expert managers than were traditional IQ measures.

An interesting footnote: Robert Sternberg was not the first person to observe these three features of intelligent behavior. In 1975, the Spanish physician Juan Huarte defined intelligence as the ability to learn, the ability to exercise judgment, and the ability to be creative (cited in Calvin, 1996, p. 13). Note the parallel of the first definition to Sternberg's componential (academic) element, the second to his contextual (street-smart) element, and the third to his experiential (creative) element.

Applications

1   In Figure 22.2, step 6 (implementation) is the aspect of intelligence usually referred to. The ability to use a great many words, numbers, and objects with masterful understanding, as measured by any of a myriad of IQ tests (Wunderlich, Schlosson, Wesman, California, Stanford-Binet, Wechsler, and so on), has served personnel and hiring managers, university admissions officers, counselors, and researchers for decades in their effort to distinguish the more intelligent from the less intelligent. In truth, all they have done is distinguish the more fluent in numbers, words, and object manipulation from the less fluent. And this is only the tip of the intellectual iceberg.

If you truly wish to identify more intelligent people, for whatever reason, you need to look for more than what we are here calling fluency of execution. Intelligence is not skin deep. You must look for the ability to establish goals for a complex project and administer it (step 1), find information relevant to the problem through appropriate research (step 2), be flexible in selecting a strategy to solve the problem (step 3), plan the steps of that strategy (step 4), and be appropriately creative in the design of the strategy (step 5). Steps 1, 2, and 4 are perhaps best measured through interviews and reference checks. Step 3, flexible strategy selection, can be measured directly by one of two tests: the Tacit Knowledge Inventory, published by The Psychological Corporation, San Antonio, Texas, under Sternberg's guidance, and AccuVision, a video-based metric distributed by Electronic Selection Systems Corp., Maitland, Florida. Flexible strategy selection can be measured indirectly through various Authoritarianism scales such as the combination of scores for the Challenger and Preserver traits on the NEO PI-R (Costa and McCrae, 1992). (See also Chapter Twenty-One.) The various situational leadership instruments from Blanchard Training and Development, Escondido, California, also provide an indirect measure. Step 5, creativity, can be assessed by tests (see Amabile, 1983), portfolios, and interviews.

Appendix I is a guide to use in evaluating tests, interviews, references, portfolios, and so on as a way of assessing a person's overall intelligence.

❷ If you are trying to hire someone, you may decide that not all of the six components of intelligence are important, or at least not equally important. In that case, you may hire someone who has less overall intelligence but who can do a special job well. Generally, those who demonstrate mastery in all six areas rise to the positions of greatest responsibility.

3 If you sense that you are lacking in one of these six areas, you can make up for that lack in one of two ways: either develop your ability through various educational opportunities or delegate tasks to others who excel in areas where you feel deficient. For example, if you tend to be rigid in selecting problem-solving strategies, then identify one or more co-workers with whom you can consult and who will be flexible in advising you to alter yourself, others, or the situation. Perhaps you are a person who consistently tries to alter the situation as a way of solving problems (spending money, rearranging, reorganizing, firing or transferring people, discontinuing products or services). Identify people who can advise you on how to develop other, perhaps more effective, strategies, such as altering yourself (changing habits, increasing communication, learning or improving a skill or body of knowledge, changing an attitude, reordering priorities) or altering others (coaching and counseling, training, disciplining).

4 Abandon the traditional management style that alters others, seeing employees as the root of all evil. Total Quality Management puts a heavy emphasis on altering the *situation;* it sees most errors as process-related, not people-related. *(Contributed by Rick Bradley)*

5 Check yourself against the list of intelligent behaviors found in Appendix J.

6 Recruit individuals for management or leadership positions who exhibit flexibility in their problem solving and a willingness to attack process issues. *(Contributed by Rick Bradley)*

7 Provide training in problem-solving techniques. *(Contributed by Rick Bradley)*

8 As a way of developing flexibility, or street smarts, study Csikszentmihalyi's concept of flow. Two of his books provide insight: *Flow* (1990) and *Creativity* (1996). The concept is briefly explained in Topic 30.3.

9 In the classroom, ensure that all three abilities are expected of students. Here is how the three might appear in two different subject areas:

Topic	Academic	Creative	Practical
Math	Find the error in this formula.	Create a formula that describes your theory.	How could this formula help traffic flow?
Business	Compare two types of report methods.	Reengineer a process.	Find a problem and apply the process to it.

TOPIC 22.4 Gardner's Content Definition of Intelligence

Howard Gardner (1983) has established eight criteria for identifying a domain of intellectual content:

1. Isolation by brain damage
2. The existence of prodigies in that domain
3. A core set of operations
4. Developmental uniqueness
5. Evolutionary plausibility
6. Validation from experimental psychology
7. Validation from psychometrics
8. The existence of a unique symbol system to communicate its content

He proposes that eight domains of intellectual content (called "talents") satisfy these criteria, as outlined and justified in his book *Frames of Mind* (1983) and later writings. In his 1993 work, *Creating Minds,* he provides in-depth biographies of people who illustrate the various talents (the category of "naturalist" was added after his book was printed, so no biographies appear for it). I have summarized them as follows:

1. *Linguistic:* Isolated in the left hemisphere, the linguistic domain performs the primary operations of semantics, grammar, phonology, and rhetoric. (*Example: T. S. Eliot*)

2. *Musical:* Isolated in the right hemisphere, the musical domain performs the primary operations of pitch, volume, rhythm, and timbre. *(Example: Igor Stravinsky)*

3. *Logical-mathematical:* Isolated in the right hemisphere for males and both hemispheres for females, the logical-mathematical domain performs the primary operations of long chains of reasoning, the capacity for abstraction, and calculation. *(Example: Albert Einstein)*

4. *Spatial:* Isolated in the posterior right hemisphere, the spatial domain performs the primary operations of correct perception of objects and the ability to transform and rotate objects in the mind. *(Example: Pablo Picasso)*

5. *Bodily-kinesthetic:* This domain is isolated in the left hemisphere in right-brain-dominant people and in the right hemisphere in left-brain-dominant people. It performs the primary operations of controlling the body and manipulating objects. *(Example: Martha Graham)*

6. *Intrapersonal:* Isolated in the right frontal area for males and the bilateral frontal area for females, the intrapersonal domain performs the primary operation of intrapersonal understanding, or knowing one's own feelings. *(Example: Sigmund Freud)*

7. *Interpersonal:* This talent involves interpersonal understanding, or knowing the moods, feelings, traits, abilities, and needs of others. *(Example: Mahatma Gandhi)*

8. *Naturalist:* The naturalist domain involves skill in observing, understanding, and organizing patterns in the natural environment, as in the recognition and classification of plants and animals. *(Examples: George Washington Carver, Charles Darwin)*

Gardner maintains that these eight domains are independent. High performance in one domain is not necessarily accompanied by equally high performance in another. Outstanding performance by one person in two or more domains is rare. While William and Henry James are both known as great writers (linguistic domain), Henry's novels are said to read like psychology texts (logical-mathematical domain) and William's psychology texts are said to read like novels (intrapersonal domain). Gardner speculates that a ninth domain— existential—may emerge, but as yet he has been unable to localize a brain function associated with this talent for speculating about the nature of the universe and existence.

In a similar vein, Robert Ornstein (1986) has developed the concept of the "multimind." At the time this book went to press, Ornstein had identified eleven such talents: activating, informing, smelling, feeling, healing, moving, locating and identifying, calculating, talking, knowing, and governing. Notice the considerable overlap between Ornstein's list and Gardner's. Gardner's approach is certainly more widely known, and I suspect that efforts such as Ornstein's will ultimately be integrated into Gardner's model.

Applications

❶ School curricula should include all of the eight domains, and teachers should be prepared to assist students in developing their strongest domains. In the early school years, children should be encouraged in all domains so that their strengths and natural talents become apparent. Howard Gardner's book *The Unschooled Mind* (1991) describes the curricular applications of his theory.

❷ Employers should expect high performance in only one domain and accept high performance in two or more domains as the exception. For example, to expect a human resources expert (interpersonal domain) to be a financial expert (logical-mathematical domain) is like expecting a starting quarterback (bodily-kinesthetic domain) to be a best-selling writer (linguistic domain).

❸ Parents should attempt to recognize the domain of excellence in each child and encourage development in it. All too often, a parent will encourage development in one domain (say, musical) when the child has a different domain of strength (say, bodily-kinesthetic). As in Application 1, parents should encourage their young children in all eight domains, with the goal of identifying one or more for special encouragement. For a parent to expect a child to have strengths in a particular domain just because the parent does is to fail to acknowledge the role of genetics in human development (see Chapter One).

4 Read Thomas Armstrong's *Seven Kinds of Smart* (1993), which contains specific recommendations for identifying and developing particular talents.

5 Read Bruce Campbell's *Multiple Intelligences Handbook: Lesson Plans and More* (1994). He also coauthored with Linda Campbell and Dee Dickinson the 1996 book *Teaching and Learning Through Multiple Intelligences.*

6 Visit the New Horizons web site's special section on Gardner and multiple intelligences, with links to Harvard's Project Zero and other related sites, at www.newhorizons.org/trm_gardner.html.

TOPIC 22.5 Structural Definitions of Intelligence

You Ming Lu and John Roder, neurobiologists at the University of Toronto, have discovered an enzyme that initiates learning and memorization. Called "Src," this neural chemical initiates the construction of neural pathways involved in the storage and processing of information. As reported in the February 27, 1998, issue of *Science,* Src stimulates phosphate in synaptic transmission and plays a significant role in keeping the synapse clear for future transmission. Referring to Src as a "smart" chemical, Lu and Roder predict that an "intelligence drug" is not far away.

In a direction of study that will proliferate as we reach the twenty-first century, Hans Eysenck has explored the neurobiological correlates of intelligence. He has identified three correlates of traditional IQ: *reaction time, inspection time,* and *average evoked potential* (AEP) (Eysenck and Kamin, 1981; Eysenck and Eysenck, 1985). The first two correlates, which are observed behaviors, are clearly less biological than the third, which is a description of brain waves, but they all have a common thread in their effort to identify the biological basis of intelligence.

In experiments on both auditory and visual reaction times, the reaction times of subjects with lower IQs—as measured by what Sternberg calls performance measures, such as the Wechsler and Stanford-Binet tests and Raven's matrices—increase as more stimuli are added. On the other hand, the more complex the stimulus, the faster the reaction of higher-IQ subjects (this is known as Hick's law). In other words, brighter people take progressively less time to react to progressively more complex stimuli. In addition, they show less variability in their reaction time. They are not only quicker; they are more consistent.

When they are asked to inspect a stimulus and provide a specific response, higher-IQ subjects take less time. An inspection test might have the following pattern: if you see a blue dot, press the button on the right; if you see a green dot, press the button in the center; if you see a red dot, press the button on the left.

The AEP is measured by the amplitude (height) of an electro-encephalogram (EEG) wave, the frequency of the wave (length of time in milliseconds between waves), and the complexity (irregularity) of the wave. According to AEP studies:

- The more intelligent the subject, the more complex the wave.

- The less intelligent the subject, the more variance there is across 100 tests.

- In studies of high- and low-income children, the AEP has been shown to be more culture-free, with less difference between classes, than the Wechsler Adult Intelligence Scale.

- Facing familiar stimuli, higher-IQ brains fire fewer neurons. Richard Haier, of the Brain Imaging Center at the University of California, Irvine, has found that positron emission tomography scans show higher brain activity while a subject is learning a game (for example, the Russian game Tetris, which has been adapted by Nintendo and Spectrum Holobyte). Later, less activity is detected, with activity decreasing as scores increase. He also confirms that the higher a person's IQ, the less brain activity there is.

- Facing novel, unfamiliar stimuli, higher-IQ brains fire more neurons (that is, they bring more resources to bear).

Figure 22.4 shows the different patterns of higher-IQ and lower-IQ subjects while performing two tests of reaction time: an auditory test and a visual test.

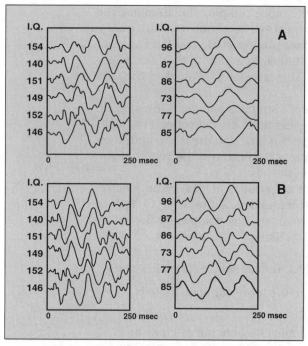

Figure 22.4. A Comparison of Evoked Potential Brain Waves in High- and Low-IQ Subjects.
Source: From *Personality and Individual Differences: A Natural Science Approach* by H. J. Eysenck and M. W. Eysenck, 1985, New York: Plenum. Reprinted with permission of Plenum Publishing Corp. and the authors.
Note: (*A*) *Auditory stimulation:* Evoked potential waveforms for (left) six high-IQ and (right) six low-IQ subjects. (*B*) *Visual stimulation:* Evoked potential waveforms for (left) six high-IQ and (right) six low-IQ subjects.

The weakness of these studies is that they relate speed to the traditional performance measures of intelligence. To my knowledge, no studies have correlated speed with, say, creativity or street smarts, Sternberg's other two major dimensions, in addition to the more traditional performance, or academic, measures.

One of the more significant physical components of intelligence is the quality of myelination. The thickness of the myelin sheath, its condition (brittle or flexible), and the effectiveness with which it grows are all associated with a variety of measures of intelligence. These relationships are summarized in an article by Edward Miller (1994). The quality of myelination is a function of diet, exercise, usage, and genetics.

Applications

❶   Where culture-free measures of IQ are critically important, consider using either a test of auditory reaction time with a supplementary test of visual reaction time (auditory tests are more reliable) or an EEG.

❷   IQ is less job-related when a worker is dealing with repetitive, familiar tasks. As tasks become more complex, IQ becomes more job-related. Don't look for bright candidates for routine work.

3 Diet, exercise, sleep, and other factors can affect the purity of the synaptic gap and the durability and firing efficiency of neurons (see Chapter Two). Don't let poor habits create a drag on your intellectual functioning.

4 In your daily approach to life, consciously try to improve your reaction time and inspection time on the tasks that are of greatest relevance to your career and lifetime goals.

TOPIC 22.6 | Intelligence and the Time Span of Work

Elliott Jaques has developed a specialized theory of intelligence as it applies to the management of work. Jaques (1994) has identified sixteen levels, or phases, of mental functioning, summarized in Table 22.2. The sixteen phases encompass brain func-

Table 22.2. An Application of Elliott Jaques's Model of Mental Processes.

	Declarative (Disjunctive)	Cumulative (Conjunctive)	Serial (Conditional)	Parallel (Conditional and Simultaneous)
Level I *Concrete Verbal*				
Level II *Symbolic Verbal*	**Stratum I** 1 day–3 months Operator	**Stratum II** 3 months–1 year First-level supervisor	**Stratum III** 1–2 years Unit manager	**Stratum IV** 2–5 years General manager
Level III *Abstract Conceptual*	**Stratum V** 5–10 years Business unit president	**Stratum VI** 10–20 years Corporate executive vice president	**Stratum VII** 20–50 years Corporate CEO	
Level IV *Universals*				

tioning that spreads from early childhood through advanced genius. Only seven of the phases are applicable to the world of work. It is these seven phases (he calls them strata) that comprise the core of his theory.

What makes Jaques's theory unique is that he has associated time spans with each stratum (phase or level). What is a time span? Put briefly, it is the length of a task an individual can handle with no help from his or her manager. For example, a Stratum II manager can handle a task that spans anywhere from three months to one year, such as the orientation and training of a new employee. A Stratum III manager can handle a task that spans from one to two years, such as the identification, purchase, installation, and training relating to a significant piece of new equipment. Jaques's recommendations are listed below as Applications.

Applications

1   Remember that people who are engaged in work that exceeds their time-span capability tend to be frustrated.

2   Be aware that people who are engaged in work that falls short of their time-span capability tend to be bored. (Notice the similarity to Csikszentmihalyi's "flow" concept in Topic 30.3.)

3   Ensure that no employee in your organization reports to a manager who is in the same time span. Managers, in order to be a resource for others, should be in the next higher time span, or stratum.

4   People should be compensated according to their time-span capability.

5   If you know a person's time span at one age, for example, at twenty-five, you can accurately predict what her or his time span will be at a later age.

6   The time span of a task is determined by interviewing people who are knowledgeable about the task, while the time-span capability of a person is determined by interviewing the person.

Table 22.3. Thinking Metaphorically About the Three Approaches to Intelligence.

METAPHOR	APPROACH		
	Domain (Field)	**Components (Mastery)**	**Biochemistry (Engine)**
Resort	Activities (golf, restaurant, swimming, tennis)	Management (advertising, planning, human resources)	Physical plant (computers, landscape, maintenance, construction)
Computer	Programs (word processing, spreadsheets)	Operating system (MS-DOS, CPM)	Central processing unit, keyboard, printer
Church	Religion or sect (Christianity, Judaism, Islam, Hinduism)	Staff and volunteers	Buildings and grounds
Business	Line departments	Staff departments	Physical plant
Military	Branch (Army, Navy)	Support and command structure	Equipment, supplies, communications
Manufacturing	Manufacturing, research and development, engineering	Sales and marketing, materials management, planning, human resources	Maintenance, purchasing, construction management

7 For a catalog of resources, contact Cason Hall & Company; Falls Church, Virginia; phone: 703-820-6200.

Some Final Thoughts on Intelligence

We humans are impelled to find the simplest explanation. Albert Einstein has cautioned us that "it is wise to express things as simply as possible, but not too simply." It appears that the twentieth century has witnessed an oversimplified understanding of intelligence. In the closing moments of the century, let us usher in a model of intelligence that is more reflective of the marvelous array of individual differences in intelligence. Paul Marciano, a young psychology professor and personal friend at Davidson College, commented to me once, "One should treat one's A students well, because they will be one's colleagues. But one should also treat one's B students well, because they will be one's doctors and lawyers and other professionals. And, alas, one should treat one's C students well, because they will endow your chair." This politic observation pays attention to the reality that there is more than one way of being smart. Earlier in this chapter, we looked at the "resort" as a metaphor for the several aspects of intelligence. Listed in Table 22.3 are several other frameworks and a description of how the various intelligences relate to them.

I propose that some enterprising soul develop a single assessment package for use in both career counseling and personnel selection. This package would need to obtain scores in all of the twenty-one elements of intelligence portrayed in Figure 22.5. In some personnel selection cases, one might only want to obtain measures that relate to a particular job in question. Table 22.4 shows how a variety of jobs fit into a matrix whose rows identify the Gardner talents and whose columns identify the Sternberg processes.

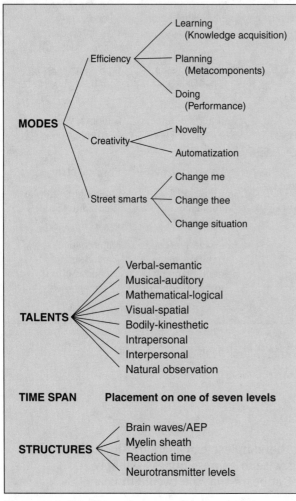

Figure 22.5. Intelligence.

Table 22.4. A Gardner-Sternberg Job Matrix.

Gardner \ Sternberg	IA. Metacomponents (Planning Ability)	IB. Performance (Vocabulary and Verbal-Numerical Reasoning)	IC. Knowledge Acquisition (Learning Efficiency)	II. Experiential (Comfort with Novel Material and Experience)	III. Contextual (Situational Flexibility, or Street Smarts)
Linguistic-Verbal ("Writing")	Book agent, publicist	Editor, speaker, actor, teacher	Critic, professor	Poet, novelist	Journalist
Musical-Auditory ("Music")	Agent, arts management	Lyricist, singer, player	Musicologist, critic	Composer, jazz musician	Accompanist, teacher
Logical-Mathematical ("Engineer")	Project manager	Systems analyst, technical writer	Purchasing agent, architect	Architect, design engineer	Project manager
Visual-Spatial ("Art")	Museum administrator	Docent, trainer	Exhibit developer	Sculptor, painter	Director of development
Bodily-Kinesthetic ("Sports")	Owner	Athlete	Sportswriter	Quarterback, point guard	Coach
Intrapersonal ("Psychology")	Chief of staff	Therapist	Researcher	Writer	Social worker
Interpersonal ("Management")	Production	Manufacturing	Quality	Research and development	Sales
Naturalist ("Biologist")	Department head	Editor	Researcher	Inventor	Environmentalist

SUGGESTED RESOURCES

Armstrong, T. (1993). *Seven Kinds of Smart: Identifying and Developing Your Many Intelligences.* New York: Plume.

Brody, N. (1992). *Intelligence* (2nd ed.). Orlando: Academic Press.

Calvin, W. H. (1996). *How Brains Think: Evolving Intelligence, Then and Now.* New York: Basic Books.

Eysenck, H. J., and Eysenck, M. W. (1985). *Personality and Individual Differences: A Natural Science Approach.* New York: Plenum.

Eysenck, H. J., and Kamin, L. (1981). *The Intelligence Controversy.* New York: Wiley.

Gardner, H. (1983). *Frames of Mind: The Theory of Multiple Intelligences.* New York: Basic Books.

Gardner, H. (1993). *Creating Minds.* New York: Basic Books.

Jaques, E. (1994). *Human Capability.* Falls Church, Va.: Cason Hall.

Ornstein, R. (1986). *Multimind: A New Way of Looking at Human Behavior.* New York: Anchor Books.

Ornstein, R. (1993). *The Roots of the Self: Unraveling the Mystery of Who We Are.* San Francisco: Harper San Francisco.

Sternberg, R. J. (1988). *The Triarchic Mind: A New Theory of Human Intelligence.* New York: Viking Penguin.

Sternberg, R. J. (1997b). *Successful Intelligence.* New York: Plume.

Part Seven

The
Brain
as
Student

Learning

23

Designing Instruction

Building Blocks for Learners

*T*he findings from cognitive research presented in this chapter all relate to how we learn. These findings will be applicable to you to the degree that you have an interest in influencing the learning of others (as well as your-self!). Clearly, not every finding and every suggested application will find its way into your learning experiences. One of the major foundations of sound learning design that should permeate your approach to learning is closely related to Addison's quote here.

> **66 What sculpture is to a block of marble, education is to the human soul. 99**
>
> —Joseph Addison

Michelangelo reputedly referred to a block of stone as "containing" the statue that he would "reveal" by chipping away the unnecessary stone. His emphasis was on intimately understanding the composition of the block, so that all he had to do as a sculptor was remove the excess, thus revealing the figure within. Each of us has a learner within that is defined by, for example, the eight Gardner talents (Topic 22.4) or the Big Five personality dimensions (Chapter Twenty-One). The experiences of an introverted intrapersonal learner will be different from those of someone who is extraverted and kinesthetic. I will not discuss this approach to learning design directly; I merely point it out and invite you to apply it in your own way.

One warning to those who design learning: Much has been said and written about the generally higher test results of Japanese schoolchildren. Apparently a major reason for this superiority is that the Japanese curriculum planners attempt a much narrower list of learning objectives than do, say, those in the United States. Where the Japanese might attempt twenty distinct mathematics skills in one year, U.S. educators might try thirty. The resulting increase in practice time per skill for the Japanese students explains much of their superiority in test performance. The lesson is clear: attempt less in breadth, demand more in depth, if what you want is higher performance in specific skills.

This chapter focuses on findings that relate to the design of learning experiences in general. Treat the chapter as a sort of cafeteria line or smorgasbord, from which you take what you need today and to which you will return later to take something different as your learning needs change. In order to help you evaluate your learning experiences overall, I have provided Appendix K, "Checklist for the Self-Evaluation of Learning Practices." Enjoy.

TOPIC 23.1 Chunking

Make an effort to limit the introduction of new information to groupings of about seven of anything. G. A. Miller (1956) has demonstrated that seven new and previously unassociated bits of information (like those found in a telephone number) are about as much as most people can work with. Once the seven or so bits of information have been mastered, they become a chunk and behave like one bit!

Applications

1   If you want people to remember a list of ten or more items, either (a) somehow reduce the list to nine or fewer items (preferably seven) or (b) break up the list into two or more units of seven chunks each, master the first list of seven before moving on to the second, and so on.

2   Where possible, take a longer list of, say, fifteen or twenty items and reduce it to about seven by identifying the biggest categories. Then learn the original list as subcategories of the shorter one. Work on the seven main categories until they have been mastered; then work on the sets of subcategories one by one until you have learned the entire list.

3   For verbal passages, start by mastering the first five to nine words or chunks. (A familiar phrase such as "Old MacDonald Had a Farm" counts as one chunk.) Then learn the next five to nine words or chunks. Put them all together and continue in the same way.

TOPIC 23.2 Testing as a Learning Process

Testing learners helps them to remember, according to Ronald P. Fisher of Florida International University. Some of his findings are summarized as follows:

- Learners who take pretests do better on their finals.

- Learners who take pretests with fill-in-the-blank questions do better on their finals than those who take pretests with multiple-choice questions.

- Learners who take pretests with inferential multiple-choice questions do better on their finals than those who take pretests with factual multiple-choice questions.

Apparently, testing gives the learner an opportunity to practice several effective learning procedures simultaneously. Tests do not have to be punitive, or even graded, to be effective. It is the act of taking the test that is helpful.

L. A. Hart (1983) argues that nondirective tests are superior to directive tests, such as multiple-choice and true-or-false exams, because learners have to identify patterns and select programs.

Applications

1 Use the beginning of a class session to review content from previous sessions. For example, in reviewing a decision-making process, you might throw out a series of questions such as "What is the first step?" "Why does it come first?" "What step is most frequently skipped?" "Why is it hard to remember?" This is a good way to use time while waiting for everyone to get back from a break.

2 Use group competition in tests. For example, divide the learners into small groups and have them make a list of the steps of a process you taught in a previous session. Let the group that finishes first recite the steps to the other groups. If they make an error, let another small group recite from that point, and so on.

3 Place learners in small groups and have each group construct a test to give to the other groups. This builds on the principle of "Handle It!" (see Topic 23.6).

4 Use card sorts to see if the steps of a process have been learned. For example, in an organization with an elaborate seventeen-step performance appraisal process, the trainer made decks of seventeen cards each, with each card containing an unnumbered step of the process. The learners had to arrange the cards in the proper sequence, as individuals and as groups. They then were allowed to review each other's work until they all thought they were right. The preferred solution was then revealed. You should be open to the possibility that in such a case the class may come up with an improvement to the process!

5 If possible, choose tests that require the learner to identify a pattern (for example, somebody doing a poor job of listening to someone else) and then to identify an appropriate program to apply (for example, a clarifying question).

6 Start a training session with a pretest that includes some of the more unusual points you will cover in your session. *(Contributed by Jane Howard)*

TOPIC 23.3 What Makes Good Textbooks?

Apart from the content of the written material used in learning, two factors seem particularly important: *style* and *organization*. In regard to style, Suzanne Wade, a professor of education at the University of Utah, reported in a presentation to the American Education Research Association in April 1993 that concrete details and visual descriptive passages are more effective in making material interesting than are amusing anecdotes and sidebars. The former make the material not only more enjoyable but more understandable, while the latter may even interfere with learning by detracting from the in-depth pursuit of information. Wade found that technical language interfered with interest and understanding at more basic levels, while concrete and visual language aided interest and understanding (*APA Monitor,* July 1993).

In regard to organization, Walter Kintsch (1994) has found that advance organizers, when they are arranged in the same way as the target text, lead to higher scores on recall of information (see Topic 24.1). However, when they are arranged differently from the target text, learners show higher scores on comprehension. Apparently, the latter condition forces more participation from the reader, hence deeper understanding. Kinsch also found that low-knowledge readers learn better from well-organized texts, while high-knowledge readers learn better from more loosely organized texts that do not spell everything out. Apparently, when more knowledgeable readers and learners see a well-organized text, they assume that they know most of it and opt not to "get involved" with the material. More loosely organized texts, such as casebooks, edited collections, and sourcebooks, are more inviting to the knowledgeable reader.

Applications

1 For beginners, prefer texts and written materials that are well organized and that employ a concrete, visual style. Avoid highly technical language. Use advance organizers that parallel the organization of the text.

2 For more advanced readers, prefer texts that are more loosely organized and that use a more technical style. Advance organizers should not be arranged in the same way as the text. Make advanced readers grapple and get involved with the material.

TOPIC 23.4 Schemas

The British psychologist Fredrick Bartlett (1932) was the first person to propose a theory of abstract cognitive structures called schemas. If schemas are similar to an experience, they render our memories accurate; if they are different, they color our memories accordingly. The biological basis of a schema is a neural pathway that represents the schematic diagram of a specific cognitive process. We have schemas for telling stories or jokes, giving directions, and solving problems. We may even have several different schemas for each task. David Rumelhart (H. Gardner, 1985, p. 125) describes the standard schema for storytelling; I have summarized his description as follows:

1. State the goal.
2. Enumerate the steps to the goal.
3. Relate the reactions along the way.
4. Describe and comment upon the success or failure in reaching the goal.

Our schemas differ from each other's just as our experiences do. Someone who has learned the Chinese language will have different schemas from someone who hasn't. In one sense, the story of our mental life is the story of either (1) forming new schemas or

(2) accommodating new experiences to old schemas. Most learning appears to be a process of fitting new information into old schemas. Our existing schemas tend to determine how we evaluate and shape new information unless we work hard to establish new schemas.

John Bransford, co-director of Vanderbilt University's Learning Technology Center, has determined that schemas play such a strong role in coloring new learning that learners can't help but modify what they hear and see according to their prior experience. Learners who hear "The doctor's son greeted his father" will typically tend to accommodate this statement to their schema about doctoring and see the son shaking hands with a father who is a doctor, rather than allowing for the possibility that the doctor is actually the mother, standing by and watching her son greet his father, who is not a doctor. Bransford says that this tendency is so strong and so pervasive that the instructor must take responsibility for listening to students discuss their newfound knowledge and clarify instances of inappropriate accommodation to previous schemas. As Hodgson's law says, we tend to remember a thing the way we want to remember it.

An example of this is a story educator John Holt tells of visiting an elementary school and observing a geography lesson. The fifth-grade teacher was pointing to a wall map of the United States and was asking the students questions dealing with points of the compass. Holt, on a hunch, asked if he might ask a question. He approached the wall map, removed it, and laid it flat on the floor. He then asked the students, "Which way is north?" All the students pointed toward the ceiling!

L. A. Hart (1983) defines learning as the acquisition of useful schemas, which he calls *programs*. He defines a program or schema as a sequence used for attaining a preselected goal. Programs are triggered when the learner recognizes a pattern. If the program works (that is, the learner achieves the goal), fine; otherwise, the learner tries another program or looks for another pattern.

Mary Crawford (1995) has clarified the influence of gender differences in learning schemas. According to her research, many females acquire certain schemas that males are less likely to acquire, such as "how to mend a shirt," while many males acquire certain schemas that females are less likely to acquire, such as "how to build a workbench." She has found gender differences in the amount of detail recalled when two groups are told the same story but given different titles, with each title representing a gender-specific schema. For example, most females will remember more detail from a story entitled "How to Mend a Shirt" than one entitled "How to Build a Workbench," even when the two stories are identical except for the title (that is, the story is about building a workbench that is used to show how to mend a shirt).

Janet Kolodnor (1997) builds on the idea of schemas by demonstrating the effectiveness of analogous situations as a teaching tool. By relating new concepts structurally to familiar situations or schemas, learners demonstrate greater understanding and retention. For example, teaching the concept of how the multiple points of view in the Continental Congress in the newly formed United States were satisfied might be simplified by convening a class meeting about a similarly divisive subject, such as how the school should or could treat the needs and desires of students and their families with respect to different religious traditions and holidays.

Applications

1 Before teaching someone a new skill or body of knowledge, first find out what the learner already knows that is similar. Then proceed with your instruction, pointing out the ways in which this new learning is similar to or different from the learner's existing schemas. For example, if the learner is to learn arc welding, find out if he or she has had experience with other kinds of welding machines, soldering irons, and so on. This is a normal part of the technical training model called job instruction training (see Eckles, Carmichael, and Sarchet, 1981, p. 340).

2 As we get older, we have more complex and more numerous schemas to build on. This is particularly helpful in the *peg-word technique* for memorizing lists. Say that you want to memorize the ten largest cities in the world. You start by making a list of rhyming words for the numbers one to ten. You then think of an association between the rhyming word (the peg word) and the name of the city; the more whimsical or outrageous the association is, the easier it will be to remember. For example:

Number	Rhyme	City	Association
One	Bun	Tokyo	*Looks like the bow on the traditional Japanese kimono*
Two	Shoe	Mexico City	*Mexico as the shoe of the body of the North American continent*
Three	Tree	São Paulo	*The land of rain forests*
Four	Door	New York	*The traditional door to the United States for immigrants*
Five	Hive	Seoul	*A beehive of political activity*
Six	Sticks	Osaka	*"O sock-a me with the sticks"*
Seven	Heaven	Buenos Aires	*Heaven is good air*
Eight	Gate	Calcutta	*"Cut a" gate into the fence*
Nine	Line	Bombay	*The coastline around the bay*
Ten	Pin	Rio de Janeiro	*Pin (blame) it on Rio*

Once you've memorized the peg words (bun, shoe, and so on), all you have to do is form good visual associations between the peg word and the related item on the list you're trying to memorize. The mind can easily relate the schema of bun, for example, to both sweet rolls and the bow on the back of the kimono. See examples in Lorayne and Lucas (1974) and Buzan (1991).

3 When you think a common schema exists for everyone in a group, you might refer to it in front of the whole class. For example, if you are talking about performance appraisal, you might discuss how it is similar to and different from traditional school report cards.

4 Ask questions and provide examples that relate to the experiences of the learners. Help them to see the connection between their experiences and what you are teaching.

5 Allow your learners time for exploration. Help them to verbalize both the patterns they recognize and the programs and schemas they choose to apply (L. A. Hart, 1983). Here's a model of the process:

- Recognize the pattern.
- Implement the program.
- Evaluate the program. If it fails, reinterpret the pattern, look for a new pattern, try a new program, or try a variation on the failed program.

6 When using familiar schemas (basketball, cars, cooking, sewing) to explain a concept (for example, how to find a percentage), remember that some students will be unfamiliar with some of the schemas. Be sure to use a representative set of schemas in order to give all the learners an equal chance to learn the concept. Try to find more gender-neutral schemas (such as eating, swimming, or reading) to use as a basis for new learning. Test the intended schema with the group by asking if everyone is familiar with it.

TOPIC 23.5 Two Modes of Processing Information

Seymour Epstein (1994), reviewing more than thirty different studies on human information processing, has identified two independent yet interactive methods that individuals use: *experiential* and *rational*. These two modes have been given various names over the last century; seeing all these different names together (Table 23.1) is a powerful argument for their prominent role in human learning.

People who are strong in one mode may be weaker in the other. Even when learners are strong in both modes, redundancy in instructional design will result in greater learning by the greater number of learners. The experiential mode is more right-brained, while the rational mode is more left-brained.

Applications

1 Ensure that your learning design contains a balance of experiential and rational learning strategies. For example, for every expository definition given to the learner, provide a story that illustrates it.

Table 23.1. Two Modes of Human Information Processing.

Mode	Experiential / Narrative (Learning Feelings and Behaviors Through Schemas)	Rational / Expository (Learning Attitudes and Beliefs Through Language)
Defining Characteristics	Unconscious, emotionally engaging, personally convincing, interpersonal, automatic, independent of intelligence and age, storylike, concrete, specific, primitive, simpler, perceptual, positive, imagistic, rapid, more effective in changing feelings and behavior	Analytical, conscious, formal, theoretical, more complex, general, removed from direct experience, capable of negation, abstract, public, logical, structural, organized, conceptual, more related to verbal, numerical, and spatial intelligence
Traditional Synonyms for Mode Title	Unconscious	Conscious
	Nonverbal	Verbal
	Procedural	Declarative
	Contextual	Propositional
	Prototypical	Logical
	Episodic/procedural	Semantic
	Tacit/implicit	Explicit
	Mythos	Logos
	Natural	Extensional
	Automatic	Reflective
	Heuristic	Effortful
	Direct, behavioral experience	Indirect, nonbehavioral experience
	Narrative	Propositional
	Biological	Conceptual
	Implicit	Self-attributed
	Biological	Linguistic
	Prewired	Intentional
Typical Learning Strategies Associated with Mode	Stories, settings, intentions, emotions, actions, scripts, narratives, plots, moods, five senses, images, pictures, acting, movement, feedback mechanisms, metaphors	Charts, tables, exposition, diagrams (nonnarrative), formulas, systems analysis, symbol systems, organizational methods, process designs

Source: Adapted from "Integration of the Cognitive and the Psychodynamic Unconscious" by Seymour Epstein, August 1994, *American Psychologist, 49*(8), 709–724.

2 For every point you explain, tell a story to illustrate it.

3 For every essay you assign, find a narrative or story to illustrate the concept, and vice versa.

4 For every drama, review criticism.

5 For every activity, talk about it (called "processing" in human relations parlance).

6 For every lecture, conduct an experiment. For example, if you are lecturing on African history, get the class to make some predictions about their peers' knowledge, and then confirm, as by asking "How many of you know where Nigeria is located?"

7 For additional ideas on how to balance the two modes, read Don Norman's *Things That Make Us Smart* (1993).

TOPIC 23.6 Handle It!

One of the best ways to learn a body of information is to manipulate it in such a way as to make it yours. I have a friend who understood this principle in undergraduate school. After each lecture, he would return to his room with his notes, then sit at his typewriter and rewrite the notes in an outline form that was meaningful to him. Four years later, he had earned his Phi Beta Kappa key! Handle it to get a handle on it.

Another dimension of this learning principle was expressed by Robert Bjork (1994, p. 192): "Manipulations that speed the rate of acquisition during training can fail to support long-term post-training performance, while other manipulations that appear to introduce difficulties for the learner during training can enhance post-training performance." I am reminded of the passage from Aeschylus's *Agamemnon* that is variously translated as "Man must suffer to be wise" and "He who learns must suffer." Nothing new, that passage by Bjork. Easy come, easy go. The easier, more pain-free the practice is in the classroom, the more difficult it will be to transfer the information to the street, home, or workplace. After students show initial understanding, the instructional design should include variations, interference, distractions, and other difficulties that will make the learner struggle with the deep, or essential, structure of a new learning and not be content with just its surface structure.

Bjork (1994, p. 188) recommends that learned material be "multiply encoded," using multiple models, paraphrases, and examples rather than a single version: "The research is unambiguous: A variety of manipulations that impede performance during training facilitate performance on the long term" (p. 192). This principle of learning is often violated for several reasons:

1. Trainers and teachers are evaluated on a short-term basis.
2. Trainers and teachers typically don't see the long-term effects of the learning.
3. Follow-up is not usually done by the original trainer or teacher.
4. Trainers and teachers often confuse current success with future success.

Applications

1 If you are a teacher and want to hand out an outline of your material, wait until after you've covered it. This forces the learners to write their own notes and struggle with the wording and outline. The act of having to "handle" the material helps the learners to build on their existing schemas.

2 If the material forms some kind of list or chart, put the elements on cards. Then have either individuals or groups arrange the cards in a correct or meaningful order.

3 Have small groups generate their own examples of the point you are making.

4 Use role playing.

5 Have the learners write their own case studies.

6 If the learners are to apply a skill (such as constructive criticism) to a job, have them write out a script to use.

7 Examine books on the subject of TRICA (teaching reading in the content areas). These texts contain hands-on activities and are meant for high school teachers with students who do not read well. The activities work well as an adult learning technique, regardless of reading level.

8 Have the learners prepare a presentation for each other. (Remember, the best way to learn something is to teach it.)

9 Suggest that the learners make a presentation back on the job to others who are unable to attend. Allow time in class to begin work on such a presentation.

10 Give the learners, alone or in groups, an unorganized list of all the elements of your presentation and let them decide how they'd like to organize it.

11 Have individuals or groups rank a list of items according to some criterion. This helps them to grapple with the concepts.

12 Vary the conditions of practice: schedule practice in a random fashion, minimize order and predictability, and vary the length, scope, distance, order, resources, context, or subject.

13 Interrupt practice with both related and unrelated events and information.

14 Introduce the model (for example, with advance organizers) by using an outline that is inconsistent with the practice model.

15 Used spaced and distributed practice rather than massed practice (see Topic 24.2).

16 Reduce feedback: use summary feedback after several trials, rather than feedback after each trial.

TOPIC 23.7 Applying Classroom Ideas to the Real World

Whenever you teach a theory or concept, give the learners time to apply it to specific situations. Many learners are unable mentally or unwilling motivationally to apply an idea to an everyday situation. Detterman and Sternberg (1993) paint a discouraging picture of training in the workplace. They distinguish between "learning" and "transfer of learning." Learning has occurred when one is able to repeat a new behavior in nearly identical situations close in time to the original learning event. Transfer of learning has occurred when one is able to repeat a new behavior in different kinds of situations that are remote in time. Detterman and Sternberg distinguish "near" and "far" transfer. Near transfer occurs when one repeats a behavior in a similar situation that is remote in time; far transfer occurs when one repeats a behavior in a different situation that is remote in time. Following a thorough review of the literature, they maintain that far transfer doesn't occur.

Roughly $100 billion is spent annually on training in the workplace. Detterman and Sternberg estimate that only about 10 percent of that training actually transfers to the workers' jobs. Baldwin and Ford (1988) confirm these numbers; in addition, they state that this 10 percent is only of the "near" variety. An example of near transfer would be learning a counseling skill in a classroom role play involving an employee who repeatedly arrives late to work, then actually using that counseling skill back on the job with an employee who is repeatedly tardy. Applying that skill to a different situation, like that of an employee who never puts her or his tools back in the right place, would be far transfer, and Detterman and Sternberg (1993) say that this just doesn't happen:

> When I [Sternberg] began teaching, I thought it was important to make things as hard as possible for students so they would discover the principles themselves. I thought the discovery of principles was a fundamental skill that students needed to learn and transfer to new situations. Now I view education, even graduate education, as the learning of information. I try to make it as easy for students as possible. Where before I was ambiguous about what a good paper was, I now provide examples of the best papers from past classes. Before, I expected students to infer the gen-

eral conclusion from specific examples. Now, I provide the general conclusion and support it with specific examples. In general, I subscribe to the principle that you should teach people exactly what you want them to learn in a situation as close as possible to the one in which the learning will be applied. I don't count on transfer and I don't try to promote it except by explicitly pointing out where taught skills may apply. . . . There is no good evidence that people produce significant amounts of transfer or that they can be taught to do so. There is, on the other hand, substantial evidence . . . that favors the idea that what people learn are specific examples. Experts are experts because they have learned many more examples than novices. . . . Current evidence suggests all that is necessary to be an expert is time, basic ability, and the opportunity to learn a large body of exemplars by experience [p. 17].

[An expert's] knowledge is so ample and elaborately structured that it is hard to present an expert with a problem that is not already represented therein [p. 174].

People who know a lot about something are not experts because of their ability to transfer but because they know a lot about something [p. 18].

The lesson learned from studies of transfer is that if you want people to learn something, teach it to them. Don't teach them something else and expect them to figure out what you really want them to do [p. 21].

Robert Bjork (1994) extends this thought by commenting that "perceived similarity, or the lack thereof, of new tasks to old tasks is a critical factor in the transfer of training. . . . To the extent feasible, a training program should provide a learned representation that permits the learner to recognize when the knowledge and skills acquired during training are and are not applicable to new problems" (p. 186). Bjork emphasizes that retrieval practice during the training session is critical in assuring future transfer and retrieval: "Retrieval information becomes more recallable in the future than it would have been without having been accessed. In that sense, the act of retrieval is a 'memory modifier.' . . . As a learning event, in fact, it appears that a successful retrieval can be considerably more potent than an additional study opportunity, particularly in terms of facilitating long-term recall" (p. 188).

Applications

1 Use printed, video, or audio examples. For example, the excellent course, "Interpersonal Management Skills" (IMS), developed at Xerox, provides printed worksheets with good and bad examples of the skills applied in different settings (plant, office, home, and so on), an audiotape with examples and practice exercises, and a videotape with both good and bad examples. The IMS program is available from Learning International, Inc.; 225 High Ridge Road; Stamford, Connecticut 06905.

2 Using your schemas, give examples from your personal experience to illustrate a concept, then ask the learners to generate other examples in small groups, building on their schemas.

3 If you want the learners to apply a concept or skill you are teaching to some situation far away from the classroom, then think up some likely scenarios and have the learners apply the concept or skill in the new settings through role play, small-group work, or individual work.

4 Whenever possible, use real situations in the classroom for the learners to copy later in other situations. Don't just use generic case studies. In my problem-solving classes, for example, I have students write up a list of problems they'd like help in solving; then we pick the ones my techniques apply to and work on them.

5 Broad and Newstrom (1992) have found that the manager, the trainer, and the learner each play an important role in transferring learning back to the job. Further, they find that the timing of the involvement of these three roles is different. Although all three should be involved with the learner before, during, and after the learning episode, it is especially critical for the learner to be involved *before* the learning (with prework and advance organizers), for the manager to be involved *during* the learning (with observation, input, feedback, and support), and for the trainer to be involved *after* the learning (with follow-through practice, support, and feedback).

TOPIC 23.8 Practice

Provide enough time for practice. Supervised practice allows for the feedback necessary to refine the learning, while practice in and of itself is crucial in the process of converting the learning from short- to long-term memory (see Chapter Twenty-Five). Practice clarifies and strengthens the neural connections that are formed while learning. But practice should not be mindless, as Topic 23.6 points out. Appropriate complications in the practice program help to build a deeper understanding of the schema underlying the new learning.

Robert Bjork (1994) comments that "people learn by making and correcting mistakes. We have known at least since [1955, in a paper by Estes] that it may be necessary to induce forgetting during training to enhance learning. Training conditions that prevent certain mistakes from happening (and give trainers a false optimism about their level of comprehension and competence) can defer those mistakes to a post-training setting where they really matter" (p. 201). Bjork warns that the principle of introducing mistakes into training is especially important in such roles as public safety officers, nuclear power plant operators, military personnel, and transportation workers. For these and other jobs, it is crucial that we look for *mistakes* during training, not the absence of mistakes.

Applications

1 Role playing is an effective way to practice, especially for interpersonal skills. Try to make it less intimidating by having several pairs or groups of three do the role play at the same time and then discuss the results together, rather than putting two individuals on the spot in front of the class.

2 Provide case studies, both off-the-shelf and real. They give learners the opportunity to practice applying their learning under your supervision.

3 Introduce appropriate distractions, irrelevant information, and other real-world properties that make practice more mindful. For example, in role-playing a seven-step counseling interview, have the interviewee intentionally lead the interviewer forward and/or backward in the process, so the interviewer develops a sense of understanding and control concerning the importance of managing the process firmly.

④ When using a simulator (such as a flight simulator) for practice, the most important element is randomness, not physical appearance. Simulators should be psychologically faithful to the real world, not just faithful in an engineering sense.

⑤ In batting practice, randomly varied pitches give better performance results than blocks of pitches (for example, fifteen curves followed by fifteen sliders).

⑥ Practice skills that require identical performance conditions in a way that varies the conditions; for example, practice free throws in basketball at varying distances and heights, practice point-after-touchdown conversions in football at different distances, timings, widths, and heights.

TOPIC 23.9 Focus and Attention

In spite of teenagers' claims that they can do homework in front of the television set, the brain cannot focus on more than one stimulus at a time. What may appear to be multitasking, or simultaneous focusing, is in fact a rapid alternation of focus. The more routine a stimulus is, the less it interferes with rival stimuli. So if you're listening to the news while driving on the interstate with moderate traffic, you will miss far less of the news than when you are driving around the Place de l'Étoile in Paris trying to maneuver across eight lanes of circular traffic. To underscore this point, University of Toronto physicians Donald Redelmeier and Robert Tibshirani report that automobile drivers are 4.3 times more likely to have an accident while using a cellular telephone than when the unit is not in use. Furthermore, they report that "hands-free" operation provides no safety advantage over hand-held sets (*New England Journal of Medicine*, February 13, 1997).

Much has been made of "information overload" in the 1990s. I don't buy it. Oprah Winfrey was concerned about forgetting the security codes to Harpo Studios in Chicago and about forgetting on Thursday the subject of Tuesday's show. Her producers called and asked if I'd care to come to the show and explain what they were referring to as "Yuppie Alzheimer's." Certainly. I explained that information overload, or Yuppie Alzheimer's, did not exist. There has always been abundant information vying for our attention. The hunter-gatherers who survived and made our existence possible were those who paid attention to the source of berries, seeds, and other nutrients. Can you imagine a gatherer in 10,000 B.C. wandering around a new terrain, finding berries, and *not* making it a point to remember the location? The next day, he'd make a beeline to yesterday's berry source. The gatherers who mindlessly skipped from bush to tree, from berry to nut, without paying effortful attention to remembering their locations, were doomed, at worst, to languish tomorrow in hunger or, at best, to waste precious time in having to relocate the stash.

So what did I tell Oprah and her viewers? "Stop and smell the roses. If you really want to remember something, make a point of remembering it. Focus, intend, practice." To make my point, I looked at her intensely and said, "I'm going to make a point of remembering exactly what you look like today. I know people will ask me. Well, you are wearing gold knot earrings with three strands woven in a pattern about three-quarters of an inch in diameter. You are wearing a two-piece tan knit suit, with the dress floor length (almost) and the jacket open and three-quarter length." By intending to remember, and by really *focusing* on her attire, I still remember it some two years later. And because so many people ask me about the show, I keep recalling it, which further reinforces the memory. Oprah can improve her recall with similar efforts at focused attention with the intention of remembering. It's funny: when we were in school, we made a point of trying to remember. As adults, we casually read or observe without similar efforts at remembering, such as taking notes or reviewing, and then we lament that we are "losing our memory" when we can't remember! Balderdash. We're expecting results like those of our schooldays without exerting a similar effort. There's something wrong with that picture.

Attention is maximized by learning design elements such as "Handle It!" (Topic 23.6) and "Practice" (Topic 23.8).

Applications

1 Avoid playing music if you want the learner to concentrate. My wife and I once attended a workshop together. The leader asked us to complete a worksheet individually and silently. As we began our seat work, the leader started to play some background music. I believe it was a fifties' tune. Well, my wife knew every word to that and each succeeding tune, silently sang along with them, and found it impossible to concentrate on the worksheet. The background music became foreground for her.

2 Don't introduce a new skill on top of a prior one until the prior skill has become routinized. Practice the skills separately until one is mastered; then you may build on it. My daughter understood this well when, at the age of eight, she took Suzuki violin lessons. One day, as I was supervising her practice, she lost patience with my approach and glared at me, saying, "I'll keep my wrist right or I'll keep my feet right. Take your pick. But don't make me do them both at the same time."

3 Try to use your car phone only when the car is not in motion.

4 When you must use your phone while driving, inform the other party that you're driving and that you may have to refrain from talking or listening if the traffic gets complex.

5 Avoid using car phones when you're approaching intersections and when you're passing or being passed. Use them instead when you're cruising down a highway or major road with moderate traffic.

6 If you're talking on the car phone and approach an intersection, simply tell the other party, "Please hold for a second until I get beyond this intersection."

7 Remember, doing two things at once is an illusion; you're actually doing the two things in alternating streams.

8 If you really want to remember something, stop and pay attention to it. Don't create competing distractions.

TOPIC 23.10   Visualization

Remember the importance and effectiveness of visual and mental rehearsal in combination with physical rehearsal and practice in preparation for an event. Visualization, also referred to as mental practice, has been demonstrated to be effective in improving motor skills, although there is no evidence that it improves cognitive and behavioral skills. See Druckman and Bjork (1991) and Gawain (1978).

Application

If you are an athlete, executive, actor—anyone wanting to achieve a smooth, masterful performance—close your eyes and internally simulate the performance in your mind. Allow yourself to accompany this visualization with approximate physical movements or pantomime.

TOPIC 23.11   Modalities

Much has been written over the last thirty years advocating the use of multiple sensory channels, or modes, for conveying instruction. Most individuals have a stronger, or preferred, mode—visual, auditory, or kinesthetic. Accordingly, if a teacher or trainer uses both visual and auditory modes to present information, the chances are enhanced that people who prefer one of these modes will learn. This is related to Howard Gardner's work on multiple intelligences (see Topic 22.4). In a recent study, researchers at the University of New South Wales reported that frequently, two simultaneous modes of presentation can enhance learning (*Journal of Experimental Psychology: Applied,* December 1997, pp. 257–287). For example, a learner could follow visual instructions and diagrams on a television monitor with auditory reinforcement of key points. The New South Wales researchers found that when two simultaneous modes each present complete details, one interferes with the other. It is better for one mode to present the complete set of instructions, with the second mode simultaneously presenting only bare, skeletal (schema-like) information that reinforces the key points of the primary mode. Two simultaneous presentation modes, each with abundant detail, violate the principle of attention (see Topic 23.9).

Applications

1   When you are lecturing or verbally presenting information, ensure that your visual aids only contain key points. Otherwise, the details in the visuals will interfere with the details in the spoken presentation. When you need to switch modes in order to present complicated visual information, as in a large row-by-column table, then you should slow your speech to make only key points while the learners focus on the details of the table.

2   When you are presenting information kinesthetically, as in demonstrating a movement with the learners moving along with you, don't be tempted to fill in the silence by talking the entire time; only speak to make key points.

3   When you are presenting information visually, as in a videotape, the most effective sound track will make sparing commentary, and only to emphasize key points in order to focus the learners' attention. Don't distract them with chatter. If you need to chatter, allow the visual mode to subside by using a freeze-frame or some repetitive action.

TOPIC 23.12   Strategies for Learning

Claire Ellen Weinstein has made lemonade of lemons. When she was a Brooklyn teacher, she found that her father and siblings were inefficient learners. In her efforts to teach them strategies they could use to improve their learning efficiency, she ultimately won a doctorate from the University of Texas at Austin that was based on her assessment of learning strategies and her accompanying developmental recommendations. Students who benefit from her model show remarkable improvements in high school and college course outcomes. The graduation rate of the at-risk students at the University of Texas at Austin who experience her model is 71 percent, compared to 55 percent for the student body at large (*APA Monitor,* April 1998, p. 36). Her instrument, LASSI (Learning and Study Strategies Inventory), is used by over half the colleges in the United States and has been translated into more than thirty languages.

The LASSI model is tripartite: skills, will, and self-regulation. The 177-item assessment measures the student learner in ten areas:

1. Information processing
2. Selection of main ideas
3. Test strategies
4. Attitude
5. Motivation
6. Anxiety
7. Time management
8. Concentration
9. Study aids
10. Self-testing

Application

Obtain a copy of LASSI and assess your learning effectiveness or that of someone close to you. Request a sample from H & H Publishing Company, Inc., in Clearwater, Florida; phone: 800-366-4079; or E-mail your request to hhservice@hhpublishing.com. Or visit their web site at www.hhpublishing.com and order LASSI in the quantity you desire.

Some Myths About Learning

Table 23.2 lists some learning methodologies that have claimed positive results but have not stood up to scrutiny. In 1984, the U.S. Army Research Institute asked the National Academy of Sciences to form a

Table 23.2. Some Myths About Learning.

Method	Conclusion and Comments
Learning during sleep	There is no evidence of this with verified sleep. There is some evidence with light sleep. It is difficult to verify sleep stages. This technique is worth a second look. Disturbing sleep raises ethical issues.
Accelerated learning (SALTT, Suggestopedia, SuperLearning)	Of eleven elements identified, only two were nontraditional and both were found to be ineffective: relaxation (too much of it causes lack of focus) and review with music (it interferes with attention). No basis was found for the high claims. Good accelerated learning is basically no different from good teaching generally. Claims of five to fifty times' improvements were based on poor research designs. The two best studies (Bush, 1986; Wagner and Tilney, 1983) found that SALTT produced 40 to 50 percent lower results than traditional methods. The other nine elements of accelerated learning were all deemed to be traditional characteristics of effective teaching already in mainstream use: advance organizers, dramatic presentation, spacing, practice, mnemonic aides, student-generated elaborations, tests, imagery, and cooperation in groups.
Altered consciousness	This is an optimal arousal concept worth further research. Devices such as Hemi-Sync that stimulate a specific hemisphere apparently do not enhance learning. A satisfactory methodology is unavailable for researching these claims.
Neurolinguistic programming (NLP)	There is no evidence that one person can influence another as a result of matching representational systems. It is difficult to isolate individual variables in NLP research. There are poor dependent variables in much of the research (for example, "client-therapist empathy" is a vague dependent variable).
Parapsychology	It doesn't work. Existing programs at Stanford University, Princeton University, and Brooklyn's Maimonides Medical Center, and in San Antonio, should be monitored. Researchers need to agree on a research methodology.
Subliminal self-help	There is no evidence, either theoretical or experimental, for the effectiveness of this technique.
Meditation	Meditation is no more effective in reducing arousal than just resting quietly. There is no evidence that soldiers can be taught "soldier-saint" superhuman skills by yogis.

committee to evaluate such "nonordinary" techniques for improving human performance. This request followed the urging of those who felt that "New Age" educational technologies that had been developed outside the mainstream might have some basis for their claims of achieving high results. The defense establishment was willing to consider any technique that might provide a competitive edge in the armed services. John Swets, a consultant from Cambridge, Massachusetts, was appointed chair of the committee, and Daniel Druckman, formerly of the consulting firm of Booz Allen and Hamilton, was appointed study director. Their results were published as *Enhancing Human Performance: Issues, Theories, and Techniques* (Druckman and Swets, 1988).

During the next two years, reaction to this publication was intense and widespread. As a result, the committee re-formed in 1990 with the purpose of evaluating additional areas that had not been included in the earlier study, as well as to address concerns in reaction to the earlier study. Robert Bjork was brought in as committee chair and Druckman was retained as study director. Their findings were published as *In the Mind's Eye: Enhancing Human Performance* (Druckman and Bjork, 1991). Several of the findings in these two books have been presented in this and other chapters.

SUGGESTED RESOURCES

Broad, M. L. (Ed.). (1997). *In Action: Transferring Learning to the Workplace.* Alexandria, Va.: American Society for Training and Development.

Broad, M. L., and Newstrom, J. W. (1992). *Transfer of Training: Action-Packed Strategies to Ensure High Payoff from Training Investments.* Reading, Mass.: Addison-Wesley.

Buzan, T. (1991). *Use Your Perfect Memory* (3rd ed.). New York: Penguin Books.

Caine, R. N., and Caine, G. (1991). *Making Connections: Teaching and the Human Brain.* Alexandria, Va.: Association for Supervision and Curriculum Development.

Druckman, D., and Bjork, R. A. (Eds.). (1991). *In the Mind's Eye: Enhancing Human Performance.* Washington, D.C.: National Academy Press.

Druckman, D., and Swets, J. A. (Eds.). (1988). *Enhancing Human Performance: Issues, Theories, and Techniques.* Washington, D.C.: National Academy Press.

Hart, L. A. (1983). *Human Brain and Human Learning.* White Plains, N.Y.: Longman.

Lorayne, H., and Lucas, J. (1974). *The Memory Book.* New York: Stein & Day.

Metcalfe, J., and Shimamura, A. P. (Eds.). (1994). *Metacognition: Knowing About Knowing.* Cambridge, Mass.: MIT Press.

Norman, D. A. (1993). *Things That Make Us Smart: Cognitive Artifacts as Tools for Thought.* Reading, Mass.: Perseus Books.

Sternberg, R. J., and Davidson, J. E. (Eds.). (1995). *The Nature of Insight.* Cambridge, Mass.: MIT Press.

24

The Role of the Teacher

Techniques for Facilitating Learning

66 *The teacher's task is not to talk, but to prepare and arrange a series of motives for cultural activity in a special environment made for the child.* 99

—Maria Montessori,
The Absorbent Mind

Not only have we all experienced classroom learning, but many of us will have the opportunity in the near or distant future to teach something to a group. Sales representatives teach their prospects as a part of their sales presentations. Other people may conduct a training class for employees, teach an elementary or secondary school class, teach at the university, conduct an evening class at the community college, give religious instruction, orient new employees, train employees on the job in new skills and technologies, or teach (that is, persuade) power brokers to pursue a certain path. This chapter is intended for the teacher in all of us.

The best lesson plan in the world is less effective than it could be if the teacher using it fails to bring to the plan what only good teachers can bring. That is the role of the teacher: to present content for learning in a way that makes students most likely to learn. I distinguish here between the design of learning experiences and the role of the teacher. Although there is some overlap, one can design learning but never teach it, and one can teach without having designed. This chapter looks at what brain research has to say about the teacher's role as a facilitator of learning, regardless of whether or not the teacher designs the learning.

> **"Those who educate children well are more to be honored than even their parents, for these only give them life, those the art of living well."**
>
> —Aristotle

L. A. Hart (1983) suggests that any educational environment should be characterized by the following four general features:

1. High expectations

2. A nonthreatening ambiance

3. A goal of 100 percent mastery

4. An air of reality (that is, it consists of more than just books)

Of course, we should all keep in mind that the learner is often the best teacher. Just because we focus in this chapter on the role of the teacher, don't ignore these principles if you're not a teacher. We are all learners, so many of these ideas apply to us as we teach ourselves.

TOPIC 24.1   Advance Organizers

Students tend to learn more when they are given some warning about what they are to learn. Perhaps this brings relevant schemas into the foreground or at least prepares them to put forth an appropriate effort to form new ones. Techniques used to alert learners about the nature of an upcoming learning episode are called advance organizers because they help them to call up relevant schemas in preparation for learning.

Applications

1 Send out preliminary reading materials.

2 Provide an outline or agenda of the learning experience both in advance of the session and at the beginning of the session.

3 Review the objectives at the beginning of the session.

4 Tell people what you are getting ready to do. Abruptly moving into an activity is disturbing to many people.

5 Have the attendees meet with their supervisor or team members before the class to agree on expectations.

6 At the beginning of the session, give the participants some kind of big-picture overview of the material to be covered; this provides a map for the terrain.

7 Ask the participants what their expectations are. *(Contributed by Jane Howard)*

8 Choose appropriate textbooks (see the Applications for Topic 23.3).

9 In Chapter Ten we learned about the Mozart effect, or how playing Mozart-type music prepares the mind for spatial reasoning tasks. That is a kind of advance organizer.

TOPIC 24.2 Spacing

In a classic 1978 experiment in educational psychology, British postal workers learned to use a new machine. Those who studied one hour a day learned twice as fast as those who studied four hours a day in two two-hour sessions. The two-hour group learned to use the machine in half as many days but spent twice as many hours learning. In other words, the more hours per day they spent in instruction, the more total time they required. Clearly this would be desirable only under a deadline. Prefer spaced to massed learning where possible. Learning is *spaced* if it is composed of multiple modules with a significant time lapse between the modules. Spaced learning for a given quantity of learning consists of shorter modules with time for practice and assimilation in between the modules.

Harry Bahrick, a psychologist at Ohio Wesleyan University, believes that teachers should institutionalize spacing concepts. His research establishes the superior effect of cumulative learning. The more that people study and review, the more they remember. He found that high school Spanish students who took five courses remembered about 60 percent of the vocabulary twenty-five years after finishing high school, while students taking only one course remembered almost none, in spite of the fact that neither group had used Spanish to a significant degree after high school. Again controlling for usage, he compared 1,726 adults who had finished high school fifty years previously and found that those who had gone on from high school algebra and geometry to take college-level math at or above the level of calculus scored 80 percent correct on an algebra test. Those who took only high school algebra and geometry and did as well as the college math group in their high school math courses managed to score only slightly better than a control group who had taken no algebra or geometry at all in high school or anywhere else! Bahrick laments that we spend millions helping people learn, then let them forget what they have learned.

Applications

1 Try to schedule learning modules of no more than two to four hours per day; allow time and space for practice between sessions. Build in frequent breaks when this isn't possible.

2 If you must have an all-day seminar, take extra care to allow participants time to read in advance and to practice and review afterward.

❸ Schools should change from the quarter system to the semester system, and from longer class periods to shorter class periods (and more of them).

❹ Schools and other learning organizations should require review of prior material both during the course and in subsequent courses.

❺ Schools should include cumulative courses that review and integrate prior courses and should give cumulative final examinations.

❻ Schools should offer courses that meet, for example, once a week for two or three years, rather than three times a week for four months. The general rule should be to spread out learning as much as possible to maximize retention.

❼ Carefully plan training for new employees to avoid overwhelming them during their first days on the job. *(Contributed by Rick Bradley)*

❽ Schedule more frequent, shorter staff meetings.

TOPIC 24.3 Breaks

Research indicates at least two good reasons to take breaks after each learning module. First, the new neural connections formed by the learning need time to fix and strengthen themselves without competition from additional novel stimuli. A simple walk around the block can serve to provide such jelling time. This is like the need in darkroom photography for a "fixing" chemical to stabilize the photographic image. Second, because of fatigue factors, errors increase as break time decreases.

Applications

❶ Some form of exercise is an excellent follow-up to a learning episode because of the impact of the extra epinephrine on the formation of neuronal connections. Perhaps you could lead your students in stretching, bending, and breathing exercises after a learning episode.

2 The best time of day to take in new material is just before going to sleep. Research indicates that material studied then tends to be remembered better. Sleep, in one sense, is another way to take a break. Encourage learners to do memory work before going to sleep.

3 In classes of adults, announce that students can leave the room whenever they wish, but also have periodic, scheduled breaks. *(Contributed by Jack Wilson)*

TOPIC 24.4 Incubation

To come up with creative responses to problems, time is needed for the information to incubate. As Louis Pasteur remarked, "Chance favors only the mind that is prepared." Do your homework; then let intuition work on it. When I was a first-year student at Davidson College, I had a tennis class under Coach Lefty Driesell. One day, after Lefty hit a ball past me, I shouted out, playfully, "LUCK!" Driesell stopped dead in his tracks, glared at me, and said, "There's no such thing as luck, Howard. It's preparation meeting the opportunity."

Applications

1 Allow for a substantial break, when possible, after problem-defining activity and before idea-generating activity.

2 Many of us participate in team-building retreats. The best use of these overnight problem-solving sessions is to present the information (attitude survey results and so on) before bedtime, then, in the morning, after it has incubated, to come up with creative responses in a planning session.

3 Teams and departments often push through meeting agendas, grasping at the first suggestion that develops in order to get to the next item. Make it a group norm to allow for more incubation time when a matter is not urgent. Better planning often results.

TOPIC 24.5 Follow-Up

The best way to ensure that classroom learning will be forgotten is to fail to provide opportunities for follow-up and follow-through. Studies show that a larger portion of the material learned in a classroom setting is retained when the learner or the teacher makes provisions for follow-up.

Applications

1 Have learners write goal letters to themselves and mail them out several months later. They all will receive letters from their conscience about what they intended to work on after the training session.

2 Make sure that after returning to the job, the learners schedule a conference with their supervisor or team to review their accomplishments and the possibilities for applying the learnings on the job.

3 Develop refresher modules of short duration for students to take periodically.

4 Have class reunions.

5 When using a series of spaced modules, provide homework assignments (practice or reading) between sessions. Review the homework, sharing the students' successes and failures at the beginning of each session.

6 Plan during class how each participant will apply new learnings to the job—for example, by writing scripts, developing implementation schedules, identifying obstacles to success, or writing personal development plans.

7 Send out audio- or videotapes that recap the major points of the training session.

TOPIC 24.6 **Control**

The teacher is the one person most able to influence the learner's sense of control over the learning process. If the learner feels in control, a wider range of learning, both rote and meaningful, can occur. If the learner feels highly controlled, only rote learning can occur. Caine and Caine (1991) call this *taxon* (list) and *locale* (map) learning. Locale learning encourages creativity, analysis, synthesis, planning, problem solving, and complex decision making. When the learner feels relaxed and in control, the cortex is fully functional, and thus higher-level, more meaningful learning is possible. When the learner feels out of control of the learning process, he or she "downshifts" (Caine and Caine, 1991) from cortical locale learning to the limbic system's taxon, or rote, learning. In this condition, the cortex essentially shuts down. The only learning possible involves rote memorization or learning of simple skills, and the only creativity or problem solving possible is that which is based on habits, instincts, or other already learned routinized behaviors.

Sometimes people appear to be able to learn only simple, routine skills because they have low ability, when in fact they can only learn routines because they are under stress. Away from the sources of the stress, they can be more creative and complex in their learning behavior. By being stressful or perceived to be stressful, the learning environment, or classroom, can itself prevent cortical learning. Make sure that your classroom does not force downshifting. (For a more extended treatment of stress and control issues, refer to Chapter Twenty.)

Applications

1 At the beginning of a class, clearly establish learner control by reviewing class norms; for example, you might say, "Feel free to take a break when you need to," "Please let me know if you're physically uncomfortable and I'll see what can be done about it," or "Please feel free to ask any questions whenever the need arises; the only dumb question is the unasked question."

2 Help learners set their own goals for learning.

3 Use effective listening techniques, such as active and reflective listening, paraphrasing, and clarifying, that have the effect of focusing on the learners and underscoring their control.

4 Ask open-ended questions; they invite the learner to be more involved in the process. Avoid questions with yes-or-no responses; they discourage involvement. And avoid questions starting with "Why . . . ?" This type of question tends to create stress in learners and make them defensive (see Flanders, 1970).

5 Use some of the Applications suggested in Topics 23.4 through 23.7. These four topics—schemas, processing modes, "handling" the material, and real-world application—place the learner in the driver's seat.

6 Respect differences in learning styles by accommodating students' stylistic differences as much as possible: their need for cool or warm temperatures, preference for dim or full light, desire for snacks, or need for physical activity.

7 Build in opportunities for participant involvement such as role plays, case studies, and small-group work. *(Contributed by Rick Bradley)*

8 Allow participants to select their own seats without assigning them. If you want to mix the learners up after a break, ask them to select new seats with new people on either side. They will still maintain the same sense of control.

TOPIC 24.7 Relaxation

As discussed in Topic 24.6, encouraging the learner to feel in control is a major strategy in preventing downshifting—that is, moving from cortical alertness to limbic arousal, or stress. Another strategy would be to help learners who are already under stress (for example, those coming into your class after a bad encounter) to "upshift"—to move from limbic fight-or-flight arousal into cortical arousal and alertness. When a person comes to your learning experience full of stress, that stress must be relieved before meaningful learning can occur. The primary strategy to use in the classroom is relaxation. However, too much relaxation is not conducive to learning. For further consideration of this point, see Topic 20.5, which discusses stress and arousal and the Yerkes-Dodson law, and the comments on accelerated learning in Table 23.2.

Applications

1 Play tapes with sounds of nature—rainstorms, desert winds, the beach, birds—before class, during breaks, or during silent individual work like reading or filling out worksheets. Nature sounds have a way of refocusing a person away from absent stress and into the here and now.

2 Play tapes with simple classical music (Mozart is a good common denominator) before class or during breaks, as a way of helping people refocus. Don't play music during individual work, however.

3 If you are the teacher, lighten up from time to time in a way that is appropriate for you. This keeps students alert and prevents them from downshifting.

4 If you are a student, practice some of the relaxation techniques described in the Applications for Topic 20.4.

TOPIC 24.8 Rapport

Researchers, particularly in the field of neuro-linguistic programming (NLP), have tried to identify why some therapists seem to work magic on clients. They have found that effective therapists tend to establish rapport with clients by matching and pacing—in other words, by mirroring the clients' posture and following their tempo. The research suggests that matching and pacing another person has the effect of establishing rapport and increasing trust and openness. Matching and pacing are discussed further in Topic 32.4.

Applications

1 Using Figure 32.1, find authentic ways of establishing rapport by matching and pacing your learners.

2 When you have a student who seems to be resisting your help, identify the biggest differences between the two of you and see if you can eliminate some of these differences or at least minimize their effects.

3 Move toward a participant who is asking a question or making a comment; establish rapport by getting closer and using eye contact. *(Contributed by Jane Howard)*

TOPIC 24.9 Positive Expectations

Rosenthal and Jacobson (1968) established that positive expectations tend to yield positive results and negative expectations yield negative results. See Topic 32.3 for more on this subject.

Applications

1 Communicate clearly to all students that you have confidence in their ability to excel.

2 Communicate to all students your confidence in your own ability to teach effectively.

3 Communicate to all students your confidence in previous students' successful application of classroom learning to the real world.

4 Resist the temptation to give up on some students; maintain high expectations for all of them. Remember, you may have some students who've been told all their lives that they're failures, so don't be discouraged if you don't make much of a dent in their self-concept.

If enough of us treat them with positive expectations, we increase the chances of their success.

5 If it is appropriate, mention other groups, classes, or organizations that have successfully completed the program.

TOPIC 24.10 **Enuf's Enuf (Habituation)**

Habituation is the psychological term for "enough is enough." Our sensory receptors become aroused when a new stimulus begins, but if the new stimulus continues without variation in quality or quantity, our sensory receptors shut down from their aroused state, having become habituated, or accustomed, to the monotonous stimulus. A change in the quality or quantity of the stimulus will arouse the receptors again. This is why, for example, it is hard to pay attention to someone who speaks in a monotone. It is also why people often add salt, pepper, or other seasoning after several bites. Druckman and Bjork (1991) stress the need to vary training conditions to prevent habituation and its attendant inefficiency in learning.

Tracey Revenson, a professor at City University of New York, attests to the value of varying presentation style by emphasizing the importance of acting ability to good teaching (*APA Monitor,* January 1994, p. 40). She constantly varies energy level, perspective and role, pace, accent, mood, and more. In the same article in the *APA Monitor,* University of Southern Indiana professor Joseph Palladino stresses the effectiveness of using appropriate humor—that is, humor that fits the context. He teaches the concept of successive approximation by getting down on all fours and bleating like a sheep until the class successfully trains him to their desired objective.

Another approach to this topic is called "mindfulness," which uses frequent changes in auditory and visual attention in order to maintain alertness. Borysenko (1987), Langer (1989), and R. Cooper (1991) each suggest specific techniques for avoiding the fatigue that results from sustained attention. A facilitator of learning should teach these techniques to the learners. Avoiding habituation, or attentional fatigue, is a two-way responsibility. The teacher can certainly provide a variety of stimuli, but the learner can also take preventive action. Mindfulness appears to be the flip side of the concept of "monkey mind," described in Topic 20.4, Application 7.

Applications

1 Have someone videotape you while you are teaching (or simply set up a videotape camera, aim it in your general direction, and let it run). Review the tape and critique yourself for signs of repetitive behaviors that might tend to lessen the alertness of your students: talking at the same pitch, the same volume, or the same speed (never even slowing down to make a dramatic point); using the same vocabulary (complex Greek- or Latin-derived words rather than simple Anglo-Saxon ones); standing or sitting in the same place; walking in the same pattern (desk to window, window to desk, desk to window, and so on); limiting eye contact (always looking at the same three or four students or from the window to the ceiling and back); or waving your arm the same way for emphasis.

2 Seek out authentic ways to vary your behavior to maximize students' alertness. Remember when the teacher played by Robin Williams in *Dead Poets Society* jumped up on his desk or walked the class into the hall to view a picture? He knew how to avoid habituation. Fight it like the pLaGuE!

3 Minimize learning tasks that exceed five to ten minutes, and search for ways to vary tasks to maximize the students' arousal: contrast lecture with discussion, whole-group or small-group learning with individual seat work, reading with writing, standing with sitting, remembering and mastering with creating, practicing with critiquing.

4 After each break, encourage the learners to take a seat in a different part of the room.

5 Jump, clap, shout, throw, wave, stomp, roll, whisper.

6 Offer graphs to trainers for feedback on how well they do with this habituation paradigm. I once was asked to observe a superintendent of schools as he conducted a staff meeting. He had a reputation for horrible meetings. The first thing I noticed was his monotone.

I charted his variation in pitch, volume, tempo, vocabulary, posture, and gesture over time. The resulting graph showed nothing but a group of flat lines. It made the point and he understood why and how to improve.

7 To avoid visual fatigue, keep shifting focus: don't focus on the same point for more than a few seconds; study an object for one minute, then close your eyes and try to reproduce it in your mind's eye, then open your eyes and compare; remember to blink frequently; practice scanning by looking for all the examples of one specific letter or number on a page; refresh your scanning skills by doing crosswords and jigsaw puzzles.

8 To avoid auditory fatigue, practice selective focus: pick out one of several auditory signals in your environment and focus on it exclusively, then pick another; when listening to music, select one instrument and focus on it for a while to the exclusion of other instruments, then shift to another instrument. When you are faced with the cacophony of two speakers blaring different voices or music, try alternating your focus between the two different signals.

TOPIC 24.11 Developing Prestige

In their research, Caine and Caine (1991) found that students perform better when they perceive the teacher to be prestigious. They further found that this prestige comes primarily from two perceptions: that the teacher has expertise and that she or he is caring. Expertise is assumed from the appearance that the teacher has mastered the subject, is not dependent on notes (except to help in sticking to the subject), and has practiced what is being preached. Caring is assumed from the appearance that the teacher accepts and values each student as a human being.

Applications

1 Practice the Applications in Topics 24.8 and 24.9.

2 Try visualizing the class process in much the same way that a skier visualizes a downhill sequence before jumping off. Keep notes on potential problems you spot while visualizing, then solve them after you finish.

3 Try a dry run in which you move through the class process rapidly, again keeping notes on potential problems.

4 Try putting notes on the borders of your transparencies to avoid the distraction of looking down at notes in your hand.

5 Try the lesson plan out first on a test group (office mates, your family, a group of employees, or even paid guinea pigs). Have them critique you or simply serve as a live test audience.

6 Arrive early and greet people by name; don't rush away as soon as the lesson is over.

7 During breaks, mix and mingle.

8 Lightly pencil your notes onto blank flip-chart pages prior to class. The notes will go unnoticed by participants and you'll be perceived as being well versed in your subject. *(Contributed by Rick Bradley)*

9 When seeking input from a group, capture their responses on a flip chart or transparency. *(Contributed by Rick Bradley)*

10 Acknowledge input from the group. *(Contributed by Rick Bradley)*

11 Work hard to understand your audience and their issues and concerns. Use this understanding to build class outlines. Use real-life examples they can relate to.

12 If you have been brought into an organization as an outside expert or guest, have someone from the organization introduce you to the group. *(Contributed by Jane Howard)*

13 Display or mention licenses, certificates, apprenticeships, degrees, and awards.

14 Whenever possible, bring current information from a recent newspaper, television show, journal, or other information source. This contributes to your learners' perception of you as keeping abreast of your field.

15 Award-winning professor Charles Brewer of Furman University says that teachers must show a "passion for their discipline, and a passion for sharing what they know about it with their classes. . . . That's what separates gifted teachers from those who merely teach" (*APA Monitor,* January 1994, p. 39).

16 Give the class a brief handout that includes a vita and other relevant information about you and your qualifications, along with a contact phone number or E-mail address, for later reference. *(Contributed by Helen Hyams)*

TOPIC 24.12 Atmosphere

Research has identified a long list of learning atmosphere variables, each of which suggests its own Applications. See more discussion of workplace design in Chapters Thirty-Three and Thirty-Four.

Applications

1 Faber Birren, in *Color and Human Response* (1978a), has suggested the many effects of color on people. See Topic 34.3 for a listing of these effects.

2 Ensure abundant light, especially at the beginning of a session, for those who may not be fully awake.

3 Remember that a moderate amount of background noise (so-called white noise) is helpful for concentration. If the room is too quiet when participants are working silently at their seats, you can run the fan of an overhead projector. *(Contributed by Jane Howard)*

Paradoxically, white noise can also be helpful in eliminating distractions when you are trying to fall asleep or stay asleep. An air filter with an audible fan works well. *(Added by Helen Hyams)*

4 You can take advantage of the knowledge that arousal (either limbic or cortical) is associated with a warmer brain, pleasant moods with a cooler brain. Robert Zajonc, of the University of Michigan, has found that slow, minor-key music warms the brain and breathing through the nose cools the brain (Izard, Kagan, and Zajonc, 1984).

5 Provide enough telephones nearby to reduce adult learners' stress at being unable to keep in touch with their offices. I've been in many workshop situations in which fifteen to twenty people had only one telephone in the building to use during breaks—not a good situation.

6 Avoid serving high-carbohydrate foods for snacks; they produce a pleasant mood and sleepiness. Choose proteins and low-carbohydrate foods like fruits, vegetables, low-fat crackers, and nonfat dips, all of which are better for mental activity. Supply juices and diet sodas rather than full-strength sugared colas.

7 Make sure that ample caffeine-free beverages are available to prevent overarousal, which makes concentration difficult.

8 Encourage participants to sit in a different place after each break; NLP research indicates that this improves participation and freshens the participants' perspective.

9 Have a no-smoking policy during class.

10 Allow fifty square feet per person in the classroom; less is stressful.

11 Plan the lighting in the room carefully when you are using slides or an overhead projector. Develop alternatives if the room must be darkened too much.

TOPIC 24.13 Richness

Mark Rosenzweig of the University of California, Berkeley, conducted a classic experiment in which two groups of rats were compared for the impact of environmental richness on brain development. One group was placed in a dull cage, the other in an enriched Disneyland-type cage. The brains of the highly stimulated rats grew larger and developed denser concentrations of synapses. Other research, including research on humans, has confirmed these findings. See particularly the work of Marian Diamond (1988), also of the University of California, Berkeley, who concludes that synaptic structures show growth from enriched environments throughout the life span, including old age.

Parallel to Diamond's work, Fred H. Gage and a team of researchers at the Salk Institute for Biological Studies report that enriched environments actually result in increases not only in synaptic complexity but also in the total number of neurons, or brain cells. Gage found a 15 percent increase in brain cells in the mice from enriched cages compared to brain cells in mice from dull cages (*Nature,* April 1997). This research, along with that of William T. Greenough of the University of Illinois, who has shown that aerobic exercise in rats increases the number of neurons (see the information on exercise in Chapter Eight), demonstrates that with proper management, we can *replace* some of the cells lost as a result of natural aging, disease, alcohol, and other brain toxins. Gage has reported that he and a Swedish team have actually observed the generation of new brain cells in humans (*Nature Medicine,* November 1998). This sets the stage for generalizing Greenough's and others' research to humans.

Applications

1 Put up a variety of posters, corporate and otherwise, such as "Today is the first day of the rest of your life," on the walls of the classroom.

2 As you complete flip-chart diagrams, lists, and so on, tear them off and tape them to the wall for visual reinforcement.

3 Place games and puzzles around the border of the room and on the students' tables for manipulation during idle moments.

4 Have a computer around for experimentation with relevant software, or for playing games during breaks.

5 Hang appropriate photographs on the walls.

6 Place artwork on the walls of the classroom and in nearby hallways.

7 Have books for browsing in the classroom.

8 Supply several daily newspapers in the classroom, such as the *Wall Street Journal* and *USA Today.*

9 Place mirrors in appropriate locations for self-stimulation. Mirrors enhance self-concept among infants and relieve boredom among adults. In one amusing incident, tenants of an office tower complained of long elevator waits. The owners installed mirrors in the elevator waiting area and the complaints disappeared. Preening makes the wait grow shorter!

10 Post information about local resources such as restaurants and shopping centers. Include maps.

11 If it is appropriate, have participants bring in and display some of their own work. As an example, in Bank of America Quality Team meetings, which bring facilitators from across the company together for two- or three-day seminars, participants are asked to show how quality is being visibly promoted in their area. The walls and tables are filled with posters, buttons, banners, T-shirts, memos, job aids, and team pictures. It creates real excitement. *(Contributed by Rick Bradley)*

12 Use graphics and color on overhead projections, slides, participant guides, and so on. *(Contributed by Rick Bradley)*

13 Ditch the black flip-chart marker. Use a variety of colors. *(Contributed by Rick Bradley)*

14 When you are headed for a particularly boring meeting, make sure to carry along at least three colors of ink pens and colored paper to take notes with. *(Contributed by Rick Bradley)*

15 Include extra, relevant reading materials such as articles for participants to read if they finish individual tasks before other people are done. *(Contributed by Jane Howard)*

TOPIC 24.14 Peer Feedback

Peer feedback has been found to be more influential than teacher feedback in obtaining lasting performance results; too much teacher feedback can be harmful (Druckman and Swets, 1988). Apparently the approval or disapproval of one's peers is the best reinforcer. Excess feedback from the teacher can be perceived as being insincere if it is too effusive or demotivating if it is too discouraging.

Applications

1 Emphasize peer feedback for student performance in small groups or one-on-one interaction.

2 One effective technique is to have graduates of a seminar meet in pairs over breakfast or lunch six months later for a follow-up session in which they discuss their successes and failures in implementing the class concepts and skills.

3 In role plays, have all the participants do the exercise at the same time in groups of three—two to actually play the roles and one to help by making suggestions to a participant who is stuck and by providing feedback. *(Contributed by Jane Howard)*

TOPIC 24.15 Self-Explanation

Michelene Chi (Chi, de Leeuw, Chiu, and La-Vancher, 1994) reported on the effectiveness of allowing learners to explain what they have learned. Learners who give explanations of what they have learned achieve at higher levels, while learners who receive explanations from the teacher achieve at lower levels. This relationship holds true regardless of ability: both high- and low-ability learners who self-explain show 30 percent increases in achievement after learning, compared to only 20 percent gains for those who do not self-explain. In addition, the more explanation that is given (people who do this are called "high explainers"), the higher the gain. So high self-explainers achieve more than low self-explainers, and low self-explainers gain more than those who do not self-explain at all. This topic actually serves as an elaboration of Topic 23.6 ("Handle It!"): verbal self-explanation is a way to personally become involved with content by handling information.

Applications

1 Ask learners to explain what they have learned both during and at the conclusion of a learning episode. Encourage them to put it in their own words.

2 A variation on Application 1 is to ask learners who've arrived at a wrong or unacceptable conclusion or solution to explain the process that led them to the wrong answer. By talking through the process, either the learner or you as the listener-facilitator can identify errors in the process that account for the unacceptable answer. The educator John Holt advocated this practice in his book, *How Children Fail* (1995). I once had the opportunity to tutor a neighbor's middle school daughter in mathematics. My strategy was simply to have her talk through the steps she had used for each of the problems the teacher had marked as wrong. In each of the wrong answers, we were able to spot an error in her process of problem solving. About halfway through the session, she remarked to me, "This is fun! I've never done this before." I asked what it was that she hadn't done before. She replied, "The teacher always goes over our wrong answers. I've never had a chance to talk about how I solve them with the teacher listening to me!"

3 Occasionally, even though a learner has arrived at an acceptable answer, you are not certain that the process that got him or her there was sound; in other words, the learner may have been lucky. In such a case, asking the student to give a self-explanation by narrating how the conclusion was reached would help to clarify whether the result was luck or skill.

4 Employ learning activities that engage the learner in writing or speaking in summaries (précis) or paraphrases.

TOPIC 24.16   Stereotypes and Performance

Claude Steele (1997), a professor in the psychology department at Stanford University, has studied the way stereotypes affect the performance of African Americans in college and the performance of females in the mathematical sciences. He has studied other stereotyped groups as well, but these two are his primary focus. Steele is interested in a particularly puzzling phenomenon: why do capable women and African Americans underperform? Or, expressed another way, why do women who are excellent at mathematics (and who positively identify with the field of mathematics) perform worse in the first two years of college than their SAT and ACT math scores would predict? In a parallel vein, why do African Americans who are high achievers in high school, and who have high SAT and ACT verbal scores, achieve a significantly lower grade point average in the first two years of college than would be predicted by their scores?

Steele hypothesized that these two groups were underperforming because of the effect of *stereotype threat*. Subtly, or not so subtly, he suspected, these two groups were receiving the message that they did not belong. To test his hypothesis, he administered difficult SAT math questions to capable college women and difficult SAT verbal questions to capable college African Americans. The experimental groups were told that the answers to the questions would in no way reflect on them as a gender or racial group. For example, students in the experimental groups might be told that the questions were being evaluated for readability in order to remove the performance threat associated with stereotyping. The control groups were allowed to complete the questions with no special instructions; in other words, they answered the questions with any assumptions they made about stereotype threat fully in effect.

The result was that the experimental groups outperformed the control groups and performed at the levels that had been predicted. Steele concluded that teachers and program administrators can remove the barriers to performance in groups affected by stereotype threat by intervening in a way that makes the students feel included, capable, valued, and successful. In a program designed to test his treatment assumptions, Steele and others carried out an intervention at the University of Michigan called "Twenty-First Century," with dramatically successful results. The Applications below list specific strategies.

Applications

① Teachers and administrators must exhibit optimistic behaviors and attitudes toward students who are subject to stereotype threat (see the discussion of optimism in Topic 20.1).

② Eliminate the stigma of "remedial" work, preferring instead programs that accept students at their current level of achievement and supportively challenge them to tackle progressively more demanding work.

③ Through a variety of means, such as posters and conversation, communicate to students that ability is not a fixed quality. Emphasize that people can incrementally increase their ability.

④ Affirm that stereotype-threatened groups (women in math courses, African Americans in college honors programs, men participating in interpersonal sensitivity training) belong in their chosen domains by providing role models and other signs of inclusion. Steele emphasizes that in this case, intellectual belonging is substantially more important than social belonging.

⑤ Value and employ a variety of approaches to the subject matter.

⑥ For students who do not positively relate to the stereotyped subject (for example, women who do not see themselves as mathematicians), emphasize nonjudgmental acceptance of their efforts, preferring a Socratic dialogue to an emphasis on right or wrong answers. Until a pattern of success emerges, prefer acceptance to praise. Above all, build the students' sense of competence, level by level.

A Final Word on the Role of the Teacher

Harvard psychologist Ellen Langer (1997) has launched a major initiative to change classroom education from a world based on right answers to one based on flexible thinking. She proposes that seven myths permeate classroom education that seriously curtails the learning process (*APA Monitor,* August 1997, p. 97). Following is my adaptation of the list of myths that she challenges:

Myth 1: The basics should be learned so well that they become second nature. (*Fact:* Overlearning stifles creativity and individual expression.)

Myth 2: Paying attention means staying focused on one thing. (*Fact:* Novelty, as in examining unfamiliar aspects of familiar objects, people, and things, holds attention.)

Myth 3: Delaying gratification is important. (*Fact:* Keeping the fun in learning leads to more meaningful learning.)

Myth 4: Rote memorization is necessary in education. (*Fact:* Students who relate material to personal experience do better than memorizers on tests of comprehension.)

Myth 5: Forgetting is a problem. (*Fact:* Memory can be a straitjacket, preventing the formation of novel uses and applications.)

Myth 6: Intelligence is knowing "what's out there." (*Fact:* Lifelong learners, not know-it-alls, are the true experts.)

Myth 7: There are right and wrong answers. (*Fact:* Correctness is dependent on context.)

Also, in a masterful summary of the effectiveness of training, Robert Bjork (1994) points out that current research challenges two traditional—and incorrect—assumptions about training: that it should be relatively risk free (that is, it should protect the learner from the pain of making errors) and that it should be orderly (with no skipping around). Bjork argues that simple and orderly learning provides good short-term results, such as A's on tests at the end of the course and high marks for the teacher. However, "simple and orderly" learning does not establish memories that last for the long term. Learners need multiple ways of experiencing a new concept or skill, and unpredictable opportunities to practice it, in order to understand it and have access to it for the long term.

Bjork supports this with two storylike experiments. A control group of batters on a California State University baseball team practiced hitting first fifteen curve balls, then fifteen sliders, then fifteen fastballs. The experimental group also practiced hitting forty-five pitches, but in random order. The latter group outbatted the group with the simple and orderly batting practice. In the second experiment, two groups of eight-year-olds practiced throwing beanbags into a bucket. They were to be tested at a distance of three feet. The control group practiced all throws from three feet, while the experimental group practiced some throws from two feet, others from four feet, and *none* from three feet. And guess what! The latter group outperformed the former, even though the experimental group had never had an opportunity to throw from the distance used in the final test.

SUGGESTED RESOURCES

Bjork, R. (1994). "Memory and Metamemory Considerations in the Training of Human Beings." In J. Metcalfe and A. P. Shimamura (Eds.), *Metacognition: Knowing About Knowing* (pp. 185–206). Cambridge, Mass.: MIT Press.

Borysenko, J. (1987). *Minding the Body, Mending the Body.* Reading, Mass.: Addison-Wesley.

Caine, R. N., and Caine, G. (1991). *Making Connections: Teaching and the Human Brain.* Alexandria, Va.: Association for Supervision and Curriculum Development.

Cooper, R. (1991). *The Performance Edge.* Boston: Houghton Mifflin.

Diamond, M. (1988). *Enriching Heredity: The Impact of the Environment on the Anatomy of the Brain.* New York: Free Press.

Druckman, D., and Bjork, R. A. (Eds.). (1991). *In the Mind's Eye: Understanding Human Performance.* Washington, D.C.: National Academy Press.

Druckman, D., and Swets, J. A. (Eds.). (1988). *Enhancing Human Performance: Issues, Theories, and Techniques.* Washington, D.C.: National Academy Press.

Hart, L. A. (1983). *Human Brain and Human Learning.* White Plains, N.Y.: Longman.

Langer, E. (1989). *Mindfulness.* Reading, Mass.: Addison-Wesley.

Langer, E. (1997). *The Power of Mindful Learning.* Reading, Mass.: Addison-Wesley.

Rosenthal, R., and Jacobson, L. (1968). *Pygmalion in the Classroom.* Austin, Tex.: Holt, Rinehart and Winston.

Sylwester, R. (1995). *A Celebration of Neurons: An Educator's Guide to the Human Brain.* Alexandria, Va.: Association for Supervision and Curriculum Development.

25

Learning That Sticks

Insights for Enhancing Memory

> **66 My memory is the thing I forget with. 99**
> —*A schoolchild*

Research on memory has taken a signifi-cant turn in the last ten years. Memory used to be regarded as a struc-ture; now it is seen as a process. A memory was thought of as a single unit with an identifiable place of residence some-where in the brain that could be recalled when necessary. Now a mem-ory is viewed as a recon-struction from many different chunks stored redundantly throughout the brain (see Topics 23.1 and 25.1). Bartlett (1932, p. 213) foresaw this development when he wrote:

> Remembering is not the re-excitation of innumerable fixed, life-less, and fragmentary traces. It is an imaginative reconstruction, or construction, built out of the relation of our attitude towards a whole active mass of organized past reactions or experience, and to a little outstanding detail which commonly appears in image or in language form. It is thus hardly ever really exact, even in the most rudimentary cases of rote recapitulation, and it is not at all important that it should be so.

This new view of memory was brought dramatically to the public's awareness after John Dean's testimony at the Watergate hearings. Viewers were initially impressed with Dean's avowed excellent memory for detail. But when his testimony was later compared to accurate records of conversations, viewers (and Dean himself) were flabbergasted to learn that most of his testimony was at best flawed and at worst made up.

Defining Memory

Memory is learning that sticks. Before memory, potential new learnings linger briefly in a kind of "scratchpad" about the size of a postage stamp that is located in the right prefrontal cortex, above the right eye and about one inch behind the forehead. This working-memory area can hold the proverbial seven plus or minus two bits of information until such time as we decide to hold onto it. When we decide to remember it, new synapses are formed, old synapses are strengthened, or both. These new or strengthened connections are the new learning. The synaptic connections are the molecular equivalent of a chunk of newly learned material, such as a telephone number. Initially, as we learn, a protein called C-kinase is deposited among certain hippocampal neurons, according to Daniel Alkon of the Marine Biological Laboratory, Woods Hole, Massachusetts. Apparently, C-kinase causes the branches of the brain cells to narrow. When they have narrowed and formed new synapses, learning has occurred. Unless the learning is converted into long-term memory, however, it will disappear, just as new muscle fiber will break down if it is not used. Again, we must use it or lose it.

Researchers on a team drawn from both the University of Texas Medical School at Houston and the University of Houston have reported the discovery of a new protein, transforming growth factor–B (TGF-B), which works as a kind of congealing agent that solidifies new synapses (*Science,* March 1997). In research with snails, the Texas team found that the presence of TGF-B was associated with substantially higher electrical charges, hence stronger responses to stimuli. The discovery of this protein shows that in addition to "Use it or lose it," we also need the proper chemical makeup. Watch this line of research; it could very probably lead to breakthroughs in the treatment of Alzheimer's disease and other memory disorders.

With continued use, the hippocampal cells extend the storage of the new learning to the cerebral cortex, which then becomes the primary location of long-term storage and retrieval. When a new learning chunk reaches the cerebral cortex, it apparently is stored for the long term. Larry Squire, of the University of California, San Diego, describes the hippocampus as a kind of broker that binds memory until the cortex takes over and becomes its handler. And Gazzaniga (1988) reports that memory occurs not just in the brain, but throughout the nervous system. In animal research, animals with no hippocampus can remember remote items but not recent items, whereas animals with intact hippocampi remember recent items better than remote items, which is the normal condition. Anders Bjorklund, of the University of Lund in Sweden, has demonstrated that aging rats with deteriorated hippocampi are unable to learn new skills, yet they are able to learn and remember after receiving transplants of good hippocampal cells from young rats.

What we know about memory formation is portrayed in Figure 25.1. The perception of an event triggers activity at the synapse. The quality of this activity is dependent on the person's readiness (fatigue, stress, medication) and volition (intention to remember, emotional arousal). If the person is ready and waiting to capture the event as a memory, C-kinase (PKC) is released and settles around the synapse, thus forming the basis of memory. With subsequent recall and practice, the new connection strengthens.

Memory appears to be fully developed by eight years of age. At that point, we remember an average of 1 bit of information out of every 100 we receive. There is some debate about the relationship of memory to IQ, but I come down on the side of those who hold that they are apparently unrelated. As I read the research, I am con-

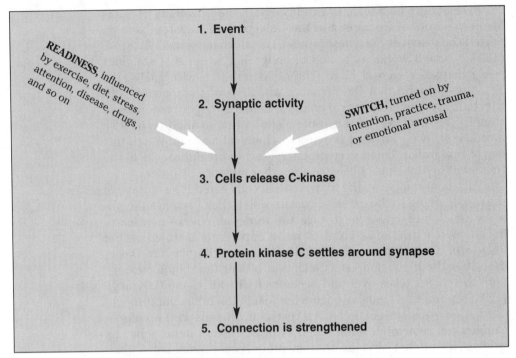

Figure 25.1. The Process of Memory Formation.

vinced that if memory and IQ appear to be directly related, it is because those with higher IQs usually attempt to acquire more learning than those with lower IQs. In a competition between adult humans and five-year-old rhesus monkeys, the University of Texas Health Science Center in Houston reported that after viewing a series of slides, humans and monkeys both got 86 percent right on a ten-item test in which they were shown the slides with new slides mixed in and were asked to press a lever when they recognized a familiar slide! One of the reasons that people who score high on conventional IQ tests also have excellent memories is that conventional IQ tests include so many questions whose correct answers rely on a good memory. A purer IQ test would separate memory as just one variable.

Remember that it is not sufficient to learn a new concept, skill, or body of information; you must convert it into long-term memory. In other words, if you take the time to read a book or article, say, on how to be a better listener, you probably will not remember the skills or concepts unless you practice one or more of the three strategies described in Topic 25.4.

TOPIC 25.1 The Three Stages of Memory Formation

Forming a chunk of memory is like making a photograph. Regard photography as a three-stage process: capturing the image on light-sensitive film, developing the film with chemicals, and fixing the image permanently with chemicals. A similar process happens in memory-chunk formation, consisting of capturing the chunk (immediate memory), developing it (short-term memory), and fixing it (long-term memory).

Immediate memory is a kind of buffer area that can hold thousands of pieces of data for two seconds or less. For example, when you look up a telephone number that you've never seen before, you'll forget it a few seconds later unless you keep repeating it. New information will push out old unless the old is paid attention to.

Short-term memory appears to function in the hippocampus as a clearinghouse that selects chunks of data to remember. A chunk is defined as an unfamiliar array of seven (plus or minus two) pieces, or bits, of information—for example, a seven-digit telephone number, a new word such as *phlyxma* (I made this up!), or a new definition composed of familiar words. George Miller (1956), in a classic article in *Psychological Review,* first identified the fact that people learn most efficiently in units of seven plus or minus two. Groups of seven occur throughout literature and history (the Seven Wonders of the World, the Seven Mortal Sins, the Seven Virtues, . . .). Interestingly, the Australian aborigines have only seven words for numbers, equivalent to one, two, three, four, five, six, and seven. Another word means simply many, or more than seven. It is perhaps because the aborigines have little or no need for long-term memory that they recall only what is reinforced daily. The word for three surely would occur every day, or at least every other day, whereas a word for sixty-three wouldn't get a chance to be reinforced every two days. Therefore, three would remain in short-term memory, but sixty-three would disappear and have to be reinvented.

More recently, Nelson Cowan has modified Miller's seven plus or minus two to the round number of four (*Trends in Cognitive Science,* March 1998, p. 77). Cowan points out that some chunks are more readily assimilated than others. For example, easily pronounced nonsense words like "wyk" are more quickly assimilated than hard-to-pronounce cousins like "wcxik." Cowan urges that four chunks (plus or minus two) are a more realistic target than Miller's seven.

Decision theorist Herbert Simon says that it takes about eight seconds of attention to add one new chunk to short-term memory. Once a chunk has been completely mastered, it becomes a bit and can then be combined with other bits to become a new chunk. In other words, a new chunk loses its identity as a chunk after it becomes second nature to us. Chunks become bits, just as images on film become printable negatives after developing.

Long-term memory appears to be located in the cerebral cortex. Apparently, hippocampal short-term memory communicates with the cortex through what we call simple human will or effort; over time, it establishes chunks in long-term storage. Using a device that measures blood flow, Henry Holcomb, a memory researcher in Johns Hopkins University's Department of Radiology, has determined that the memory for a new motor skill takes five to six hours to move from temporary storage in the front of the brain to permanent storage in the rear of the brain. Attempting to learn another new skill before this five- to six-hour period is up will cause problems for the prior learning. Holcomb recommends that new learnings be followed by more familiar, routine activity. Much more research is required before we know if this principle also applies to nonmotor memory.

A key to the formation of long-term memory is the level of the neurotransmitters epinephrine and norepinephrine. James McGaugh, a psychobiologist at the University of California, Irvine, showed that rats with low epinephrine levels had poor recall ability but booster shots of epinephrine after they had learned something improved their retention. He further found that injecting older rats after they had learned a maze improved their memory. Larry Stein, also at Irvine, shocked rats when they stepped off a platform that was surrounded by water. Weeks later, when the rats were put back on the platform, they remembered and didn't step off. However, when he blocked their norepinephrine, he found that although they could *learn* not to step off, they couldn't *remember,* and they stepped off into repeated shocks. When we have a strong experience, norepinephrine tells the brain to print it, and we hang on to the memory.

Apparently, trivial experiences, about which we don't get juiced up, are lost. Blocking norepinephrine prevents us from remembering new information. This is why some people with amnesia can remember distant events but not recent ones.

Epinephrine and norepinephrine are released by the adrenal medulla when the body is subjected to physical or emotional stress. In addition to increasing blood flow, this release causes extra glucose production. The rate of glucose breakdown is a measure of cortical activity. So although you can relax when you are reading, you need to put in a little sweat equity (known as grunting and groaning) in order to convert what you learn into long-term memory.

We acquire one or two bits of information per second during concentrated study; by midlife we have acquired roughly 10^9 bits. Our average brain capacity is 2.8×10^{20}, or approximately ten million volumes (books) of a thousand pages each. This outrageous capacity mandates humility. I've heard people lament that they couldn't learn anymore, that their "brain is full." Yeah, right! There is no way that their brain is full. They have simply reached a point of fatigue and need a break for things to settle. Then, just as our last meal is digested and our body yearns for more, we are ready to learn more. I've never met the person who has reached the limits of her or his capacity to learn. I *have,* however, met plenty of folks who have quit learning.

Daniel Alkon (1992, p. 208) writes: "Once a memory link is formed, there is a short period of perhaps hours to days during which the responsible cellular changes can reverse. Then the cellular changes become permanent." In other words, if we fail to review the learning, it will likely disappear, or reverse. Once the memory or learning has become firmly established, however, "the old memory cannot be erased. Instead, to modify the meaning of the older memory, new memories must be added." As a bleak testimony to the persistence of memory, Alkon laments that memories of early painful and intense abuse are doomed to be permanent. He does not foresee any surgical, pharmacological, or psychotherapeutic cure. Instead, he finds that victims must comfort themselves with three common strategies for avoiding such memories: compulsive behavior, fantasizing, or dulling the senses (p. 213).

Forget about forgetting: life is a constant struggle of new learning striving to coexist with the old. Sometimes it appears to us that old memories have been lost, but Alkon points out that "when they are forgotten, the records are not erased but inhibited" (p. 209). Further, he suggests that "the brain is not like a computer that can be reprogrammed after the deletion of old programs. The new programs have to be reconciled with the old. . . . Whatever pharmacological tools we can devise to facilitate remembering, forgetting, and learning anew, they will not replace the memory banks themselves, or the steps by which they are acquired" (pp. 224–225). Because of this persistence of memory (remember Salvador Dali's "wilting watch"?), some of us will succumb to its familiar voice and give up on new learning.

Karl Pribram, Psychiatry Professor Emeritus at Stanford University, writes of the holographic structure of long-term memory. Each memory seems to be stored throughout the brain, rather than in a single confined location. Apparently, memories hook onto related networks of other memories, so that, for example, redheads are all somehow loosely tied together in your storage, and you can dump out a long list of redheads upon request. These networks become diffuse and interdependent. Neal Cohen, an associate professor at the University of Illinois at Urbana's Beckman Institute, trained rats to learn a maze, then operated on them. If less than one-fifth of the cortex was removed, regardless of where it came from, the rats exhibited no memory loss. If more than one-fifth of the cortex was removed, a proportional loss of memory occurred. So there appears to be no one location within the cortex for memory storage; instead, each memory seems to have an extensive set of backups.

Applications

1   After a learning episode of an hour or so, take a break and do something to pump up your epinephrine levels: walk about, do isometrics, climb some stairs, do laundry, move some boxes—anything that will generate epinephrine and norepinephrine to help fix the memory. Then go back and review the old material before going on to something new.

2   Making the effort to reorganize new material you've read or heard about is, in itself, a form of stress that will help you to convert the material to long-term memory.

3   Take notes on material you wish to remember. *(Contributed by Rick Bradley)*

4 In order to retrieve inhibited memories—ones you know are there but can't find—try some method that "uninhibits" the mind, such as hypnosis, relaxation exercises, free-association techniques, or visualization.

5 Attempt to organize your day so that new learnings occur at one of three times: shortly after first waking, shortly before sleeping, and approximately halfway in between. Caution: Remember that exactly halfway between waking and sleep onset is the low point in your circadian rhythm, so you'll be better off timing the new learning a couple of hours before or after that point. For example, if I rise at 7:00 A.M. and retire at 11:00 P.M., my low point—and a good time for a nap— would be around 3:00 P.M. New learnings could be timed for around 8:00 A.M., 1:30 P.M. (or 4:30 P.M.), and 9:00 or 10:00 P.M., depending on when the afternoon session occurred.

TOPIC 25.2 Maintenance Requirements

Once a long-term memory has been formed, three major factors interfere with retrieving it: clogging at the synapse, deterioration of the neuronal pathways involved, and stress. Clogging at the synapse occurs over time as protein particles accumulate on both sides of the synaptic gap; it consists of pregap or *dendritic* clogging and postgap or *axonic* clogging. This clogging is similar to the protein accumulation on contact lenses. Just as this protein accumulation can be removed by soaking and baking, synaptic clogging is removed by the neurotransmitter calpain, found in calcium. Another finding, by Richard Wurtman, director of the Clinical Research Center at Massachusetts Institute of Technology, is that Alzheimer's patients have buildups of rock-hard amyloid protein and a deficiency of acetylcholine, which is necessary to break down amyloid protein.

Some deterioration of the neuronal pathways occurs naturally through aging (see Topic 11.1 for a list of factors that contribute to the deterioration of neurons), but there is one source of deterioration over which we have control: the lack of production of the neurotransmitter acetylcholine, whose presence is crucial to the maintenance of neuronal membranes. With insufficient acetylcholine, these cell membranes become brittle and fall away. The dietary source of acetylcholine is fat. Diets with levels of fat below the recommended daily allowance represent a threat to acetylcholine levels. Normal or even high fat content in your diet, however, does not ensure sufficient acetylcholine. Other factors, such as genetics, disease, medication, and stress, can influence acetylcholine levels downward.

Stress causes the limbic system to work in the foreground, thus drastically reducing the availability of the cortical system. As a result, memory retrieval is highly ineffective and unreliable. For example, when I make a presentation, I experience stress. If I am prepared and speak from well-organized notes, the presentation goes well. On the other hand, if I haven't organized the material, have no notes or outline, and am winging it, I do less well. The difference is not how thoroughly I know the material—I know it equally well in both cases. The difference is that under stress, I cannot access or retrieve the material as effectively. The notes help to guide the retrieval, and this has the added effect of reducing the stress.

Electroshock can improve memory by approximately 300 percent, with effects that last for about three weeks. Apparently electroshock shakes some of the protein off the synapse. Some improvement of memory is possible with the drug physostigmine, which inhibits the formation of cholinesterase, an enzyme that breaks down neurotransmitters such as acetylcholine. Improvements have also been seen in studies at Northwestern University Medical School with a drug called nimodipine, which appears to inhibit calcium buildup in people who consume too much calcium. In experiments, older rabbits learned more quickly after taking nimodipine. More recently, researchers at Northwestern University Medical School found that cycloserine and monoclonal antibodies appear to have profoundly positive effects, improving and speeding up memory as well as improving memory in Alzheimer's patients. These two chemicals act on the nimodipine receptors in the hippocampus, allowing calcium to enter and help in forming new synapses.

Older citizens often lament what they perceive as deteriorating memory. Grandparents can sit around reminiscing about World War II, yet they can't remember to fulfill a recent request. They say they just can't make new memories. But the real difference between short-term and long-term memory is the difference between learning a telephone number long enough to dial it immediately and learning it long enough to dial it a week later. That distinction is often confused in people who seem to remember remote events but can't remember something they were told yesterday. Bolles (1988, p. 234) writes: "Memories for recent and for long-ago events depend on the same constructive abilities and the same emotional, factual, and interpretive levels of memory. If a person can still remember past events well and still tell interesting stories about the long ago, he has the equipment to do the same for more recent events. Failure to remember the present in such cases suggests a failure to pay attention to the present, not an inability to learn new details." This suggests that for many, what may appear to be poor short-term memory may in fact be a symptom of depression. Depressed people may not pay sufficient attention to events or care enough about them to remember them. Short-term memory problems can also be a symptom of stress. John Newcomer, along with other researchers at Washington University in St. Louis, administered glucocorticoids (stress hormones) for four days. Subjects were not aware of their ensuing memory dysfunction, but the researchers observed a sharp drop in memory. After they discontinued administration of the stress hormones, the memory dysfunction disappeared within one week.

Applications

1 If you want others to think they have your attention, focus on what they are telling you, including their name. Saying "I have to hear a name three times before I remember it" just doesn't wash; it simply leaves you sounding like someone who doesn't pay attention. If you don't want to forget a name, keep saying it to yourself, associate it with other images, and ask questions about it, such as "Is it a popular name in your family?" "What part of the world does it come from?" and "Is it a nickname?"

2 If someone, particularly an older person, appears forgetful, remember that it could be something as simple as his or her mind having wandered momentarily or something as major as depression.

3 When problems with short-term memory appear, look for possible stressors that could be chemically interfering with memory formation. Engage in activities that either remove the source of stress or combat the symptoms (see Chapter Twenty).

4 Maintain the recommended daily allowances for fat and calcium (see Appendix A).

5 Remove (or minimize as much as possible) the stress in your life (see Topic 20.4).

6 Consult your neurologist for possible experimental drug treatment of memory problems.

7 If someone you know, especially an older adult, seems confused or is having memory problems, check for an excess or deficiency of dietary calcium.

TOPIC 25.3 The Two Kinds of Memory Chunks

Richard Hirsh (1990), of McGill University in Montreal, describes two kinds of memory chunks: *facts* and *skills*. Fellow Canadian Endel Tulving calls them *semantic* and *episodic* units, while others have labeled these memory chunks *declarative* and *procedural, conscious* and *nonconscious, perceptual* and *conceptual, perceptual* and *tacit,* or *explicit* and *implicit.* Facts are more discrete chunks of memory, such as word definitions, symbol meanings, and associations with dates, places, and faces—hence Tulving's reference to them as semantic. Skills are more continuous chunks of memory, such as stories and kinesthetic sequences (tying shoes or riding a bicycle). Skill learning is primarily associated with the limbic (animal) brain, whereas fact learning is primarily associated with the cerebral cortex, which develops after the limbic area does. Perhaps this is why we can't remember much from the first several years of life. Hirsh reports that damage to the hippocampus prevents learning of new facts but allows learning of new skills.

The ability to learn facts and skills may be associated with hemispheric specialization. The area devoted to fact learning may be a kind of articulation apparatus located in the verbal area of the cortex (see Topic 12.1), while the area devoted to skill learning may be a kind of visual-spatial notepad located in the visual-spatial area of the cortex (in the right hemisphere for males and both hemispheres for females). I know of no research to back this up, but it would seem to be a logical inference from existing studies.

Application

It is possible that you have more strength in one kind of memory unit than in another. If so, emphasize your strength rather than regretting your weakness. I am sure that my skill (visual-spatial) memory is superior to my fact (language) memory. So I should abandon the frustrating pastime of trying to keep my foreign language ability up and enjoy my ability to learn to play new musical instruments.

TOPIC 25.4   The Three Strategies for Remembering

Minninger (1984) has categorized the many memorization gimmicks into three categories: *intend, file,* and *rehearse.* This approach has been around for some time. Erasmus wrote in 1512, "Though I do not deny that memory can be helped by places and images, yet the best memory is based on three important things: namely study [rehearse], order [file], and care [intend]." Intend to remember something; that is, don't assume that it'll just stick after exposure—you need to make a point of wanting to remember it. File it by organizing it and playing with it in your own special way. And rehearse it, or practice it, as a way of showing that you intend to remember it. Do it and say it repeatedly. These three generic strategy types are the means by which we convert short-term memory to long-term memory.

Applications

1 Here are some ways to apply the *intend* strategy:

- Before reading an article or book, preread it by reviewing the section headings, pictures, charts, graphs, figures, appendixes, and bibliography to get a feeling for how it is laid out and what it covers. This will serve as a kind of advance organizer that will make the reading more meaningful.

- Before taking a course or workshop, do all you can to be ready to receive the material: review the course syllabus if it is available; familiarize yourself with the course outline, agenda, handouts, or bibliography if you can; and read relevant material suggested by a librarian, the instructor, the bibliography, graduates of the course, or common sense. Contact other prior participants to discuss what they learned.

- Consciously decide to remember something; then select a way to file it (see Application 2 below). D. J. Herrmann (1991) provides many good suggestions in his book *Super Memory: A Quick-Action Program for Memory Improvement*. His approach is not as technical as those of Buzan (1991) and Lorayne and Lucas (1974).

- Once you've decided to memorize information, one way to show your intention is to chunk it (see Topic 23.1) and learn the chunks. Divide and conquer.

- Understand and practice the concept of state dependence described in Topic 25.5.

2 Here are some ways to apply the *file* strategy:

- Make a flowchart, Pareto chart (see Topic 31.3), or any other kind of organizational chart that structures what you've learned in a way that's meaningful to you.

- Using self-sticking notes or a material like flannel board, write out a single chunk of what you've learned on its own separate sheet. Then arrange the chunks on a wall in a way that makes sense to you. Restudy the arrangement from time to time and rearrange the notes as needed. When you've fixed the organization the way you like it, make a flowchart or some other kind of chart or outline and put it away for easy review or retrieval. Keep it in your portable notebook for frequent rehearsal.

- Describe the person or object you want to remember in a way that evokes the name of the object. For example, you might associate the name Ann Woodward with this description: "She who keeps the extra timber for repairs to Green Gables."

- Substitute words (perhaps with rhymes) as an aid to remembering a name. Try to make the words graphically visual. For example, if Harvey Darrow has bad acne, associate the name with the substitutes "larvae barrow" while visualizing a wheelbarrow containing dirt filled with larvae (acne). At a party, if you want to remember the name Ted Miller, and Ted is extremely lacking in personality, remember him as the Dead Miller. I invite folks who reverse my first and last names to remember my name as rhyming with the "fierce coward" (Pierce Howard). See *The Memory Book* (Lorayne and Lucas, 1974) and *Use Your Perfect Memory* (Buzan, 1991) for many ideas on visualization techniques for memory. These authors remind us that our memory for images is better than our memory for words, and our memory for concrete words is better than our memory for abstract words.

- Lorayne and Lucas (1974) recommend another technique called *linking,* which is a way to remember a list of things. If you need to stop by the grocery store to pick up milk, bread, hose, and shrimp, link each word to the next one on the list by some exaggerated visual connection. For example, a huge carton of milk has a loaf of bread for a stopper, with a pair of hose connected to the loaf to pull it out in order to pour the milk in a saucepan to boil the shrimp. Once you've made these linking associations, all you have to remember is the first image—the big bottle of milk—and the rest follows.

- Use the peg-word technique, described in Topic 23.4, Application 2. The peg-word technique is actually a variation on the loci technique of Simonides, the ancient Greek orator. Simonides associated parts of a speech with parts of familiar places (loci); for example, each spot in a familiar walkway or building would be associated with a paragraph or subtopic of the speech.

- To remember a number, such as a telephone number, substitute the phonetic consonant equivalents for the numbers and fill in with vowels to make up words. To substitute consonants, try these possibilities:

  1 = *d* or *t* or *th* (one vertical stroke)

  2 = *n* (two vertical strokes)

  3 = *m* (three vertical strokes)

  4 = *r* (last letter of the sound of four)

  5 = *L* (Roman numeral for 500; five fingers spread out look like an *L*)

  6 = *j,* soft *g, sh,* or *ch* (*J* and *6* are mirror images; the others sound like the *s* or *x*)

  7 = *k,* hard *g,* or hard *c* (angular, like a *7; g* and *c* sound like *k*)

8 = *f, v,* or *ph* (cursive *f* looks like an *8; v* and *ph* sound like *f*)

9 = *b* or *p* (*b* looks like an upside-down *9* and *p* like a backward *9; b* and *p* sound alike: they are labial consonants)

0 = *z, s,* or soft *c* (first letter in zero)

So, to remember the telephone number for our favorite Indian restaurant, I came up with Lub Duk Tiki-Ba, or 591-7179 (LBD-KTKB). Leave out the vowels and substitute numbers for consonants according to the above list (or think up your own). See Lorayne and Lucas (1974), Buzan (1991), and Minninger (1984) for more examples. Try to create outrageous, gruesome, or bawdy images—they're easier to recall and can be your private joke on the world.

❸ Here are some ways to apply the *rehearse* strategy:

- Obtain or create the material on audiotape and review it while driving, jogging, walking, or riding the bus.
- Create a tickle file. Assign a file folder for each month, week, or day and insert any notes you would like to review in the appropriate folder.
- Use a highlighter or pen while reading to note sections for review; then periodically review the highlighted sections.
- When you are idle (stopped at a red light, walking, and so on), recall recently memorized material and rehearse it. Review this material with a walking or jogging partner.
- Make a set of flash cards of the steps in a process or some other sequential list of items you want to remember, with the correct sequence of each card indicated on the back side. Shuffle the cards and sort them.
- For many additional suggestions, information, and training opportunities, get on the mailing list of The Buzan Centre of Palm Beach, Inc.; 415 Federal Highway; Lake Park, Florida 33403; phone: 800-964-6362 or 800-Y-MINDMAP.

TOPIC 25.5 **State Dependence**

People recall information more readily when they can remember the state in which they learned that information. This is the basis of the old advice to play back in your mind everywhere you've been in the last thirty minutes when you want to find an object you've lost in that time period. In one research study, subjects memorized a list in the basement of a building and were tested. When they were moved to one of the upper floors of the building and were given the same test, they scored poorly. They then were asked to visualize the basement in which the memory task occurred, and their scores improved; when they were returned to the actual basement room where they had memorized the list and were tested again, their scores improved even more. This phenomenon is called *state dependence,* the theory that recall of learning can depend on the state or other situation that existed when the learning took place.

State dependence is reported to hold true for place (as in the basement example), mood (if you were angry when you learned, remember the anger), odors (remember that the olfactory sense is located in the limbic system), and physical condition (if you were drinking coffee while you were learning, you will remember better if you drink coffee). Why? Apparently, the synapses formed to create a specific memory are connected to neural networks that form the basis of the conditions associated with the time and place of learning. Recalling the place (for example, a specific room in a house) in which you learned a person's name will help you to access the name, because the two are connected by neural networks. This is similar to taking a photo of a person against a distinctive background.

Applications

1 When you are with someone who is having a hard time remembering something you both want to remember, get the other person to focus on the place, the mood, and her or his physical condition when the information was learned. The same goes for you if you're trying to remember something.

2 Make an effort to learn things under conditions that are easy to replicate when you need to remember what you've learned.

❸   When you are trying to teach job-related skills, create a learning environment that approximates the conditions on the job. *(Contributed by Rick Bradley)*

TOPIC 25.6   **Memory and Emotion**
_____

The role that emotion plays in the formation and recall of memory is not clear. We know that some minimal level of arousal, hence emotional activity, is necessary to pump sufficient adrenaline and noradrenaline into one's system to cause a memory to "take." On the other hand, we know that intense emotional experiences appear to interfere with memory formation. Marcia Johnson, a professor of psychology at Princeton University, has found in her research that experiences with emotional components appear to be remembered with fewer perceptual details (*APA Monitor,* October 1995). She also has found that focusing on the emotional aspect of a memory results in recall of less detail. More importantly, she has found that focusing on the emotional aspect of both real and imagined memories blurs the source of the memory.

Applications

❶   When you are attempting to reconstruct a memory that has a strong emotional component, be aware that you may have a tendency to "supply" details that are not, in fact, details of the experience (the emotions block acquisition of the actual details). Where possible, seek corroboration from another person.

❷   In an emotionally intense situation in which memory is important, attempt to find a moment of composure to focus on elements you need to remember.

TOPIC 25.7 Real Versus Imagined Memories

Elizabeth Loftus and Katherine Ketcham, in their 1994 work *The Myth of Repressed Memory,* have offered a damning indictment of psychotherapists and others who engage in what the authors refer to as "iatrogenic implantation," in which a healer or therapist plants the seed of a memory in a patient and, through a process of suggestion, assists the patient in creating a full-blown "recovered memory." The result is not a memory, nor is it recovered.

Memory is malleable. The authors lay a solid background composed of vignettes that illustrate the malleability of memory processes:

- Ulrich Neisser of Cornell University's psychology department interviewed and recorded the circumstances of forty-four students at the time of the January 1986 *Challenger* explosion. Two and one-half years later, the memories of where they were had changed: not one was 100 percent accurate and over one-third were severely inaccurate. The students with inaccurate memories couldn't recognize or accept the authenticity of the written records from only two and a half years earlier.

- Pitcher Jack Hamilton of the California Angels threw a ball that crushed the left side of Boston's Tony Conigliaro's face. Neither Conigliaro nor Hamilton were the same after this life-changing event. Though we usually believe that our memories of such experiences are accurate, Hamilton's memory of the event twenty-two years later was severely flawed. In an interview with the *New York Times* upon Conigliaro's death in 1990, Hamilton relayed the wrong inning for the bad pitch, the wrong score, the wrong position in the batting order, and the wrong time of year and recalled it as a day game when in fact it was a night game!

Searching for ways to establish the malleability of memory in order to lay a groundwork for discrediting the "recovery" movement, Loftus recounted the now well-known "lost at the mall" story. She asked a friend if he could convince his eight-year-old daughter that she had been lost in a mall at the age of five, when in fact she had never been lost. The friend said that his daughter would never go along with such a "planted" memory. But to the friend's amazement, after some encouragement, his eight-year-old bought the implanted memory hook, line, and sinker, so much so that she pointed out to her father that he had been "not as scared as I was."

Loftus and Ketcham conclude that there is no such thing as repression, that people don't conveniently select traumatic episodes to be removed from conscious memory and file them away in "special, inaccessible memory drawers." There are three kinds of amnesia, but they differ significantly from so-called repression:

1. *Anterograde amnesia,* in which patients exhibit a reduced ability to recall events after injury to the brain, as in the famous Central Park jogger rape case.

2. *Retrograde amnesia,* in which patients exhibit a reduced ability to recall events preceding brain injury.

3. *Psychogenic amnesia,* in which a traumatic event interferes with memory storage and results in fragmentary recall.

None of these three forms of amnesia show anything like the selective elimination of complete episodes claimed by "recovery" therapists. Loftus and Ketcham conclude that repression is nothing more than the invention of the therapist in forced cooperation with the patient. The result of a highly trusting patient in the hands of a suggestive therapist is *pseudomemories.* These "recovered" memories of early abuse have a way of blossoming from nowhere. They spring from the same therapists and their "support" groups, like children who are always sent to the principal's office by the same teachers. These therapists and their ongoing groups have a vested interest in uncovering new supplies of "repressed" memories.

The scientifically accepted phenomenon closest to what is called repression is psychogenic amnesia. But, as the authors point out, in psychogenic amnesia memories are fragmented, not completely eliminated, and over time they tend to clear up. Loftus and Ketcham tell the story of a daring attempt to document "iatrogenic implantation," or therapist-induced "memories," by a journalist (I think it was a journalist!) who had himself wired (I think it was a male!) and then went to a therapist who had a reputation for recovering memories of childhood abuse among patients. The resulting transcriptions clearly documented the therapist's leading questions and suggestions. With a patient suffering from depression or anxiety, these implantations could easily form the core of a constructed "memory." Just as lawyers may not lead witnesses, so therapists may not lead patients.

Marcia Johnson (see Topic 25.6) has found that real memories tend to have significantly more detail than imagined ones. Memories founded in actual perception usually have more sensory detail; memories originating in the imagination have more information about thoughts and feelings. An individual can develop a knack for identifying memories that possess more perceptual detail, lending more credence to their having a basis in real experience. Johnson calls this process "source monitoring" (*APA Monitor,* October 1995, p. 31). Stephen Kosslyn (1994), a professor of psychology at Harvard University, has determined that these two processes, which he calls *perception* and *imagery,* occur in the same area of the brain. This helps to explain why some subjects may think they actually witnessed an image when in fact they only imagined it, which is of interest to those who study the reliability of eyewitness testimony.

Eric and Minouche Kandel (*Discover,* May 1994) report that the release of the body's natural painkillers—the opioids—interferes with memory formation. They further speculate that under certain circumstances, as in early abuse, when the pain from an experience becomes so intense that it triggers the release of opioids, the memory formation associated with that event is impeded by the painkillers. Under such circumstances, they maintain, memories of early abuse may never become strongly established. The result is not repression or forgetting, but rather weak or nonexistent neural pathways.

One recent line of research by Daniel Schacter of Harvard University has established that positron emission tomography (PET) reveals a distinct pattern for "true" memories that distinguishes them from false memories. True memories are associated with a higher level of brain activity than false memories. This higher level results from the greater detail associated with real memories and is clearly visible in PET scans in the hippocampal and temporoparietal regions. This finding, reported in the August 1996 issue of *Neuron,* is regarded as a major breakthrough in understanding false memory, but the process is complex and costly and it will probably not be available for everyday verification in the near future. However, it is conceivable that we may eventually ascertain the veracity of memories through such brain scans. In fact, Lawrence Farwell (see Topic 19.10, "A Note on Deception") has developed such a technique—Farwell Brain Fingerprinting—but it is not yet admissible in the courts.

Applications

1 When you are in doubt about the veracity of a memory, compare the perceptual details in your mind's eye to the details of a memory for which you have corroboration. If the doubtful memory has fewer perceptual details (such as colors, smells, and shapes) than confident memories, be distrustful of it.

2 In attempting to manage the testimony of an eyewitness, establish baseline levels of perceptual detail (by having the eyewitness relate details from memories known to originate in perception) before exploring the eyewitness testimony. Comparison of the two levels of detail should help in establishing the degree of reliability of the testimony.

3 The best way to establish the veracity (or falseness) of a memory that is uncertain is to corroborate it through the testimony of other reliable observers—memory partners, as it were. I have seen several references in the literature to the healthful habit of ceasing to rely solely on one's own memory or reconstruction of events, instead soliciting the complementary support of a memory partner in the form of a family member, friend, or co-worker.

4 If you become involved in a serious charge that concerns an unverifiable memory, consult a neurologist to see if PET technology is an option for clarifying the nature of the memory.

5 For an excellent review of the literature on false memory syndrome, read Kenneth S. Pope's "Memory, Abuse, and Science" (Pope, 1996).

TOPIC 25.8 Helping Others Remember

Research into witness management has led to several interesting techniques for eliciting latent memories from others. For example, build on a witness's schemas (see Topic 23.4) by identifying something in the witness's background that she or he can relate to the scene of the memories in question. A witness who likes working with wood should focus on the qualities of the wooden furniture in the scene about which he or she is trying to recall details. The witness is likely to have paid close attention to the wood and is then more apt to recall other details. Another witness management technique is to minimize questions, asking only a few open-ended questions from which the witness can reveal his or her schemas. The interviewer then builds on the information the witness has volunteered.

Weingardt, Leonesio, and Loftus (1994) write about "eyewitness metacognition" and form several conclusions about the actual and perceived accuracy and trustworthiness of eyewitness testimony:

1. Peripheral details are more likely to be contaminated by misleading postevent information than is central detail.

2. Misleading information is more damaging or influential when it is related in complex sentences than when it is stated simply and obviously.

3. People who receive misleading information make more errors in memory and are overconfident about the misinformation compared to the original information.

4. The more spatial, temporal, sensory, and semantic details that are provided, the more likely a memory is to be based on perception and not on imagination, and the more likely it is to be perceived to be based on perception.

5. People who see their memory as poor tend to put more faith in written accounts.

6. People tend to think that they're good at remembering what they said in the past (even if they aren't), so if they don't remember it, they tend to think that someone else said it.

7. Juries report a greater belief in witnesses who seem confident.

8. Weingardt, Leonesio, and Loftus's meta-analysis based on thirty-five studies shows that the correlation between witness confidence and accuracy is only +.25.

9. The major factors associated with accurate self-confidence in identifying a criminal are the personality of the witness, previous feedback to the witness on his or her accuracy, and the perpetrator's use of disguise.

Applications

1 Use a person's interests to elicit memories. For example, if the person is a soap opera addict, ask first, "Was there a television set in the room? Describe it. What was on top of it? Beside it? On the wall above it?" Use the TV set to retrieve images of the rest of the room. If you start with an impersonal question that the person cannot immediately relate to her or his experience, you are less likely to get the desired level of detail. Ask someone who's bookish about printed matter, an artist about artwork, a musician about a piano, and so on.

2 Ask open-ended questions beginning with words like *when, where, how many, how long,* and *what.* These types of question starters are more likely to get people talking and to exploit their memory than closed-ended questions that typically elicit yes-or-no responses, such as "Did you arrive before 8:00 P.M.?"

3 In preparing witnesses, develop written accounts when possible.

4 To maximize perceived credibility, develop as much spatial, temporal, sensory, and semantic detail as possible.

5 Key witnesses whose credibility may be strained should be coached in nonverbal presentation of self-confidence (eye contact, speaking out, a comfortable posture).

Some Final Thoughts on Memory

Bolles (1988, p. 23) describes the process of memory like this: "We remember what we understand; we understand only what we pay attention to; we pay attention to what we want." In other words, experience arouses emotion, which fixes attention and leads to understanding and insight, which results in memory. Bolles continues: "Attention is like digestion. We do not store the food we eat; we break it down so that it becomes part of our body. Attention selects parts of experience and uses [them] to nourish our memories. We do not store this experience, we use it. Of course, we eat many things that we do not digest and we also experience many things without paying them any attention" (p. 183).

SUGGESTED RESOURCES

Alkon, D. L. (1992). *Memory's Voice: Deciphering the Brain-Mind Code.* New York: HarperCollins.

Bolles, E. B. (1988). *Remembering and Forgetting: An Inquiry into the Nature of Memory.* New York: Walker.

Buzan, T. (1991). *Use Your Perfect Memory* (3rd ed.). New York: Penguin Books.

Edelman, G. M. (1987). *Neural Darwinism: The Theory of Neuronal Group Selection.* New York: Basic Books.

Gordon, B. (1995). *Memory: Remembering and Forgetting in Everyday Life.* New York: MasterMedia.

Loftus, E., and Ketcham, K. (1994). *The Myth of Repressed Memory.* New York: St. Martin's Press.

Lorayne, H., and Lucas, J. (1974). *The Memory Book.* New York: Stein & Day.

Schacter, D. (1996). *Searching for Memory.* New York: Basic Books.

Weingardt, K. R., Leonesio, R. J., and Loftus, E. F. (1994). "On Eyewitness Metacognition." In J. Metcalfe and A. P. Shimamura (Eds.), *Metacognition: Knowing About Knowing* (pp. 155–184). Cambridge, Mass.: MIT Press.

26

A Matter of Style

How We Differ in Our Approaches to Learning

> **Learning is not attained by chance, it must be sought for with ardor and attended to with diligence.**
>
> —Abigail Adams

The second half of the twentieth century has seen a virtual alphabet soup of personal learning style models, variously called learning styles, thinking styles, teaching styles, and cognitive styles, with cognitive styles typically viewed as the most inclusive category. Thinking styles typically include both learning styles and teaching styles as subsets. For the purpose of this chapter, I will use the term *learning style,* and I will include thinking,

Table 26.1. Models for Differences in Learning Style.

Name of the Model	How the Model Names the Style	Source
Conceptual Tempo	Reflectivity Impulsivity	Kagan (1966)
Psychological Differentiation	Field dependence Field independence	Witkin and Goodenough (1981)
Theory of Types	Extraversion/Introversion Sensing/Intuition Feeling/Thinking Judging/Perceiving	Myers and McCaulley (1985)
Gregorc's Energic Model	Use of space (concrete/abstract) Use of time (sequential/random)	Gregorc (1982)
Teaching Methods	Projects Drill and recitation Peer teaching Discussion Teaching games Independent study Programmed instruction Lecture Simulation	Renzulli and Smith (1978)
Scope	Deep/depth Elaborative/breadth	Schmeck (1983)
Dunn and Dunn	Environmental (sound/light) Emotional (motivation/responsibility) Sociological (peers/self) Physical (perceptual/mobility)	Dunn and Dunn (1978)
Holland Hexagon	Realistic Investigative Artistic Social Enterprising Conventional	Holland (1985)
Kolb	Converging/Diverging Assimilating/Accommodating	Kolb (1978)
Teaching Range	Wide/Narrow	Joyce and Hodges (1966)
Teaching Styles	Task-oriented Cooperative planner Child-centered Subject-centered Learning-centered Emotionally exciting	Henson and Borthwick (1984)

Table 26.1. Models for Differences in Learning Style.		
Name of the Model	**How the Model Names the Style**	**Source**
Kirton	Adaption/Innovation	Kirton (1977)
Achievement Pattern	High honors Subject cup Extracurricular Getting by	Howard and Howard (1993)
Social Style	Independent study Contract learning Tutorial Traditional classroom	Howard and Howard (1993)
Honey and Mumford	Activists Reflectors Theorists Pragmatists	Honey and Mumford (1982)
Whetten and Cameron	Receptive/Preceptive Systematic/Intuitive Active/Reflective	Whetten and Cameron (1984)
Modalities	Visual Auditory Kinesthetic Olfactory Gustatory Tactile Group/Alone	Griffin (unpublished)

teaching, and learning as changing aspects of the characteristic way that individuals go about processing new information. Table 26.1 lists some of the more frequently cited models that have been proposed to explain individual differences in learning style.

It is clear that the domain of learning styles has been shaped and reshaped in many ways. What has been missing is a grand theory that integrates this domain. Just as I was dreading this chapter and its multiplicity of models and attendant absence of consensus, I picked up my July 1997 issue of *American Psychologist* and found that Robert Sternberg (see Topic 22.3) had come to the rescue. In an article entitled "Are Cognitive Styles Still in Style?" Sternberg and Elena Grigorenko describe their "theory of mental self-government" approach to learning style. They present a model that builds on Sternberg's triarchic theory of intelligence (see Topic 22.3), employing a metaphor derived from government, with executive, legislative, and judicial branches.

TOPIC 26.1 The Mental Self-Government Model of Learning Style

Sternberg and Grigorenko (1997, p. 707) portray the domain of learning style with a five-part model, shown in Table 26.2. They clearly assume that the way people manage their learning is similar to the way the government runs the country. They find that every individual "possesses every style to some degree."

Table 26.2. Sternberg and Grigorenko's Learning Style Model.

Aspects of the Model	Specific Styles for the Aspect	Characteristics of Each Style
Functions	Legislative	Creates one's own rules, formulates one's own structures and approaches; avoids the prestructured
	Executive	Is an implementer; follows rules; relies on existing structures and predefined rules
	Judicial	Prefers to evaluate, judge, and analyze existing rules and ideas
Forms	Monarchic	Focuses on a single goal or task until it is completed
	Hierarchic	Has multiple goals with varying priorities; is comfortable with systematically getting things done
	Oligarchic	Has multiple goals with equal priorities; has difficulty setting priorities for getting things done
	Anarchic	Does not like to be tied down to the current way of doing things; tends to be opposed to existing systems or ways without always having an alternative; has a random approach that often leads to unusual connections
Levels	Local	Prefers specific, concrete details that require precision in execution
	Global	Prefers general problems that require abstract thinking and conceptualization in the world of ideas
Scope	Internal	Prefers working alone, independently of others and on one's own
	External	Prefers to work with and interact with other people
Leanings	Liberal	Goes beyond the current way and permits change from traditional methods (as opposed to the Legislative style, the new ideas do not have to be one's own)
	Conservative	Prefers to follow the traditional and the familiar (may think up one's own ideas, but they are consistent with custom)

Some people are more flexible than others. Although the styles are not fixed, but fluid, some individuals persist in a style when one would expect them to alter their style according to the circumstances. This resistance to changes in circumstances suggests that "there may be preprogrammed dispositions that are difficult to change" (p. 708). In other words, learning styles have both a genetic and an environmental component, and the environmental part is most subject to change.

We can see that Sternberg and Grigorenko have incorporated many of the models shown in Table 26.1 into their integrative approach. The test that is used to measure the presence of these styles is the Thinking Styles Inventory (Sternberg and Wagner, 1991; Sternberg, 1997c). This is a self-report instrument that employs a nine-point scale. In addition, Sternberg and Grigorenko have devised a series of instruments for use by educators (the Thinking Styles Questionnaire for Teachers, Set of Thinking Styles Tasks for Students, and Students' Thinking Styles Evaluated by Teachers—all unpublished but available from the authors: Robert Sternberg and Elena Grigorenko; Department of Psychology; Yale University; P.O. Box 208205; New Haven, Connecticut 06520; phone: 203-432-4633; E-mail: robert.sternberg@yale.edu). All of these tests have good reliability and validity. They correlate with neither traditional IQ measures nor grade point averages, so they appear to be measuring something different from intelligence or aptitude.

Sternberg and Grigorenko conducted a series of studies in which they correlated scores on the Thinking Styles Inventory with other measures using a number of analyses. They compared students and faculty from four different kinds of schools: urban public, prestigious traditional private, Catholic parochial, and progressive avant-garde private. The Applications listed below are based on the findings from these studies.

Applications

1 Teachers in the lower grades are more legislative and less executive. Hence, they must find ways that may not be natural for them to work with students who have an executive (structured) style; teachers in the upper grades are more executive than legislative and hence must find ways that may not be natural for them to work with students who have the legislative (creative) style.

2 Older teachers are more executive, local, and conservative. Hence, they typically must work harder to find ways to appeal to students who are legislative, judicial, global, and liberal, whereas younger teachers, who are more legislative, judicial, global, and liberal, must work harder to find ways to appeal to students who are more executive, local, and conservative.

3 Science teachers tend to score as more local, while humanities teachers score as more liberal. Thus, science teachers must typically work harder to appeal to students who are more global (abstract), and humanities teachers must typically work harder to appeal to students who are more conservative.

4 Teachers' styles have a tendency to match the style of their school. Therefore, school leaders need to be aware of the stylistic profile of their overall program and pay special attention to students who clearly do not fit that profile. The faculty will not naturally design learning experiences that these atypical students will find comfortable.

5 There is a strong inclination for students' styles to match their teachers' styles, which suggests that students recognize their teachers' styles and adapt to them. Teachers need to make a special effort to include or accommodate students whose styles clearly depart from theirs. Being aware of stylistic differences and communicating a knowledge of those differences to the students can lead to successful adaptations.

6 The lower the educational and occupational levels of the students' fathers, the more likely the students are to be judicial, local, conservative, and oligarchic. In schools where parents are predominantly less educated and less successful, a curriculum should be designed that appeals to those four styles. In schools where parents are better educated and more successful, the curriculum should primarily appeal to the legislative, global, and liberal styles.

7 Later-born siblings tend to be more legislative in style (creative), while earlier-born siblings tend to be more judicial and executive. Teachers and parents need to understand that siblings naturally differ in their styles. Therefore, teachers should not always expect a child to match the style of a sibling they taught earlier.

8 Teachers are inclined to evaluate and grade more favorably students who match their styles. Schools as a whole grade students higher whose styles match that of the school. Teachers and schools, then, should be mindful of their tendency to downgrade and devalue students whose styles differ from their own. Philosophically—yes, even ethically—teachers and school administrators need to be aware of this tendency to devalue nonmatching students. To compound this effect, Sternberg and Grigorenko also found that teachers often over-estimate how close their students are to them in style. As a result, they may encourage students in teacher-compatible stylistic patterns that are based on projections rather than on reality. Teachers must be diligent in adjusting for this blind spot. In support of this pattern, consider that across schools, grade point averages do not correlate with any of the styles. However, within each school, strong correlations exist between grade point averages and styles. These correlations range from −.42 to +.58.

TOPIC 26.2 The Relation of Learning Style to Personality

I have a special interest in the way in which personality traits relate to other constructs. Upon close inspection of the definitions for Sternberg and Grigorenko's styles, I have tried my hand at estimating the Big Five infrastructure that underlies learning style. I am at present conducting ongoing research that will confirm or clarify these associations. The associations in the following list are based on the personality factors and facets in the NEO-PI-R (Costa and McCrae, 1992) as described in Topic 21.3 and Table 21.3. The intent of this list is to suggest the probable personality trait infrastructure that is associated with each of the learning styles. A plus sign in the list indicates that the style is associated with high scores for a factor or facet and a minus sign with low scores.

Learning Style	Five-Factor Infrastructure
Functions:	
Legislative	O+C–
Executive	O–C+
Judicial	O–A–C+
Forms:	
Monarchic	O–C+
Hierarchic	O+C+
Oligarchic	O+C–
Anarchic	N+O+A–C–
Levels:	
Local	O1–O5–
Global	O1+O5+
Scope:	
Internal	N–E–E1–E2–A–
External	N+E+E1+E2+A+
Leanings:	
Liberal	O1+O4+O5+O6+
Conservative	O1–O4–O5–O6–

The degree of flexibility for each set of attributes can be associated with the actual scores on the specified NEO PI-R factors and facets: midrange scores (45–55, on a scale of 1 to 100) would be more flexible and fluid, while extreme scores (below 45 and above 55) would be more fixed, less situational, and less adaptive to pressure. I remember a professor in graduate school who, on the first night of class, revealed that he was extremely executive and conservative, and that students veering from his requirements would find it tough going. I, being legislative, judicial, and liberal, refused to stay in the course, yet it was required for graduation. Luckily, and due to my persistence and that of several of my cohorts, we were able to form an ad hoc independent study group under the tutelage of a less rigid professor.

Applications

1 If you have NEO PI-R scores available on teachers and students, try using them to estimate learning styles. The Center for Applied Cognitive Studies (800-BIG-5555, or visit our web site at www.centacs.com) has a software program ("The Learner") that estimates scores on the Sternberg-Wagner model as well as on other learning style models. These estimates are based on NEO PI-R scores.

2 Be aware that personality traits as measured by the Big Five are associated with differences in learning style. If you know your Big Five profile, use that knowledge to assess your blind spots as a facilitator of learning. Be aware that you are most likely to undervalue the performance of learners who are different from you.

A Note on Genetics and Learning

Researchers are discovering specific genes that affect various aspects of the learning process (*APA Monitor,* May 1997, p. 29). For example, the gene named Linott is associated with the ability to form a new learning. Fruit flies (drosophila) whose Linott gene has been removed are unable to form new learnings, while flies whose Linott was removed in infancy are able to learn new tasks when the gene is restored in adulthood. In addition, the gene called Creb is associated with the ability to retain a new learning over the long haul—that is, to store it in long-term memory. Fruit flies with Linott but without Creb can form new learnings but cannot remember them. Intensive research is under way for possible applications to human learners. It is not clear at this time whether these genes affect the learning styles presented earlier. Certainly, how one goes about learning, and the relative effectiveness of one's learning styles, must be considered to be a combination of genetic (nature) effects on the one hand and environmental (nurture) effects on the other.

SUGGESTED RESOURCES

Sternberg, R. J. (1997c). *Thinking Styles.* New York: Cambridge University Press.

Sternberg, R. J., and Grigorenko, E. L. (1997, July). "Are Cognitive Styles Still in Style?" *American Psychologist, 52*(7), 700–712.

Sternberg, R. J., and Wagner, R. K. (1991). "MSG Thinking Styles Inventory Manual." Unpublished test manual, Yale University Department of Psychology, New Haven, Conn.

Web Sites

Learning Styles Resources for K12 site:
http://falcon.jmu.edu/~ramseyil/learningstyles.htm

27

Giftedness

Letting the Genius Out of the Bottle

> 66 *Stupid is as stupid does.* 99
> —Forrest Gump

Responding to the gifted individual is a dilemma for a democracy. The desire to treat each individual the same and to provide equal resources for all has been the hallmark of societies that wish to abandon the elitist aristocracies of yesteryear. In a pure democracy, in the tradition of the U.S. experiment called the American Dream, each individual is to have an equal opportunity to achieve. None are to be given special advantages by the government (though that is not to say that parents can't provide special advantages for their children). The turf must be even, at least with respect to government's role.

In spite of this philosophical commitment in our democracy, voices have been raised in advocacy for special groups, and the gifted are a particularly problematic special group. Parents who lobby to have different or extra attention paid to their exceptionally intelligent children are frequently viewed as elitist or pushy, as self-indulgently bragging, or as seeking attention.

> **"If a man has a talent and cannot use it, he has failed. If he has a talent and uses only half of it, he has partly failed. If he has a talent and learns somehow to use the whole of it, he has gloriously succeeded, and won a satisfaction and a triumph few men ever know."**
>
> —Thomas Wolfe,
> *The Web and the Rock*

Gifted children are a problem. Easily bored and immensely talented in one or more fields, they often languish in the typical classroom. Because they represent only a small tail in the normal distribution of ability, they usually are one of a kind in their classes. All too often, unmoved by their ennui, other students and teachers will respond, "If they're so smart, let them find a way to make the humdrum interesting."

Ellen Winner, of Boston College's Department of Education and the Harvard Graduate School of Education's Project Zero, accepts the societal commitment to children with special needs, as long as the resources do not exceed those that are available to others. Winner (1997) points out that giftedness is troublesome to define. As Robert Sternberg and Howard Gardner portray intelligence (see Chapter Twenty-Two), giftedness can be understood as *modular*. With modular gifts, an individual might be gifted in one or more of several areas, such as verbal, musical or auditory, or kinesthetic skills, or in one or more of several aspects of intelligence, such as creativity, street smarts, or informational encoding. But as tradition would have it, intelligence, and hence giftedness, is a unitary concept called "g," for general. This traditional definition of intelligence is used by Winner and most other writers on the subject of giftedness; we will use it here for the convenience of understanding the research findings.

Traditional intelligence and giftedness are made up of verbal, numerical, and spatial reasoning. One's ability to solve problems in these three areas is referred to as IQ. IQ tests report 100 to be the average score. A score of 100 suggests that an individual's verbal, numerical, and spatial abilities are comparable to those of most people in his or her cohort, or age group. Winner identifies two levels of giftedness: being moderately gifted or profoundly gifted. Moderately gifted schoolchildren have measured IQs somewhere around 130–150 and typically perform about one to two years in advance of their cohort. The primary difference between average children and moderately gifted children appears to be one of degree: moderately gifted children remember more, calculate faster, and solve problems more quickly.

Profoundly gifted children have IQs in the region of 180. They are not only different from average children; they are different from moderately gifted children. Winner suspects that profoundly gifted children are different in kind, not just in degree, from both average and moderately gifted children. Examples of feats performed by the profoundly gifted include situations in which four-year-olds, unaided, have figured out the rules of algebra, memorized an entire musical score in a moment, or discovered how to identify all the prime numbers. The profoundly gifted, according to Winner, would appear to have two markers: an intrinsic drive to master a particular domain and a prodigious problem-solving and memory apparatus that, unaided, has the capacity for breakthrough thinking.

TOPIC 27.1 Recognizing Giftedness

Children with either moderate or profound giftedness usually show early signs, including the following (Winner, 1997, p. 1072):

- A long attention span

- A preference for novelty

- Overreactivity to physical sensations

- A good memory for recognition of previous experience

- Early onset of language

- Intense curiosity, drive, and persistence

- Obsessive interests

- Metacognitive ability (that is, the gifted think about how they think and can talk about their learning and problem-solving strategies)
- Typically, the ability to read one or two years before beginning kindergarten
- The ability to excel at abstract logical thinking
- A fascination with numbers and numerical patterns
- Typically, a more solitary or introverted nature
- A preference for older children
- Difficulty finding compatible peers of any age
- Twice as many social or emotional problems as average children
- A fiercely independent and nonconformist nature
- The ability to derive pleasure from work
- Positive self-esteem about their intellectual ability

Winner points out that not all gifted children follow the same developmental story line. Many hide their talents until they are older (she cites Charles Darwin as an example). Often parents or the school fail to stimulate a child with challenges, and some gifted children who are more needful of external guidance languish until such a challenge appears. Also, although many children are gifted globally, not all are. In one study of a thousand gifted teenagers, over 95 percent showed a marked discrepancy between their math and verbal performance. Moreover, gifted children who have creative strength in a particular domain need to be treated differently from those who have analytic strength in the same domain (give the former the challenge of inventing a new formula, the latter a tough problem to solve). Finally, a child gifted in one domain can have a learning disability in another.

Applications

1 Review the kinds of intelligence in Chapter Twenty-Two. Find a way to provide challenging experiences—in school, outside of school, or both—for children who demonstrate a strong interest and quick learning ability in one or more of the modules in the Gardner-Sternberg Job Matrix (see Table 22.4). At a minimum, find a mentor.

2 Consult with a local education professional who specializes in the academically gifted for suggestions about resources to use with your child.

3 Explore the Gifted Resources home page at www.eskimo.com/~user/kids.html.

4 Read Sternberg's *The Triarchic Mind* (1988; see also Topic 22.3) and Armstrong's *Seven Kinds of Smart* (1993; see also Topic 22.4). (It is hoped that Armstrong will come out with a new edition to cover Gardner's eighth talent.)

TOPIC 27.2 Supplementing the Curriculum for Gifted Children

Two different kinds of supplementary programs are available for gifted children: pullout programs and summer and weekend programs. Three-fourths of all school districts in the United States use pullout programs, in which children experience regular classrooms for most of the day and are "pulled out" into special enrichment classes with other gifted children. Pullout programs typically emphasize one of three areas: *process, content,* or *project.* Process courses train students in problem solving and critical thinking and typically do not emphasize a specific subject matter such as math or history. Content courses offer advanced study in a specific subject, such as literature or biology. Project courses focus on completion of a project that might culminate in a presentation or other tangible product. Winner observes that pullout enrichment programs are often criticized for being superficial and unsystematic, yet the research does show modest gains in achievement scores for gifted children who participate.

The other supplementary intervention, consisting of summer and weekend programs, is called talent search. This process selects high scorers on normally administered achievement tests, then administers the Scholastic Aptitude Test to these youngsters. Those who do well are invited to attend special weekend and summer programs. Julian Stanley developed the first program, in mathematics, at Johns Hopkins University. Today, programs are available at Duke University, Northwestern University, and the University of Denver. These talent search programs yield impressive results. In one study, 85 percent of talent search graduates finished college with an excellent record and attitude.

Applications

1 Encourage regular classroom teachers to incorporate the best features of pullout programs into the standard classroom. There is no reason, for example, that a regular classroom teacher cannot design a long-term project on which a gifted child can work along with her or his nongifted peers.

2 Check with the Department of Education at your local college or university and inquire about special weekend and summer programs for gifted youth.

TOPIC 27.3 Changing the System of Education for Gifted Children

The system in which a gifted child receives an education can be changed in three ways: *ability grouping, special schools,* and *acceleration*. Ability grouping needs to be contrasted with tracking. In tracking, students are permanently placed in classes along with peers of similar ability levels. In ability grouping, the grouping is ad hoc and not rigid. A special one-semester course in advanced science might be offered, then disbanded. Ability grouping can include within-class arrangements, in which students at similar levels in the same classroom work together. These groupings are flexible and can change from subject to subject. Winner reports that 90 percent of U.S. elementary schools use such groupings.

A variant of ability grouping, cooperative learning, places a gifted child with several nongifted children. Research reports are not kind about the effects of cooperative learning on the gifted child.

Although cooperative learning appears to work well with many students, gifted children tend to prefer more solitary, independent, and competitive styles. In addition, gifted students frequently lament that they end up doing most of the work while less gifted class members remain passive. They also report being bored and/or resentful at having to constantly explain subtleties to less able students. Another form of ability grouping clusters gifted students from different grades and classes in a special class that is only for the gifted. The research shows that ability grouping per se achieves only modest gains. However, when it is accompanied by an appropriately challenging curriculum for the gifted students, more dramatic gains emerge.

The second method of systemic change is the special school for gifted children. Private schools have long sought out more intelligent students, but public schools for the gifted are rare except at the senior high school level. The North Carolina School for Math and Science, founded in 1980, is a model for such schools, with "imitators" in Texas, Illinois, and Louisiana. Although no research is available to assess the effect of these programs (research would require random assignment to these schools and to control groups, which Winner points out would be politically horrendous), the dramatic success of their graduates speaks well for their effectiveness.

The third method of systemic change is acceleration. The theory behind acceleration is that moderately gifted students work more quickly than others, so they should be given a course that advances them at an accelerated pace—a year of math in a quarter, for example. Other forms of acceleration include allowing students to enter school early or skip grades. These techniques all seem to work well for moderately gifted students, but placing profoundly gifted children with average children several years older results in matched speed but unmatched ability in critical thinking, insight, and memory. Some gains in the speed of mental processing come with age, and putting faster young kids with older kids makes sense in that case. But the profoundly gifted are not just faster, like a computer with more processing speed. They have a different "operating system," like a computer that can perform operations, independent of speed, that lesser computers can't fathom.

Grade skipping is risky. Although some studies do show modest gains in gifted children who've skipped grades, studies also reveal an alarming number of cases in which these students develop depression and extreme stress through being placed among older students who are physically and emotionally more mature. Also, the more creative form of giftedness is not based on speed of processing, but rather on *uniqueness* of processing. So grade skipping for many gifted children does not accomplish anything.

Applications

1 The single-shot strategy most likely to benefit all students—the gifted included—is the promotion of higher standards. Both average, moderately gifted, and profoundly gifted students at all levels would benefit from the challenge of overall higher standards of performance. Far fewer programs for the gifted are found in many Western European and East Asian school systems. These countries have generally higher standards, hence less need for gifted programs.

2 Another strategy that benefits all students, including the gifted, is flexible ability grouping. Winner (1997) calls for flexible ability grouping across grade levels, with changing placements based on need, interest, and performance.

3 Abandon the elitist term "gifted class," preferring the term "advanced class" for such students.

4 Abandon IQ testing as a criterion for placement in advanced groupings, preferring evidence of interest and ability observed in the student's initial curricular experiences.

5 Encourage the formation of special schools and programs that bring the profoundly gifted together in similar age groupings.

6 On an individual level, find mentors and after-school programs that challenge young people in their area of talent.

Giftedness, Adulthood, and Eminence

Unfortunately, giftedness does not necessarily lead to eminence in adulthood. A high IQ in youth does not automatically translate into major contributions to one's field as an adult. Barron and Harrington (1981) have found that when IQ scores exceed 120, they fail to predict adult eminence. To quote Winner: "[People] with IQs of 170 or above were no more likely to become eminent than were those with lower IQs. . . . Most gifted children do not grow into eminent adults and do not ever make major contributions to the way people think about a particular domain" (Winner, 1997, p. 1073).

Why? Two explanations push to the fore. First, eminence is based on more than verbal, numerical, and spatial reasoning, which is the bulk of what traditional IQ tests measure. What Sternberg calls "successful" intelligence does not require profoundly high scores on verbal and numerical reasoning. Rather, it requires a profound ability to sense the unique needs of a situation and to arrive at the interventions that will advance toward the goals implicit in that situation. So the first explanation has to do with the narrow definition currently used for giftedness: we do not identify as gifted, for example, young people who have profound gifts on the leadership scale.

Second, again quoting Winner, eminence requires "creativity, dissatisfaction with the status quo, and a desire to shake things up, and these personality traits are not necessarily reflected in high academic achievement or high IQ" (p. 1073). Often, the problems gifted children have in social development lead them wide of the path of social contribution.

SUGGESTED RESOURCES

Barron, F., and Harrington, D. M. (1981). "Creativity, Intelligence, and Personality." *Annual Review of Psychology, 32,* 439–476.

Rogers, K. B. (1986). "Do the Gifted Think and Learn Differently? A Review of Recent Research and Its Implications for Instruction." *Journal for the Education of the Gifted, 10,* 17–39.

Winner, E. (1996). *Gifted Children: Myths and Realities.* New York: Basic Books.

Winner, E. (1997, October). "Exceptionally High Intelligence and Schooling." *American Psychologist, 52*(10), 1070–1081.

28

Building Babel

The Acquisition and Development of Language

> **66 Sticks and stones may break my bones,**
>
> **But words will never hurt me. 99**
>
> —Nursery rhyme

> **66 Words are heavy things. If birds talked, they couldn't fly. 99**
>
> —Marilyn, in "Northern Exposure"

The two opposing attitudes expressed in the opening quotations for this chapter reflect the old dualistic thinking. From what we know today about the mind-body relationship, language clearly has the force to alter the physical composition of the body. Malevolent, adulatory, and romantic words alike have the power to alter the balance of chemical neurotransmitters. Stroking words provide the glue that holds groups together. In fact, Robin Dunbar, in his book *Grooming, Gossip, and the Evolution of Language* (1996), proposes that by measuring the size of the neocortex in various mammals, we can estimate the maximum-size group in which a mammal can sustain enough grooming behavior to keep the group cooing. He estimates that according to his formula, the human's neocortex can handle a group of about 150. Beyond that size, he maintains, an individual would have to spend an inordinate amount of time making lubricative chitchat. Chitchat, of course, is the human equivalent of chimps looking for nits. Threatening and hateful words can so disorient the hearer that poisonous toxins affect the sense of balance and timing, leading to accidents that break bones. Indeed, words can be heavy things.

If the eyes are windows to the soul, then words are windows to the self. In fact, the Five-Factor Model (see Chapter Twenty-One)—the current paradigm for personality traits that is sweeping the field of personality research—is based on the assumption that there is enough information in language to describe individual differences in personality. That is, the synonym clusters found by factor-analyzing language can adequately describe similarities and differences in personality. Other theories are in fact nothing more than interacting patterns of synonym clusters, and any theory of personality must take these clusters into account.

This chapter serves to highlight current knowledge about how we acquire and develop language. Before presenting specific findings, let's take a brief look at the physical structures that are responsible for language. Most of the action occurs in the perisylvian area of the left hemisphere. The front of this area (the so-called Broca's area) is primarily responsible for grammar and speech, while the rear area (the so-called Wernicke's area) is primarily responsible for word sounds and meanings. This holds for sign language as well as spoken language. Because the right hemisphere is the site of visual-spatial activity, one might logically (but incorrectly!) assume that sign language is associated with right-hemisphere activity. However, as Stephen Pinker (1994, p. 302) puts it, "Language, whether by ear and mouth or by eye and hand, is controlled by the left hemisphere."

Traditionally, philosophers and artists have proclaimed that language was what made us uniquely human. In recent years, animal trainers have asserted that chimps and other primates can be taught both sign language and spoken language. Pinker evaluates these claims with a resounding *Nyet!* and declares that chimp talk is now a "thing of the past" (1994, p. 341). At some point in our ancestry, around 200,000 years ago, a series of minute changes over time resulted in our gift of language: "the ability to dispatch an infinite number of precisely structured thoughts from head to head by modulating exhaled breath" (p. 362).

TOPIC 28.1 How Language Grows Up

Pinker (1994) writes that live spoken language is critical to the child's learning. In studies where deaf parents had their hearing children listen to television, the children did not learn the language. "Motherese" is best; it is slower, more grammatical, more varied in pitch, and pointed more directly to the here and now of the child than is "televisionese." The language does not have to be mother's speech, however: in some cultures, older children are expected to train the wee ones, with the mother putting off her chat with the new child until it can hold its own.

Betty Hart, an assistant professor of human development, and Todd Risley, an adjunct professor of human development, both at the University of Kansas at Lawrence, studied forty-two children of welfare, professional, and working-class parents (reported by Sandra Blakeslee in the *New York Times,* April 17, 1997, p. 21D). They describe the following patterns occurring during the first two and a half years of life:

- Children of professional parents hear an average of 2,100 words per hour.

- Children of working-class parents hear 1,200 words per hour.

- Children of welfare parents hear 600 words per hour.

- Professional parents talk directly to their children three times as much as parents in the other two categories.

- Children of professional parents get positive feedback ("Atta-kid!") thirty times per hour, twice as frequently as working-class children and five times more than welfare children.

Hart and Risley conclude that these language patterns account for much of the large gap that favors children of professional parents in measurements of mental ability at age three.

Although human talk is mandatory for language learning in infants, apparently the correction of grammatical mistakes is not a requirement. Pinker reports that the research leaves no doubt that children tune out others' evaluation of their grammar. The primary corrective role of the parent appears to be to clarify the truthfulness and propriety of what the child says. In response to a child's "She not here—she gone," for example, a parent might respond either "Yes" or "No, I think *she's* in the bedroom." Apparently, explicit corrections do not affect the learning of standard forms; it is the effect of hearing the standard form enough times for it to stick.

Well, let's start at the beginning of language acquisition. The following list traces the significant steps involved in the development of individual language ability:

In the womb: Pinker (1994, p. 264) cites evidence that the embryo learns the prosody (melody and rhythm) of its mother's tongue while in the womb.

Birth: Children are born with the ability to discriminate phonemes (p. 264); they must babble in order to ultimately be able to match the sounds their parents make. Peter Jusczyk, a Johns Hopkins University professor of psychology, has established that infants in the first year learn to recognize and then store names (or words) before actually associating them with particular objects (Beth Azar, in *APA Monitor,* January 1996, p. 20).

Twelve months: Children begin to learn and use single words (half are for objects, the remainder for actions and social routines). The one-word stage lasts from two months to a year. Some infants show a preference for object words, others for social-routine words. (This is probably related to personality traits.) Phonetic discrimination begins to decrease (see Topic 16.1 for a discussion of neuronal commitment).

Eighteen months: Children begin to learn and use two-word phrases; they are now learning words at a minimum of one every two hours.

Thirty-three to forty-two months: Sentence length increases, and sentence types increase exponentially, with children attaining several thousand sentence types by the age of three. Pinker says, "For any [grammatical] rule you choose, three-year-olds obey it most of the time" (1994, p. 271).

Four years: Every language—whether German, Chinese, Thompson, English, or Arabic—is acquired by a native language learner with ease by the age of four.

Six years: Children have an average vocabulary of thirteen thousand words, with a word being equal to one root (*sail, sailboat,* and *boat* would count as two words) or one derivative (a word that cannot be understood from the root alone, as in *forestaysail,* a type of triangular sail); this is a rather conservative estimate.

Seven years: Immigrants joining a new language culture up to the age of seven can learn the new language's grammar like a native. From age eight onward, performance steadily decreases. For phonetics, decreases in performance begin at around ten months to one year. According to University of Chicago researchers Peter Huttenlocher and Arun Dabholkar, however, the auditory cortex continues with a high level of activity until around the age of twelve. They have found that young people can learn to speak a language accent-free until then, with, of course, a range of individual differences. Using functional magnetic resonance imaging techniques, Joy Hirsch, a neuroscientist and head of the fMRI Lab at Memorial Sloan-Kettering Hospital, found that bilingual adults who learned two languages as infants had one single brain area—Broca's area—for both languages, while those who learned two languages at age eleven had two separate areas, one Broca's area for each language, although they were similar in size and near each other (*Nature,* July 1997).

Eighteen years: The average high school graduate knows sixty thousand words (with probably twice as many for brighter students who read more); this pace would entail learning about ten words each day, or roughly one each hour and a half (excluding sleep).

The University of Kansas conducted a study in which parents tape-recorded all of their interactions with their children from infancy (*Science,* August 17, 1996, pp. 100 ff.). Researchers measured the children's intelligence at ages three and nine. They found that "total talk time" was a better predictor of children's IQ than parents' socioeconomic status, employment status, or degree of education.

Applications

1 In order to learn a language (spoken or signed) like a native, the learner must start by the age of six.

2 Do not rely on television, radio, or other electronic media to teach language to your children. Talk with them and allow them to be around others who will talk with them.

3 Realize that children learn a new word every 1½ to 2 hours. Don't rest on your laurels when your child learns a new word. You've got about nine more to go for the day!

4 When a child makes a grammatical error, do not make a point of correcting the error. Simply continue to speak correctly and the child will pick it up. If you cannot resist the urge to correct a child's grammar, try restating the error in a low-key, correct manner. For example, when a child says, "The cat goed away," say matter-of-factly, "Yes, the cat went to find a rat." Only make explicit corrections for errors of fact ("No, the cat is in the corner") or propriety (if the child says, "I pulls the tail on the cat," say, "No, don't pull the cat's tail. It might hurt him"). Priorities become obvious when the child makes an error in grammar and fact or propriety at the same time, as in "I wants to play in the oven." Clearly you shouldn't confuse the child by replying, "No, you *want* to play in the oven."

5 Support any legislation or other social initiative that increases the quality and quantity of adult language that children of working-class and welfare parents hear and interact with.

TOPIC 28.2   The Case for a Universal Grammar

Stephen Pinker (1994) makes a compelling case for a single universal grammar that explains how all languages work with just two rules. The first rule states: "A phrase consists of an optional subject, followed by an X-bar, followed by any number of modifiers" (p. 110). The second rule states: "An X-bar consists of a head X [noun, verb, preposition, or adjective] and any number of role-players, in either order" (p. 111).

These rules are true for every language (p. 111), according to Pinker. And, although this suggests a universal genetic predisposition toward these two rules for the human species, there is no relationship between genetic structure and the ability to learn a specific language. Up through the time of neuronal commitment (see Topic 16.1), any child can learn any language, given a normal brain. As Pinker enjoys commenting, much to the chagrin of Francophiles, French genes are not required for learning French! The learning of a specific grammar is purely environmental. Or, as Pinker puts it: "People store genes in their gonads and pass them to their children through their genitals; they store grammars in their brains and pass them to their children through their mouths" (p. 258).

Application

Be assured that any child can learn any language, independent of the child's genetic makeup. All children have a language instinct based on a universal grammar, and all languages reflect this universal grammar.

TOPIC 28.3 Teaching Reading

Two rival approaches to the teaching of reading—phonics and whole language—have struggled for ascendancy in the form of publishers who wish to dominate the textbook market. Current research slightly favors the whole-language approach, yet an enlightened approach would appear to use a combination of word-attack skills (phonics, in which students are taught, for example, that "p" is said as "puh") and word-recognition (whole-language) skills. A recent research project conducted by Jenifer Katahira of Pasadena, California (who teaches kindergarten as well as teachers of reading), and psychologist Virginia Berninger of the University of Washington established the superiority of the whole-language approach in raising student achievement. Berninger is teaming up with Wendy Raskind, a geneticist at the University of Washington School of Medicine, to investigate the possibility of identifying potentially poor readers through brain scan techniques and treating them with gene replacement therapy. Look for the results!

Application

When teaching reading, emphasize word-recognition (whole-language) techniques, but teach word-attack skills (phonics) to the students who respond well to it. Don't browbeat kids who find phonics aversive; just focus on whole-language techniques.

TOPIC 28.4   "Speed" Reading

Back in the 1950s, the U.S. Department of the Navy studied the effectiveness of so-called speed reading programs and found that they were no more or less than skimming techniques. Students were trained to read topic sentences (the first and last in the paragraph), and the comprehension tests used to evaluate the training only questioned the content in these sentences. When students were tested on material that was scattered randomly throughout the reading passages, comprehension plummeted.

More recently, University of Missouri at Kansas City educational psychologist Ronald Carver (1990) published a review of research on reading speed. Several findings emerged:

- The normal reading speed is 200 to 300 words per minute.
- Faster speeds involve skipping words.
- Skipping words results in decreased comprehension.

Applications

1 When you are reading only to find new information on a subject you are already familiar with, then reading, or skimming, faster than 300 words per minute makes sense.

2 When you are reading for detailed understanding of a more unfamiliar subject, you should slow down your reading, probably below 200 words per minute.

3 For most other reading, accept the typical rate of 200 to 300 words per minute.

4 Don't claim to read at a thousand or more words per minute. That's not reading, according to research; it's skimming. Calling it speed reading is like referring to microwaving a dinner-in-a-box as "cooking." It's not; it's nuking, or warming.

TOPIC 28.5 | Ebonics

Standard American English (SAE) is the dominant version of English spoken in the United States. Black English Vernacular (BEV) is a variant of English that is also spoken in the United States. Stephen Pinker makes the case that BEV, also called Ebonics, has integrity as a language and adheres to the logic and traditions of good linguistics (1994, pp. 29–31). Here is an example: "You ain't goin' to no heaven" employs two negatives in the same fashion as the "*ne . . . pas*" construction in French. "Ain't . . . no" differs from SAE, but it is not ungrammatical, bad grammar, or ignorant. It is a logical part of its own language. It is not SAE, nor does it intend to be.

Robert Williams, the father of Ebonics, has presented research that demonstrates that BEV students score higher on IQ tests when their language is employed. Largely as a result of his work, the Oakland (California) Unified School Board has recognized Ebonics as the primary language of black students. Their expectation is that if BEV is accepted in the curriculum, black students who are not versed in SAE will perform better in all subject areas. Realistically, however, in the United States, certain doors will be closed to those who do not know SAE.

Applications

1 For an excellent treatment of the integrity of BEV, read William Labov's "The Logic of Nonstandard English" (1969). And, of course, consult Pinker's *The Language Instinct* (1994).

2 Regard BEV as a language in its own right, not to be replaced by SAE or French or Quebecois or Spanish or any other language, but certainly able to exist simultaneously with them. The truths described in Topic 28.1 about nonnatives who are learning a new language apply equally to the native BEV speaker who is learning

SAE. SAE should be regarded as a second language for native speakers of BEV, as well as for native speakers of French, Spanish, and Vietnamese.

TOPIC 28.6 **Plain English and the Tradition of Legal Redundancy**

The U.S. government has a department whose mission is to serve as a guardian of "plain English." In fact, many state governments have passed a so-called plain English law. This law requires, among other things, that those who draft contracts and other legal documents write in a manner that is direct and understandable by the reader and signer of the contract. In states that are governed by a plain English law, obfuscatory language in a legal document can establish the innocence of a defendant who is found to be in violation of the terms of the contract. If the defendant can establish that the language is not plain English, then he or she is excused. You cannot be bound to terms that you cannot understand.

One of the more interesting features of plain English is the move away from "legal redundancy": *meet and proper, last will and testament, cease and desist,* and so on. In a classic from the plain English movement, *Plain English for Lawyers* (1994), author Richard C. Wydick explains the historical background that resulted in legal redundancy. An understanding of this background clearly removes any need for legal redundancies in the 1990s. During the Old English period in Britain (roughly the seventh through twelfth centuries), residents spoke two languages side by side: Anglo-Saxon (also called Old English) and Latin (which had been spoken by the Roman legions and was still used in the church).

After the Normans, who spoke French, defeated the English at the Battle of Hastings in 1066, the French language dominated court life. Not until William Caxton printed the first book in England in 1477, the first of a hundred or so that he printed, did the English language begin to stabilize into what we now know as Modern English. For eight centuries in England, workers and rulers could not understand each other's language. The workers spoke English (Old or Middle), and the rulers spoke Latin or French. With some exceptions, a thoroughgoing language barrier permeated England. In order for contracts to be binding, they had to be drafted with their key words written in both of the two languages. Hence *meet* (from Old English *metan* or *gemāéte* and Middle English *mete*) and *proper* (from Middle French *propre* and Latin *proprius*). Try your hand at looking up the derivation of other legal word pairs. You'll find that in all cases, one is English and the other French or Latin (with the older words Latin, the newer words French). For the last five hundred years, there has been no need for legal redundancy. Its persistence is not mandated by linguistic clarity, but by either ignorance of history or slavish adherence to tradition.

Applications

1 Learn to write in plain English. The Information Design Center of the American Institutes for Research in Washington, D.C., has designed an excellent workshop: "Reader-Focused Writing Tools." Call them at 202-342-5000 for more information.

2 If your state does not have a plain English law, create interest in your legislative delegation. Information is available on two web sites: www.plainlanguage.gov (a U.S. site) and www.wordcentre.co.uk (a site in the United Kingdom).

3 When you encounter a legal document that employs legal redundancies, ask the attorney to remove them and thus simplify the language. Often, lawyers will reply that the redundancies convey essential meanings and must be retained. If that is the case with your encounter, ask the attorney just what the differences in meaning are. Often, when asked, lawyers will hem and haw and refer to arcane subtleties that those who haven't attended law school just wouldn't understand. At this point, the time has arrived for you to pull out your knowledge of English history and the plain English laws. Enjoy. And, of course, if *you* are an attorney who employs legal redundancies, let today be the first day for a new you who writes plain English. Not boring or dull English, just English that is plain and understandable.

4 An excellent document with suggestions on how to advance the cause of plain English is Joseph Kimble's article, "Plain English: A Charter for Clear Writing" (1992). Contact him at kimblej@cooley.edu.

TOPIC 28.7   E-Prime: To Is or Not to Is

David Bourland, Jr., argues that the verb "to be" has misled us into the harmful habits of (1) unequivocally absolute statements ("Russia is the evil empire") and (2) inflammatorily ambiguous statements ("My way is better than yours") (reported in Bois, 1966). Bourland believes that we should banish the verb *to be* from the language, forcing ourselves to use more descriptive and less judgmental statements. Compare "Thou art a hot number" to "Shall I compare thee to a summer's day?" or "He is lazy" to "His breaks average thirty minutes, and he produces 80 percent of his quota." Bourland refers to English without *to be* as E-Prime. He has developed the following formula to describe it: $E' = E - e$, where E is the traditional, intact English language and e is the verb *to be* with its many inflections.

Applications

1 On official documents such as performance appraisals, contracts, or memos of record, prefer action verbs to the verb *to be*. By eliminating words like *is* and *are* (and hence the passive voice and subjunctive mood), your writing will be more descriptive and informative and less blameful and judgmental.

2 When you catch yourself in an argument with someone, try talking in E-Prime. First, it slows you down and leads to more thoughtful language. Second, it eliminates many phrases that tend to alienate and offend people, such as "That's a stupid thing to say" or "You're just plain wrong."

3 Use E-Prime in developing course outlines, scripts, speeches, and presentations.

TOPIC 28.8 **Myths About the English Language**

Myths about language abound. They are perpetuated by popular pundits of the press whom Pinker calls "language mavens": William Safire, Richard Lederer, Theodore Bernstein, William Espy, Dimitri Borgman, and Gyles Brandreth, just to name a few. Pinker dates the emergence of the language mavens to the eighteenth century, when England had established its colonial tentacles throughout the world. Traders were clamoring for English language learning materials. The authors of these texts were accomplished Latin students. Consciously or unconsciously, with no historical or scientific foundation, they transferred rules of Latin grammar to English grammar. Pinker's Chapter Twelve, "The Language Mavens," is an entertaining summary of this misapplied logic. Pinker sees most of the mavens' rules as shibboleths: tests to see if you belong to the in-group (have you mastered your Latin?). Here is a list of some of the more familiar myths, rules that have no basis in English linguistic science and that should not be held as a yardstick for judging language:

- Don't split an infinitive. (You may; Latin infinitives *can't* be split.)

- Don't end a sentence with a preposition. (Prepositions are perfectly good words to end a sentence with. However, like any stylistic device, overuse may become monotonous.)

- Two negatives make a positive. (Mick Jagger laments that he "can't get no satisfaction.")

- Do not convert nouns into verbs, as in changing *priority* to *prioritize*. (How else does language change and grow and enlarge its rich texture? However, such neologisms are generally unwelcome in formal prose.)

- Don't begin a sentence with a conjunction. (This is OK, but don't overdo it.)

- "She out-Sally-Rided Sally Ride" is an incorrect construction. (It is fine; verbs formed from nouns are inflected differently from standard verbs.)

- Watch your *who* and *whom*. (This is a gasping, dying vestige of the Old English case system; *ye* and *thou* are already dead and reduced to *you*. Let *whom* die. That is not a question, but a request.)

I will not try reporting on the "me and my friends . . ." discussions in Pinker's book. If you love language, *The Language Instinct* is a must-read. Pinker offers a final dismissal of the language mavens by attributing the majority of their misadvice to two "blind spots": "One is a gross underestimation of the linguistic wherewithal of the common person. . . . The other . . . is their complete ignorance of the modern science of language" (p. 398). Pinker laments that more members of his profession have not written for the popular market. The exceptions—those American linguists who have written for the mass market—include Joseph Emonds, Dwight Bolinger, Robin Lakoff, James McCawley, Geoffrey Nunberg, and, of course, Stephen Pinker.

My editor, Helen Hyams, of Austin, Texas, points out that "language does change and grow, but until the new words are accepted by dictionaries, they're not 'correct'; they're considered colloquial, informal language or even jargon or slang. I don't use formal language in speech or letters, but if I didn't use it in material intended for publication, both the author and I would be criticized. I love it when authors use language in original ways, and no publisher minds either, but it's usually easy to tell creativity from laziness or an inability to use the language. Perhaps it's better not to encourage the latter" (personal communication, March 1999). Touché!

Applications

❶ Pinker recommends two style manuals that are highly readable and essentially devoid of myth: William Strunk, Jr., and E. B. White, *The Elements of Style* (1979), and Joseph M. Williams, *Style: Toward Clarity and Grace* (1990).

❷ Trust your language instincts. Listen to advice, but eschew what offends your ear. Read *The Language Instinct* by Pinker if you want to see how language science should shape language usage.

❸ Agree on standards, then let go of your early childhood training. A couple of years back, I taught an effective business writing seminar for a Big Eight accounting firm. After hearing me assert that it is permissible to end sentences with prepositions, begin them with conjunctions, and split infinitives, they rebelled. As break time was imminent, I suggested a challenge: "What would you accept as standards for your firm's usage?" They suggested two: the *Wall Street Journal* and their own annual report. Over the break, I checked over their most recent annual report and the front page of the *Wall Street Journal.* The annual report contained a dozen split infinitives along with a couple of dozen sentences beginning with a conjunction or ending with a preposition. The *Wall Street Journal* followed suit. They grudgingly acknowledged that their high school mavens' advice was not consistent with accepted standard practice.

TOPIC 28.9　Writer's Block

The principle of focused attention (see Topic 23.9) applies to the common problem of "writer's block"—the experience of wanting to write yet failing to come up with the requisite words. Albert Joseph, in his popular business writing workshop entitled "Put It in Writing," advises the would-be writer that this inability to get words to flow can be attributed to the attempt to do two things at once—namely, to determine both the *how* and the *what.* The *what* is the content—facts, concepts, and stories—while the *how* is the style—word choice, sentence structure, and point of view. Joseph argues that the brain is trying to do two things at once, similar to listening to the radio and trying to read a book. Joseph suggests that first establishing the *what* will remedy the problem.

Application

When you face a writing task and can't quite get started, try making a list of all the subjects you want to cover. Then sequence the items in the list. The "mind map" (see Topic 31.3) is an effective technique for this kind of outlining. It employs a much more forgiving format than the traditional outline (Ia, Ib, IIa, IIb . . .).

TOPIC 28.10   Language and Mood

Activity in the left hemisphere of the brain (measured as glucose consumption) accompanies positive emotions such as cheerfulness and approach behaviors (see the closing comments in Chapter Two). Negative emotions and avoidance behaviors are associated with right-brain activity (Fox, 1991; Gazzaniga, 1985). The language region of the brain is located in the vicinity of the left perisylvian fissure, and the evidence points to the positive effect of talking on mood.

Application

Try writing (letters, a journal, your autobiography, a biography, or some other genre) or talking (to a friend, family member, child, stranger in a pub, or other person) as a way to improve a mood you do not wish to perpetuate. Talking or writing gets you out of the blues.

TOPIC 28.11   Language and Memory

William Levelt, director of the Max Planck Institute for Psycholinguistics in Nijmegen, the Netherlands, has identified three interactive networks that account for the process of thinking up words to use in everyday speech (reported by Sandra Blakeslee in the *New York Times,* September 26, 1995, p. Cl). He calls these three systems the *lexical network,* the *lemma network,* and the *lexeme network.* The lexical network is the first to activate as we think up what we want to say. This node stores meanings, or definitions, but not the words themselves. That is why, when we are trying to think up a word, we can see, smell, or hear what the word we want is associated with. Speakers who use gender words (*le* and *la; der, die,* and *das*) can even know the gender without knowing the word! This lexical node includes links with synonyms.

The second network is the lemma system; it applies the speaker's language syntax rules (such as verb form, case, and gender) to the meaning. Often, when we have many associations with the sought-after word, we experience the "tip of the tongue" (or, for the deaf, the "tip of the finger") sensation. Competition occurs, and the word we want does not always make it to consciousness. Then we have to "reboot" in hopes that a fresh start will permit the desired word to surface.

The third network, the lexeme network, applies phonemes, or sounds, to the word-meaning that win the competition, and—voilà—we say the word. This helps to explain how, when we are unable to form a word, we can run through the alphabet and often the right word will pop up. This alphabet run-through helps us to tag the right phoneme to the one word-meaning of several that are vying for attention. Levelt argues that the speed of neuronal transmission does not slow down as we age, but the larger number of associations we have, combined with some loss of connections and remoteness of the use of a given word, typically requires more processing time. Levelt finds that a speaker can generally form two to three words per second, containing a total of ten to fifteen syllables. The average time required for naming is seventy one-thousandths of a second.

Application

Don't worry when you can't form a word; just be amused at the silent competition being waged in your left hemisphere. Often, just giving it time will work. If not, leave it and come back to it. If all else fails, silently say the letters of the alphabet slowly from *a* to *z* (or whatever the letters are in your current language) once, then a second time if necessary. These silent phonemes act like magnets to draw out the word-meanings vying for recognition. Be patient: remember that more commonly used words take less time and effort to form. As we age, the number of our associations, hence the scope of the competition, becomes immense, so the processing time is longer.

SUGGESTED RESOURCES

Carver, R. (1990). *Reading Rate: A Review of Research and Theory.* Orlando: Academic Press.

Dunbar, R. (1996). *Grooming, Gossip, and the Evolution of Language.* Cambridge, Mass.: Harvard University Press.

Hart, B., and Risley, T. (1995). *Meaningful Differences in the Everyday Experiences of Young American Children.* Baltimore: P. H. Brooks.

Labov, W. (1969). "The Logic of Nonstandard English." *Georgetown Monographs on Language and Linguistics, 22,* 1–31.

Pinker, S. (1994). *The Language Instinct.* New York: Morrow.

Part Eight

*Making
Mountains
Out of Hills*

Creativity and Problem Solving

29

Getting to New You

The Psychobiology of Creativity

> 66 *'Tis wise to learn; 'tis godlike to create!* 99
>
> —*John Godfrey Saxe*

*T*he call for creativity strikes fear in some while arousing enthusiasm in others. Why? This chapter addresses that question, based on the current state of research on creativity.

TOPIC 29.1 The Creative Act

Teresa Amabile, a leading researcher in creativity, has defined creativity conceptually as follows: "A product or response will be judged as creative to the extent that (a) it is both a novel and appropriate, useful, correct or valuable response to the task at hand, and (b) the task is heuristic rather than algorithmic" (1983, p. 33). She then identifies three criteria for distinguishing more creative contributions from less creative ones: (1) novelty (we haven't seen or heard this before), (2) relevance (it relates to satisfying the need that originally prompted the contribution), and (3) spontaneity (the contributor didn't use a formula to "mechanically" come up with the contribution).

Margaret Boden (1990), thinking in parallel with Amabile, distinguishes between psychological creativity and historical creativity. The first is merely something new for the individual doing the creating; the second is something new for humanity. To quote Boden: "A merely novel idea is one which can be described and/or produced by the same set of generative rules as are other, familiar ideas. A genuinely original, or creative, idea is one which cannot" (p. 40).

How do we know whether or not a contribution possesses these three features? Amabile (1983, p. 31) proposes a consensual definition: "A product or response is creative to the extent that appropriate observers independently agree it is creative. Appropriate observers are those familiar with the domain in which the product was created or the response articulated." Her definition reflects Aristotle's comment in the *Rhetoric* that he can't tell how to make good art; he can only describe the art that observers over the ages have agreed upon as good.

Application

The merely novel is often represented to us as being creative. Novelty by itself, however, is an insufficient basis on which to judge something as being creative. Novelty without relevance falls somewhere between whimsy and the psychotic. Novelty without spontaneity is tiresomely formulaic; it leads viewers to respond, "I could have done that myself"—for example, after seeing a painting with a repeating pattern of colors and squares or hearing a twelve-tone-row composition. The classic example of nonspontaneous art is "painting by the numbers." Stress the necessity for all three elements, either in your own creative processes or in those of your students, co-workers, and children.

TOPIC 29.2 The Psychology of the Creative Personality

Amabile (1983) identifies three components of creativity in individuals: *domain-relevant skills, creativity-relevant skills,* and *task motivation.* These three components must all be present for an individual to be fully creative.

To have *domain-relevant skills,* the individual must possess the knowledge, technical skills, and special talents peculiar to the domain in which she or he wishes to be creative. Without this, it may be easy for a person to create novel and spontaneous contributions, but relevance will be, at best, random. The presence of these skills is dependent on innate logical ability and information-processing skills, as well as on formal and informal education. Amabile defines a talent as a skill in which an individual has an apparently natural ability. Thus, someone can play the piano technically well but have no talent for it, leaving listeners less than impressed. Or a person can master the technical side of a welding process but, without a talent for it, can be frustratingly error-prone. This definition of talent fits well with Gardner's definition of the eight domains of intelligence summarized in Topic 22.4.

Amabile identifies *creativity-relevant skills* as occurring in three different areas:

1. *Cognitive style:* This area includes the ability and willingness to break perceptual sets (as opposed to functional fixedness), be comfortable with complexity, hold options open and not push for closure, suspend judgment rather than reacting to things as good or bad, be comfortable with wider categories, develop an accurate memory, abandon or suspend performance scripts, and see things differently from others.

2. *Knowledge of heuristics:* Heuristics are insightful tips for coming up with new ideas (for a more complete treatment of heuristics, see Topic 31.4). Probably the most famous heuristic comes out of the neurolinguistic programming literature: "If what you're doing is not working, try something different." This is based on the axiom: "If you always do what you've always done, you'll always get what you've always gotten." A dated but highly effective introduction to heuristics is Zuce Kogan's *Essentials in Problem Solving* (1956). Also full of insightful tips are Adams (1980), Bandler and Grinder (1982), de Bono (1967), M. Fisher (1981), P. Goldberg (1983), and von Oech (1983).

3. *Work style:* A positive work style consists of the ability to sustain long periods of concentration, the ability to abandon nonproductive approaches, persistence during difficulty, a high energy level, and a willingness to work hard.

Amabile finds that two prerequisites determine our level of performance in these three areas of creativity-relevant skills: *experience* and *personality traits*. Experience in generating ideas in and out of the classroom contributes heavily to a person's creativity. You can't do it unless you've done it! Among the personality traits critical to creativity-relevant skills are

- Self-discipline

- Delay of gratification

- Perseverance

- Independent judgment

- A tolerance for ambiguity

- Autonomy

- The absence of sex-role stereotyping

- An internal locus of control

- A willingness to take risks

- The ability to be a self-starter

- The absence of conformity to social pressure

Amabile has found that the creative personality must also have *task motivation,* or a positive attitude toward the task—that is, he or she must want to do it. An unwillingness to do a task results in measurably lower creativity, using the parameters of novelty, relevance, and spontaneity. In addition, research has conclusively demonstrated that internal motivation (see Topic 32.2) is a prerequisite for creative behavior. Internal motivation (doing something because we want to) produces greater novelty, domain relevance, and spontaneity than external motivation (doing something because a boss, spouse, or teacher wants us to). If we perceive that we are doing something because we want to, even if another person wants it too, then creativity is enhanced. The highest creativity occurs when we discover the need for a creative response ourselves and choose to contribute independent of any possible external constraints. When external constraints, such as deadlines, rewards, or punishers, are imposed on a personally desirable task, creativity can still flourish if we are able to cognitively minimize the constraints. When we are unable to forget about them, creativity suffers.

Eisenberger and Cameron (1996) offer a different view on the subject of rewards. Their analysis suggests that the only detrimental effects of rewards on creative behavior occur when the rewards are handed out regardless of the quality of the creative output. I must qualify their finding, however, by observing that their article reads more like a diatribe against cognitive science and an apologia for behaviorism.

The one exception to the negative effect of external motivation is a situation in which the guidelines for success are carefully spelled out. For example, a school art contest or a sales force contest with specific rules and guidelines can generate creative behavior. The guidelines can free us to be spontaneous and novel within a clearly defined playing field. Apparently, the rules have the effect of increasing both the perceived fairness of the contest and our perceived chances of winning.

More recent research has clarified Amabile's findings. Eisenberger and Cameron (1996) report that rewards for excellent performance do not act as a deterrent to creativity. It is the less discriminating rewards for daily effort that deter creative achievement. Carol Dweck, a psychologist at Columbia University, has found that rewards for effort are more encouraging in the long run than rewards for success. Research suggests that no one general rule defines the best way to encourage creative excellence. People are different.

Do what works. To encourage creativity in a person, match her or his personality and its attendant values. Reward extraverts with a party, introverts with a good book! However, if I had to state a general rule, it would go something like this: avoid overly controlling other people, emphasize verbal encouragement, and time encouragement for exceptional occasions (of either effort or achievement).

Applications

1 If you expect others to be creative, take the time to develop their buy-in. Negotiate with them until you perceive that they want to do the task and feel in control of the process. Avoid setting goals and methods *for* others if you expect creative behavior; set them *with* others, in joint discussions and mutual agreements. Setting goals unilaterally typically breeds fears and resentments that stifle creativity.

2 In looking for creative talent, value technical expertise (domain-relevant skills) as much as the more creative behaviors.

3 In looking for creative talent, look for indications that the individual is a self-starter who can work without close supervision.

4 Reward creativity after the fact rather than before. Working to obtain a reward generally stifles creativity, whereas unexpected rewards encourage further creativity. On the other hand, always rewarding creativity after the fact will stifle it in the long run, because the reward becomes expected. Usually, it is best to just be comfortable accepting creative people's own satisfaction with their contribution. Many creative people report discomfort, even resentment, when a to-do is made over their contribution. It is the creative process itself that is rewarding, and they are eager to return to it.

5 If you are commissioning a problem-solving team, ensure that they understand their goal and have management support to implement their solution. If their solution has limits (for example, the project can't cost over ten thousand dollars), state them up front. *(Contributed by Rick Bradley)*

TOPIC 29.3   The Biology of the Creative Personality

Whatever finally comes to be established as the biological basis of creativity, it will certainly be a composite of three of the Big Five personality factors (see Chapter Twenty-One): the Explorer, the Challenger, and the Flexible. Although the precise biological foundation has not been finally defined, many elements of that foundation have been tentatively identified. The Explorer trait (high in Openness) is probably related to higher acetylcholine, calpain, and C-kinase levels, with the key biological difference between Exploring and Preserving lying in the degree of complexity of the synaptic connections. Inasmuch as the corpus callosum is thicker in right-brain-dominant people, we will probably find it thicker in creative minds. The Challenger trait will probably be found to have as its basis low serotonin and endorphin levels. In fact, many creative personalities (see Amabile, 1983) report the need to do something special to calm down for work, such as meditation or music. This suggests less active opioid receptors than the norm. Finally, the Flexible trait is related to lower testosterone and higher dopamine levels (Geen, Beatty, and Arkin, 1984). Candace Pert, who led the Johns Hopkins University team that isolated endorphin receptors in the brain, is reported to be at work on receptors for the hallucinogen PCP (phencyclidine). One possible outcome of her research would be "creativity pills" that could enhance one's ability, for example, to bisociate—that is, to combine features of two distinct objects to form a third, new one, as when Gutenberg formed the printing press from features of the grape press and the coin stamp.

On a molecular plane, creativity can be described as a function of alpha waves, which occur somewhere between alertness and sleep (Goleman, Kaufman, and Ray, 1992). Thomas Edison built this fact into his Menlo Park invention center in the following manner: he would sit in a comfortable chair, holding heavy metal balls draped over the side of the chair in each hand and poised directly above two pans positioned on either side of the chair. He would attempt to doze, until he was startled into waking by the sound of the balls landing in the pans. At this moment, he reports, he had his best creative insights. Robert Epstein (1996) relates that Salvador Dali would lie on a sofa, hold a spoon so that it balanced lightly over the edge of a glass on the floor, then try to reach the "hypnagogic" state. When the spoon clanked into the glass, he roused himself and captured any ideas that had been generated. I wonder if one learned from the other! At any rate, we relinquish control of our mental processes in this brain state. On the continuum from tight mental self-control to the loss of control we experience in sleep, creativity occurs toward the sleep end of the continuum.

Applications

1   The diet to increase creativity is no different from the diet recommended for overall good health (see Appendix A). A word of warning, however: consumption of simple carbohydrates and fats tends to interfere with creative activity by reducing arousal, while consumption of proteins and complex carbohydrates, unless it is excessive, has no apparent negative impact on arousal.

2   Creative episodes are most productive when they are preceded by some form of meditation or aerobic exertion. Richard Restak (1991) calls this an *attentional*—as opposed to *intentional*—mental space.

3   Plan a physical group activity (team building, an icebreaker, an Outward Bound type of initiative) prior to a brainstorming session; see Fluegelman (1976) for ideas. *(Contributed by Rick Bradley)*

4   More introverted people will probably be at their creative best in the mornings, while more extraverted people will probably be at their creative best in the evenings (see the discussion of extraversion, arousal, and caffeine in Topic 6.3).

5   When you are trying hard to come up with a new idea and are feeling frustrated by it, try letting go of your control by walking, dozing, or relaxing in other ways.

TOPIC 29.4   The Four Stages of the Creative Process

Graham Wallas (1926) identified four phases of the creative process, which have lasted to the present day. Using the common language of more recent writers, I would summarize them as follows:

1. *Preparation:* Doing research, gathering facts, assembling people or materials—whatever is needed to have all domain-specific information at our disposal before the creative act. Chick Thompson (1992) reports that Yoshiro NakaMats, a professional Japanese inventor and the holder of 2,300 patents, sees memory work as the basis of the freedom necessary for creativity.

2. *Incubation:* Allowing the collected materials to gestate, to be assimilated into our preexisting schemas, and to inter-play unconsciously or consciously in our minds without the stress of having to produce. Incubation can be as short as a fifteen-minute break or as long as a lifetime. It asks us to let go of the data long enough to gain some perspective. A commonly reported form of incubation is dreaming. Elias Howe dreamed of primitives with spears that had eyes at the end, which led to the invention of the sewing machine; Friedrich August Kekulé's dream of snakes biting their own tails led to the discovery of the benzene molecule.

3. *Inspiration:* The actual "Aha!" or "Eureka!" moment when preparation and incubation produce inspiration. This stage has also been called illumination and discovery. It can take the form of focusing our attention on coming up with a solution through the sheer force of our will, or it can consist of merely participating in a structured idea-generating session such as brainstorming.

4. *Evaluation:* The attempt to verify that the proposed solution is domain-relevant and logically fits the requirement of the original need or stimulus. This stage is also called confirmation. The question asked is "Will it work?"

Mihalyi Csikszentmihalyi illustrates these phases by portraying several contemporary creative geniuses at work (1996). One particularly illuminating example is that of physicist Freeman Dyson:

"It was the summer of 1948, so I was then twenty-four. . . . And at that time the big problem was called quantum electrodynamics, which was a theory of radiation and atoms, and the theory was in a mess and nobody knew how to calculate with it. It was a sort of a logjam for all kinds of further developments. . . . At that moment there appeared two great ideas which were associated with two people, Schwinger and Feynman. . . . Each of them produced a new theory of radiation, which looked as though it was going to work, although there were difficulties with both of them. I was in the happy position of being familiar with both of them and I got to know both of them and I got to work. [*Beginning of Phase I, Preparation*] I spent six months working very hard to understand both of them clearly, and that meant simply [the] hard, hard work of calculating. I would sit down for days and days with large stacks of papers doing calculations so that I could understand. . . . [*Beginning of Phase II, Incubation*] And at the end of six months, I went off on a vacation. I took a Greyhound bus to California and spent a couple of weeks just bumming around. . . . [*Emergence of Phase III, Inspiration*] I got on the bus to come back to Princeton, and suddenly in the middle of the night when we were going through Kansas, the whole sort of suddenly became crystal clear, and so that was sort of the big revelation for me, it was the Eureka experience or whatever you call it. Suddenly the whole picture became clear, and Schwinger fit into it beautifully and Feynman fit into it beautifully and the result was a theory that actually was useful. That was the big creative moment of my life. [*Beginning of Phase IV, Evaluation*] Then I had to spend another six months working out the details and writing it up and so forth. It finally ended up with two long papers in the *Physical Review,* and that was my passport to the world of science" [p. 82].

Amabile integrates these four stages of the creative process into a flowchart that includes the three components of creativity: task motivation (incubation), domain relevance (preparation and evaluation), and creativity skills (inspiration). This flowchart is shown in Figure 29.1. The solid lines indicate the sequence of events of the creative process, while the dotted lines indicate where each of the three components of creativity have their greatest impact on the process.

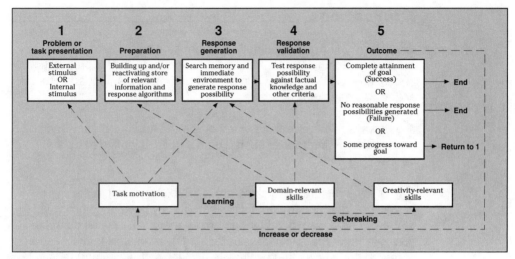

Figure 29.1. The Componential Framework of Creativity.
Source: From *The Social Psychology of Creativity* by T. M. Amabile, 1983, New York: Springer-Verlag. Reprinted by permission of Springer-Verlag.

Csikszentmihalyi (1996) adds a fifth stage to Wallas's four: *elaboration*. Based on Thomas Edison's quip that "genius is one percent inspiration and ninety-nine percent perspiration," elaboration involves the painstaking process of taking the evaluated idea and converting it in all of its detail into a fully realized entity.

Chick Thompson (1992, pp. xi–xviii) tells the story of Yoshiro NakaMats and his three-phase philosophy of creativity:

1. *Suji (knowledge),* similar to Wallas's preparation step

2. *Pika (inspiration),* similar to the incubation and illumination steps combined

3. *Iki (practicality),* similar to the evaluation step

Thompson describes this process as "Ready, Fire, Aim." NakaMats has a static room consisting only of natural materials (plants, natural fibers, and wood, but no plastic) and a dynamic room with music, video, and other media for stimulation. After spending *pika* time in these two rooms, he goes for a swim, during which he expects to have his inspiration, much like Thomas Edison's ball-in-the-pan method (see Topic 29.3).

Applications

1 When you expect yourself or someone else to come up with a creative contribution, be sure to allow adequate time for preparation and incubation. Ask "What information or material is needed before action can be taken?"

2 Always take a break between preparing for your creative act and actually trying to execute it. There's good scientific evidence for sleeping on it!

3 Many structured exercises are available to assist in the process of idea generation. One element they have in common is that they find a way to hold judgment in abeyance until all contributions are on the table for consideration. These exercises are based on research that shows that evaluative activity is stressful and thus activates the limbic system (see Chapter Two). When the limbic system is activated, the cerebral cortex is significantly shut down, inhibiting creative production. Two of the more common exercises are *brainstorming* (excellent for extraverts) and *brainwriting* (excellent for introverts); they are included as Appendixes L and M.

4 Identify your places of greatest inspirational moments and keep paper and pencil in each location ready for quick recording. For me, these locations are the bathroom, car, and bedroom.

TOPIC 29.5 Creative Giants

Mihalyi Csikszentmihalyi, in his book *Creativity* (1996), reported on the findings from interviews with ninety-one individuals—from physicists to sculptors—who had made exceptional contributions to their fields. He defined exceptional creative contributions as the interaction of a system with three elements:

1. A "culture" (such as genetics or symphonic composition) with an identifiable set of symbolic rules that govern participation in that culture

2. A person with the capability of interacting with the culture in a novel way

3. Experts who recognize and place their stamp of approval on the innovation of this exceptional person

This interaction results in changing the culture in a significant way, so that subsequent participation in the culture is no longer what it used to be. Csikszentmihalyi distinguishes this paradigm-shifting, culture-changing contribution from the merely brilliant or insightful behavior of scintillating conversationalists who are able to see the world in new ways.

The personalities of these creative giants—Stephen Jay Gould, Jack Anderson, Nadine Gordimer, and John Hope Franklin, to name but four—require a singular commitment to mastering the domain, as Amabile described it in Topic 29.2. Other than hard work and dedication to one's domain, Csikszentmihalyi found two significant features that distinguished these giants from the merely brilliant and insightful: curiosity and complexity. Listen as he describes the first: "Each of us is born with two contradictory sets of instructions: a conservative tendency, made up of instincts for self-preservation, self-aggrandizement, and saving energy, and an expansive tendency made up of instincts for exploring, for enjoying novelty and risk— the curiosity that leads to creativity belongs to this set. We need both of these programs. But whereas the first tendency requires little encouragement or support from outside to motivate behavior, the second can wilt if it is not cultivated" (1996, p. 11).

The second feature, complexity, is described at greater length:

> By this I mean that they show tendencies of thought and action that in most people are segregated. They contain contradictory extremes—instead of being an "individual," each of them is a "multitude." Like the color white that includes all the hues in the spectrum, they tend to bring together the entire range of human possibilities within themselves.
>
> These qualities are present in all of us, but usually we are trained to develop only one pole of the dialectic. We might grow up cultivating the aggressive, competitive side of our nature, and disdain or repress the nurturant, cooperative side. A creative individual is more likely to be both aggressive and cooperative, either at the same time or at different times, depending on the situation. Having

a complex personality means being able to express the full range
of traits that are potentially present in the human repertoire but
usually atrophy because we think that one or the other pole is
"good," whereas the other extreme is "bad" [p. 57].

Csikszentmihalyi identifies ten polar opposite personality traits
that creative giants hold in a "dialectical tension" (p. 58). Adherence
to these traits is not merely "wishy-washy," as in being moderately
nurturing and moderately competitive, but both fiercely competitive
and intensely nurturing; not just a midpoint on a continuum, but an
alternating embrace of the extremes. Whereas much of the population exhibits a preference for one end of the continuum over the
other, this embracing of polarity makes creative giants more complex. Csikszentmihalyi's ten pairs of antithetical traits (pp. 58–76) are

1. Energy versus rest

2. Smart versus naive

3. Disciplined versus playful

4. Fantasy versus realism

5. Extraversion versus introversion

6. Humble versus proud

7. Masculine versus feminine

8. Traditional versus rebellious

9. Passionate versus objective

10. Enjoyment versus suffering

To translate this model into a simpler format, it would appear
that Csikszentmihalyi could describe his curiosity component as a
high score on Openness in the Five-Factor Model of personality (see
Chapter Twenty-One), with the ten polarities representing equal
tendencies at the two extremes of each of the other four Big Five
personality dimensions (Negative Emotionality, Extraversion, Agreeableness, and Conscientiousness). With the exception of the second
pair of antithetical traits—smart versus naive—which relates to
intelligence rather than being a personality trait, each of the other
nine relate clearly to Big Five traits:

Negative Emotionality	9, 10
Extraversion	1, 5, 10
Openness (facet 1: Fantasy)	4
Openness (facet 6: Values)	8
Agreeableness	6, 7
Conscientiousness	3

The curiosity component relates to the fourth and fifth facets of the Openness dimension: Activities and Ideas. See Topic 4.4 and Chapter Twenty-One for more discussion of the Big Five. By understanding the basic structure of personality and how it relates to the dynamics of the creative giant, we may gain greater understanding, acceptance, and control of the drive toward creative greatness in ourselves and others.

Csikszentmihalyi summarizes his extended discussion of the ten polarities in this manner: "Therefore, the novelty that survives to change a domain is usually the work of someone who can operate at both ends of these polarities—and that is the kind of person we call 'creative'" (p. 76).

Application

If you aspire to make great contributions or intend to live around someone who does, make your peace now with these many conflicting demands.

TOPIC 29.6 Creativity and Madness

Throughout history, writers have linked creativity and mental derangement. Consider:

"[People] outstanding in philosophy, poetry, and the arts are melancholic."

—Aristotle

> *"Great wits are sure to madness near allied,*
> *And thin partitions do their bounds divide."*

—John Dryden

> *"The lunatic, the lover, and the poet,*
> *Are of imagination all compact."*

—William Shakespeare

Ruth Richards, in the April 1992 *Harvard Health Letter,* reviews studies that show a high incidence of mood disorders among more creative personalities. There is growing evidence that creative outlets in and of themselves have a therapeutic benefit for those with mood disorders. Mood disorders represent a loss of self-control, just as creativity is associated with a loosening of self-control.

Applications

❶ Encourage creative responsibilities for those with bothersome mood swings.

❷ Do not insist that creative personalities have perfect mood control.

TOPIC 29.7 Assessing for Creativity

Amabile (1983) reviews the various personality, biographical, and behavioral inventories that have purported to measure aspects of creativity. Most measure aspects of only one component: creativity-relevant skills; for the most part, they do not measure either domain-relevant skills or task motivation (see Topic 29.2 for definitions).

Applications

❶ The NEO Five Factor Inventory and NEO PI-R, described in Chapter Twenty-One, can give as good a profile of the personality traits relevant to creativity as any other inventory. Most multifactor personality tests today have "creativity" scores that are derived from scores on the individual scales related to creativity.

2 Global Creativity Corporation (P.O. Box 294; Mill Valley, California 94942; phone: 415-331-4823) has developed the Innovation Styles Profile, a brief, twenty-eight-question questionnaire that yields a descriptive profile of how the respondent might typically approach the creative act. The same information could be derived from a multi-factor inventory, but if all you want to do is measure creativity styles, this is an effective instrument. Other brief instruments are included in many of the books written about creativity, such as Milton Fisher's "Test Your Intuitive Quotient" in his book *Intuition* (1981).

3 If you want to measure creative behaviors (the tests in Applications 1 and 2 only measure traits), then you must turn to the Torrance Tests of Creative Thinking (also called the Minnesota Tests of Creative Thinking), developed by E. Paul Torrance (1974).

4 Martin Seligman (see the discussion of his learned-optimism theory of motivation in Topic 20.1) has developed the Seligman Attributional Style Questionnaire, available by calling Martin Seligman or Peter Schulman at 215-898-2748. In my judgment, this is the best instrument available for measuring extrinsic and intrinsic motivation. Another version of the test is available in his book *Learned Optimism* (1991).

5 I know of no one test that purports to measure completely all three components of creativity as Amabile has described them. I suggest that you review the specific facets of the three components listed in Topic 29.2 (and in Amabile, 1983) in order to identify which of them are most relevant to your measurement problem. Then piece together a testing protocol to measure those facets.

6 Daniel Cappon measures intuition in his Intuition Quotient Test in his book *Intuition and Management* (1994a).

7 Weston H. Agor includes an assessment instrument for intuition in the book *Intuition in Organizations: Leading and Managing Productively* (1989). He includes national norms by management level, gender, ethnic background, and occupational specialty.

8 In their review of creativity research, Sternberg and Lubart (1996) recommend several different approaches to the measurement of creativity.

SUGGESTED RESOURCES

Amabile, T. M. (1983). *The Social Psychology of Creativity.* New York: Springer-Verlag.

Boden, M. A. (1990). *The Creative Mind: Myths and Mechanisms.* New York: Basic Books.

Csikszentmihalyi, M. (1990). *Flow: The Psychology of Optimal Experience.* New York: HarperCollins.

Csikszentmihalyi, M. (1996). *Creativity: Flow and the Psychology of Discovery and Invention.* New York: HarperCollins.

Eisenberger, R., and Cameron, J. (1996). "Detrimental Effects of Reward: Reality or Myth?" *American Psychologist, 51*(11), 1153–1166.

Goleman, D., Kaufman, P., and Ray, M. (1992). *The Creative Spirit.* New York: NAL/Dutton.

Koestler, A. (1964). *The Act of Creation.* Old Tappan, N.J.: Macmillan.

Sternberg, R. J., and Davidson, J. E. (Eds.). (1995). *The Nature of Insight.* Cambridge, Mass.: MIT Press.

Sternberg, R. J., and Lubart, T. I. (1996, July). "Investing in Creativity." *American Psychologist, 51*(7), 677–688.

Thompson, C. (1992). *What a Great Idea! The Key Steps Creative People Take.* New York: HarperCollins.

30

Chipping Off the Old Block

Removing Barriers to Creativity

> **One must be something to be able to do something.**
>
> —Johann Wolfgang von Goethe

Chapter Twenty-Nine was concerned with the definition and measurement of creativity. For many people, the greatest obstacle to creativity is simply not knowing how to access their creative potential. Creative people know that their ideas don't just always pop into consciousness. An element of intention helps to lubricate the idea pathway. This chapter will address the "how-to" of accessing one's creativity.

TOPIC 30.1 General Principles for Developing Creativity

The presence of creativity in individuals will, of course, be founded on the development of their domain-relevant skills, creativity-relevant skills, and task motivation. The methods for developing domain-relevant skills are well known: schoolwork, reading, professional associations, mentoring, training classes, and coaching and counseling. The material in Chapters Twenty-Three through Twenty-Eight described the most effective ways to use these methods. The methods for developing intrinsic motivation are also covered in some detail in Topic 32.2.

Amabile (1983, pp. 161–164) discusses several principles concerning the development of creativity in young children, which are summarized here:

- Ability grouping benefits only higher-ability students.

- Parents' and teachers' expectations significantly determine creativity (see Topic 32.3 for Rosenthal's work on the self-fulfilling prophecy).

- Teachers tend to wrongly perceive boys as having the greatest variability in creativity—that is, they see them as having both the most and the least creativity, with girls seen as having average creativity. If you are a teacher, beware of this tendency!

- More informal classrooms generate more creativity.

At the university level, Amabile identifies the differences between professors who are successful in facilitating creativity and those who inhibit it. I summarize her discussion (p. 164) as follows:

Facilitating Professors	**Inhibiting Professors**
See students as individuals	Discourage students' ideas
Encourage independence	Are insecure
Model creative behavior	Have low energy
Spend time with students outside class	Emphasize rote learning
Expect excellence of students	Are dogmatic
Maintain enthusiasm for the subject and learning	Are not up-to-date

Facilitating Professors (cont.)	**Inhibiting Professors (cont.)**
Accept students as equals	Have narrow interests
Recognize student competence	Are unavailable outside the classroom
Are interesting lecturers	
Are good one-on-one	

Amabile also identifies several guidelines for establishing an environment in the workplace that will result in increased creativity (pp. 166–167). I summarize them as follows:

- Give employees the responsibility for initiating new activities.

- Empower employees to hire assistants (allow a budget for doing the less creative work, such as number crunching or assembly).

- Provide freedom from administrative interference.

- Provide job security.

Combine the following Applications with the suggestions in Chapters Twenty-Three through Twenty-Eight for developing creative behaviors.

Applications

1 When working with groups, use techniques for suspending judgment such as brainstorming (instructions are given in Appendix L) and brainwriting (see Appendix M).

2 To get unstuck and find inspiration for the moment, use heuristic techniques, such as those in Adams (1980), Bandler and Grinder (1982), De Bono (1967), M. Fisher (1981), P. Goldberg (1983), Kogan (1956), Senge (1990), and von Oech (1983).

3 Explore the works of writers who deal in paradox and perceptual flexibility, such as Escher (1983), Falletta (1983), M. Gardner (1979), Hofstadter (1979), Korzybski (1948), Michalko (1991), Polya (1971), Poundstone (1988), and Zdenek (1985). These are only a few of many such works, but they represent an excellent start. Digesting these volumes will result in an impatience with conventional assumptions and a greater tolerance for ambiguity.

4 Allow yourself and others long periods of uninterrupted concentration. Constant disruption is the enemy of creativity. Quality circles are an attempt to provide workers with periods of concentration so that they can creatively solve nagging problems in the workplace.

5 Develop the habit of bringing your assumptions to the surface and questioning them. Three excellent readings in this area are Kuhn (1970); Senge (1990); and Watzlawick, Weakland, and Fisch (1974).

6 Develop the practice of exploring the ways in which two or more ideas or objects can be combined to produce new ideas or objects. Koestler (1964) calls this *bisociation,* while Robert Epstein (1996) calls it *generativity.* Some examples of bisociation from the history of invention are listed in Table 30.1.

7 Build the habit of playing creative games such as charades, Facts 'n' Five, or Pictionary; ask at your library, bookstore, or game store for help in identifying more such games and learning how to play them. Many books for children are filled with creative games and exercises.

Table 30.1. Examples of Bisociation.

Person	Idea A	Idea B	Result of Bisociation
Archimedes	How to measure gold content of Tyro's crown	Overflowing bathtub	Displacement theory
Pythagoras	Musical pitches	Blacksmith forging iron rod	Discovery of relation of length to pitch in music
Alexander Fleming	Mucus from nose falls into culture	Spore flies in window and lands in culture dish	Penicillin
Blaise Pascal	Mathematics	Gambling	Probability theory
Friedrich August Kekulé	Chemistry	Dream of snakes swallowing each other's tails	Benzene ring
Johannes Gutenberg	Grape press	Coin stamp	Printing press

8 Many books provide specific methods for lessening dependence on so-called left-brain activity. Chick Thompson (1992) describes techniques that are helpful for developing creativity in a wide range of business and personal settings. Betty Edwards (1989) provides hints on more right-brained approaches to learning to draw.

9 Get on the mailing list of the Global Intuition Network. Write to: Dr. Weston H. Agor; Global Intuition Network; P.O. Box 614; University of Texas at El Paso; El Paso, Texas 79968-0614.

10 Mihalyi Csikszentmihalyi concludes his book *Creativity* (1996) with a chapter entitled "Enhancing Personal Creativity." The steps he urges are an excellent summary of much of what is known about developing creativity in oneself and others. For the full meaning of these steps, I recommend that you read the chapter. Otherwise, this simple listing will give you a hint as to the demands he makes on someone who would aspire to creative greatness:

- Try to be surprised by something every day.
- Try to surprise at least one person every day.
- Write down each day what surprised you and how you surprised others.
- When something strikes a spark of interest, follow it.
- Wake up in the morning with a specific goal to look forward to.
- Commit to doing things well.
- Continually increase the level of challenge.
- Take charge of your schedule.
- Make time for reflection and relaxation.
- Shape your space.
- Start doing more of what you love, less of what you hate.
- Develop what you lack and want.
- Shift often from openness to closure, closure to openness.
- Find a way to express what moves you.
- Look at problems from as many viewpoints as possible.

TOPIC 30.2 Obstacles to Creativity

Over the years, I have maintained a list of what I call obstacles to creative behavior, which I have used with various workshop populations. Each obstacle can be evaluated in many ways. For example, fear is a known obstacle to creativity. But fear can emanate from any one of many sources: ourselves, our co-workers, our spouse, our boss, the corporate culture, the neighborhood, and more. To deal with fear as an obstacle, we must first be clear as to its source. Following are specific obstacles to creativity:

- *A critical nature:* An overly critical nature serves as an inhibitor of creativity. Goleman, Kaufman, and Ray (1992) call this psychosclerosis, or hardening of the attitudes! It is especially active during the preparation phase and is often referred to as the voice of judgment or functional fixedness.

- *Personality type:* Creativity is minimized among the Preserver ("Stick with what works"), Adapter ("Don't rock the boat"), and Focused ("We need it yesterday") personality types. See Chapter Twenty-One for information on these personality types.

- *Poor diet:* A normal, healthy diet is imperative (see Topic 5.1 and Appendix A), with a special caution against excessive simple carbohydrates and fats and insufficient protein and complex carbohydrates.

- *Poor physical condition:* Although you don't have to be a marathoner to be creative, you must be sufficiently active and healthy to maintain the alertness necessary for creativity.

- *Fear:* Fear activates the limbic system and proportionally shuts down the cerebral cortex, the center of creative activity. Fear is often accompanied by lack of faith in one's ability. The relationship between fear (and other stressors) and creativity is portrayed in the performance cycle in Figure 30.1. Cortical-state high performance is downshifted into limbic-state lower performance by stress, but it can be upshifted again into high performance by relaxers such as aerobic exercise and meditation.

- *An unproductive conflict style:* Negotiators who look for win-win situations breed more creativity than those who tend to avoid conflict or thrive on it (see Chapter Twenty-One).

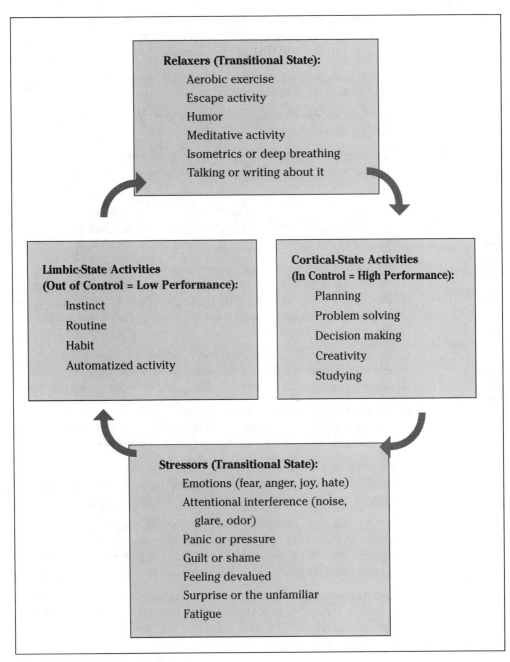

Figure 30.1. The Performance Cycle.

- *Poor group health:* If the team with which you are involved (a work group, your family, and so on) is functioning poorly, your creativity and that of the team will be inhibited.

- *A highly developed superego:* An overly active conscience (full of don'ts) inhibits creativity.

- *Left-hemisphere dominance:* All logic and no play makes Kelly a dull person.

- *A conservative culture:* If your organization's culture is characterized by celebration of the status quo, creativity is inhibited.

- *Inappropriate questioning skills:* Closed-ended (yes-or-no) questions inhibit creativity, while open-ended questions encourage creativity.

- *Perceptual fixedness:* If you continue to see what you've always seen, you'll continue to get what you've always gotten. Perceptual fixedness can only be helped by extraordinarily close and precise observation—by seeing what is there, not what you expect to be there.

- *An unchanging perspective:* If you continue to look at the mountain from the same side, you'll always see the same mountain.

- *A need for power and control:* Control freaks, those who must always be right ("My way or the highway"), are the ultimate obstacle to creativity, both for others and for themselves.

- *Pessimism:* Seligman (see Topic 20.1) has demonstrated conclusively that personal, pervasive, and permanent pessimism results in less productivity, including creative productivity.

- *Time pressures:* Amabile (1983) warns that one of the biggest killers of creativity is unnecessary time constraints. This is a special problem if you're trying to encourage creativity during a brief period of time during a school day.

- *External rewards:* Enticing someone with external rewards to produce creative results tends to be less effective than encouraging creativity for its own sake. See the discussion on the psychology of creativity in Topic 29.2.

Application

Identify the obstacles to creativity in your life. Develop a plan to eliminate or minimize these obstacles in areas where you wish to be more creative.

TOPIC 30.3 Csikszentmihalyi on Flow

Mihalyi Csikszentmihalyi (pronounced "Mee-high Chick- sént-mee-high"), a University of Chicago philosopher, has identified a state of mind that he calls "flow" (1990). Flow refers to a condition in which the individual experiences intense enjoyment, losing all sense of time, place, and extraneous physical sensations. In such a state, the individual is so absorbed in the event at hand that nothing else intrudes into awareness. Csikszentmihalyi (1990, pp. 49 ff.) enumerates eight ingredients that comprise this flow state:

1. The individual feels that he or she has a chance of successfully completing the event; this requires a sense of having sufficient energy and skill for the event.

2. The individual is able to concentrate and become one with the activity.

3. The individual's goals are clear.

4. The individual receives immediate feedback.

5. The individual engages in a deep, effortless involvement that pushes away everyday cares.

6. The individual has a sense of control over her or his actions.

7. The concern for self disappears, but the self feels stronger afterward.

8. Time is altered: minutes seem like hours and hours seem like minutes.

Csikszentmihalyi has identified two factors that influence the flow state. One factor is the level of proficiency of the individual;

the other is the level of difficulty of the activity in which the individual is engaged. The chances of being in a flow state are optimum when the skill level and difficulty level are properly matched. The flow state is uncommon when skill exceeds or falls below the level of difficulty. Excess skill leads to boredom; deficient skill leads to frustration. Csikszentmihalyi (1990, p. 52) describes the relationship this way: "Enjoyment [flow] appears at the boundary between boredom and anxiety, when the challenges are just balanced with the person's capacity to act." This relationship is illustrated in Figure 30.2.

Applications

❶ When an event bores you, realize that your skill level most likely exceeds the demands of the situation. One way to relieve the

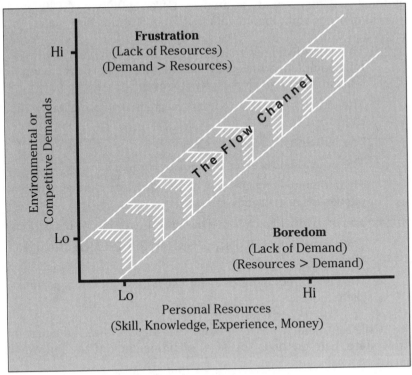

Figure 30.2. Csikszentmihalyi and the Ingredients of Flow.

boredom is to reduce your skill, as in handicapping yourself. For example, I get bored folding clothes, so I time the event to match something of interest on television. Many a sock has found its mate during the news hour or a ball game. Another way to relieve the boredom is to increase the demands of the situation by raising the level of difficulty or competition. For example, if you are writing a long memorandum whose subject bores you, try putting high standards on your writing to create interest in the task: use only the active voice, sentences of fewer than twenty words, concrete figures of speech, or some other characteristics of fine writing that you might not normally use with such a piece.

② When an event frustrates you, realize that your skill level most likely is too low for the situation. You can remedy this by either increasing your skill or reducing the level of difficulty. I remember that one day in the library, when I was reading a research report, I became frustrated. I realized that the frustration stemmed from a statistical term that I didn't understand and that was central to the report. I got out of my chair, found a statistics text, looked up the term, and returned to my chair. When I resumed my reading, the frustration was gone. Flow, and the possibilities for ensuing creativity and enjoyment, followed.

TOPIC 30.4 The Persistence of the Past in Present Creative Acts

In a series of experiments, Thomas Ward of Texas A&M University; Cristina Cacciari of the University of Bologna, Italy; and Raymond Gibbs of the University of California, Santa Cruz, have established that people invariably create "new" concepts that are based on their old concepts (*APA Monitor,* August 1995, pp. 1, 20). Gibbs calls the elements of old concepts that persist in the formation of new ones "image schemas." As an example of this phenomenon, consider the invention of the streetcar. The first streetcar designers had the stagecoach firmly in their minds—it was the basis of their image schema for mass land transit in the city. Failing to consider the uniqueness of the streetcar in contrast to the stagecoach, the designers carried forward the schema so that the conductor was seated forward and on top of the streetcar. As a result, several conductors died when they were thrown from their perch after braking. In another example, when schoolchildren are told to create a completely new, imaginary, and different kind of house or animal, they always include the central elements of their image schemas for a house and animal: windows, door, and chimney for the one and four legs, tail, and head for the other.

Application

When you ask people to create a completely new concept, help them to become aware of possible schemas that might keep them from arriving at concepts that are truly novel, then focus on the key principles involved in the creative act.

TOPIC 30.5 The Influence of Social Networks on Creativity

Dean Keith Simonton, a psychologist at the University of California, Davis, has studied the lives of scientists, artists, philosophers, and composers in order to determine the influence of social factors on their creativity. His research has led to the discovery that mentors play a critical role in the development of creative talent (*APA Monitor,* August 1995, p. 21). The artists he studied were exposed to role models at an early age. In adulthood, these creative talents thrived most when they were around colleagues and competitors who could "feed off each other." Simonton points to the absence of mentors as the primary reason for low creative output during the Dark Ages. Kevin Dunbar, a psychologist at McGill University in Montreal, extends this finding by pointing out that researchers in the more creative scientific laboratories thrive in the presence of colleagues with dissimilar backgrounds and specialties. Dunbar argues that this diversity of researchers allows reasoning from analogous situations. Analogous situations suggest novel approaches, whereas laboratories that are staffed with researchers who have similar backgrounds and specialties lack this fecund source of insights.

Applications

1 Expose your children to role models with talents that you suspect the children possess.

2 Where creative output is necessary, ensure that diverse resources are allowed to mingle. Don't put a team composed only of electrical engineers together to create a new electrical design; include diverse perspectives so team members will feed off each other's ideas.

3 Join the De Bono listserver and newsgroup:
        Address: LISTSERV@SJUVM.STJOHNS.EDU
        Message: subscribe DEBONO <firstname lastname>

TOPIC 30.6   Hypnosis and Creativity

Weston Agor, founder of the Intuition Network (see more at www.intuition.org), has used hypnosis to access creative ideas among business leaders. In controlled experiments, he divides a group into *intuitives* and *analyticals,* with the intuitives excelling in brainstorming. He then introduces an audiotape for the purpose of inducing a hypnotic state. Both groups have claimed to be exhausted of ideas; however, the members of both groups supply substantially more ideas after the tape, with the intuitives again excelling. The use of the terms *intuitive* and *analytical* may be explained by reference to the Big Five personality dimensions (see Chapter Twenty-One). Intuitives are high in Openness and low in Conscientiousness, while analyticals are higher in Conscientiousness and lower in Openness.

Application

In situations that demand greater creativity, if the stakes are high and the people involved have given it their all, try importing a clinician who is properly trained in hypnosis. You may obtain guidelines for using hypnosis from the American Society of Clinical Hypnosis; 2200 East Devon Avenue, Suite 291; Des Plaines, Illinois 60018.

TOPIC 30.7 Epstein on Barriers to Creativity

Robert Epstein (1996) insists that no ideas are new, in the sense that all ideas build on previous knowledge. He believes that everyone can be creative, and that four obstacles account for most of the blocked creativity:

1. The lack of a method or habit for capturing creative ideas when they occur

2. Reticence about taking on challenging, creative tasks that seem impossible or overwhelming

3. Failure to learn any significantly new subject matter (the more you know, the more likely it is that bisociation will occur)

4. Living and working in environments that do not inspire

Applications

1 Keep tape recorders, pads and pencils, or other recording devices with you in places where you tend to lose the most ideas. I keep dozens of notepads at my desk, more at my bedside, in the bathroom, and in the cars. As I write this, I'm at the end of a roughly two-hour drive from Charlotte to Durham, North Carolina. I had six notepads on the front seat with me, and the first two or three pages of three of them are full. By the time I return home tomorrow, all six will probably have served faithful duty.

2 From time to time, take on an "impossible" problem in need of new ideas, not necessarily with the hope of finding the right idea, but to take pleasure in practicing idea generation. Occasionally, my wife and I will enjoy coming up with bizarre ideas on how to change someone's bad habit.

3 Learn a new subject from time to time. Or learn a new aspect of a familiar subject. I learned to play classical trumpet several years ago. Recently, I've tried learning to play jazz trumpet. Learning jazz improvisation and technique is a significantly different experience from playing and reading classical music.

4 Change your environment occasionally by adding, changing, or removing something in a way that modifies your daily perspective.

TOPIC 30.8 Using Synesthesia to Move from the Humdrum to the Creative

Diane Ackerman (1990) points out that creative people throughout history have used a variety of gimmicks to force their minds from the ordinary concerns of daily living into more creative realms. The common thread among these gimmicks is the use of *synesthesia,* the phenomenon whereby immersing oneself in one of the senses tends to stimulate associations with the other senses. As an example, low sounds tend to elicit visual images of dark colors and high sounds tend to lead one to images of light, bright colors. I had read about the use of these synesthetic transport techniques: for example, William Faulkner took a jug of whiskey into the hayloft to inspire him. To help me get into a writer's mood, I used to wear a garish pink baseball cap that my wife, Jane, gave me on my fiftieth birthday with the phrase "50-Year-Old Kid" printed on the front. I had to quit wearing it when, upon picking me up for a business lunch after a morning I had spent writing, she observed my "hat hair." So I switched to burning a big, fat, red candle—it was the holiday season, so it was ready at hand. I've been using the candle ever since as a gimmick to transport me into the writing world.

The following Applications are examples of synesthetic transport gimmicks used by writers throughout history, as listed by Diane Ackerman.

Applications

1 Dame Edith Sitwell lay in a casket.

2 William Wordsworth, A. E. Housman, and Bertrand Russell were walkers.

3 Friedrich von Schiller placed rotten apples in his desk drawer.

4 Amy Lowell and George Sand smoked cigars (Lowell once ordered ten thousand from Manila). George Sand also wrote right after making love.

5 Samuel Johnson and W. H. Auden drank tea.

6 Victor Hugo and Benjamin Franklin worked in the nude (Franklin sat in a tub).

7 Colette picked fleas from her cat.

8 Hart Crane listened to Latin music.

9 Willa Cather read the Bible.

10 Stendhal read relevant books for the novels he wrote (as in the French Civil Code for *The Charterhouse of Parma*).

11 Alexandre Dumas père wrote nonfiction on rose paper, fiction on blue, poetry on yellow; he ate an apple daily at 7:00 A.M. under the Arc de Triomphe.

12 Rudyard Kipling had a fetish for the blackest of India inks.

13 Voltaire used his lover's naked back as a writing desk.

14 Robert Louis Stevenson, Mark Twain, and Truman Capote all wrote lying down.

15 Karl Marx, Ernest Hemingway, Thomas Wolfe, Virginia Woolf, and Lewis Carroll all wrote while standing.

16 Hemingway sharpened a bunch of pencils first. (My friend Sandy Welton does this too.)

17 Edgar Allan Poe perched his cat on his shoulder.

18 Aldous Huxley wrote with his nose.

SUGGESTED RESOURCES

Amabile, T. M. (1983). *The Social Psychology of Creativity.* New York: Springer-Verlag.

Csikszentmihalyi, M. (1990). *Flow: The Psychology of Optimal Experience.* New York: HarperCollins.

De Bono, E. (1967). *New Think.* New York: Basic Books.

De Bono, E. (1970). *Lateral Thinking: Creativity Step by Step.* New York: HarperCollins.

De Bono, E. (1994). *De Bono's Thinking Course.* New York: Facts on File.

Goleman, D., Kaufman, P., and Ray, M. (1992). *The Creative Spirit.* New York: NAL/Dutton.

Koestler, A. (1964). *The Act of Creation.* Old Tappan, N.J.: Macmillan.

Michalko, M. (1991). *Thinkertoys: A Handbook of Business Creativity for the '90s.* Berkeley, Calif.: Ten Speed Press.

Seligman, M.E.P. (1991). *Learned Optimism.* New York: Knopf.

Sternberg, R. J., and Davidson, J. E. (Eds.). (1995). *The Nature of Insight.* Cambridge, Mass.: MIT Press.

Thompson, C. (1992). *What a Great Idea! The Key Steps Creative People Take.* New York: HarperCollins.

Torrance, E. P. (1974). *Torrance Tests of Creative Thinking.* Bensenville, Ill.: Scholastic Testing Service.

Web Sites

Brain Store site (Eric and Diane Jensen's catalog):
    www.thebrainstore.com

De Bono site:
    www.edwdebono.com

Intuition Network:
    www.intuition.com

31

Creating Leverage

A Guide to Problem-Solving Breakthroughs

> **"Difficulties strengthen the mind, as labor does the body."**
>
> —*Seneca*

*T*he word *problem* comes from the Greek *pro-*, "forward," and *ballein,* "to throw or drive"; it means something thrown forward, as when we put something on the table for inspection. A question asked, a diseased animal being inspected, and an unidentified fingerprint at a crime scene all have been "thrown forward," or singled out from the ordinary for our inspection and consideration. *Webster's New World Dictionary* defines a problem as "anything requiring the doing of something." In other words, when you have a problem, you can't just keep doing business as usual. You must do something that is not normally a part of your routine; special attention is required.

Before plunging into the details of problem-solving styles, definitions, and techniques, I want to make one point perfectly clear: the best problem solver is an expert in the subject involved. An expert might be an engineer, a consultant, a professor, a competitor, or even someone who knows the task intimately—the worker. No technique is as good as an expert. So, depending upon the seriousness of the problem, consult an expert before trying one of these techniques. For example, if you've got a cold, treat yourself, but if the symptoms are more complex, consult an expert—your doctor. The techniques mentioned in this chapter are intended to serve either (1) when relevant expertise is unavailable or (2) when the experts have been stumped. I was once called in to help solve a problem that had plagued the experts for about nine months. A $500,000 machine had been failing in the field 50 percent of the time. By applying the right technique (root-cause analysis, described by Plunkett and Hale, 1982), I led a group of ten experts and we found the cause of the problem in six hours.

TOPIC 31.1   Styles for Approaching Problems

In the last ten years, attempts to define problem-solving styles have flourished. These styles are all based on various combinations of personality traits (see the Big Five traits discussed in Chapter Twenty-One). The literature on problem-solving styles is extensive, and I will not treat it here. Suffice it to say that all the attempts at defining styles are based on extreme scores on the Big Five. Four of the ten possible Big Five extreme scores appear to be most commonly associated with problem-solving style:

1. *Preserver (low Openness):* The Preserver aims at a quick solution based on tried-and-true principles.

2. *Explorer (high Openness):* The Explorer aims at an innovative solution based on a new insight.

3. *Challenger (low Agreeableness):* The Challenger aims at the truth by using unrelenting logic.

4. *Adapter (high Agreeableness):* The Adapter aims at harmony and buy-in by building consensus.

Basadur, Graen, and Wakabayashi (1990) offer an alternative based on one of these dimensions (Openness) and one different one (Conscientiousness). According to their model, four problem-solving styles emerge based on the combination of extreme scores:

1. *Implementor:* Low Openness + high Conscientiousness

2. *Generator:* Low Openness + low Conscientiousness

3. *Optimizer:* High Openness + high Conscientiousness

4. *Conceptualizer:* High Openness + low Conscientiousness

Applications

❶   When you are faced with a problem of some magnitude, consider which style is most relevant to understanding and solving it. For many complex problems, a combination of all the styles is particularly powerful.

❷   To assess your own style and the styles of those around you, use the worksheet in Appendix E to find the Big Five trait descriptors most typical of you and yours, or you might contact the publishers of the tests and models identified in Table 31.1.

❸   When you are assembling teams to solve problems, encourage diversity—in personality, styles, expertise, departmental experience, and so on. *(Contributed by Rick Bradley)*

❹   The diversity recommended in Application 3 may also help with general acceptance of the team's solution to the problem afterward. *(Contributed by Jane Howard)*

Table 31.1. Appropriate Techniques for Different Types of Problems.

Kind of Problem	Appropriate Technique	Where to Learn Technique
Problem with unknown cause	Root-cause analysis	Education Research (1987) Kepner and Tregoe (1981) Plunkett and Hale (1982)
Problem with known cause or cause irrelevant	Creative problem solving (assorted varieties)	Bransford and Stein (1984) Hayes (1989) Nadler and Hibino (1990) Nierenberg (1985) Prince (1970) Rickards (1974)
Decision between solutions with certain outcomes	Matrix-decision analysis	Education Research (1988) Hayes (1989) Kepner and Tregoe (1981) Moody (1983) Plunkett and Hale (1982)
Decision between solutions with uncertain outcomes	The decision tree (based on probability theory)	Behn and Vaupel (1982) Hayes (1989) McGuire and Radner (1972) McNamee and Celona (1987) Moody (1983)
A jumbled list	The analytic-hierarchy process (also called scaled comparison)	Moody (1983) Saaty (1982)
Adversarial problem solving	Explanatory coherence	Thagard (1992)

TOPIC 31.2 Types of Problems

Ideally, problems lead to solutions. In light of that, I think in terms of two types of problems:

1. Problems for which the possible solutions are unknown

2. Problems for which the solutions are known, but the best solution is not obvious

The goal in solving the first type of problem is to generate ideas, whereas the goal in solving the second type is to make a decision.

Problems for which the solution is unknown can be further subdivided into two categories:

1. Problems where the cause is unknown and must be discovered

2. Problems where the cause is known, or is unknown and irrelevant

An example of the first category would be a blown fuse or a tripped circuit breaker. If you do not discover the cause of the electrical overload, you risk fire (at most) or the unavailability of that electrical circuit (at least). An example of the second category would be having a flat tire in the desert with no jack available. The cause of the flat is most likely irrelevant; you just need some good ideas.

Problems for which the best solution is not obvious can be subdivided into three categories. Although these situations are frequently referred to (erroneously, I think) as problems, they are more aptly called decisions. The verb *decide* comes from the Latin *de-* ("off") and *caedere* ("to cut"), or "to cut off." In other words, decision time is the time to cut off debate and affirm the solution to the problem at hand. In its purest form, then, a problem is a mess without a solution, and a decision situation is a mess with two or more possible solutions. The three classes of solution are

1. Solutions with certain outcomes

2. Solutions with uncertain outcomes

3. Solutions in need of being prioritized

An example of the first type is deciding which home to buy; the outcomes are certain, in the sense that their features are plain to the eye. An example of the second type is deciding whether or not to risk major surgery; the outcomes are unknown, although to some degree they are predictable. An example of the third type is having a list of twenty projects that need to be undertaken, yet having a budget for only a few of them.

Applications

① When you commit to trying to solve a problem, first determine what kind of problem it is. Once you know that, you will know your objective. This information is summarized in Table 31.2.

② Often, it is not enough to figure out what kind of problem you are facing. You must also determine an appropriate technique to use in solving that problem. Refer to Table 31.1 for the names of possible techniques to use in solving each kind of problem and resources for learning these techniques.

TOPIC 31.3 Describing the Problem

The first step in any problem-solving process is taking time to describe the problem as presented. All too often, in the American "pioneer" spirit, we concentrate on the quick fix and take pride in coming up with solutions as soon as we discover a problem. But research continues to support the thesis that the time taken to plan at the front end is inversely proportional to the time required for execution. In other words, the effectiveness of

---

Table 31.2. Kinds of Problems and the Nature of Their Solutions.

Kind of Problem	Nature of Appropriate Problem-Solving Activity
Problem with unknown cause	Finding the cause
Problem with known cause or cause irrelevant	Generating ideas that could fix the problem
Decision between solutions with certain outcomes	Deciding on one best solution
Decision between solutions with uncertain outcomes	Deciding which solution has the highest probability of success
A jumbled list	Determining priority order

problem solving is enhanced by the time you spend understanding and gaining consensus about the problem at the front end.

Lemieux and Bordage (1992) make the case that time taken in medical diagnosis, especially, helps to eliminate nonrelevant problem information. They distinguish between *linear* (or horizontal) and *semantic* (or vertical) problem solving. Linear problem solving is a logical, "if-then" type, where one piece of information is supposed to lead inferentially to the next. They propose that semantic problem solving, although it is perhaps a bit more unwieldy, is more thorough in leading the diagnostician toward the most relevant problem information and away from irrelevant information. This semantic process is based on the use of *continua* (also called axes or opposites). They find that better medical diagnosticians use a series of continua to describe a specific medical problem and then base their diagnosis on whether or not the diagnosis fits the description.

The first five of the following Applications present the more popular and effective techniques for describing problems.

Applications

1 *Mind mapping* (see Figure 31.1) is a technique attributed to Tony Buzan (1991). You start by writing down the main problem you're trying to describe in the middle of the page. Circle that problem, then think of everything that might be related to the problem, jotting down words and phrases around the page and linking smaller concepts to bigger concepts. This is a free-form method of outlining that is modeled on the image we have of neural networks in the brain.

2 The *Ishikawa* or *fishbone diagram,* also known as the cause-and-effect diagram, has become popular in world business through the total quality revolution. A simple treatment of it is available in Walton (1986); see also Gitlow, Gitlow, Oppenheim, and Oppenheim (1989). The fishbone chart is a cross between traditional outlining and mind mapping; it is not as logically restrictive as outlining and not as free-form as mind mapping. The chart assumes that any given problem will have about four major areas (commonly, but not always, identified as people, methods, machinery, and materials). These four areas become the fins of a fishbone. Ideas related to the big ideas become bones on the fins (see Figure 31.2).

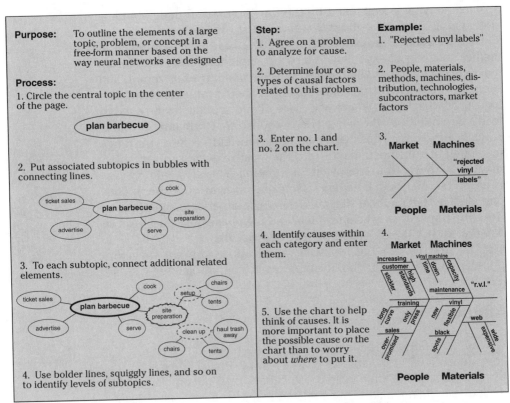

Figure 31.1. Mind Mapping.

Figure 31.2. Fishbone Diagram.

❸ The *Pareto chart* is also known as the Eighty-Twenty Rule, or the law of the mighty few. Simply put, it is a frequency distribution of problems that enables you to identify the mighty few (usually about 20 percent of your problems) that could give you the maximum payoff (that is, reduce your problems by about 80 percent) if they were fixed. Other common phrasings of the Pareto principle are "Which 20 percent of your sales prospects could get you 80 percent of your sales goals?" and "Which 20 percent of your quality problems account for 80 percent of your cost variances?" For examples of the Pareto principle, see Walton (1986).

❹ The comparison of *actual versus ideal*, also referred to as *current state versus desired state, is versus should*, and *performance versus standard*, has become the most common way of beginning a problem-solving process. Simply put, you first list all the details associated with the current problem (the actual problem situation). Second, you describe what the situation would look like (or sound like or smell like) if the problem were fixed (the ideal). This contrast between actual and ideal provides the focus for generating ideas that might solve the problem, allowing you to move from the actual to the ideal state.

❺ The *Cause and Effect Diagram with the Addition of Cards (CEDAC)* was developed by Productivity Design, Inc., in Boston. It is a variation on the Ishikawa diagram (see Application 2) in which cards or self-sticking notes are used for greater ease of movement. For information, contact: Nate Apkon, President; Productivity Design, Inc.; 648 Beacon Street, Sixth Floor; Boston, Massachusetts 02215; phone: 617-262-1717.

❻ Describe a problem, particularly a medical problem, using continua like those that follow:

Local < ·······················> General

Slow < ·······················> Fast

Gradual < ·······················> Abrupt

Peripheral < ·······················> Central

Recent < ·······················> Distant

Constant < ·······················> Intermittent

Superficial < ·······················> Deep

Regular < ·······················> Irregular

Bilateral < ·······················> Unilateral

Focused < ·······················> Diffuse

❼ Many software programs have emerged in the last five years that assist in "process mapping." Some of the program names to look for are Decision Explorer, Inspiration, Visio, IDEF-O, and COPE. For information on Inspiration plus links to other tools and sites, visit the Computer Assisted Qualitative Data Analysis Software network web site at www.soc.surrey.ac.uk/cagdas/. For information on Decision Explorer, visit www.banxia.com. In a recent Internet inquiry, I found that a majority of respondents pointed to Inspiration as the best value: it has a moderate price, is relatively easy to use, and is not as complex or sophisticated as some of the other software.

TOPIC 31.4 Reaching Solutions: Algorithms and Heuristics

Research on human attention throughout the years has demonstrated strongly that we cannot concentrate on more than one focal point at a time. This truth can be built into our approach to problem solving if we focus on one aspect of the problem at a time. Algorithmic problem-solving methods naturally do this by dividing problem solving into steps.

Many will argue that the practice of proceeding one step at a time kills creativity. These people use heuristic problem-solving methods to approach a problem more globally. For example, "If pushing doesn't work, try pulling" is a classic heuristic approach to problem solving. It encourages a big-picture approach in which we think about all aspects of the problem at once. This works best for experts who are intimately familiar with the technical details of the problem and can draw on extensive mental networks.

The word *heuristic* comes from the Greek *heuriskein,* meaning "to find or discover"; Archimedes supposedly said "Eureka!" or "I found it!" when he discovered the specific-gravity method for determining the purity of gold. When heuristic methods fail to yield a solution, an algorithmic (stepwise) approach should be tried. Ellen Langer, a professor of psychology at Harvard University, proposes a compromise between the algorithmic and heuristic approaches that she calls "mindfulness" (*APA Monitor,* September 1994, p. 28). Mindfulness allows the individual problem solver or decision maker to remain in control of the process, rather than being passively led through the stepwise sequence of an algorithm. We accomplish this by collecting a reasonable amount of information (or thinking up some on our own), stopping short of certainty, and then actively making a decision. She cautions, however, against "cognitive commitment," which can cause a person to rigidly hold beliefs without modifying them when new relevant data emerge.

Applications

1 Of the many problem-solving methods identified in Table 31.1, four are particularly noteworthy for their attention to breaking the problem-solving process down into discrete parts: root-cause analysis, matrix-decision analysis, the decision tree, and the analytic-hierarchy process.

2 The more familiar you are with the details of the problem, the more likely you are to have success with heuristic approaches. Heuristic techniques are really just rules of thumb for approaching problems. Here is an assortment of these rules of thumb:

- To detach something, attach it to something else.
- If you can't remove it, counteract it.
- Find a similar problem. Is its solution applicable?
- Reframe the problem. A different definition can yield new possible solutions.
- Simulate the problem to understand it better.
- Work backward from the actual state to the former ideal state.
- Remove the unnecessary.
- Dream: fantasize a solution assuming that all restrictions have been removed.
- Simplify by removing some variables.
- Establish subgoals; break the problem into smaller ones.
- List your assumptions and challenge them.
- Study, then incubate.
- Expand, reduce, reverse, substitute, rearrange, regroup, and alternate.
- Make overt the covert.
- Try less of the same.
- Try advertising instead of concealing.
- When one way fails, try the opposite.

③ For more heuristic techniques, see Adams (1980, 1986), Bandler and Grinder (1982), de Bono (1967), M. Fisher (1981), P. Goldberg (1983), Kogan (1956), and Nierenberg (1985). Also get yourself on the mailing lists of these excellent resources for problem solving:

> Mindware (catalog); 1803 Mission Street, Suite 414; Santa Cruz, California 95060; phone: 800-447-0477

> Shamrock Press (catalog); 1277 Garnet Avenue; San Diego, California 92109; phone: 619-272-3880

④ When heuristic techniques don't work, try a more algorithmic approach.

TOPIC 31.5 Games and Problem-Solving Ability

A wide variety of games, puzzles, and toys come under the heading of brainteasers, including such items as Rubik's Cube, the tangram, the Tower of Hanoi, Jim Fixx's word-game books, and Martin Gardner's math and logic puzzle books. These games are helpful in maintaining flexibility in approaching problems. People who report that they enjoy and play these games also score higher on problem-solving tests.

Robert Sternberg discusses at length the role of puzzles, games, brainteasers, and insight-oriented exercises in *Intelligence Applied: Understanding and Increasing Your Intellectual Skills* (1986).

Applications

① Make a habit of giving games and puzzles to your children starting at an early age, with the games becoming gradually more sophisticated.

② Do not tease adults for being attracted to brainteasers; they are avoiding perceptual fixedness and developing their mental flexibility.

③ If you work in a facility with a waiting area, consider putting out games and puzzles as well as magazines.

4 Encourage the appropriate use of games, puzzles, and other brainteasers in the workplace.

TOPIC 31.6 Sleep, Relaxation, and Problem Solving

Often, a problem on your mind interferes with sleep and relaxation. One way to eliminate this bother is to do a mental dump: write down everything in your mind related to the problem or concern. By writing it down, you will be able to rest, knowing that the elements will not be forgotten.

Sleep also serves as a good break between the data collection and solution aspects of problem solving. By collecting all relevant data and then sleeping, you allow unconscious forces to develop a pattern, insight, or inspiration relative to the data.

If sleep time is not available, simply engage in a relaxing activity after finishing the preliminary problem solving and before trying to come up with a solution. Patterns will emerge in this gestation period.

Applications

1 Keep writing materials at your bedside in case you need to do a mental dump.

2 When you are trying to solve a problem, take a break (sleep, nap, walk, have lunch) before trying to come up with a final solution.

TOPIC 31.7 Trust the Experts

As I pointed out at the beginning of this chapter, research on the effectiveness of various problem-solving techniques suggests that experts are generally better than techniques. In other words, before you take the time to learn a problem-solving technique to solve an electrical engineering problem, first go to an electrical

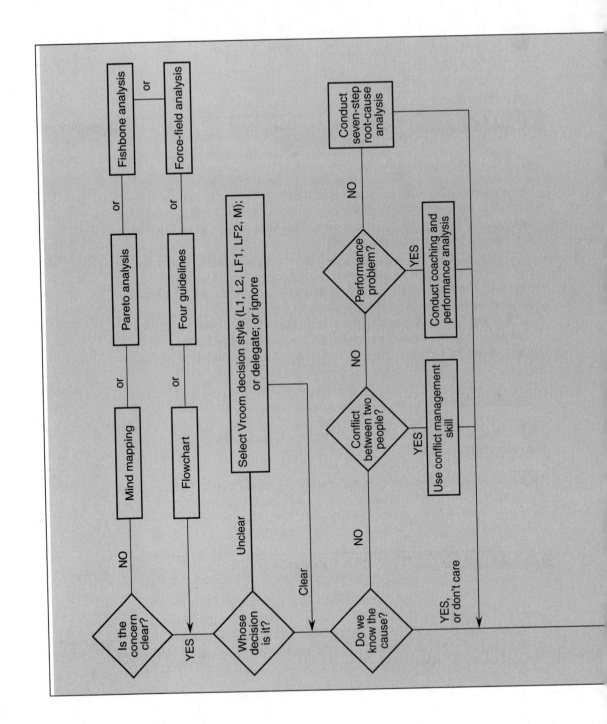

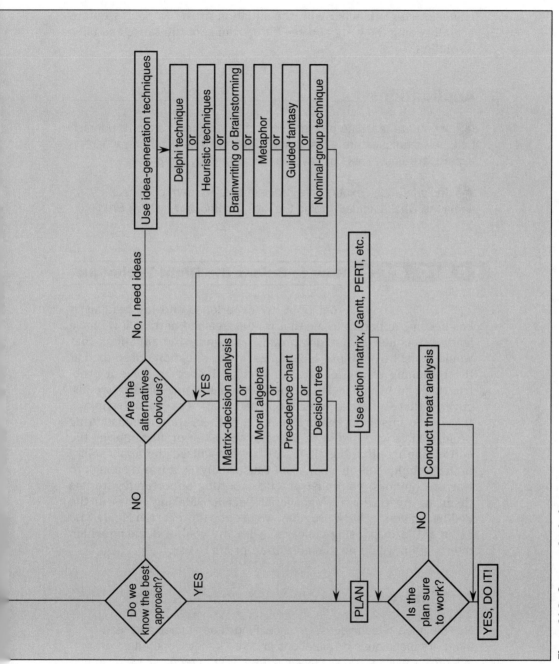

Figure 31.3. Concern Analysis.

engineer who is familiar with the situation or the workers who are actually doing the work and see if they can spot the cause and offer a solution.

Applications

1 If you are teaching problem-solving techniques, caution students that the techniques are a last resort and should be used only when experts are unavailable or have been stumped by the problem.

2 Include a task expert on a problem-solving team or consult someone who is actually doing the job. *(Contributed by Rick Bradley)*

TOPIC 31.8 How to Select the Right Technique

From both my experience and my reading, it has become apparent to me that we have gained nothing if we have learned techniques but not how to recognize the situations that would benefit from those techniques. In the situation I described at the beginning of this chapter in which I helped to solve a problem that had been nagging a manufacturer for nine months, we discovered that six people in the group had studied the same technique that I used in solving the problem. All of them were manufacturing professionals who had been trying to solve the problem during the entire nine months, but they had not recognized the applicability of the technique in question: root-cause analysis. It is not enough to learn techniques; you must practice spotting opportunities to use them. In my graduate "Managerial Decision Making" class in the Pfeiffer University MBA program, we use the flowchart in Figure 31.3 as an aid in diagnosing concerns, with the goal of deciding which intervention would be the most appropriate to use.

Application

Don't just learn techniques. Practice. Find case studies and read them. Try techniques on situations and see if they work. After considerable practice, you will develop the ability to recognize situations that would benefit from specific techniques.

Some Final Thoughts on Problem Solving

Problem solving is made up of many elements. If I were forced to recommend an overall approach—one that would fit most situations—it would be the following one:

1. Ask an expert. Consider carefully who the possible experts are (a worker on the job, a consultant). If no one is available or helpful, then . . .

2. Decide what kind of problem it is (see Table 31.2).

3. Select a method to use for that kind of problem (see Table 31.1). If you are an expert on the subject, first try a more holistic approach (see the list of heuristic tips in Topic 31.4, Application 2). If heuristic techniques don't work, or if you're not an expert, then try an algorithmic approach.

4. Evaluate your recommended solution in light of Sternberg's flexible domain of intelligence (see Topic 22.3). Remember that you can change yourself, the other person, or the situation. If one approach doesn't work, shift to another venue!

SUGGESTED RESOURCES

Adams, J. L. (1980). *Conceptual Blockbusting: A Guide to Better Ideas* (2nd ed.). New York: Norton.

Adams, J. L. (1986). *The Care and Feeding of Ideas: A Guide to Encouraging Creativity.* Reading, Mass.: Addison-Wesley.

Bandler, R., and Grinder, J. (1982). *ReFraming: Neuro-Linguistic Programming and the Transformation of Meaning.* Moab, Utah: Real People Press.

Basadur, M., Graen, G., and Wakabayashi, M. (1990). "Identifying Differences in Creative Problem Solving Style." *Journal of Creative Behavior, 24*(2), 111–131.

Buzan, T. (1996). *The Mind Map Book.* New York: Plume.

Gitlow, H., Gitlow, S., Oppenheim, A., and Oppenheim, R. (1989). *Tools and Methods for the Improvement of Quality.* Burr Ridge, Ill.: Irwin.

Hayes, J. R. (1989). *The Complete Problem Solver* (2nd ed.). Hillsdale, N.J.: Erlbaum.

Metcalfe, J. (1994). *Metacognition: Knowing About Knowing.* Cambridge, Mass.: MIT Press.

Moody, P. E. (1983). *Decision Making: Proven Methods for Better Decisions.* New York: McGraw-Hill.

Plunkett, L. C., and Hale, G. A. (1982). *The Proactive Manager: The Complete Book of Problem Solving and Decision Making.* New York: Wiley.

Sternberg, R. J. (1986). *Intelligence Applied: Understanding and Increasing Your Intellectual Skills.* Orlando: Harcourt Brace.

Part Nine

*The Brain
in the
Workplace*

Working Smarter

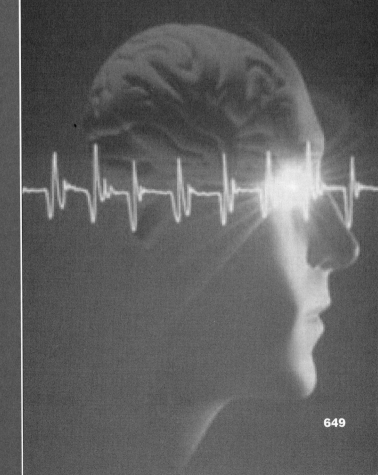

32

From Waltz to Tango

Brain-Friendly Approaches to Change

> 66 *International government does not mean the end of nations, any more than an orchestra means the end of violins.* 99
>
> —*Golda Meir*

C hange. Without it there is only death. Life is change. Cell division, new synapses, digestion. Growth is not possible without change, whether we talk of individuals or organizations. The organization is an extension of the individual. The health of the organization, whether it is a marriage, a business, a team, or a bridge club, is directly related to the health of the individuals within it. Peter Senge (1990, p. 139) writes, "Organizations learn only through individuals who learn. Individual learning does not guarantee organizational learning. But without it no organizational learning occurs."

Without learning there is no growth. Japanese entrepreneur Kazuo Inamori, founder and chairman emeritus of Kyocera Corporation, asserts: "If employees themselves are not sufficiently motivated to challenge, there will simply be no growth" (Senge, 1990, pp. 139–140). To decide that we have arrived at the right answers for all time is to decide that growth is no longer important. In fact, our pronouncements are at best only approximations of the truth. Every day we do what we can to get one micron closer. The quest is eternal. We should, and will, never arrive at any final answers. Bernard Phillips, a Quaker preacher, once gave a sermon entitled "The Search Will Make You Free." Personal mastery is one of Senge's five disciplines necessary to the learning organization. He writes, "People with a high level of personal mastery live in a continual learning mode. They never 'arrive'" (p. 142). John Kotter, a Harvard Business School professor and researcher on leadership, identified twelve crucial ingredients of successful leaders. Some years later, he acknowledged an oversight and added a thirteenth: lifelong learning. In some ways, it is silly to write a chapter on change, because change is incessant.

One of the motives that drives conscious individual and organizational change is the pursuit of the ideal, of utopia, of perfection. Of course, there is a sense in which we will never know the secret truths of the universe. Cautions against the scientist's arrogant presumption of omniscience are spelled out by Capra (1984), Gleick (1987), and Heisenberg (1962). We can never know with certainty; at best we can estimate probabilities. We can continually improve these estimates, but when we tamper with a system to improve it, our intervention can cause an unforeseen, unpredictable turbulence in the system. We must learn to be comfortable with chaos. Control is an illusion. In Michael Crichton's apocalyptic novel *Jurassic Park* (1990, p. 313), the scientist Malcolm says:

> "And now chaos theory proves that unpredictability is built into our daily lives. It is as mundane as the rainstorm we cannot predict. And so the grand vision of science, hundreds of years old—the dream of total control—has died, in our century. And with it much of the justification, the rationale for science to do what it does. And for us to listen to it. Science has always said that it

may not know everything now but it will know, eventually. But now we see that isn't true. It is an idle boast. As foolish, and as misguided, as the child who jumps off a building because he believes he can fly."

I do not mean to sound the death knell of science—only an end to the illusion of omniscience. Between the extremes of Aristotle and Plato there is the voice of W. Edwards Deming. Aristotle would confine us to the realities of the way things are, while Plato would propel us toward the clouds of the unknowable. In between, Deming urges that we ask daily, "What can I do to improve, today?"

The first part of this chapter will describe findings from brain research that are relevant to facilitating change and that would appear to hold true for both individuals and organizations. I have sequenced them in a somewhat logical order:

32.1	Kuhn: The Shifting Paradigm
32.2	Empowerment: Extrinsic Versus Intrinsic Rewards
32.3	The Pygmalion Effect: Rosenthal and the Self-Fulfilling Prophecy
32.4	Establishing Rapport: Neurolinguistic Programming and Nonverbal Behavior
32.5	Using Gap Analysis to Define Goals
32.6	The Importance of Choice in Selecting Strategies
32.7	Increments Versus Leaps

In addition to these seven ingredients of change, I have identified five factors that primarily affect organizational change:

32.8	Chaos Theory and the Role of Information
32.9	Group Size and Cohesion
32.10	The Ideal Manager of Change
32.11	Appreciative Inquiry Versus Problem Solving
32.12	Yali's Question and the Nature of Progress

I will close the chapter with a brief treatment of ancillary factors in facilitating change.

TOPIC 32.1 Kuhn: The Shifting Paradigm

It has become the vogue to talk about paradigm shifts. Thomas Kuhn started it all in *The Structure of Scientific Revolutions* (1970). In this insightful study of the history of science, he gave the world a new verbal toy to play with. The word *paradigm* comes from the Greek *para* ("beside") and *deigma* ("shown"). A paradigm is something shown beside the real thing; it is a pattern or model, like a set of drawings that explains the structure underlying specific phenomena. Kuhn gets more specific when he defines paradigms as "universally recognized scientific achievements that for a time provide model problems and solutions to a community of practitioners" (p. viii). New paradigms emerge because of their capacity to solve more problems, especially problems that the old paradigm couldn't solve. As Kuhn writes: "The failure of existing rules . . . is the prelude to the search for new ones" (p. 68). A paradigm shift is generally preceded by a proliferation of theories that try to explain what the old paradigm can't. Kuhn traces in some detail the shift from Priestley's phlogiston theory to Lavoisier's oxygen theory, from Newton's ether to Einstein's relativity, from corpuscular theory to wave theory.

Because paradigm shifts generally require major "retooling," the people affected by the potential shift tend to resist strongly. They wish to forestall the expense and learning curve associated with accepting a new paradigm. Retooling is an extravagance, so when it takes place, it suggests that a new paradigm has emerged. This perfectly explains the transition from the assembly-line production paradigm, which held strongly around the world through the 1950s, to what now appears to be the continual improvement paradigm of the 1990s. Over the last forty years, gurus have proposed a variety of theories to explain what the old production paradigm couldn't. Theories such as Theory X-Y, Theory Z, statistical process control, and DIRTFOOT (Do It Right The First Time) have all vied to replace the time-and-motion studies of the production paradigm in the business world.

Kuhn points out that new paradigms tend to be defined by (1) younger people and/or (2) people who are new to the field. In both cases, the pushers of the new paradigm are not wedded to the conventional ways of doing things. Hence, the Japanese, with a past record of poor quality in manufacturing, have pushed the quality paradigm.

Lance Morrow wrote a feature essay in *Time* magazine entitled "Old Paradigm, New Paradigm" (January 14, 1991, pp. 65–66), in which he listed examples of old and new paradigms. Here are several of his plus several of mine:

Old Paradigms	New Paradigms
Fidel Castro	Vaclav Havel
Apartheid	F. W. de Klerk and Nelson Mandela
The American Century	The Pacific Rim
Cigarette smoking	Smoke-free spaces
Labor unions	Self-directed work teams
CBS News	Cable News Network
Charisma	Teamwork
Knowledge	Information
Northern Ireland	The new Germany
Letter writing	E-mail and faxing
Nationalism	Pluralism
Communism	Democracy

Applications

1 Paradigms are useful frameworks for solving problems. Be open to the possibility that a new paradigm may emerge in your lifetime that will increase your effectiveness. It doesn't matter whether you invent or discover the new paradigm yourself or follow another person's lead; just don't get caught holding on to an old paradigm for loyalty's sake. If a new set of guidelines appears able to answer more questions than the current set, go for it.

2 Paradigms will shift more frequently now and in the future than in the history that Kuhn described. W. Edwards Deming's dictum of continuing improvement is a paradigm in and of itself and calls for constant attention to opportunities for modifying paradigms.

3 In problem-solving situations, allow your paradigms to surface and be examined. *(Contributed by Rick Bradley)*

4 View the series of five videos narrated by Joel Barker: *Paradigm Mastery,* available from the publisher, StarThrower, at www.starthrower.com. Show this series to a group that needs to change and discuss it with them. It stresses the importance of questioning our assumptions by taking a fresh look at things.

TOPIC 32.2 Empowerment: Extrinsic Versus Intrinsic Rewards

The apparent consensus of current thinking on motivation revolves around the question of who sets a course of action: *external* (or *extrinsic*) *motivation* refers to courses of action set by others, while *internal* (or *intrinsic*) *motivation* refers to courses of action set by oneself. Listed in Table 32.1 are some examples of motivational situations (those in which an individual is expected to act in some way), with both external and internal versions of the motivational stimulus.

Consistently, internal motivators yield higher performance than external motivators. Amabile (1983) notes one exception: when clear

Table 32.1. External Versus Internal Motivation.

Call for Action	External Version	Internal Version
Sales goals	Manager or company sets goals for representatives	Manager and representative set goals together and mutually agree on them
Incentives	Company announces incentives	Employees negotiate incentives
Child discipline	Parent determines consequences of misbehavior	Child and parent together negotiate appropriate consequences
Class award	Teacher announces award before competition, presents award afterward	Award is announced only after work is completed
Work design	Management designs and monitors	Workers design and management supports

guidelines are presented that call for essentially rote performance, then external motivators yield superior results. She also identifies a variation on this principle—rewards that convey competency information, as in "A panel of art experts mistakenly judged the copy of the Van Gogh you painted to be the original." External motivators are more effective with algorithmic, or step-by-step, tasks, while internal motivators are more effective with heuristic, or experimental, ones. I am reminded of a now-discontinued (I hope) incentive program by an NFL team in which thousand-dollar bonuses were allegedly handed out after each game for every player on the opposing team who was put out of commission (for example, if a tackler broke the leg of a pass receiver).

Caine and Caine (1991) point out that under conditions of continuous stress, internal motivation becomes more and more difficult to generate as people begin to see themselves as fulfilling only goals formed by others. Amabile (1983) extensively documents the harmful effects of extrinsic motivation on creativity and problem solving. Gazzaniga (1985) has found that people who are learning to perform a skill under external conditions begin to perform that skill only when the reward possibilities continue to be presented. If you give a person a day off for a job well done, his or her future good performance will tend to become tied to continuing rewards. Give what you've always given, and you'll get what you've always gotten. Stop giving, and you stop getting. Research supports the benefits of mutually discussing possible rewards, rather than paternalistically doling out what you think people want.

Internal motivators are developed when people participate in goal setting and problem solving, as opposed to allowing others to set their goals, make their decisions, and solve their problems. In the summer of 1990, while my wife and I were walking down the coast of Sunset Beach, North Carolina, we asked each other what bothers could be removed to make life more enjoyable. Jane's top bother was feeling guilty about not providing her share of the caregiving for her parents, who were living six hours away by car in Opelika, Alabama. I suggested that she make a conference call to her two sisters—one lived in Alabama, the other in Minnesota—and discuss the problem. I remember that we emphasized the wisdom of trying to figure out a solution before her parents experienced another crisis (her mother had recently broken a hip) and our options became severely limited and, in fact, thrust upon us.

The call and subsequent research resulted in several options that were mutually agreeable to the three sisters. Jane, as spokesperson, called her parents to discuss the options, one of which was to maintain the status quo. They were also invited to identify other possible options. As it turned out, her parents became very excited about one particular option: to move to a retirement community in Charlotte located about five minutes from our home, with the two sisters retiring to our region (one to the mountains, the other to the beach) within about five years. My wife's mother brightly queried, "When do we leave?"

Although the move and settling in did not happen without some sadness, regret, and fear, my wife's parents did settle in and make new friends and new church homes. My wife's mother, a former church organist, played more piano than ever and entertained almost daily in the parlor after dinner. At the age of seventy-seven, she gave a one-hour organ recital for over forty residents of the retirement community. The health and vigor of Jane's parents improved by this change, and Jane's guilt disappeared. If our hand had been forced by a crisis, like a massive stroke, it is highly possible that guilt would have been transmogrified into resentment and anger. I see this episode as a testament to participation in internal motivation.

Gazzaniga (1985), Caine and Caine (1991), Amabile (1983), and Seligman (1991) all call for an end to external motivators. We have been operating under the paradigm of the behavioral contingency model of externally imposed rewards and punishments since the 1940s. Now the time has come to eliminate them, to encourage the new paradigm of empowerment through self- or mutually developed action planning. Gazzaniga goes so far as to decry bureaucracy and institutionalization as the enemy of internal motivation. He sees institutional relief of the symptoms of social ills as the opposite of caring: "I am claiming that a culture becomes more caring and humane the more its citizens feel themselves to be part of the problems that beset their lives. The only sure way to bring them close to such problems is to structure a culture where they deal with the problems at a personal level" (1985, p. 198).

From a societal perspective, what these researchers are saying is consistent with the current preoccupation of many social philosophers with treating root causes, not symptoms. In a recent task force on our aging population, the group coalesced around the need to address causes but agreed that we can't ignore symptoms. For example, to ensure that each senior citizen gets at least one hot meal a day, we need to back up and treat the causes of malnutrition among that population. Our inability to provide such meals is actually both a symptom and a cause—a symptom of poor public transportation and a cause of malnutrition. The resources are there, but access is limited. So we must fix the infrastructure.

Applications

❶ If you are a parent or a teacher, don't assume that you always know the right rewards and punishments. When appropriate, consult with your children or students. Read Glasser (1990) and Dreikurs and Cassel (1972) for ideas.

❷ If you are a manager who is responsible for the performance of others, talk with them to learn what's important to them and what their career goals are. Don't assume that you know the best way to reward them or the best direction for them in their careers. A former manager of mine assumed that I was motivated by the desire to earn more and more money, even after I explained that I was more motivated by challenging projects than by big bucks. My ultimate departure from that company was largely based on his failure to abandon his externally imposed rewards for me (higher salaries) and accept my need for challenging and interesting projects. Bucks don't always have bang!

❸ Build an empowered workforce. If you are part of a management team, take time to explore ways to give people increasing responsibility and opportunities to solve their own problems, make their own decisions, formulate their own plans, establish their own goals, negotiate their own rewards, and even describe their own jobs. Mutually agree on goals, then get out of their way. Don't be an intervener with your people, coming down like an avenging god. Instead, be a supporter, and be there when they need you for resources and consultation. For further ideas on empowerment, read *The Empowered Manager* by Peter Block (1987) and *Developing Superior Work Teams* by D. C. Kinlaw (1990).

❹ As a spouse and friend, help people understand dilemmas rather than "fixing things" for them. Long term, these externally imposed solutions tend to lose their power. If your friend or spouse can participate in formulating her or his own solutions, these internally generated solutions are more likely to hold their power. Be more of a consultant than a boss. "Teach a person how to fish and . . ."

5 Do not protect alcoholics or other addictive personalities from the consequences of their binges. Such protectors used to be called patsies and are now called enablers. A considerable litera-ture has emerged on this subject as a part of the Adult Children of Alcoholics movement. Write for information, a bibliography, catalogs, and reading material to the following groups:

National Association for Children of Alcoholics; 31582 Coast Highway, Suite B; South Laguna, California 92677; phone: 714-499-3889

Adult Children of Alcoholics; P.O. Box 3216; Torrance, California 90505; phone: 213-534-1815 (send a stamped, self-addressed envelope for a schedule of meetings)

6 Amabile (1983) identifies several indicators for judging whether or not a person is intrinsically motivated. I summarize four of them as follows:

- The individual is curious or stimulated by the task.
- The individual gains a sense of competence from the task itself.
- The individual perceives the task as being free of strong external controls.
- The individual feels as if he or she is at play, not at work.

7 In one corporation where I am currently consulting, management doles out recognition cards as rewards. Employees then exchange the cards for a gift of their choosing. Many employees have confided that they would much rather receive a verbal recognition statement speci-fying what they did well and the impact it had on the company. Stay close enough to the people around you to know what rewards they really value.

8 In training classes, don't use "off-the-shelf" cases exclusively. Build in opportunities for trainees to identify real-time, back-home cases where they can apply their newly acquired skills, concepts, knowledge, or attitude.

TOPIC 32.3 The Pygmalion Effect: Rosenthal and the Self-Fulfilling Prophecy

Many regard Robert Rosenthal as the prophet of the Pygmalion effect (also known as the self-fulfilling prophecy). According to the myth, Pygmalion created a female statue and treated it with such affection that, through Aphrodite's intervention, the statue came to life and responded to him. Such is the essence of the self-fulfilling prophecy: what we expect tends to come true. In a famous report (Rosenthal and Jacobson, 1968), Rosenthal describes a case in which a researcher told teachers that a testing program had identified some students as having high potential and others as having low potential. In fact, the students had been picked randomly and assigned to one of the two groups. The results after a year in school: the so-called high-potential group showed significant gains in achievement and ability as measured by standardized tests, while the so-called normal group showed no significant gains.

Rosenthal's initial report has been followed by twenty years of research exploring the limits of the self-fulfilling prophecy. According to today's thinking, although we can't think a statue into coming alive, we can certainly influence our level of performance and that of others by our expectations. Cousins (1989) includes positive expectations as one of the four key ingredients of hardiness as it relates to psychoneuroimmunology. The concept of the self-fulfilling prophecy is also very close to Seligman's concept of the optimistic explanatory style; in some ways, Seligman's research has subsumed Rosenthal's. Rosenthal identifies six ways to communicate expectations. I have summarized them and provided examples in Table 32.2.

Table 32.2. Rosenthal's Six Methods for Communicating Expectations.

Communication Method	Positive Versions	Negative Versions
1. *Expressing confidence in my ability to help you*	"I know I can train you." "Stick with me—I make winners." "I've got the Midas touch."	"I'm not sure I know how to train you." "I'm not very good at training."
2. *Expressing confidence in your ability*	"I know you can do it."	"I'm not sure if you can do it."
3. *Nonverbals: tone of voice, eye contact, energy level*	Smile, nod, pat, eye contact, upbeat energy	Looking away, tentative tone of voice, distant
4. *Feedback: specific and ample; mentioning the good with the bad*	"Good coverage, yet a couple of technical flaws."	"Try harder." "All wrong." "Reread it; you'll see what I mean."
5. *Input: amount of information given to person*	"Let's go over it in detail."	"I don't have time to go over it."
6. *Output: amount of production encouraged*	"Here's a new challenge."	"Better try the same thing again."

Applications

1   Be aware that negative expectations of yourself or others are likely to produce negative results. Although positive expectations ("I think I can" or "You can do it") cannot guarantee success, they certainly increase its chances.

2   Think of a particular person in your life who performs at a lower level than you'd like to see. Examine the six communication methods in Table 32.2 and see if you may be communicating negative expectations without meaning to. Work on being as positive with this person as you can in each of the six ways. Write out a script for yourself with sample comments in each of the six areas.

3   View the award-winning video *Productivity and the Self-Fulfilling Prophecy,* second edition, available from CRM Films; 2215 Faraday Avenue; Carlsbad, California 92008; phone: 800-421-0833. Check with your regional media distributor for ordering information. Discuss

its implications for your situation. A video with implications for
race relations is *The Eye of the Storm,* produced in the 1970s by the
American Broadcasting Company and distributed by the Center for
Humanities, Inc.; P.O. Box 1000; Mount Kisco, New York 10549.
It shows how the self-fulfilling prophecy works in conjunction
with prejudice.

4 Keep the idea of a self-fulfilling prophecy in mind when you
are working with teams. Be positive in your approach to problem
solving and work toward win-win situations or compromises. Keep the
team asking "How can we make this work?" In many situations, one
positive person can turn the entire team around. *(Contributed by
Jane Howard)*

TOPIC 32.4 **Establishing Rapport:
Neurolinguistic Programming
and Nonverbal Behavior**

The most readable treatment of neurolinguistic
programming (NLP) is Genie Laborde's *Influencing with Integrity*
(1983). NLP originated when some psychotherapists began to wonder how the great therapists—Frederick Perls, Virginia Satir, Milton
Erickson—worked their magic with patients. They concluded that
these outstanding therapists demonstrated the ability to consciously
or unconsciously establish a deep rapport with their patients, leading to trust, disclosure, openness to change, and receptivity to the
therapist. Through extensive observation, the researchers concluded
that this rapport was established when the therapists matched
content and paced tempo with the client.

Matching content has been made popular through the "VAK" concept of visual, auditory, and kinesthetic matching. In *visual* matching,
the patient says, "I can't see what she means," and the therapist
responds, "What she wants is hazy to you." By matching the visual
imagery contained in the patient's language, the therapist builds rapport. If the patient's language contains *auditory* imagery ("I hear
what you're saying"), the therapist can respond with an auditory
image ("I'm coming through to you loud and clear"). *Kinesthetic*
matching ("I'm struggling to understand you") might be answered
with "You're trying to grasp what I mean." Pacing involves matching

the tempo of the patient's speech, movements, and breathing: the therapist talks more slowly when the patient does, synchronizes his or her breathing, and matches fidgeting with fidgeting. Figure 32.1 is a guide to the many possible ways to match and pace as a way to establish rapport.

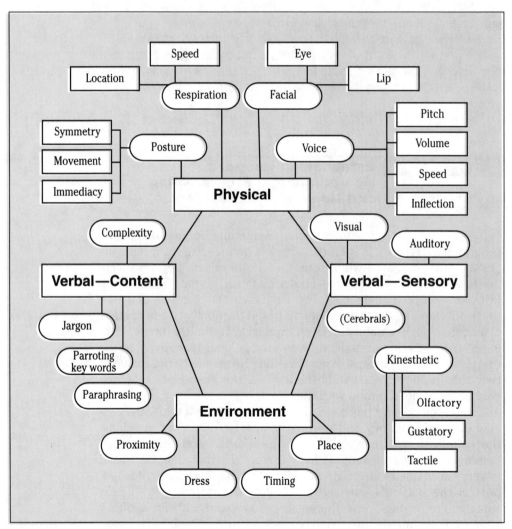

Figure 32.1. The Elements of Rapport.

I do need to point out, and not assume that it is obvious, that matching and pacing are situational and not continuous. To continue to match and pace hour after hour, day after day, would be inauthentic and unhealthy.

Mehrabian (1971) has identified three ways in which people consciously or unconsciously send nonverbal messages by pacing and positioning their bodies during normal interactions. The three modes represent distinct clusters of physical behaviors, each of which has a unifying feature, with each cluster having its own unique "message."

Cluster 1: Physical Immediacy

The more physically immediate we are to another person, the more liking we tend to communicate to that person. The less immediate we are, the less liking we communicate. Immediacy is conveyed by these behaviors:

Vis-à-vis orientation

Eye contact

Distance

Touching

Cluster 2: Activity Level

The more active we are in the presence of another person, the less attentive that person perceives us to be. Activity is conveyed by these behaviors:

Foot movements

Leg-swinging movements

Head nods

Arm movements

Hand movements, including holding objects

Self-manipulation, as in adjusting glasses, scratching, playing with hair

Cluster 3: Relaxation

The more symmetrical our body is, the more tension we communicate, while the more asymmetrical we are, the more relaxation we communicate. Relaxation in the presence of another person communicates superior status, or superiority. Tension in the presence of another person communicates inferior status, or inferiority. Here are the ways we portray symmetry and tension:

Leg symmetry (for example, not crossed)

Foot symmetry (parallel, not askew)

Arm symmetry

Hand symmetry

A forward lean, like that of a suppliant (as opposed to a backward lean)

Neck tension, with the chin up

Interestingly, Mehrabian finds that mirroring another person's behavior is effective for communicating acceptance rather than superiority or inferiority. So if someone seated before you appears tense and symmetrical and you want that person to relax and feel accepted, you should sit in a symmetrical manner yourself until she or he begins to relax. This is consistent with the NLP practice of matching and pacing.

When I was working on my doctoral dissertation during the fall of 1971, a graduate student from Wake Forest University was helping me to analyze the nonverbal behavior of teachers shown on videotapes. My dissertation (Howard, 1972) involved the nonverbal language of teachers toward students. To repay my graduate assistant, I offered to help her with her master's thesis, which also involved Mehrabian's body language model. One Saturday afternoon, she called almost in tears to inform me that her Wake Forest faculty adviser had virtually canceled her thesis project. Could I drive out to the campus and intervene? I arrived at the professor's office and took a seat on a small sofa opposite his desk. I sat back, crossed my legs in a relaxed manner, and unconsciously communicated my superiority. I got nowhere in my rational pleadings, and after about fifteen minutes, I thought to myself, "Use nonverbal behavior, stupid!"

I immediately moved into a symmetrical position, leaned forward with my hands clasped in my lap, and looked up to him in the classic, and inferior, position of the suppliant, not unlike that of prayer. I maintained this posture while I continued my conversation, and within ten minutes we had his approval. I think what happened is that he saw me, a non-faculty member, as a threat, and my relaxed, superior posture reinforced his feelings. By moving into the inferior, tense, symmetrical position, I communicated to him that, after all, he was the boss. With that role reestablished, he showed appropriate magnanimity and approved the thesis project.

Applications

1 Pick a person you need to influence. Peruse Figure 32.1 and identify one or more channels through which you might try to establish rapport in an acceptable way.

2 Read Laborde's *Influencing with Integrity* (1983) and *Fine Tune Your Brain* (1988). In addition to ample explanatory material, Laborde provides an excellent bibliography.

3 Observe and model yourself after an influential person.

4 Watch for demonstrations of rapport that you have established with someone you've been talking with. If one of you shifts position and you notice that the other one shifts too, you have probably established rapport. *(Contributed by Jane Howard)*

5 Use immediacy to convey liking. If you need to convey dislike without being verbally explicit, you can use the opposite behaviors: avoid eye contact, increase the angle from a vis-à-vis orientation to 90 or 180 degrees, and stand or sit farther away.

6 Reduce your activity level to communicate to others that they have your undivided attention. When our younger daughter was about six years old, she came up to me as I was stretched out on the sofa one evening reading the paper. She tugged on my arm to get me to answer a question. I took my glasses off, held them and the paper in my hands, and looked at her, hoping she would accept my answer with alacrity and I would soon be back in my world of current events.

But she stayed and kept tugging and asking more questions. Finally, I decided to give her my full attention. I put my glasses back on, laid the paper down completely, and looked her squarely in the eye. Satisfied that she had "won," she completed her inquiry and left me to the headlines.

7 Remember that an asymmetrical, relaxed posture communicates superiority. Mirror other people's behavior to communicate that you accept them and regard them as being of equal status and worth.

TOPIC 32.5 Using Gap Analysis to Define Goals

Festinger (1953) and others have built a solid tradition of research on the subject of cognitive dissonance. In a nutshell (the pathway of this book is littered with many nutshells—hope you're not allergic!), this tradition has established that human organisms naturally work to reduce any discrepancy between the way they perceive themselves (for example, smart, attractive, and capable) and the way their significant others perceive them. In the world of work, an industry has emerged out of this tradition, commonly referred to by two labels: *gap analysis* and *the 360°*. The term *gap analysis* is used to refer to the measurement of two gaps: the discrepancy between how people see themselves and how others perceive them and the discrepancy between the importance of a specific performance competency to a person's job and how well the person actually performs that competency. So two kinds of gaps may emerge: perception gaps and performance gaps. The inclusion of other raters in addition to the person being rated makes it a 360°, because the subject is in essence encircled, surrounded by people who are knowledgeable about his or her performance—a boss, peers, subordinates, customers, and the like. Without the other raters, the perception gap cannot be measured. I should point out that although the performance gap *can* be measured by questioning only the subject of the analysis, the concepts of performance gap and perception gap are normally combined; this requires a small group of raters as well as the subject.

People receiving feedback from such gap analysis and 360° tools typically form action plans aimed at reducing both the perceptual and actual performance gaps.

Applications

1 An excellent introduction to the "how to" of gap analysis is found in Tornow and London (1998).

2 Visit the web site of Mediappraise, a company located in the "research triangle" of North Carolina that conducts 360°s on-line at www.mediappraise.com.

3 Other resources include Brutus, Fleenor, and London (1998), Fleenor and Prince (1997), and Leslie and Fleenor (1998).

TOPIC 32.6 **The Importance of Choice in Selecting Strategies**

Change is a source of stress for most people in most situations. Why? As we saw in Chapter Twenty, stress occurs when people feel out of control or when their pursuit of a goal has been obstructed. The key to stress reduction is finding a way for them to regain a sense of control over their destiny.

So when we must force change on others, whether as parents, partners, managers, or professionals, we must deal with the stress that is likely to accompany that change. The best way to accomplish this is to involve the "victims" of change in planning and selecting the strategy for accomplishing the change. For a review of the literature on managing change through employee participation, see Chapter Ten in Cummings and Worley (1997).

Applications

1 When you are responsible for implementing a change project, first get clear on the goal, or purpose, of the project (for example, "We are at present averaging fifty-five days per outstanding receivable. Our industry standard is twenty. We would like to get our average down to at least thirty in the next six months"). Once you are clear on the goal, communicate it to the people who must accomplish the work and involve them in creating and selecting the strategies by which the goal can be accomplished. If the "victims" have also been involved in defining the goal, so much the better (for example, "Our outstanding receivables are averaging fifty-five days and the industry standard is twenty days. Clearly we must get our average down. Let's talk about a target or goal that is attainable, even if it is a bit of a challenge").

2 The same process works when you are trying to get a child to change an undesirable behavior. A popular treatment of discipline that involves the child in selecting a strategy is given in Dreikurs and Gray (1993).

TOPIC 32.7   Increments Versus Leaps

In his Pulitzer-prize-winning work *Guns, Germs, and Steel* (1997a), Jared Diamond describes the course of most major changes, discoveries, and inventions. Let us listen to Diamond: "My two main conclusions are that technology develops cumulatively, rather than in isolated heroic acts, and that it finds most of its uses after it has been invented, rather than being invented to meet a foreseen need" (pp. 245–246). In support of this, he recounts a series of incremental technology developments. For example, James Watt gets the credit for patenting the steam engine in 1769, but he only improved on a version by Thomas Newcomen some six decades earlier, which in turn was an improvement on Thomas Savery's steam engine of 1698, which was preceded (this is beginning to sound like "begats") by steam engines built by the Frenchman Denis Papin, the Dutchman Christiaan Huygens, and others. Or consider Thomas Edison, who was displeased when entrepreneurs debased his phonograph by using it to play recorded music! Diamond goes on: "But the question for our purposes is whether the broad pattern of world history would have been altered significantly if some genius inventor had not been born at a particular place and time. The answer is clear: there has never been any such person. All recognized famous inventors had capable predecessors and successors and made their improvements at a time when society was capable of using their product" (p. 245).

Application

In planning individual and organizational change, think of increments and not of leaps. Increments of change are based on current technology or ideas that have an immediate new use: the chances of success are maximal; the chances of backsliding are minimal. Leaps, on the other hand, are based on untested technologies or ideas that might satisfy a long-standing need, but the chances of success are minimal; the chances of backsliding maximal.

TOPIC 32.8 Chaos Theory and the Role of Information

Chaos theory maintains that life, in its minute detail, is essentially chaotic and without order. It is only when we back away from the detail that we can find patterns. This new theory, which is well described in Gleick (1987), is integrated, along with several major breakthrough scientific theories, into a work that examines their implications for leadership. This work, *Leadership and the New Science,* by Meg Wheatley (1994), argues that leadership for the twenty-first century has a different priority than it had in the past. According to past theories, leadership (or management) served the task of "getting things done through other people." The new task of leadership, according to Wheatley, is to maximize the flow of information (or pile on the details). Only through observing the massive storms of information that surround us can we see the "strange attractors" and "turbulence" among the data. It is from such massive displays of data that patterns emerge. Identification of these patterns leads to improved planning, decision making, problem finding, and problem solving.

Applications

1 Keep all of your significant interpersonal relationships in good condition. Wheatley observes that information flows out of healthy relationships, whereas damaged relationships hamper the flow of information. When people who work and live with you harbor resentment, fear, or anger, they tend not to open up to you. To that extent, you will be making decisions with less than complete information. Check regularly with each key associate to take a reading on the quality of your relationship. Your questions could be as simple as "How are we doing?" or "What are some ways we could improve the way we work together?"

❷ Regularly survey your customers, employees, suppliers, and other stakeholders to see what the health of their relationship is with you and your company. This is the psychological version of an annual physical.

TOPIC 32.9 Group Size and Cohesion

Robin Dunbar has reported on research that relates brain size to group size. He identifies four interrelated findings from animal and human research (1996, p. 192):

1. Among primates, social group size appears to be limited by the size of the species' neocortex.

2. The size of human social networks appears to be limited for similar reasons to a value of around 150.

3. The time devoted to social grooming by primates is directly related to group size because it plays a crucial role in bonding groups.

4. It is suggested that language evolved among humans to replace social grooming because the grooming time required by our large groups made impossible demands on our time. Language evolved to fill the gap because it allows us to use the time we have available for social interaction more efficiently.

Dunbar's theory accounts for previous research that estimated between 100 and 150 as the maximum size of a cohesive human group. It also explains why most employee opinion surveys tend to fault communication practices in their organizations; you can never communicate too much, especially when the size of the work group is too large.

Applications

1 Every organization should be organized into communities of no more than about 150 people. Schools, churches, banks, and plants should evolve in a manner that permits each member to feel a part of a group with no more than 150 members. Each of these communities should be allowed to develop its own identity through workplace design, social and recreational practices, carpools, and internal communication organs.

2 Every organization should have a process that continually monitors the effectiveness of communication practices (newsletters, bulletin boards, meetings, and so on) through all the communities within the organization.

TOPIC 32.10 The Ideal Manager of Change

Robert McDaniel (1992) studied sixty-two managers of change projects in a West Coast electronics firm of some eight thousand employees. A clear pattern emerged that differentiated effective managers of change from ineffective ones. The effective managers were socially confident (they were not easily embarrassed), assertive (one didn't have to try to read their minds), open to new ideas (they were not tied to the tried-and-true), and conscientious (they were reliable, prepared, ambitious, disciplined, cautious, and well organized). These qualities are measured, respectively, in the NEO PI-R Five-Factor Model dimensions called N4, E3, O5, and C (see Chapter Twenty-One).

Elliott Jaques (see Topic 22.6) has found that effective managers must have sufficient mental complexity, as measured by the time span of work, to be a resource to those who report to them. If a manager cannot handle a longer, more complex time span than her or his reports, the manager may flounder, unable to be a resource because of an inability to see how all the issues interrelate.

Application

When you must find an individual or a team to lead a change project, ensure that the appropriate personality qualities and mental capabilities are present. If one or more qualities are absent, plan how you will compensate for their absence.

TOPIC 32.11 **Appreciative Inquiry Versus Problem Solving**

David Cooperrider and others argue that when people need to change, they work better with an ideal model than without one (Cooperrider and Dutton, 1998; Hammond, 1996). Traditional methods of problem solving do not customarily use ideal models; instead, they focus on what is wrong and how to fix it. Cooperrider has encouraged a kind of "best practices" approach, in which people who are responsible for a process that is not doing well are exposed to a model of a group that is performing the process in a satisfactory manner. Thus the name of this approach, "appreciative inquiry"—that is, appreciating someone else's excellent performance and inquiring as to what his or her keys to success might be.

For example, I once read a case study in which a hospital-related hotel (for families of patients) failed to make a profit. The change agent identified a noncompeting hospital hotel in another part of the country that was successful and secured permission for representatives of each department of the nonperforming hotel to visit the model hotel for several days. After a day or so of observation, the visitors sat down with the model hotel's employees and each other and created an agenda for taking home the best of what they saw.

Application

Read Cooperrider and Dutton (1998) and Hammond (1996) to learn more about appreciative inquiry. And visit Sue Hammond's Thin Book Publishing Company site at www.thinbook.com.

TOPIC 32.12 Yali's Question and the Nature of Progress

In what I deem the most significant book ever written on human relations, Jared Diamond (1997a) argues that societies have progressed at different rates throughout history not because of different mental ability, but because of different geography. Diamond, a physiology professor at the University of California, Los Angeles, is known as an anthropologist. He began his fieldwork in New Guinea in the late 1960s, where he developed a friendship with a New Guinean named Yali. One day, Yali asked Diamond, "Why is it that your people export more to my people than my people export to yours?" Diamond could not give the stereotypical answer, "My people are biologically superior to your people," because he knew it wasn't so. Yali's mental capability was equal to his. Diamond responded, "I don't know, but I'll find out." His book *Guns, Germs, and Steel* is the answer to Yali's question.

How to do justice to such a masterpiece? In short, Diamond found that civilization is impossible without farming. And farming is impossible without animals and plants that can be domesticated. Some peoples remained hunter-gatherers for substantially longer periods of time than others because of the absence or severely restricted range of domesticable plants and animals.

Thus, we must approach our advanced state of progress or civilization with humility and gratitude for being in the right place at the right time. Differential levels of societal progress do not have to do with mental capability, but rather with resources.

Applications

1 Understand that, for example, aboriginal peoples are hunter-gatherers not from lack of ability, but from lack of resources. Read *Guns, Germs, and Steel* to understand the subtleties of this powerful principle.

2 If you are involved in designing and planning a school curriculum, please encourage the use of Diamond's work as a model for teaching the history of civilization.

The Elements of Successful Change

To help organizations go through a major change process, it is necessary to find outside change agents who know how to put all the research together and facilitate effective change programs. One such consulting firm is Rapid Change Technologies of Sedona, Arizona. Magaly D. Rodriguez, the company's CEO (E-mail her at magaly@sedona.net), follows brain research discoveries and integrates them into her intervention model. She describes this model in her promotional material as "experiences designed to stimulate imagination, reduce stress, bond teams and clear toxic relationships." Specifically, she works with her clients through a five-phase process:

1. Relieve distress by creating emotional safety.
2. Enrich "people environments."
3. Grow leaders bigger.
4. Commit to sound management of business *and* people.
5. Take ideas to action quickly.

Programs like that of Rapid Change Technologies incorporate not only the explicit change elements discussed in this chapter; they also incorporate ancillary elements such as approaches to stress reduction (see Chapter Twenty), emotional intelligence (see Chapter Nineteen), and communication skills. What effective change programs have in common is the ability to help people set aside business as usual and think freshly about tapping their inner resources to identify what it takes to move to the next level.

Evolution involves three elements: variation, replication, and differential "fitness" (Dennett, 1995, p. 343). Genes mutate, the mutations are reproduced, and those that are more compatible with the current environment survive and continue to replicate. In organizations, the equivalent of genes is ideas. If an organization is to evolve, ideas must change and replicate throughout the organization. Those that are most compatible with the current organization's needs will survive and continue to replicate. In order for new and potentially beneficial ideas to emerge, language must flow freely in the organization. Language is the medium of ideas. When language is constrained, ideas are stillborn. Language breeds change and life, just as silence is the agent of stasis.

From Chapter Twenty, we know that stress is the symptom of an individual's loss of personal control, and prolonged stress leads to burnout. Organizational stress is the result of large-scale constraints intentionally or unintentionally placed on the flow of ideas; long-term organizational stress leads to organizational failure. Organizational constraints on the flow of information could be the result of something as benign and simple as the inertia of people who are just doing their individual jobs forty hours a week without ever stopping to talk about how they are doing, or the constraints could result from something as complex and sinister as managers who are control freaks and deeply afraid of change.

I cannot imagine a relationship that is more full of growth and ever changing than the one I have with my wife, Jane. She is totally courageous, unafraid of new ideas, totally loving yet absolutely free of the urge to put constraints on me. I work hard to be as freeing with her as she is with me. Recently, I discovered William Blake's four-line gem "Eternity," a perfect summary of how I feel about Jane, the ideal relationship, the ideal organization, and the prerequisite for change:

Eternity

He who binds to himself a joy

Does the winged life destroy;

But he who kisses the joy as it flies

Lives in eternity's sun rise.

SUGGESTED RESOURCES

Amabile, T. M. (1983). *The Social Psychology of Creativity.* New York: Springer-Verlag.

Cooperrider, D. L., and Dutton, J. E. (1998). *Organizational Dimensions of Global Change.* Thousand Oaks, Calif.: Sage.

Cummings, T. G., and Worley, C. G. (1997). *Organization Development and Change* (6th ed.). Cincinnati: South-Western.

Dennett, D. C. (1995). *Darwin's Dangerous Idea: Evolution and the Meanings of Life.* New York: Simon & Schuster.

Diamond, J. (1997a). *Guns, Germs, and Steel: The Fates of Human Societies.* New York: Norton.

Dunbar, R. (1996). *Grooming, Gossip, and the Evolution of Language.* Cambridge, Mass.: Harvard University Press.

Kuhn, T. S. (1970). *The Structure of Scientific Revolutions* (2nd ed.). Chicago: University of Chicago Press.

Rosenthal, R., and Jacobson, L. (1968). *Pygmalion in the Classroom.* Austin, Tex.: Holt, Rinehart and Winston.

Senge, P. (1990). *The Fifth Discipline.* New York: Doubleday/Currency.

33

Brain Ergonomics

Workplace Design for Quality and Productivity

> 66 *God obligeth no man to more than he hath given him ability to perform.* 99
>
> —The Koran

*E*rgonomics is the study of how to adapt the workplace to the worker. It comes from the Greek root *ergon*, or "work," and is also referred to as human-factors engineering. Its efforts are aimed at making the workplace more user-friendly for human workers by minimizing or eliminating harmful stress on their bodies and minds. An ergonomics specialist, for example, would figure out how to make my keyboard bend outward from the middle in a way that would eliminate the stress on my wrist that causes tennis elbow.

This chapter deals with one specific domain of ergonomics: how the brain responds to the workplace. Here we are looking at the elements of workplace design that specifically affect the brain and nervous system. We will not talk about the proper shape of a chair for optimal back support, but about such things as the effect of light on mood and wakefulness. Remember that many of the findings in this chapter are equally applicable to the home, which is a workplace of sorts for all of us.

Temporal Considerations

The mind is like a moving picture: you can't stop it. If you stop a moving picture, you have a photograph; if you stop your mind, you have a corpse. Time is inextricably woven into the fabric of mental activity. Some even define intelligence as speed of response. Several aspects of time affect the functioning of the brain at work.

TOPIC 33.1 Time Out!

We have long known the importance of breaks for minimizing error and fatigue and maximizing productivity, quality, and morale. A recent study (Okogbaa and Shell, 1986) summarizes this research. In addition, the authors offer specific guidelines for minimizing fatigue in computer operators.

As a general rule, workers need five- to ten-minute breaks every one to two hours. The frequency and duration of these breaks will depend on the nature of the work and the worker. To determine the need for breaks, try (1) asking the worker and (2) keeping error logs.

Breaks also support the need in thought processes for "chunking" (see Topic 23.1) and spacing (see Topic 24.2). Work involving higher mental functions such as analysis and synthesis needs to be spaced out to allow new neural connections to solidify. New learning drives out old learning when insufficient time intervenes.

Applications

1 Allow yourself and your workers to establish optimal periods for breaks. As a simple guideline, when you become aware of more errors or fatigue, take a break.

2 Keep records on error rates over time. Talk with your workers, sharing these records with them. Establish a mutually agreeable policy for taking breaks.

3 Where possible, avoid rigidly mandating the length of time between breaks. Fatigue may set in earlier or later than your fixed work period, and workers need to recognize it and respond to it promptly. Workers differ: some require longer work periods with longer breaks, while others require shorter periods with shorter breaks. Workers need to feel that they have the authority and responsibility to take a break when they feel the onset of fatigue, particularly where safety issues are involved (for example, driving, operating heavy equipment, or lifting loads).

4 The ideal break involves some level of exercise, such as throwing horseshoes, walking, or playing basketball. This can either dissipate the results of overarousal or stimulate people out of boredom or underarousal.

5 During breaks, mind workers should avoid simple carbohydrates and fats (this includes most candy bars and other sweets), which cause sleepiness; proteins and complex carbohydrates such as fruits are fine.

6 Too much caffeine (more than one serving every six hours) causes errors of commission; mind workers are more subject to this phenomenon than muscle workers, who burn off excess caffeine more quickly. On the other hand, too little caffeine can cause drowsiness and errors of omission. This could be a serious safety issue for operators of heavy equipment.

7 Display signs like the following ones in break areas to remind workers of the guidelines in Applications 3–6:

"Been sitting all day? Take a stroll outside!"

"Been standing all day? Take a load off your feet!"

"Feeling tense and shaky? Get some exercise."
  (Show pictures of people throwing horseshoes or darts or jumping rope.)

"Feeling drowsy? Try exercise, fresh air, light, caffeine."

"Try these foods when you feel nervous:"
  (Show pictures of carbohydrates and fats.)

8 Offer a lunchtime training program to give information on breaks to people.

TOPIC 33.2 Shift Work

For workers who must work a night shift, such as midnight to 8:00 A.M., two issues are important: (1) ensuring good sleep and (2) ensuring alertness at work. Because the body appears to work on a twenty-five-hour cycle (see Topic 7.2), shifts should advance forward, not backward. In other words, day shifts should be followed by afternoon shifts, then by night shifts. Following a day shift with a night shift fights against the natural body clock.

Timothy Monk, a psychiatry professor at the University of Pittsburgh School of Medicine, has identified eight common risks associated with shift work (Slon, 1997):

1. Chronic fatigue

2. Depression and loneliness

3. Susceptibility to colds and flu

4. Stomach problems

5. Erratic menstrual cycles

6. Obesity

7. Heart disease

8. Accidents

Long term, the best remedy is to relieve your body of the stress of night work. Ichiro Kawachi, an associate professor of health and social behavior at the Harvard School of Public Health, has found that working the night shift for more than six years nonstop results in a 50 percent increase in the risk of heart disease (Slon, 1997). In addition, Monk reports that many career night-shift workers "hit the wall" and lose their adaptability to night work. When this happens, they should find day work.

For the many other factors that affect the quality of sleep, browse through Chapter Seven.

Applications

1 Monk has a variety of recommendations for helping shift workers to maximize the chances of a good night's sleep, including the following:

- Take sleep seriously: avoid TV, don't fall asleep on the couch, and so on.
- Prepare a quiet room. Ensure total darkness: use blindfolds; avoid clocks that glow in the dark or tape over the glow; use black window shades, even black garbage bags and duct tape if necessary. Use earplugs (the new foam rubber plugs are form-fitting and unnoticeable); disable telephone and doorbell ringers; buy a "white noise" machine to mask a variety of sounds; listen to a tape recording of waterfalls or something equally soothing.
- Use a "do not disturb" sign (or a sign that says, "Quiet! Shift worker sleeping inside").
- Set the thermostat so the bedroom is 65 to 68 degrees Fahrenheit when you try to sleep; cooler temperatures make sleeping easier.
- If you don't sleep a full episode, try napping during the afternoon lull between 2:00 and 4:00 P.M. (15 to 30 minutes if you've slept four cycles or about 6 hours; 1½ hours if you've only slept 2 to 3 cycles or about 3 to 4½ hours).
- Avoid exercising just before going to sleep; instead exercise upon waking. The exercise makes you alert, not sleepy.

- Expose yourself to bright lights while at work at night; full-spectrum light is best (see a discussion of full-spectrum light and the Color Rendering Index in Topic 34.2, and especially in Application 1).
- Don't drink caffeinated drinks after midnight or less than six hours before trying to sleep; it takes that long for the caffeine to metabolize.
- Eat your largest meal at "lunch" during the night shift, then eat a light "dinner" with carbohydrates and your daily fat allowance (see the discussion of nutrition and alertness in Topic 5.7). If healthy snacks are unavailable, take small portions of fresh fruits and vegetables, low-fat yogurt, air-popped popcorn, or some other snack that does not contribute to the tendency to gain weight during night work.
- Try taking a ten-minute brisk walk during breaks. You will burn calories and increase alertness, rather than consuming them and getting sleepy, even around 4:00 A.M., when circadian rhythms foster sleepiness.
- Avoid sunlight on the drive home in the morning as much as possible (try to drive on shady streets), so daylight doesn't get a foothold on your biorhythms. Monk recommends welder's goggles, but they are unsafe, so try close-fitting wraparound sunglasses.
- Resist eating a big meal in the morning before going to bed. It interferes with sleep, causes indigestion, and leads to weight gain (you have no exertion afterward to burn off the calories).
- Go straight to bed. Don't do chores or watch TV; instead, read something with the aid of a weak light.
- Avoid alcohol as a sleep inducer: it deprives you of rapid-eye-movement (REM), or dream-stage, sleep, and although you might get to sleep more quickly, it prevents the most relaxing form of sleep.

2 Wake up to bright lights to help reset your body clock. (See Topic 7.2 for the recommended light strength and pattern.) Work areas, break areas, and toilets should all be especially well lit for shift workers.

❸ For an ideal twenty-one-day shift progression built on the twenty-five-hour cycle, refer to Table 7.1 in Topic 7.2, "The Circadian Rhythm."

❹ Monk recommends going to bed the same time every night (or day). If you are working nights during the week and you want to catch a daytime activity with your family on Saturday, then go to bed on Saturday morning at the regular time, get up for the event, then take a long nap. That way, your body doesn't have to keep resetting its clock.

❺ Monk says that the ideal shift work is "rapid change forward" shifts: two on days, two on evenings, two on nights, then several days off, but make sure to go to bed the same time every night and catch up on the sleep you miss on the two night shifts.

❻ The French have a reputation for treating night workers well. One key, apparently, is their tendency to ask night workers what would help to reduce their stress. The workers ask, for example, to have more flexibility in taking time off for vacations and holidays. This gives them a greater sense of control (and we know that this is a major stress reducer).

❼ Provide protein snacks for night workers to minimize the drowsiness that results from consuming fats and simple carbohydrates.

TOPIC 33.3　Naps at Work

Rossi and Nimmons (1991) cite support for two or three twenty-minute naps per day. That is the ideal number for maximum quality, productivity, sense of well-being, and overall health and longevity. Studies show that nappers outproduce non-nappers; however, a goal of three naps a day is out of reach for most people. Perhaps a minimum of one fifteen- to thirty-minute nap per day should be voted a basic human right.

Neurologist Roger Broughton of the University of Ottawa concludes from his twenty years of sleep research that "humans are born to nap" (*BrainWork: The Neuroscience Newsletter,* March–April 1998). He suggests about a twenty-minute timed nap that occurs about twelve hours after the midpoint of the previous night's sleep. The improvement in alertness from such a brief nap is being acknowledged by the corporate world, as witnessed by the *Wall Street Journal*'s report that several companies are providing employee nap rooms. See more in Chapter Seven.

Applications

1   Many companies have official policies that prohibit employees from napping during the workday. These policies serve public relations purposes and are not consistent with research on productivity. Don't associate reasonable napping with laziness; associate it with productivity.

2   Some people should not be permitted to nap for safety reasons, but even they would be safer workers if they were allowed to nap while off-duty.

3   If you are a citizen and spot a public worker napping, resist calling in to report it as laziness and a waste of the taxpayers' dollars. Appreciate the productivity, quality, safety, and health benefits associated with a nap. Of course, if you see a public worker snoozing the day away, that's another matter!

Nontemporal Considerations

The mind not only works over time: it works in the context of the quality of the moment. The immediate quality of the environment can significantly affect mental function. This section explores some environmental qualities that have an immediate impact on the brain.

TOPIC 33.4 Negative Ions

The atmosphere we breathe normally is full of positive and negative ions. Air conditioning, lack of ventilation, and long dry spells remove negative ions, which usually serve to latch onto airborne dirt particles and wrestle them to the floor, rendering the air purer. Roughly one-third of the population seems to be particularly sensitive to negative-ion depletion. The proportion of negative ions is highest around moving water (storms, oceans, rivers, waterfalls)—it's no wonder that we feel so energized at the beach. The best ratios of negative to positive ions are associated with waterfalls and the time before, during, and after storms. The worst are found in windowless rooms and closed, moving vehicles. Air purifiers typically work by emitting negative ions, which purify room air by attaching to impurities and sinking them.

High concentrations of negative ions are essential for high energy and positive mood (Thayer, 1996). In fact, Marian Diamond, a professor of neuroanatomy at the University of California, Berkeley, has found that levels of negative ions are inversely related to levels of serotonin in the brain. Negative ions suppress serotonin levels in much the same way that natural sunlight suppresses melatonin. Hence the invigorating effect of fresh air and sunshine and the correspondingly depressed feelings associated with being closed in and dark. If you deplete the air of negative ions, you experience an increase in serotonin and its attendant drowsiness and relaxation— not what you want when mental agility is demanded. Diamond's research (1988), along with other information on ions, is summarized in Yepsen (1987).

In an interesting twist, Josh Backon, a member of the Department of Cardiology, The Hebrew University of Jerusalem, writes in an Internet posting (his E-mail address is backon@vms.huji.ac.il) that in order to increase left-hemisphere activity (linear, language, logical), one can block the left nostril and engage in "forced unilateral nostril breathing." Likewise, to increase right-hemisphere activity (creative, holistic, emotional), the right nostril should be blocked. This practice increases the supply of negative ions to a specific hemisphere.

Applications

1 Don't live or work in a space with no fresh air unless the air conditioning system contains an ion generator.

2 Purchase a room ion generator to keep in the room in which you spend the most time, and run it when you are not getting any outside air.

3 Take frequent breaks in fresh air, and when you can't, open the window!

TOPIC 33.5 | Stress in the Workplace

J. Donald Millar, director of the National Institute of Occupational Safety and Health, in a presentation at the 1991 American Psychological Association convention in San Francisco, reported that workers' compensation claims for stress-related problems rose 700 percent in California from 1979 to 1988. Nationally, stress-related claims have recently comprised 12 percent of all workers' compensation claims. During the 1980s, roughly one-fourth of all Social Security disability claims were for mental disorders—that's 600,000 people each year.

Millar cites several sources of this increase of stress in the workplace, including an unpredictable economy, conversion from manufacturing jobs to service jobs, and the increasing role of computers (Bales, 1991, p. 32). He also refers to a greater use of contract workers as a way to beat rising medical costs. His recommendations are listed below as Applications. Additional information on the causes and remedies of stress is given elsewhere in this chapter as well as in Chapter Twenty.

Bond, Galinsky, and Swanberg (1998) reported in *The 1997 National Study of the Changing Workforce* that extensive research using three thousand interviews identified workplace stress as the primary cause of home stress, and not the other way around. In fact, they found that stress tends to originate at work, spread to the home, then boomerang back to the workplace in an intensified form. Interviewees reported that poor working conditions were more stressful than poor pay and benefits. In addition, job stress has had a greater negative effect on productivity than stress caused by child care or eldercare. The four most significant requirements for job satisfaction emerged as

1. Job autonomy

2. Learning opportunities

3. Supportive supervisors

4. Flexible work arrangements

Women, as a group, have special work-related stress concerns. For example, Amy Wolfson of the College of the Holy Cross, Worcester, Massachusetts, found that in a survey of 184 professional women, 92 percent failed to get a good night's sleep during the week, reporting at least one hour less per night than optimum (*APA Monitor,* November 1996, p. 41). In addition, she found that women who worked thirty-five hours or more each week slept less and rose earlier than women who worked less. The women reporting sleep loss also reported associated physical complaints and decreased alertness. As a result of her interviews, the women perceived that they had to cut back on sleep in order to work longer hours.

Paralleling Wolfson's study, researchers at the Center for Health Promotion and Disease Prevention at the University of North Carolina at Chapel Hill studied women's health habits at eight factories across the state. Here are some of their findings:

- One-third of the women smoked.

- Around 70 percent ate no low-fat foods.

- Ninety percent failed to eat the daily minimum of five servings of fruits and vegetables.

- Fifty-three percent said that they had too little time to exercise.

- Forty-three percent lacked the will to go to a gym after work.

The women cited lack of time, support, and education as the primary reason for their poor health habits. Time and support both played a role in a common complaint, that as working mothers, they simply didn't have the time or energy to cook healthy meals and exercise.

The Chapel Hill group designed an intervention customized for these women. They have, for example, published a personalized magazine based on the information from the survey, with specific recommendations on how to find time, will, support, education, and energy. The program, entitled "Health Works for Women," was presented at the American Psychological Association's Women's Health Conference in 1996; it was summarized in the *APA Monitor* (November 1996, p. 41).

Applications

1 Design healthy jobs. This includes everything from applying principles of ergonomics to asking workers how their jobs could be improved.

2 Monitor jobs to ensure that workers stay healthy. This includes conducting attitude surveys and employing a variety of participative management techniques.

3 Educate managers and the public on the causes and consequences of stress in the workplace.

4 Improve the availability of mental health services.

5 Notify management about stressors on the job. *(Contributed by Rick Bradley)*

6 Be as concerned about the job-related stress of your employees as you are about their stressors off the job, such as those addressed by employee assistance programs. Some kind of grievance procedure, whistle-blower policy, or other recourse for employees who are experiencing various forms of job stress should be available.

7 Encourage the use of gym facilities by employees during the workday. Better yet, provide workout facilities and showers in the workplace.

TOPIC 33.6 **Testosterone and the Achievement Syndrome**

Moir and Jessel (1991) summarize the research on the relationship between testosterone level and what might be called the achievement syndrome. They find that automatized behaviors—repetitive behaviors that require little mental or physical effort—drop off over time because of fatigue or boredom. The performance level for these behaviors does not drop over time in people with higher testosterone levels (they make fewer mistakes and don't tire as quickly). Examples of such behaviors are math computation, walking, talking, keeping balance, maintaining observation, and copying. In several controlled studies, subjects injected with testosterone showed significantly less decline in skill performance as time passed. Those who were not injected showed an increase in mistakes and fatigue. No level of testosterone is directly related to degree of persistence, which is defined as a combination of focus and energy. This phenomenon equates to the Five-Factor Model personality trait of high Conscientiousness (see Chapter Twenty-One).

Applications

1 Testosterone level can be increased by participating in a competitive sport and winning. So if you feel you need a boost in testosterone and resist the idea of injections, try finding a tennis opponent you can beat before automatized behavior is required.

2 Redford Williams's research (R. Williams, 1989) showed that two kinds of arousal can be generated by the mind's reaction to the environment: energy to focus and concentrate, which results from increased testosterone production, and energy to fight, flee, or freeze, which results from increased cortisol (from the epinephrine-norepinephrine chain). The latter suppresses the former; in other words, as cortisol production increases, testosterone decreases. So if automatized behavior is important to you, you need to dissipate the cortisol, or stress, in your body.

TOPIC 33.7 Temperature and Mood

Craig Anderson writes that hot temperatures affect mood (*APA Monitor,* February 1998, p. 8). Whether it is a hot day in the plant (defined as a day when the temperature reaches at least ninety degrees Fahrenheit) or a hot day on the streets, hot temperatures are associated with hot tempers. More precisely, Anderson reports, as global warming occurs, for every one-degree increase in average daily temperature in the United States, we can expect an increase in murders and assaults of 3.68 incidents per 100,000 of population.

Applications

❶ Make special provisions for workers who must experience temperatures in excess of ninety degrees Fahrenheit. I know a plant in Kentucky where, when temperatures reach the boiling point, the human resources manager instructs the neighborhood grocer to send over enough ice cream to give all the workers as much as they want, as long as the temperature exceeds ninety, at no cost to the workers.

❷ Discipline yourself to practice and encourage lower fossil fuel consumption and be willing to pay extra for cleaner energy and fuel-efficient transportation.

TOPIC 33.8 Handedness

About 10 percent of the population is left-handed, a proportion that appears to persist across generations, socioeconomic conditions, and race. Of these left-handers, 60 percent are male and 40 percent female. Handedness appears to be related both to our specific genetic inheritance and to the stress and trauma associated with pregnancy and birth. On one "hand," if both parents are left-handed, one out of two offspring will be left-handed; if one parent is left-handed, the ratio will be one out of six; and if neither parent is left-handed, only one out of sixteen offspring will be left-handed. On the other hand, because the left brain is more sensitive to oxygen deprivation in the womb, functions such as handedness may be shifted to the right hemisphere, causing left-handedness.

Left-handedness is associated with right-brain qualities: lefties tend to be more creative and imaginative, better at visual-spatial tasks, and better at mathematics. Left-handedness is also associated with a higher accident and injury rate; left-handers have 20 percent more sports-related injuries, 25 percent more work-related accidents, a 49 percent higher risk of home accidents, a 54 percent higher risk while using tools, and an 85 percent higher risk while driving a car. Gerald Larson of San Diego's Navy Personnel Research and Development Center studied 2,379 Navy enlisted men and found that the lefties among them reported a significantly higher incidence of "mental lapses" (Associated Press release, August 23, 1993). These lapses include moments when one loses focus or attentiveness, as in not seeing something in plain view; forgetting a well-known name; or forgetting why one moved from one room to another. Larson attributes lefties' higher accident rate to the same biological infrastructure that resulted in these lapses.

This accident-proneness may explain why righties outlive lefties by five years (females) to ten years (males). Challenging these statistics, Stanley Coren (1992), a member of the University of British Columbia's psychology department, says that they're based on the old days when lefties were forced to be right-handed; therefore, there are simply not as many left-handers proportionately among seniors today as there will be in several decades. In fact, Lauren Julius Harris, a professor of neuropsychology at Michigan State University, reported the results of a survey that showed an increase in left-handedness in North America from 4 percent in 1928 to 13 percent in 1983 (*APA Monitor,* April 1997, p. 13). And in a 1993 *Neuropsychologica* study of the elderly, many respondents indicated that because of urging by teachers and parents, they switched early on from left- to right-handedness. The true relationship between handedness and longevity will not be known until such time in the twenty-first century as the effects of the stigma against left-handedness have disappeared.

It's not easy being left-handed in a right-handed world! Interestingly, some parts of our environment favor left-handers. The standard "qwerty" keyboard, for example (*qwerty* stands for the sequence of letters on the left side of the top row), places the most frequently used letter, *e,* on the left side, as well as other highly popular typing letters: *a, r, t, s, d, c,* and *b.* Maybe that's why I (a rightie) developed tendinitis in my left arm from keyboarding and had to wear a brace on my left wrist when I was going to be typing for more than thirty minutes. Since I began using an "ergonomic keyboard" that entails almost no bending at the wrist, I no longer have to use the brace.

Applications

1 If you are left-handed, learn to shop for and use tools and equipment that are user-friendly for lefties. If you are responsible for buying things for lefties or training them, put yourself in their position before making purchasing decisions. Better yet, ask them! Too many of us make decisions affecting left-handers without assessing their strengths and weaknesses.

2 For further ideas and information, call or write: Lefthanders International; P.O. Box 8249; Topeka, Kansas 66608; phone: 913-234-2177. This organization boasts of over thirty thousand members and publishes *Lefthander Magazine,* which is organized from back to front.

3 If you're a right-handed keyboarder, use a left-wrist brace to minimize stress on the left arm while keyboarding for long periods of time. You might also try using a Dvorak keyboard, in which the most frequently used keys are assigned to the strongest fingers, rather than a qwerty keyboard. If you're a leftie, stick with qwerty.

4 Check out the Usenet bulletin board at alt.lefthanders.

5 Begin using an ergonomic keyboard at your computer. I've been using one now for three years—awkward at first, but soon comfy.

TOPIC 33.9   Workplace Design: Using the Principles of Feng Shui

Evalee Harrison (E-mail: HMI_Evalee@hotmail. com), executive director of the Health and Movement Institute in Emeryville, California, espouses the *feng shui* (pronounced fung shway) approach to space design. Feng shui, which literally means "wind and water," or one's natural surroundings, is the ancient Chinese art and science of placement. Its purpose is to optimize well-being, energy, productivity, and wealth. Also known as *geomancy*, feng shui is based on a balance of yin and yang, mixtures of the five Eastern elements (earth, fire, water, metal, and wood). Good mixtures bring Chi, or the cosmic breath of good energy, while imbalances bring "sha," or cosmic bad breath. Harrison quotes Deborah McDonald, founder of the Feng Shui Design Group, as proposing that one's environment "be a metaphor for who you are and what you want to achieve in the workplace" (*San Francisco Examiner,* May 31, 1998, p. J5). Simplified, feng shui encourages you to underscore your goals with relevant design elements. If you want growth, then fill your space with growing plants. If you want riches, use colors with symbolic associations with richness, such as gold, silver, and purple. If you are a health professional, decorate with items that reinforce good health practices, such as posters with large, bright, glossy photographs of fresh fruits and vegetables.

The active principle of feng shui is to think about whether your environment supports who you want to be. If you want to be spontaneous and chaotic, then permit clutter. If you want to be focused and disciplined, then eschew clutter. The senses—what you see, hear, touch, smell, and taste—should be in harmony with your core identity—what you believe in, your values, and your goals.

Actually, feng shui is not as accepting of individual differences as I make it sound. As you read the literature, a clear preference for discipline, productivity, achievement, pride, and orderliness emerges. While I have found no hard research evaluation of feng shui, the proposition that one's values should be aligned with one's environment has a certain intuitive appeal. I read K. M. Lagatree's *Feng Shui* (1996) as a primer and, although I found many of the principles inspirational and clearly worth trying, some of them must be taken with a grain of salt. For example, the elaborate symbolism associated with the eight points of the compass (and also associated with the geographical regions of China) fall apart when you try to implement them south of the equator! The fact that southeastern China is associated with trade doesn't translate to southeastern Everywhere (Kansas, Ecuador, Ghana, and so on) being associated with trade. The following Applications provide specific suggestions for the use of feng shui principles.

Applications

① Clutter diffuses energy and creativity. Spend a small portion of every day reducing clutter.

② Prepare an "abundance corner," similar to the Buddhist shrine often seen in Asian-style workplaces, that clearly identifies who you are and where you are headed. Awards, symbols (for example, a fancy quill pen for a writer), and other paraphernalia create a kind of personal shrine that reinforces your momentum.

③ Furniture and equipment with sharp edges and straight lines support work that emphasizes detail and precision, while curves and free-form shapes support more creative tasks.

④ Arrange your work space so that you always have a clear view of your entrance or door. This minimizes surprise, anxiety, and uncertainty.

⑤ Large or tall work furniture that totally encloses a person can be overcome by the selective use of mirrors that enable otherwise impossible eye contact.

⑥ The center floor space of a room is the "place of perfect balance; walking through or just standing in it nourishes us by allowing us to experience this balance" (Jody Hymes of Oakland, California, cited by Evalee Harrison, *San Francisco Examiner,* May 31, 1998, p. J5).

⑦ Have an abundance of basic tools: pencils for writers, disks for computer operators, folders for organizers, rags for cleaners. When workers have to search for basic tools, it "undermines their confidence and constricts their flow" (Jody Hymes, cited by Evalee Harrison, p. J5).

⑧ Fix anything that is broken immediately; letting the problem linger (especially squeaks, grating noises, or drips) will "dissipate your energy [and] rob you of your peace of mind and creativity" (Jody Hymes, cited by Evalee Harrison, p. J5).

9 Clearly identify your work space as yours: put your name, title, and room number outside your office or space, and put a nameplate on your desk.

10 To increase your command over a meeting, sit in a chair facing the entrance or door. You will have a better feel for the dynamics of the meeting.

SUGGESTED RESOURCES

Bond, J. T., Galinsky, E., and Swanberg, J. E. (1998). *The 1997 National Study of the Changing Workforce.* New York: Families and Work Institute. (See also www.familiesandwork.org.)

Coren, S. (1992). *The Left-Hander Syndrome: The Causes and Consequences of Left-Handedness.* New York: Free Press.

Druckman, D., and Swets, J. A. (Eds.). (1988). *Enhancing Human Performance: Issues, Theories, and Techniques.* Washington, D.C.: National Academy Press.

Lagatree, K. M. (1996). *Feng Shui.* New York: Villard.

Rossi, E. L., and Nimmons, D. (1991). *The 20-Minute Break: Using the New Science of Ultradian Rhythms.* Los Angeles: Tarcher.

Slon, S. (1997, June). "Night Moves." *Prevention,* pp. 106–113.

Thayer, R. E. (1996). *The Origin of Everyday Moods: Managing Energy, Tension, and Stress.* New York: Oxford University Press.

Yepsen, R. B., Jr. (1987). *How to Boost Your Brain Power: Achieving Peak Intelligence, Memory and Creativity.* Emmaus, Pa.: Rodale.

34

Stop, Look, and Listen

The Five Senses in the Workplace

> **❝It is shameful for a man to rest in ignorance of the structure of his own body, especially when the knowledge of it mainly conduces to his welfare, and directs his application of his own powers.❞**
>
> —Philipp Melanchthon

The five senses all directly affect our presence of mind. Diane Ackerman has provided an entertaining summary of research on the five senses in *A Natural History of the Senses* (1990). This chapter explores how the input of our five sensory channels affects our minds at work and play. In turn, we will examine the impact on the mind of the visual; auditory; olfactory, or smell (see Topic 5.4 for gustatory, or taste); and kinesthetic senses.

Kinesthetics is the study of touch, space, and motion. You've often heard that you can learn by hearing, by seeing, and by doing. Kinesthetic learning is learning by doing. We will look at four specific aspects of kinesthetics in the workplace: proxemics, room arrangement, touch, and temperature.

TOPIC 34.1   Sensory Input in the Workplace

Each of us is constantly taking in sensory data as the afferent nerves send visual, auditory, olfactory, tactile, and gustatory messages to the brain. These messages vie for attention with other mental activities such as creativity, analysis, and inspection, all of which can be interrupted by sensory data. Make sure that sensory input in your workplace is not driving productive mental activity out of your workers.

As a general rule, extraverted people have a higher threshold for sensory stimulation, while introverted people prefer less stimulation. See Chapter Twenty-One for further discussion of personality dimensions.

Applications

1   Talk with your workers to find out if they have noticed any sensory distractions in the workplace that make their work unnecessarily complicated, including noises, glares, smells, tastes, or other physical discomforts that take their mind off the task at hand, however momentarily. Distractions beget errors.

2   Include questions about sensory distractions in your annual employee attitude survey.

3   When you conduct walkthroughs, imagine yourself in the workers' shoes and try to identify sensory distractions that might cause them to make errors.

4   Identify and remove any sensory distractions that hinder your own performance. *(Contributed by Rick Bradley)*

⑤ More introverted people are highly sensitive to input through the five senses; hence, they require relatively little sensation before they've had enough. Moreover, they are easily distracted by the senses. Bright lights and loud noises can wear out introverted people, whereas extraverted people typically can take much more of the "madding crowd" before they feel a need to be "far from" it. The peripheral nervous systems of these two extremes in personality have different thresholds for sensation. Keep the workplace quiet and still for more introverted people such as engineers, computer professionals, bookkeepers, and librarians. More extraverted people tend to be comfortable with a moderate hubbub around them.

TOPIC 34.2 The Effect of Light

Light affects mood and alertness by shutting down the production of melatonin, the sleep inducer. Darkness triggers the pineal gland in the base of the brain to secrete melatonin (see the discussion in Topic 7.9). Because alertness is important for safety and productivity, the work environment should be well lit. If a low degree of alertness, or even drowsiness, is acceptable, then brightness is not as important. Full-spectrum lights are best. Weatherall (1987) points out that most lights are concentrated in the wrong part of the spectrum (orange-red-violet), although blue-green is the most vital part. Absence of this part of the spectrum leads to measurable fatigue and eyestrain.

Light deprivation not only affects performance; it can also lead to a form of depression. So-called winter depression, or seasonal affective disorder, which is associated with the shorter days and longer periods of darkness of winter, has recently been successfully treated with light therapy (see Topic 18.5).

For travelers passing through several time zones, exposure to bright lights several "mornings" in a row in the new time zone can reset the body clock. In September 1991, our family hosted the matron of the King's College Chapel Choir from Cambridge, England. Charlotte was the choir's first stop in the United States. The group was whisked from the airport to our church, and then straight to our several homes. We arrived at our home around 9:00 P.M. (which was about 2:00 A.M. for Dorothy, the matron). We had a full schedule the following day, so we called Dorothy to tea at 7:30 A.M., turning on every light in the house to help her reset her body clock. We didn't tell her why we were so light-happy, but she reported later that this was one of her best trips ever, and that she had felt unexpectedly refreshed.

In an unusual experiment, Timothy Monk and Julie Carrier of the Western Psychiatric Institute and Clinic in Pittsburgh had young adults stay awake for thirty-six hours beginning at 9:00 A.M. (*Sleep,* September 1997). Although the researchers found that the subjects' measured accuracy was stable from day to night (with night performance somewhat slower), they were surprised to discover that the subjects performed more speedily on cognitive tasks during the second day, after having been up all night, than they did during the prior night. They concluded that the mind is generally sharper during daylight hours than during the night.

Architects now refer to the incorporation of natural sunlight into work and learning environments as "daylighting." Architectural schools such as the one at the University of North Carolina at Charlotte are building "daylighting rooms" for research and teaching. Three elementary schools in Johnston County, North Carolina, have all-natural lighting and report 5 to 14 percent higher scores on standardized tests than traditionally designed and lighted schools.

Further discussion of light and sleep may be found in Chapters Seven and Thirty-Three.

Applications

1 Ensure adequate lighting in the workplace. Skimping on lighting can affect morale, quality of work, and productivity. Weatherall (1987) suggests using the Color Rendering Index (CRI) as a measure of the adequacy of artificial light. In this index, natural light equals 100; the higher the numerical light rating, the lower the need to take a physical sample to a window to determine its correct color. Ask at your local lighting supply company for fluorescent or incandescent bulbs with a CRI of 90 or higher.

2 Provide extra lighting for workers on night shifts. This lighting can be turned off during the day, but on dark, overcast days, use it to help them to shake off the doldrums.

3 In training sessions, plan carefully when you use transparencies or slides requiring subdued lighting. If it is not possible to lower the lights, plan a break or activity immediately following the presentation to rest the audience's eyes.

4 If your employer doesn't see fit to provide you with full-spectrum light when natural sunlight is unavailable, you can purchase your own high-intensity light box for maximum alertness. For information, contact the Society for Light Treatment and Biological Rhythms at 303-424-3697.

5 A catalog including full-spectrum lamps is available from Frontgate in Cincinnati, Ohio. Call 800-626-6488 to order a catalog.

6 Visit the web site for Vita-Lite at www.backbenimble.com/office/vitalite.htm.

7 In designing new buildings or renovating old ones, maximize the use of natural sunlight.

TOPIC 34.3   The Effect of Color

Faber Birren, in his book *Color and Human Response* (1978a), reports specific tendencies in people's responses to various colors. I summarize them as follows:

Color	Response
Red	*Good for creative thinking, short-term high energy*
Green	*Good for productivity, long-term energy*
Yellow, orange, or coral	*Conducive to physical work, exercising; elicits positive moods*
Blue	*Slows pulse and lowers blood pressure; conducive to studying, deep thinking, concentration; accent with red for keener insights*
Purple	*Tranquilizing; good for appetite control*
Pink	*Restful; calming*
Light colors	*All-purpose; provide minimum disruption across all moods and mental activities*
White	*Disrupting, like snow-blindness; avoid*

Birren recommends light colors for most situations and warns against all-white schemes, which can be disruptive.

Following are some other points of general interest taken from Birren's studies:

- Most people like primary colors.

- More discriminating people like purple, blue-green, and pink.

- Brown, white, gray, and black are the least preferred colors; they tend to attract the mentally disturbed.

- Extraverts, brunets, and Latins prefer warmer colors such as red or orange. (Red is "warm" because the lens adjusts to red shapes at a closer distance than with other colors, so they appear to leap out at us.)

- Introverts, blonds, and Nordics prefer cool colors such as blue or green. (Blue is "cool" because the lens adjusts to blue objects farther away than it does with other objects, so blue objects appear to recede.)

I recommend that you approach these findings with caution. Birren does not offer detailed research citations in support of his conclusions, and some of the color research is contradictory. For example, according to some reports, yellow walls elicit positive moods; another report finds that yellow walls in hospital rooms are associated with patients who require more pain-killing medication.

Application

Evaluate the colors used throughout your workplace in terms of the nature of the work performed in each area. Here are some apparently winning combinations:

Cafeteria	Purple
Sales room	Yellow, orange, or coral
Conference rooms	Red
Offices	Blue with a tinge of red
Production areas	Green

Rooms with overly active children	Pink (it tends to calm them)
Waiting areas	Green (it's restful)
Alleviation of tremors	Blue lighting
Need to increase strength	Red lighting

T O P I C   3 4 . 4   The Effect of Shapes and Designs

Beginning in the crib, all humans benefit from a visually enriched environment, with mirrors, artwork, posters, games, colors, and diverse shapes. To the degree that your workforce will benefit from cortical alertness, provide them with food for the eyes, but consult with them to determine the practicality of your ideas. I remember the choral rehearsal room in the Cunningham Fine Arts Building on the Davidson College campus in Davidson, North Carolina. It was beautifully designed, with black wire mesh on the wall behind the conductor, punctuated with thin, vertical teak strips, but we singers developed headaches from the dizzying effect created when the conductor moved back and forth in front of the strips.

When the eye sees an unfamiliar shape or scene, it automatically corrects it to some more familiar schema. This happens regardless of the background. As a result, we often think that we see something familiar when in fact we don't. The wider our range of experience, the more likely we are to have these mistaken impressions.

Applications

1 Dot the walls of your meeting rooms with appropriate posters containing philosophical or other thoughtful or amusing statements. IBM has done a good job of this, with posters reminding workers that "The individual comes first" or "Today is the first day of the rest of your life." These posters are available free from the IBM Gallery of Science and Art; 590 Madison Avenue; New York, New York 10022. *(Contributed by Jack Wilson)*

② Provide a budget for artwork and allow employee participation in making selections.

③ Put yourself in the position of your workers and identify overly distracting or boring visual areas in their workplace. Better yet, ask them how to improve the view that meets their eyes at work.

TOPIC 34.5 Differences in Visual and Auditory Perception

Research has shown that males, with their larger right hemisphere, tend to demonstrate better visual perception and discrimination, which is centered in the right hemisphere. Females tend to demonstrate greater auditory perception, which is centered in the left hemisphere.

Applications

① In setting up work assignments, remember that females tend to make fewer errors in auditory tasks, such as talking on the telephone, taking dictation, interviewing others, or listening for malfunction indicators in machinery. Males tend to make fewer errors in visual tasks, such as proofreading, visual scanning, or looking for malfunction indicators in machinery.

② Also remember that because they are more sensitive to auditory stimuli, females become fatigued more readily in a noisy environment. Males don't, but they do become fatigued more readily in a visually chaotic environment.

TOPIC 34.6 The Relation of Sounds to Concentration

The brain responds to organized and unorganized sounds. The first we call music; the second, noise. One person's music can be another's noise. As a general rule, neither music nor noise should be present where careful mental work is required. As Robert Pirsig comments in *Zen and the Art of Motorcycle Maintenance* (1974), don't trust a mechanic who listens to music while working on your car. If you're listening to music, then you're not listening to the engine. So-called background music does not stay in the background. I find that I write more quickly and effectively when the stereo is off, because I can't create a sentence and listen to a passage of Tchaikovsky at the same time. If I'm trying to do both, then I'm actually alternating between the two, inevitably adding time and errors to my writing and thinking. See Chapter Ten for further discussion of music and the brain.

Applications

1 Background music should only accompany routinized tasks and other situations in which the mind is not actively engaged. I've seen it used effectively in manufacturing assembly operations and in elevators. But don't provide background music for mental work, because it will inevitably occupy the foreground. For example, when I'm placed on telephone hold, I prefer that no music be piped into my ear. Why? Because I try to do miscellaneous paperwork while I'm waiting, and the music is distracting.

2 Remember that people have different tastes in music. What is satisfying for one person may be intrusive for another. I've known retail workers who came to hate holiday music when their stores played the same tapes repeatedly for a month.

3 See Chapter Ten for a discussion of music and the mind.

TOPIC 34.7 Noise in the Workplace

Noise can be the bane of a mind worker's existence—from conversation to clacking equipment, from dripping water to occasional footsteps. Research indicates that so-called white noise, a low-pitched, sustained noise of low volume, serves to mask all other noises. Such an effect can be created by fluorescent light fixtures! One day, in the Davis Library on the campus of the University of

North Carolina at Chapel Hill, I was totally absorbed in reading a series of journal articles back in the bowels of the stacks. Just as I finished an article on the positive effect of white noise in masking out distractions, I became aware of a low, sustained buzz emanating from somewhere above. I wondered—did the designer of this library know about white noise, or was this just a lucky accident?

Continued exposure to loud noise, especially a chronic noise, damages the cochlear hairs in the ear (Ackerman, 1990). Limiting fat in the diet, reducing caffeine, and avoiding smoking will improve such hearing loss. And, of course, avoiding continued exposure to the loud noise! In addition to damaging the hearing mechanism, continual noise increases aggressive behavior and reduces healthy behavior. In one elementary school experiment, children sent to a remedial reading teacher who were eleven months behind in their reading scores found that the gap disappeared after being away from constant noise.

The Occupational Safety and Health Administration (OSHA) recommends wearing safety earplugs when one is exposed to noise levels above 89 decibels. Listed below are some common sounds and their decibel levels (Yepsen, 1987):

Sound	Decibel Level
Dripping faucet	40
Moderate rainfall	40
Chirping birds	60
Vacuum cleaner	70–75
Cocktail party (100 people)	70–85
Busy traffic	75–85
Diesel truck	80
Window air conditioner	80
Electric shaver	85
OSHA threshold	*89*
Screaming child	90–115
Amplified rock music	90–130
Chainsaw	100
Jackhammer	100
Motorcycle	100
Inside of a subway train	100
Power mower	100–105
Hockey game crowd	120

Loud thunder	120
Jet engine at takeoff	120–140
Air-raid siren	130

In contrast to noise, listening to our favorite music triggers endorphin release. In studies where endorphins were blocked with nalaxone, listening to one's favorite music failed to produce pleasurable results.

Application

Consult with an acoustical engineer about the proper way to mask noises that represent potential distractions for your mind workers. Machines are available that generate white noise.

TOPIC 34.8 A Warning About Music at Work

In August 1997, Bob Pike of Creative Learning Techniques in Minneapolis wrote this note in response to an Internet query about using music as a part of corporate training programs:

> About four years ago I was cautioned by our copyright attorneys that the use of music in a training program without a license was a copyright violation. In fact I had heard several horror stories about companies playing themes like "Rocky" as walk-in music to a sales meeting being fined $10,000. Until that time I had played a variety of music and carried lots of tapes and CDs . . . and had a lot of people asking me for titles and then purchasing them on their own. I thought (and still think) that I was doing the music industry a favor by promoting their music.
>
> My attorneys said that whether the session was paid or free, internal or external, it still constituted a public performance and was therefore a copyright infringement. Since that time BMI and ASCAP, who collect these performance fees and distribute them to those due the royalties, have actually hired people who do nothing but check meeting rooms and if they hear music they ask to see the performance license. Some of you remember that last year the Girl Scouts' camps were sued for singing "Happy Birthday" without a performance license! (BMI and ASCAP later

backed down and said they had really only planned to go after the rich kids' type of camps!)

As a result of all this I went back to a book that I had read by Steven Halpern called *The Human Instrument*. Steven is a marvelous composer (his most famous album is *Spectrum Suite*) who has done years of research on the impact of music on people physiologically and psychologically. He has even composed music he calls the "anti-frenetic" alternative to listen to while driving in freeway traffic to reduce the stress. Based on his book I went to my tape producer and listened to literally hundreds of music cuts and put music into six categories for my training purposes: Intro/Exit/Discussion/Reflection/Break/Games. I combined pieces to come up with thirty minutes of music in each category. I paid the tape producer a substantial fee to own the rights to use and allow others to use . . . this music. For over a year my trainers and I used these tapes exclusively in our seminars. We then started marketing them at a reasonable price to others. Since then we have developed a second volume based on the same principles incorporated in the first volume.

Info on availability can be obtained by E-mailing a request to custsvc@cttbobpike or by calling 800-383-9210.

Hope this helps.

Applications

❶ If you use recordings or perform current music as a part of your workday, run it by your company lawyer to assess your potential liability and proceed accordingly. Otherwise, try using a tape like Bob Pike's that has paid the piper.

❷ In response to Pike's Internet posting above, Randy Buerkle of the Workplace Music Factory (phone: 937-335-0797; E-mail: flagship@wesnet.com) wrote:

> Bob Pike made some good points about copyright infringements while using music in training. Better to be safe than sorry. However, I'd like to suggest that the passive use of music in training is but the tip of the iceberg. There are certainly many more training applications than the use of musical recordings which are very safe and legal.

Based on Howard Gardner's seven basic intelligences, our company presents a workshop for facilitators and trainers which incorporates adult learning activities using music. For instance, we have a song title activity which illustrates diversity; a case study which puts music to organizational change; a team-building activity based on percussion (using real instruments); and a group problem-solving session using a micro-opera. These activities are designed to *involve* the learner with the musical medium. And little or no musical ability is required, which makes them inviting to apprehensive learners.

We also have a tape which we use in our training sessions. Included in the eleven titles are "Do the Paradigm Shift," "Performance Appraisal Blues," "Canon for Technical Support," "Buzzwords for Me—Confusion for You," and "Phantom of the Classroom." They can be used for topical discussion or warm-up after breaks. Most are original tunes, but those which use popular melodies have been licensed through ASCAP or BMI by the Harry Fox Agency in New York.

Why music? Because it is appealing to most adults when used intelligently and in a nonthreatening manner. Music also adds playfulness to otherwise serious training issues. But on a more scientific basis, music taps a part of our consciousness which facilitates learning. By integrating melody, rhythm, and rhyme, adult learners are more apt to link the musical experience to retention. Think of all the Mother Goose rhymes and holiday songs people remember from childhood. Compare that to the number of people who cannot cite even their own organization's mission statement. Hmmm—maybe this has given you some ideas!

❸ Give Randy's material a try.

❹ Even better, try developing your own musical material for use in training and other settings.

TOPIC 34.9 The Relation of the Sense of Smell to the Limbic System

The conventional view until 1995 was that the sense of smell was the only one of the five senses with a direct link to the limbic system. However, in the October 1995 issue of *Scientific American,* Richard Axel pointed out that we have two noses: the smell nose and the sex nose. The vomeronasal organ ("sex nose"), which detects pheromones, the scent essential for mating, is attached directly to the limbic system. The other, nonsexual, smell organs are connected to the higher cognitive centers, hitting the limbic system only after they've passed through the higher centers. Thus, they are under greater control.

Axel, in his excellent summary of research on how we perceive scents, points out that in humans, one thousand genes encode one thousand distinct odor receptor systems (each system containing thousands of neurons) that enable us to recognize some ten thousand different odors. In contrast, we have only three color receptors on the retina that work together to discriminate between several hundred hues.

Ackerman (1990) identifies seven categories of smell: minty, floral, ethereal (for example, a pear), musky, resinous (for example, camphor), foul or putrid (for example, rotten eggs), and acrid or pungent (for example, vinegar). These compare to four taste categories: sweet, sour, salty, and bitter. The rest of the taste sensations are actually attributable to smell. Ackerman suggests that in order to determine the basic taste of something, one should try exhaling while chewing.

Humidity and low barometric pressure heighten the sense of smell. So in stormy, inclement, or pressure-inverted weather, wear and use less perfume and other odors; they can become offensive, especially to people with particularly sensitive schnozzes (like me).

Applications

1 Be particularly sympathetic to others' complaints about bothersome smells, such as perfume, food, or smoke. Not all people are sensitive to the same odors, and sensitivities can be extremely disruptive.

2 In Topic 25.5, I wrote about state dependence, the phenomenon whereby people tend to remember more effectively if they recall the state they were in when the memory was acquired. This principle holds true for smell. In order to remember the details of a passage you were reading, for example, recall the odor of the leather chair in which you reclined while reading.

3 Alan Hirsch, director of the Smell and Taste Treatment and Research Foundation in Chicago, has found that the odor of barbecue smoke makes a room seem smaller than it is. On the other hand, the odor of green apples tends to make the same room feel larger.

TOPIC 34.10 The Effect of Odors on Productivity

Fragrances improve performance at about the same rate as a cup of coffee, according to William Dember, a professor of psychology at the University of Cincinnati, and Raja Parasuraman, director of the Cognitive Science Laboratory at the Catholic University of America. At a meeting of the American Association for the Advancement of Science, they reported that on a forty-minute test of vigilance (like the test needed for air traffic control or distance driving), thirty-second bursts of peppermint or muguet (lily of the valley) scent every five minutes resulted in a 15 to 25 percent improvement in performance. One interesting aspect of the study is that workers who received scented bursts showed less decline in performance as the task continued over time. In other studies, lavender scents have been associated with increases in metabolism and alertness.

In the same meeting at which Dember and Parasuraman presented their findings, Robert Baron, a professor of psychology at Rensselaer Polytechnic Institute in Troy, New York, reported that pleasant fragrances cause people to be more efficient, increase their risk level, form more challenging goals, negotiate more agreeably, and behave less combatively.

Along the same lines, Shimizu Technology Center reported that keypunch operators improved 21 percent with lavender bursts, 33 percent with jasmine, and 54 percent with lemon. Similarly, Robert Baron reported that pleasant cooking odors (baking cookies, perking coffee) elicit higher helping behavior in a mall (for example, people are more likely to respond when someone asks, "Hey, buddy, do you have change for a dollar?") (*Personal and Social Psychology Bulletin,* May 1997, pp. 498–503).

Aroma-Sys of Minneapolis and Holmes Products Corporation of Milford, Massachusetts, have each developed scent technologies. Aroma-Sys sells the EPA-1000 aroma diffusion system, which is used by retail stores, corporate offices, beauty salons, spas, health care facilities, and numerous fine hotels. Their device takes a scent cartridge of your choice and emits bursts in your large air distribution system. Holmes sells the Indoor Quality System, or "I.Q. System." It is a freestanding appliance based on a device patented by Robert Baron. The Aroma-Sys device is intended for larger industrial systems, while the Holmes appliance is designed for personal use.

Research continues on the effectiveness of these scent distribution systems. In an article in the March 1995 *APA Monitor,* Susan Knasko of the Monell Chemical Senses Center in Philadelphia spoke of eleven studies that reported on attempts to establish a connection between scents and productivity: five showed no influence, three had positive results, and three had negative results. Apparently, many variables affect the influence of scents, including the nature of the work performed, competing aromas, a tendency to become accustomed to scents, and individual differences among customers and workers.

Applications

1 For larger system uses, as in office buildings, hospitals, or plants, call Mark Peltier at Aroma-Sys (phone: 612-924-0336) for more information on the EPA-1000.

2 For personal, single-room use, call Holmes Products at 508-634-8050 for more information on the I.Q. System, or call the inventor, Robert Baron, at Rensselaer Polytechnic Institute (phone: 518-276-2864). Baron is selling his own version by mail order; it's called the PPS, for Personal Productivity/Privacy System.

3 In Japan, Shimizu Corporation sells a process that emits bursts of fragrance through existing ventilation ducts. The system, which has been sold to Japanese hotels, banks, nursing homes, and offices, sells for ten thousand dollars.

4 In designing fragrances for entertaining particular nationalities, employ these known associations:

Germans	Pine
French	Floral
Japanese	Delicate
North Americans	Strong
South Americans	Stronger (for example, Venezuelan floor cleaners contain a pine odor that is measurably ten times stronger than that of floor cleaners used in the United States)

TOPIC 34.11 Proxemics

Proxemics is the study of how people physically distance themselves from others. Here are several general rules:

- Generally, women are more comfortable at close distances from other women; men are more comfortable at greater distances from other men. This is probably a relic dating from a time when men were genetically selected for their ability to function as isolated hunters outdoors, whereas women were genetically selected for their comfort in more crowded conditions back in the cave and when nursing and caring for their young.

- The smaller the enclosed space, the farther people will want to sit or stand from each other. The larger the enclosed space, the closer they will choose to sit or stand from each other.

- When two people stand face-to-face, they communicate that they like each other. As the imaginary angle between them increases through a right angle to 180 degrees, less liking is communicated.

- The closer two people stand to one another, the more they communicate mutual liking.

- Moderate eye contact communicates liking, while excessive eye contact communicates hostility (as in staring your opponent down); sparse eye contact communicates apathy or aversion.

- Cultural differences exist concerning comfortable distances and gazing patterns. If people from a different culture from yours appear to be standing farther or closer than is comfortable for you, the chances are that it's more comfortable for them. If you adjust the space between you, they will immediately return to the previous distance. I once taught with a man from Jamaica who would talk to me standing closer than was comfortable for me. At first I interpreted this as a sexual advance. After learning that Jamaicans generally stand closer to others, I felt more comfortable.

- Anthropologist Ray Birdwhistell (1970) has established that in American culture, masculinity is communicated nonverbally by standing with arms akimbo, feet parallel in the same plane, and pelvis rotated forward (tummy in), while femininity is communicated nonverbally by arms folded together, feet planted asymmetrically, and pelvis rotated backward (tummy out).

Applications

1 Generally, men require a larger work space than women (see Topic 12.8). If you allow people to self-select how much space they need to perform their work, women will select less space, men more.

2 In small offices, meeting rooms, or waiting areas, place chairs and sofas as far apart as possible to give people more space. Using wider chairs accomplishes a similar purpose.

3 When you desire to communicate explicitly to people that you like them (for instance, in a performance appraisal or sales call), stand or sit face-to-face at a minimal comfortable distance with moderate eye contact. Avoid either staring them down or excessively gazing away (for example, looking out the window).

4 If a person of the opposite sex is coming on to you in an unwanted manner, try using the three nonverbal sexuality communicators of your opposite sex: a woman, for example, to "turn off" a man, would stand with feet planted parallel, arms akimbo, and pelvis rotated forward.

TOPIC 34.12 Room Arrangement

C. L. Williams and others (1985), in *The Negotiable Environment,* demonstrate that different personality temperaments respond better to different room or office arrangements. Shown in Figure 34.1 are office arrangements for the Preserver, the Explorer, the Challenger, and the Adapter (these personality temperaments are described in Chapter Twenty-One). See if you can identify which is which.

Application

When you are designing office environments, take into account the preferences of people with differing personality temperaments:

- Explorers generally prefer more books and artwork.

- Preservers generally prefer more action-oriented pictures and objects (cars, airplanes, horses).

- Challengers generally prefer computers and other sources of data.

- Adapters generally prefer to have an area set aside for group meetings (a round table, a corner sofa).

- Flexibles generally prefer lots of surface space for all their piles of stuff.

- Focused people generally prefer elaborate storage equipment; staying organized is a must.

- Extraverts generally like lots of eye contact; they prefer windows, open offices, and low walls.

- Introverts generally like to be able to close the door and isolate themselves for extended periods of time.

- Reactives will let you know their wants, which will probably change from time to time.

- Resilients will probably not care that much about their office arrangement.

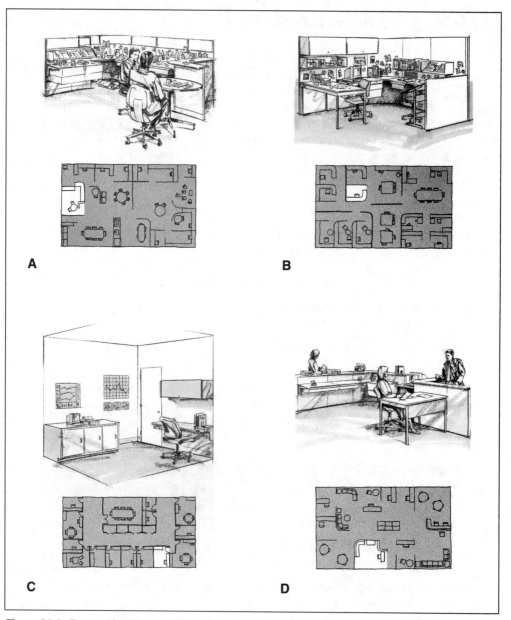

Figure 34.1. Personality Type and Office Arrangement.
Source: From *The Negotiable Environment: People, White-Collar Work, and the Office* by C. L. Williams and others, 1985, Ann Arbor, Mich.: Miller, Herman. © 1985 by Miller, Herman, Inc. Reprinted by permission.
Note: (*A*) Preserver; (*B*) Explorer; (*C*) Challenger; (*D*) Adapter.

TOPIC 34.13 **The Sense of Touch**

For some people, the sense of touch is an important element of motivation for work. Be aware that artificial touch sensations can demotivate some workers. For some, glass is preferable to plastic, wood or metal to plastic, wood to metal, natural fibers to synthetic fibers, natural plants to artificial plants, china to plastic or paper plates, leather to plastic, and so on.

Touch is particularly important among infants. Premature infants who receive massages grow 50 percent faster, have a calmer temperament, are discharged earlier, and perform better on a variety of tests (Ackerman, 1990). The primary touch receptors are those for pressure, pain, and temperature.

Dudley Flood, a human relations consultant in the North Carolina public schools during school integration in the 1960s and 1970s, used to lament the prohibition against touch at school and work. Trying to find a safe middle ground with the "PC" police, Flood opined that it is OK to touch the "hard areas," such as the top of the shoulder, the elbow, the kneecap, the top of the head, and the hands. Touching the other, softer areas is unwelcome except in more intimate relationships. Diane Ackerman (1990) writes about "unnoticed touching," as in the touch of wait staff when handling the bill, of a librarian when handing over a book, or of a phone booth patron brushing someone as she or he leaves the booth. In these three circumstances, unnoticed touching results in a better outlook, including higher sympathy, on the part of the touched person toward the toucher. Wait staff who touch get higher tips, librarians who touch get more smiles from patrons, and phone booth users who touch or brush are more likely to get money they left in the booth returned to them.

In what amounts to a review of the research in this area, the University of Miami School of Medicine's Tiffany Field establishes the basis for the healthful effects of touch in her article "Massage Therapy Effects" (1998).

Applications

❶ Consult with workers about what's important to them in their work environment. Specifically ask about what materials they prefer and the importance of tactile sensations to them. If how their materials, equipment, and furniture feel to their touch is not important to them, then there is no need to change them.

2 Find appropriate ways to touch that are "unnoticed," or natural and momentary. Limit yourself to the "hard areas."

TOPIC 34.14 Temperature

The cooler your brain is, the more relaxed you are. The warmer your brain, the more aroused you are (this arousal can be either limbic or cortical). Hence the stereotypes of the cool, unflappable British subject and the passionate, hot resident of the equatorial zones. Robert Zajonc, professor emeritus of psychology at the University of Michigan, reports that higher temperatures can affect the level of neurotransmitters in the neurocirculatory system, especially the level of norepinephrine (*APA Monitor,* October 1990). Interestingly, Zajonc reports that breathing through the nose cools the brain.

Applications

1 One simple way to try relaxing at work is by breathing through your nose.

2 In areas where cortical alertness is necessary, keep temperatures in the upper range of the comfort zone. Too cool a meeting room shuts down cortical functions.

3 In areas where you want people to be relaxed (waiting areas, sales presentation rooms, cafeterias, break areas), keep temperatures in the lower range of the comfort zone.

SUGGESTED RESOURCES

Ackerman, D. (1990). *A Natural History of the Senses.* New York: Random House.

Axel, R. (1995, October). "The Molecular Logic of Smell." *Scientific American,* pp. 154–159.

Vroon, P. (1997). *Smell: The Secret Seducer.* New York: Farrar, Straus & Giroux.

Yepsen, R. B., Jr. (1987). *How to Boost Your Brain Power: Achieving Peak Intelligence, Memory and Creativity.* Emmaus, Pa.: Rodale.

Part Ten

*Looking
Beyond
Appearances*

Schemas, Reality, and Spirituality

35

Epistemology

Finding Common Denominators

> **If believers could come to realize there isn't ten cents worth of difference in their substantive plans, perhaps they might then begin to see the magical part for what it is.**
>
> —*Michael Gazzaniga,*
> **The Social Brain**

The word *epistemology* comes from the Greek *epi-* + *histanai,* meaning "to cause to stand upon," or "to set." This strong image suggests the essence of empiricism, which maintains that if the majority of people can agree during their waking hours that something exists, then it does. It can stand the test of time. It can stand up on its own, without crutches. The phrase "to cause to stand upon" is close to the more contemporary test: "Will it fly?" Can it hold its own? This rings of rugged empiricism, a radical practicality. It suggests the structure that lies at the core of a thing. There it is. Therefore we know it.

Epistemology is defined as the study of the origin, nature, methods, and limits of knowledge. The word *knowledge* derives from the Middle English *knowen,* meaning "to know as a fact." It is interesting to note the similarity of "to know" (Old English *cnāwan*) and "to gnaw" (Middle English *gnawen*). We gnaw something until we get to the bone, the core. To gnaw something is to know it. We know by gnawing. We pry until the bare bones stand there before us, and then we accept what we see as knowledge—we acknowledge it.

Epistemology, then, is looking beyond the appearance to find the core, beyond the clothes and flesh to find the skeleton, beyond the words to find the idea. It is the habit of mind that sees the infrastructure behind, under, within the external structure; outlines within the complete thing; skeletal figures within physical figures. The current plaything of epistemologists is the discussion of "metacognition," or thinking about thinking. Diagramming the flow of a negotiation is an example of thinking about thinking. Of all the branches of philosophy, epistemology should be the most visual, as words give way to structures.

> "Most people would die sooner than think—in fact, they do so."
>
> —Bertrand Russell

And of all the branches of philosophy, epistemology is the most closely linked to cognitive science, the study of the mind-brain. How do we come to accept something as knowledge? What are the methods by which we determine what is knowledge? How is knowledge recognized? And how do we distinguish what is knowledge from what is not? These are some of the questions we will explore in this chapter.

TOPIC 35.1   Bartlett: Schema as Reality

Fredrick Bartlett (1932; see Topic 23.4) sees the schema as the ultimate basis of our personal reality. Hence, our individual knowledge is a collection of schemas. While reviewing my French language ability in preparation for a trip to Paris, I was aware that as an American-born English speaker I have no built-in schema for the French medial consonant construction (*va t'il, y a t'il*); thus it is extremely difficult for me to recognize it in spoken form. In a less technical vein, I was reared with a strong schema for reciprocity, so I feel unsettled until I have returned a good deed and, yes, until someone else has returned my good deed! My schema "Eat to show Mama you love her" has led to a pesky tendency to overeat as an adult.

Applications

1 Know your schemas. Be aware that we tend to see reality through the filtering effect of our schemas. We screen out what doesn't fit. Forming new schemas takes conscious effort.

2 Be aware of others' schemas. Know that their disagreements with you are probably due to conflicting schemas. Peter Senge (1990) calls these schemas "mental models"; he asks us to take the time to identify our assumptions with our significant others at work or home, then use them to make decisions, solve problems, and make plans. By getting these assumptions out into the open, we may be able to pursue the mature approach of selecting the assumptions that seem most effective for the occasion at hand. Maybe your assumption is more appropriate than mine. Maybe we'll find a schema we both possess that allows a win-win situation.

3 Practice Senge's "left-hand-column" method (Senge, 1990). After a significant interchange with one or more people, try writing out the key statements you made in the right-hand column, labeled "What I Said." In the left-hand column, labeled "What I Was Thinking," enter the thought that lay behind your words. This is a helpful process for checking out your assumptions and paradigms and getting them on the table. Here are a couple of examples:

What I Was Thinking	What I Said
"The bottom may fall out any day."	"Yes, I think we're right on target."
"Courtesy will soften the blow."	"May I take your coat?"

4 Practice the art of thinking in metaphors or analogies. By comparing a present subject to a remote one that is similar in structure, you will find that new insights emerge. Observing that my love is like a red, red rose can lead to the insight of accepting the painful along with the pleasurable. The "synectics" approach to problem solving (Prince, 1970) employs the use of metaphor for gaining insight into problems. The essence that related metaphors have in common is what we call a schema.

❺ Practice the art of visualizing a subject or concept. Don Norman (1993) points out that we make models (graphs, charts, calendars) of things in order to understand, to communicate, and to improve. By reducing a subject to a visual representation, we focus on the essence, or schema, underlying the subject. That is the purpose of a flowchart. A manufacturing company once came to me lamenting that they were wasting twenty-seven cents out of every dollar of raw material, while the industry standard was twelve cents of waste. I had them make a flowchart of the process they used, and they identified some two dozen trouble spots in the process. This directly led them to improve their waste to only fourteen cents on the dollar.

Listed below are two types of visualization patterns: *representational* and *organizational*. Representational visuals attempt to draw the actual physical structure of a subject in outline form, as in the stick figure of a human. Organizational visuals only attempt to highlight the categories and relationships, without focusing on surface recognition. I am in the process of preparing examples of each of these visualization tools for publication separate from this book. If you are interested in obtaining a copy, contact me. I'll be able either to send you a copy of the draft or refer you to the published version. Meanwhile, two good references for visualization tools are Hyerle (1996) and Walton (1986).

Representational Visual Tools

Diagram (generic)

Domain-specific tools:

      Chemistry: equations, molecule models, bonding diagrams

      Language: sentence diagrams

      Movement: Labanotation

      Music notation

      Philosophy: truth tables, Venn diagrams, Euler's notations

      Physics: Niels Bohr's particle state notation

Flowchart (process flow diagram)

Gantt chart

Organizational charts (deployment chart or relationship diagram)

Program Evaluation and Review Technique (PERT) chart

Rough sketch

Scale drawing

Star or network diagram

Surface maps

System flow

Organizational Visual Tools

Act III (action plan)

Brace map

Bridge map

Bubble map (also double bubble map)

Card sorts (plain, sticky)

Cause and Effect Diagram with the Addition of Cards (CEDAC)

Character diagram

Circle map (similar to Venn diagram)

Circular flow

Classification tree

Compare-and-contrast process map

Concept map

Control chart

Feynman diagram

Fish chart (Ishikawa, cause-and-effect)

Force field

Graphs (pie, line, bar, scatter)

Histogram

Human interaction outline

Inductive tower

Matrix, or row-by-column (also weighted matrix)

Metrics (Likert scale, comparison, anchors, continuum)

Mind map

Pareto chart (80-20 chart)

Planning wheel

Pyramids

Run chart (trend chart)

Scattering-matrix diagram (S-matrix)

Semantic maps

Sorting tree

Stepwise listing

Time line

Tree diagram or map

Venn diagram

X-Y function graph

TOPIC 35.2 Healy: Reality as Schema

Jane Healy (1990) reports that excessive television watching by children produces adults who have failed to develop schemas for active engagement with their environment. By viewing a world (television) in which no time or need for reflection (or internal talking) exists, children build only minimal skills for listening and responding. Their answers become formulas based on their favorite programs. So, for example, if you have a child who often watches soap operas, he or she stands a strong chance of developing the schema "disappointment leads to crying, which leads to restoration," as opposed to "disappointment leads to thinking through the cause and working toward restoration." Obviously the first schema is part of a fantasy world and will normally lead to frustration in the "real" world.

Applications

1 Withhold all television watching until reading, mathematics, learning, and interpersonal habits are firmly established.

2 Find a way to get children (or, increasingly, adults) who've succumbed to the "entertain me" syndrome of the TV addict into a long-term, intensive, small-group experience. This could be anything from a volleyball team to a support group.

3 Watch television with your children to compare your version of reality with what the television programming is offering. Discuss how you, your children, and the television characters see the world differently and similarly.

TOPIC 35.3 Critical Thinking

Diane Halpern defines critical thinking as "the use of those cognitive skills or strategies that increase the probability of a desirable outcome—in the long run, critical thinkers will have more desirable outcomes than 'noncritical' thinkers (where 'desirable' is defined by the individual, such as making good career choices or wise financial investments)" (*American Psychologist,* April 1998, p. 450).

Critical thinking is the habit of mind that resists being deceived by appearances. Critical thinking says, "All that glitters is not gold," and asks, "What are some other ways of explaining what has happened?" Critical thinking hesitates, where fools rush in. In the same article, Halpern relays that in a college survey, just over 99 percent of students expressed a belief in at least one of the following ideas and over 65 percent reported having a personal experience with one of them:

- Astral travel

- Auras

- Bermuda triangle mysteries

- Channeling

- Clairvoyance

- Ghosts

- Healing crystals

- Levitation

- Plant consciousness

- Precognition
- Psychic healing
- Psychic surgery
- Psychokinesis
- Telepathy
- UFOs

Clearly a need exists for developing critical thinking skills from an early age onward! Programs should contain training including, but not limited to, the following topics:

- The purpose and nature of critical thinking
- The qualities of the critical thinker
- Obstacles to critical thinking
- Logic and deductive reasoning
- Inductive reasoning (how to generalize)
- Visual tools
- Verbal tools
- Process and policy tools
- Common logical fallacies
- Resources for critical thinking

Applications

1 I have developed a PowerPoint presentation on critical thinking for use with my MBA course in managerial decision making at Pfeiffer University. You are welcome to view it by visiting www.pfeiffer.edu/~phoward and clicking on "Critical Thinking Presentation." Feel free to use these slides in working out your own presentations on critical thinking (credit is always nice, however!).

2 Explore the additional web resources for critical thinking listed in the Suggested Resources at the end of this chapter.

SUGGESTED RESOURCES

Hyerle, D. (1996). *Visual Tools for Constructing Knowledge.* Alexandria, Va.: Association for Supervision and Curriculum Development.

Korzybski, A. (1948). *Science and Sanity: An Introduction to Non-Aristotelian Systems and General Semantics* (3rd ed.). Lakeville, Conn.: International Non-Aristotelian Library.

Lakoff, G. (1987). *Women, Fire, and Dangerous Things: What Categories Reveal About the Mind.* Chicago: University of Chicago Press.

Norman, D. A. (1993). *Things That Make Us Smart: Cognitive Artifacts as Tools for Thought.* Reading, Mass.: Perseus Press.

Sagan, C. (1995). *The Demon-Haunted World.* New York: Random House.

Senge, P. (1990). *The Fifth Discipline.* New York: Doubleday/Currency.

Walton, M. (1986). *The Deming Management Method.* New York: Dodd, Mead.

Web Sites

allCLEAR 4.5 flowcharting software home page:
www.clearsoft.com

Decide Right 1.2 for Windows 95; individual decision matrix tool:
www.avantos.com

Decision Explorer software home page:
www.banxia.com

Institute for Professional Education problem-solving seminars:
www.theIPE.com

Laban symbol system, software for notating movement:
www.dance.ohio-state.edu/files/LabanWriter/index.html

Mind map software (Tony Buzan):
www.mindman.com

STELLA system process flow software:
www.hps-inc.com

SureFire Decisions for Windows 95; decision matrix for groups or individuals:
www.beaconrock.com

36

States of Consciousness

Phases of the Mind

O n October 30, 1998, Vilayanur Ramachandran, a senior scientist at the Center for Brain and Cognition at the University of California, San Diego, addressed the first Learning Brain Expo in San Diego. In describing the many possible combinations of information substances and neural pathways, Ramachandran made the astounding comment that there are more possible brain states than there

> **There are brute, blind neurophysiological processes and there is consciousness, but there is nothing else.**
>
> —John Searle,
> The Rediscovery of the Mind

are particles in the universe. With that said, I humbly attempt to execute a chapter on consciousness!

To begin: what is consciousness? David Chalmers, a member of the philosophy department at the University of California, Santa Cruz, calls it "the subjective, inner life of the mind" (1995, p. 80). Gerard Edelman (1987), in elaborating his theory of neuronal group selection, talks of two kinds of consciousness: primary consciousness, which involves an awareness of the present, and higher consciousness, which involves awareness of the past, projection into the future, and the ability to see patterns in the totality of one's behavior, past, present, and future. Francis Crick (1994), co-discoverer of DNA's structure and now a neuroscientist with the Salk Institute in La Jolla, California, calls it "no more than the behavior of a vast assembly of nerve cells." In a fairly readable summary, John Horgan reviewed these and other approaches to consciousness in the July 1994 issue of *Scientific American.*

> Buddhist monk to hot dog vendor: "Make me one with everything."

What to make of it all? The problem with the term *consciousness* is its all-inclusiveness. To say that there are more brain states than particles in the universe is to suggest that there are uncountable states of consciousness.

TOPIC 36.1   What Is Consciousness?

In order to render the subject more manageable, I have toyed with the work of Harvard University's J. Allan Hobson. In *The Chemistry of Conscious States* (1994), he proposes three primary variables that underlie the many kinds of conscious states: *source, mode,* and *level of activation.*

Source

Consciousness is neural activity, and this activity can be initiated from an internal source (for example, "will" or "instincts") or an external source (for example, a conversation or a concert). The source is not either-or in nature. In fact, much of the time we experience both internal and external sources. As I keyboard at this moment, I am both referring to my written notes (external) and making connections to other ideas (internal). In fact, source is a continuum, ranging from the purely internal source of the dream state to the purely external source of a blaring rock band.

Mode

Hobson sees two primary modes of chemical activity as being associated with neural activation: the aminergic system (including norepinephrine and serotonin) and the cholinergic system (including acetylcholine). The amines are associated with wakefulness and with managed, or controlled, neural activity that is subject to one's effort of will. Acetylcholine, on the other hand, is associated with unmanaged neural activity, such as the activity that occurs during REM sleep or delirium states. Volition inhibits acetylcholine and enhances the amines, while absence of volition releases acetylcholine and suppresses the amines. During normal, non-REM sleep, these two chemical systems are in balance. At other times, the two systems are always operating, but one of them will tend to be more dominant than the other.

Level of Activation

The nervous system transmits electrical signals. One way of describing the level of electrical activity is by categorizing the frequency of the "waves" that are generated in an electroencephalograph:

Beta waves: Above 11 cycles per second; associated with the wakeful alertness known as attention and arousal

Alpha waves: About 9 to 11 cycles per second; associated with resting quietly and meditating with the eyes closed; alpha waves typically move back up to beta waves when eyes reopen

Delta waves: About 4 to 8 cycles per second; associated with light sleep

Theta waves: Below 4 cycles per second; associated with deep sleep

States of consciousness can be described in terms of these three variables. For example, REM sleep has high activation, a cholinergic mode, and an internal source. In order to view how these three variables might interact to explain discrete states of consciousness, I have prepared a three-dimensional drawing, shown in Figure 36.1. It is actually a cube, but it is meant to represent the brain and nervous system as a whole. Do not attempt to see "left brain, right brain" or "cortex versus limbic system" in this drawing. Think holistically when you view it.

According to Allan Hobson, we can throw away all terms like *preconscious, subconscious, unconscious,* and their kith and kin. Only two terms are needed to describe this terrain: *conscious* and *nonconscious.* To the degree that the mind refers to the brain's collection of information, consciousness is one's awareness of the portion of the information that is accessible at any one time; nonconsciousness is all of the information that is inaccessible at any particular time. Information moves from consciousness to nonconsciousness, and this movement is essentially ruled by chance, with the illusion of minimal guiding by something called the will.

Applications

1 Understand that to some degree, states of consciousness are subject to manipulation. By controlling internal sources of stimulation as opposed to external ones, by controlling stimulants such as caffeine, and by controlling depressants such as alcohol, we can influence our states of consciousness.

2 Make peace with difficult philosophical terms. For example, how does this definition jibe with religion and the concept of soul? If "neurons 'r' us," then what is the role of spirit? In the spirit of the times, we would not distinguish between body and soul. To the degree that soul outlasts body, we can understand the soul as the essence of a person that remains as a memory among others. We have eternal life to the degree that others keep our memory alive.

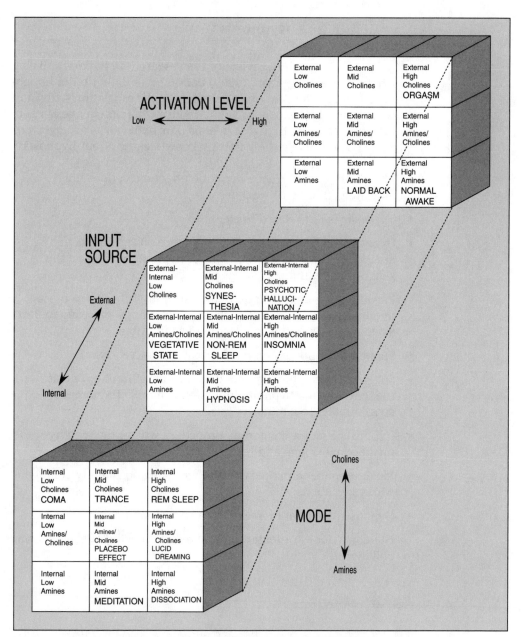

Figure 36.1. Split Three-Dimensional Model of States of Consciousness.
Source: Based on *The Chemistry of Conscious States* by J. A. Hobson, 1994,
New York: Little, Brown.

TOPIC 36.2 Hypnosis

In a review of the research on hypnosis, Irving Kirsch and Steven Jay Lynn (1995) endorse the definition of hypnosis proposed by the American Psychological Association's Division of Psychological Hypnosis as "a procedure wherein changes in sensations, perceptions, thoughts, feelings, or behavior are suggested" (p. 846). They propose the following known truths about hypnosis:

- The ability to experience hypnotic phenomena does not indicate gullibility or weakness.

- Hypnosis is not related to sleep.

- Hypnotic responsiveness depends more on the efforts and abilities of the person who is being hypnotized than on the skill of the hypnotist.

- Participants retain the ability to control their behavior during hypnosis; they are aware of their surroundings and can monitor events outside of the framework of suggestions.

- Spontaneous posthypnotic amnesia is relatively rare.

- Suggestions can be responded to with or without hypnosis; the function of a hypnotic induction is merely to increase suggestibility to a minor degree.

- Hypnosis is not a dangerous procedure when practiced by qualified clinicians and researchers.

- Most hypnotized people are neither faking nor merely complying with suggestions.

- Hypnosis does not increase the accuracy of memory.

- Hypnosis does not foster a literal reexperiencing of events from childhood.

Applications

1 Psychologist Judy Lasher and surgeon Anne Ouellette of Jackson Memorial Hospital in Miami, Florida, team to use hypnosis in lieu of general anesthesia for hand operations. Because they use only local painkillers and sedatives along with the hypnosis, the patient can move during the surgery, providing helpful feedback to the surgeon on the effectiveness of the operation. The hospital's staff have found significant reductions in postoperative complications and length of hospital stay as a result of the new practice.

2 Hypnosis has been found to be an effective supplement to other pain management therapies. Its effectiveness relies on the hypnotic relationship's power to enable the subject to switch from external to internal sources of consciousness.

TOPIC 36.3   The God Module

Vilayanur Ramachandran of the Center for Brain and Cognition at the University of California, San Diego, presented findings at the October 1997 meeting of the Society for Neuroscience that couple temporal-lobe activity with mystical religious experience. This so-called "God module" is common among people who suffer a unique kind of epilepsy that is typically accompanied by visions of God and feelings of being at one with the universe.

Application

Research is under way aimed at clarifying the extent of the temporal lobe's activity during moments of reported religious experience. It remains unclear which came first, the vision or the memory, or whether nonepileptic people show the same temporal-lobe activity during such visions and feelings. Watch for further reports.

TOPIC 36.4   The Efficacy of Prayer

In 1988, physician and author Larry Dossey read about a ten-month-long computer-assisted review of 393 cardiology patients, half of whom were prayed for by home prayer groups and half of whom were not prayed for. It turned out that the prayed-for group was five times less likely to require antibiotics and three times less likely to develop fluid in the lungs (pulmonary edema). As a result of reading about this study, Dossey engaged in a five-year exploration of more than 130 scientific studies that resulted in the book *Healing Words* (1996). His conclusion: praying for someone's health makes a positive impact on that person's recovery in a significant number of the cases. Although skeptics abound, some impressive results have been reported, including one study in which ten people focused their prayers on retarding the growth of a laboratory fungus while they were fifteen miles from the cultures. Over 70 percent of the cultures showed retarded growth, with the same results occurring sixteen times out of sixteen. (No mention was made of a control group.)

Application

Why not cover your bases and offer prayer for those who might benefit from it. Although I am not a prayerful person myself, I do have a strong belief in the power of positive personal regard. When my wife or a friend is making a presentation, I focus my positive attention on that person in a supportive manner. It can't hurt, and it seems to be well taken.

SUGGESTED RESOURCES

Chalmers, D. J. (1995, December). "The Puzzle of Conscious Experience." *Scientific American,* pp. 80–86.

Crick, F. (1994). *The Astonishing Hypothesis: The Scientific Search for the Soul.* New York: Scribner.

Cytowic, R. E. (1993). *The Man Who Tasted Shapes.* Los Angeles: Tarcher.

Edelman, G. M. (1992). *Bright Air, Brilliant Fire: On the Matter of the Mind.* New York: Basic Books.

Hobson, J. A. (1994). *The Chemistry of Conscious States.* New York: Little, Brown.

Kirsch, I., and Lynn, S. J. (1995, October). "The Altered State of Hypnosis: Changes in the Theoretical Landscape." *American Psychologist, 50*(10), 846–858.

37

Updating Your Owner's Manual

Continuing the Search for New Mind-Body Applications

66 *We should live for the future, and yet should find our life in the fidelities of the present; the last is the only method of the first. 99*

—Henry Ward Beecher

From the gaping head wounds of World War II to the drug-sizzled brains caused by poison-trafficking cartels, we try to learn from our misery. A recent television program described how doctors, noticing that the symptoms of crack cocaine addicts resemble those of patients with Parkinson's disease, have made advances in the treatment of Parkinson's disease. But we do not have to wait for tragedy in order to make progress. Scientific exploration and discovery today make the 1990s an exciting time to be alive. And the more open we are to learning the work of others, the more exciting the twenty-first century will be.

While I was working on the first edition of this book, my wife and I overheard our daughter Allegra talking with a girlfriend who was lamenting her steady boyfriend's unwillingness to talk seriously about their relationship. Allegra told her friend that she had learned in her dad's book about females being wired to talk and males being wired to do, and that she had tried the suggestion of getting a boy to do something so that talking would become an accompaniment to the activity rather than an activity in and of itself. "And you know?" she added to her friend. "It really worked! He talked while we were walking and didn't seem to mind it at all. Give it a try."

What I like about this story is that (1) it shows an experimental, evaluative approach in responding to research and (2) it builds on differences rather than using differences to blame and justify resentments. I hope that this book will become something of a cafeteria for you. By that I mean that you can come to it for nourishment and ideas and take what appears to be helpful to you. Return to it when you are baffled by a concern that is covered by one of these chapters—for example, problems related to aging parents or friends; concerns about an unmotivated child, friend, or co-worker; or a gnawing dissatisfaction with your ability to memorize. This book should yield up to you a specific practical idea or at least suggest relevant resources.

In a sense, I have been sowing seeds, and I'm inviting you to reap one or more of the many I have thrown out. My observation is that the Age of Research is alive and well. From the health and fitness enthusiasts to the corporate quality gurus, people are spreading the gospel of continuing improvement. But you can't continually improve without doing, following, and evaluating research and then implementing the findings appropriately in your own life. I emphasize, however, the need to be critical. Just as I included the Caveat Box in Chapter Three, I urge you to keep your nonsense detector turned on whenever you encounter suggestions for improvement. While perusing futurist magazines, I often see advertisements for pills "to make you more intelligent." Amused and alarmed, I call the telephone number provided and ask them to send me a copy of the research results of the product testing. They never have any. All they can send me is a somewhat more lengthy version of the advertisements I have read. I'm still waiting for a get-smart pill with sound research behind it. I decline, incidentally, to accept various offers of a free thirty-day supply.

This kind of irresponsible advertising will confront us with more frequency, more force, and more marketing savvy. We must all do what we can to be as informed as possible about what works, what's dangerous, and what's simply inert. In that spirit, I have included in the back of the book a Reader Participation Card, which I hope you will use to let me know what works, what doesn't, and what new ideas you'd like me to add (citing you as the source) in subsequent editions of this book. As an alternative, you may E-mail me at pjhoward@centacs.com.

The advances in brain research are breathtakingly rapid. Even as I write and you read, some piece of information in this book is being challenged or enhanced. Who knows where the next major advance will be and what difference it will make in our lives? Just this morning I read about a high-fat diet as a treatment for epilepsy!

As research expands our sense of what is true and what is real, paradigms begin to shift, sometimes imperceptibly, sometimes earthshakingly. In looking over the ways in which cognitive science affects our lives, I see ten paradigms that seem to me to be in the middle of major shifts:

Traditional Paradigm	Emerging Paradigm
1. Motivators are external.	Motivators are internal.
2. There are four personality traits.	The Five-Factor Model emerges.
3. Aging lowers ability.	Use it or lose it!
4. IQ is a single-faceted, academic concept.	IQ is a multifaceted, street-smart concept.
5. There are no sex differences.	The sexes are wired differently.
6. Nurture is the main factor.	Nature is the main factor.
7. Germs cause disease.	The mind controls disease.

8. Diet is unrelated to the brain.

    Diet influences mental function.

9. The brain is seen as a computer.

    The brain is seen as a pharmacy.

10. Memory is retrieval of complete episodes.

    Memory is construction of episodes from pieces of information.

Perhaps these ten perceived shifts will form the basis of another book! Until then . . .

Appendixes

Eating Right

Limit
Egg yolks
Organ meats
Fried foods
Fatty foods (pastries, spreads, dressings)
Animal protein (has no known benefits and may cause cancer)
Alcohol
Certain shellfish (there is some debate over which; scallops are apparently okay)

Emphasize
Fish
Skinless poultry
Lean meats
Low- or nonfat dairy products
Complex carbohydrates (fruits, vegetables, starches)

Eliminate
Dietary supplements (megadoses have no known benefits and may be toxic)
Calcium, fish oil, or fiber supplements (they have no known benefits and must be taken in food)

Specific Limits
Fat
No more than 30 percent of daily calories
(1 tablespoon of peanut butter = 8 grams = 90 calories)
Saturated fats
Less than 10 percent of the fat allowance
(includes coconut oil and animal fat)
Complex carbohydrates
At least 55 percent of daily calories
Vegetables
Five or more servings, especially of green and yellow vegetables (1 serving = ½ cup)
Fruits
Five or more servings, especially of citrus fruits
(1 serving = 1 medium-sized fruit or ½ banana)
Starches
Six or more servings; includes rice, potatoes, pasta, legumes, and whole-grain bread and cereal (1 serving = 1 slice of bread)
Protein
Eight grams per kilogram of body weight (for a 180-pound man, an 8.4-ounce hamburger patty; for a 120-pound woman, a 5.6-ounce hamburger patty)
Alcohol
Less than 1 ounce daily (2 cans of beer or two small glasses of wine; *none* for women who are pregnant or trying to conceive)
Salt
Six grams a day (about 1 teaspoon)

Note that in general, Americans eat too much fat, cholesterol, and protein and too few complex carbohydrates.

Source: Based on *Diet and Health: Implications for Reducing Chronic Disease Risk* by National Research Council, Committee on Diet and Health, 1989, Washington, D.C.: National Academy Press.

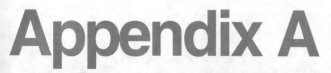

Appendix A

A Listing of Sex and Gender Differences

Males	Females
Have better general math ability	Have better general verbal ability
Are better at spatial (three-dimensional) reasoning	Are better in grammar and vocabulary
Are better at chess	Are better at foreign languages
Are better at reading maps	Have better fine-motor (hand-eye) coordination within personal space
Are better at reading blueprints	Have better sensory awareness
Have better vision in bright light (see less well in darkness)	Have better night vision (are more sensitive to bright light)
Have better perception in blue end of spectrum	Have better perception in red end of spectrum
Have more narrow vision (tunnel vision), but better depth and perspective	Have wider peripheral vision for "big picture"; have more receptor rods and cones
Have more stuttering and speech defects	Perceive sounds better
Enroll more in remedial reading (4:1)	Sing in tune more (6:1)
Take more interest in objects	Are more interested in people and faces
Talk and play more with inanimate objects	Read character and social cues better

Preschoolers:
- Average 36 seconds for goodbyes
- Occupy more play space
- Prefer blocks and building
- Build high structures
- Are indifferent to newcomers
- Accept others if they are useful
- Prefer stories of adventure
- Identify more with robbers
- Play more competitive games, such as tag

- Use dolls for "dive bombers"
- Are better visual-spatial learners

Preschoolers:
- Average 93 seconds for goodbyes
- Occupy less play space
- Prefer playing with living things
- Build long and low structures
- Greet newcomers
- Accept others if they are nice
- Prefer stories of romance
- Identify more with victims
- Play less competitive games, such as hopscotch

- Use dolls for family scenes
- Are better auditory learners

Males	Females
Require more space	Require less space
Have a better aural memory	Have a better visual memory
Are more easily angered	Are slower to anger
Talk later (usually by four years of age)	Talk earlier (99 percent are understandable by three years of age)

Appendix B

Males	Females
Are more sensitive to and prefer salty tastes	Are more sensitive to bitter tastes; prefer sweets and more subtle tastes
Have relatively insensitive skin	Have extremely sensitive skin
Have right hemisphere larger than left	Have left hemisphere larger than right
Favor right ear	Listen equally with both ears
Solve math problems nonverbally	Tend to talk while solving math problems
Handle multitasking more easily	Are less at ease with multitasking
Have better memory for relevant or organized information	Have better memory for names and faces and for random and irrelevant information
Use less eye contact	Use more eye contact
Have a shorter attention span	Have a longer attention span
Don't notice the smell of Exaltolide (a musklike odor)	Are especially sensitive to the smell of Exaltolide, especially before ovulation
Are more sensation-seeking	Are less sensation-seeking (but American females are more sensation-seeking than English females)
Are more frequently left-handed	Equal numbers are right- and left-handed
Use left hemisphere in spelling	Use both hemispheres in spelling
Have differentiated hemispheres: right for math and spatial skills, left for language	Have undifferentiated hemispheres
Have corpus callosum that shrinks about 20 percent by the age of fifty and is thinner relative to brain size	Have corpus callosum that is thicker relative to brain size and doesn't shrink over time
Have left hemisphere that shrinks with age	Have left hemisphere that shrinks symmetrically and minimally
Prefer greater distance from same-sex others	Are more comfortable than males are when they are physically close to same-sex others
Are three times more likely to be dyslexic or myopic	Are less likely to be dyslexic or myopic
React to pain slowly	React to pain more quickly; can tolerate long-term pain or discomfort better
Report feeling less pain	Report feeling more pain
Cope with pain less well	Cope with pain better
When left alone, tend to form organizations with hierarchical, dominant structures	When left alone, tend to form informal organizations with shifting power sources
Interrupt to introduce new topics or information	Interrupt to clarify or support

Source: Based on *Brain Sex: The Real Difference Between Men and Women* by Anne Moir and David Jessel, 1991, New York: Carol Publishing/Lyle Stuart.

Aerobic Versus Nonaerobic Exercise

Aerobic Exercises:
Minimum Required Times for Health Effects

Twelve Minutes	*Fifteen Minutes*	*Twenty Minutes*
Jumping rope	Jogging	Walking
Running in place	Running	Outdoor bicycling
Jumping jacks	Dancing	Stationary bicycling
Chair stepping	Mini-trampoline	Ice skating
Rowing	Treadmill	Roller skating
Cross-country skiing		Swimming

For the above, add several minutes for warming up.

Nonaerobic Exercises:
Why They Are Nonaerobic

Stop and Go	*Short Duration*	*Low Intensity*
Tennis	Weight lifting	Golf
Softball	Sprinting	Canasta
Football	Isometrics	Frisbee
Calisthenics	Square dancing	
Handball	Downhill skiing	
Racquetball		
Basketball		

Source: Adapted from *The New Fit or Fat* by Covert Bailey, 1991, Boston: Houghton Mifflin. Copyright © 1977, 1978, 1991 by Covert Bailey. Reprinted by permission of Houghton Mifflin Co. All rights reserved.

Appendix C

Human Universals

This appendix presents Steven Pinker's (1994) summary of anthropologist Donald E. Brown's list of patterns underlying the behavior of all documented human cultures (D. E. Brown, 1991). Pinker points out that this list neither condones nor advocates specific patterns. Neither is it an explicit argument for the innateness or instinctiveness of specific patterns. For whatever reason, these patterns are simply evidence of a universal human nature. Finally, the fact that the patterns are universal does not mean that they are inevitable. We do, after all, have some degree of control over our choices.

1. Value placed on articulateness
2. Gossip
3. Lying
4. Misleading of others
5. Verbal humor
6. Humorous insults
7. Poetic and rhetorical speech forms
8. Narrative and storytelling
9. Metaphor
10. Poetry with repetition of linguistic elements and lines separated by pauses
11. Words for days, months, seasons, years, past, present, future, body parts, inner states (emotions, sensations, thoughts), behavioral propensities, flora, fauna, weather, tools, space, motions, speed, location, spatial dimensions, physical properties, giving, lending, eliciting emotional reactions, numbers (at least "one," "two," and "more than two"), proper names, and possession
12. Distinctions between mother and father
13. Kinship categories, defined in terms of mother, father, son, daughter, and age sequence
14. Binary distinctions, including male and female, black and white, natural and cultural, and good and bad
15. Measures
16. Logical relations, including "not," "and," "same," "equivalent," "opposite," general versus particular, and part versus whole
17. Conjectural reasoning (inferring the presence of entities from their traces)
18. Nonlinguistic vocal communication such as cries and squeals
19. Interpretation of intention from behavior
20. Recognized facial expressions of happiness, sadness, anger, fear, surprise, disgust, and contempt
21. Use of smiles as a friendly greeting
22. Crying
23. Coy flirtation with the eyes
24. Masking, modifying, and mimicking facial expressions

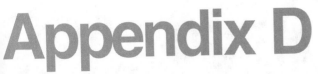

Appendix D

25. Displays of affection
26. Sense of self versus other, responsibility, voluntary versus involuntary behavior, intention, private inner life, and normal versus abnormal mental states
27. Empathy
28. Sexual attraction
29. Powerful sexual jealousy
30. Childhood fears, especially of loud noises and, at the end of the first year, strangers
31. Fear of snakes
32. "Oedipal" feelings (possessiveness of mother, coolness toward her consort)
33. Face recognition
34. Adornment of bodies and arrangement of hair
35. Sexual attractiveness, based in part on signs of health and, in women, youth
36. Hygiene
37. Dance
38. Music
39. Play, including play fighting
40. Manufacture of, and dependence upon, many kinds of tools, a large number of which are permanent, made according to culturally transmitted motifs, including cutters, pounders, containers, string, levers, and spears
41. Use of fire to cook food and for other purposes
42. Drugs, both medicinal and recreational
43. Shelter
44. Decoration of artifacts
45. A standard pattern and time for weaning
46. Habitation in groups that claim a territory and have a sense of being a distinct people
47. Families built around a mother and children, usually the biological mother, and one or more men
48. Institutionalized marriage, in the sense of a publicly recognized right of sexual access to a woman eligible for childbearing
49. Socialization of children (including toilet training) by senior kin
50. Imitation by children of their elders
51. Distinction between close kin and distant kin and favoring of close kin
52. Avoidance of incest between mothers and sons
53. Great interest in the topic of sex
54. Status and prestige, both assigned (by kinship, age, sex) and achieved
55. Some degree of economic inequality
56. Division of labor by sex and age
57. More child care by women
58. More aggression and violence by men
59. Acknowledgment of differences between male and female natures

60. Domination by men in the public political sphere
61. Exchange of labor, goods, and services
62. Reciprocity, including retaliation
63. Gifts
64. Social reasoning
65. Coalitions
66. Government, in the sense of binding collective decisions about public affairs
67. Leaders, almost always nondictatorial, perhaps ephemeral
68. Laws, rights, and obligations, including laws against violence, rape, and murder
69. Punishment
70. Conflict, which is deplored
71. Rape
72. Seeking of redress for wrongs
73. Mediation
74. In-group/out-group conflicts
75. Property
76. Inheritance of property
77. A sense of right and wrong
78. Envy
79. Etiquette
80. Hospitality
81. Feasting
82. Being active primarily during daylight hours (a diurnal pattern)
83. Standards of sexual modesty
84. Sex that generally occurs in private
85. A fondness for sweets
86. Food taboos
87. Discreetness in elimination of body wastes
88. Supernatural beliefs
89. Magic practiced to sustain and increase life and to attract the opposite sex
90. Theories of fortune and misfortune
91. Explanations of disease and death
92. Medicine
93. Rituals, including rites of passage
94. Mourning of the dead
95. Dreaming, interpreting dreams

Source: Adapted from *The Language Instinct* by Steven Pinker, 1994, pp. 413–415, New York: Morrow.

Big Five Feedback Form

Name: Date:

Negative Emotionality Scale

	Resilient				Responsive			Reactive			Negative Emotionality Scale
20	25	30	35	40	45	50	55	60	65	70	75	80

Positive descriptors: Secure, calm, Rock of Gibraltar, concentrating, steady, unflappable, stress-free
Negative descriptors: Lethargic, laid-back, unresponsive, unaware, insensitive, tunnel-visioned

Positive descriptors: Alert, aware, empathetic, expressive, energetic
Negative descriptors: Tense, high-strung, depressed, neurotic, restless

Extraversion Scale

	Introvert				Ambivert			Extravert			Extraversion Scale
20	25	30	35	40	45	50	55	60	65	70	75	80

Positive descriptors: Private, reserved, serious, works alone, self-minimizing, prefers writing
Negative descriptors: Seclusive, fearful, submissive, retreating, eccentric, loner

Positive descriptors: Conversational, energetic, assertive, confident, happy, optimistic, sociable
Negative descriptors: Outspoken, talkative, overbearing, aggressive, exhibitionistic, heedless, shallow

Openness Scale

	Preserver				Moderate			Explorer			Openness Scale
20	25	30	35	40	45	50	55	60	65	70	75	80

Positive descriptors: Seeks depth, practical, expert knowledge, down-to-earth, efficient, traditional, practice until perfect, conservative
Negative descriptors: Narrowness, no big picture, misses new opportunities, lacks perspective, set in ways, rigid to new experiences, closed

Positive descriptors: Broad interests, curious, likes novelty/variety, chases ideas/theory, imaginative, liberal, understands big picture
Negative descriptors: Dabbler, amateur, easily bored, impractical, head in clouds, lacks detail, lives in fantasy

Agreeableness Scale

	Challenger				Negotiator			Adapter			Agreeableness Scale
20	25	30	35	40	45	50	55	60	65	70	75	80

Positive descriptors: Independent, skeptical, direct, self-interested, competitive, questioning
Negative descriptors: Rejecting, hostile, rude, self-centered, combative, argumentative

Positive descriptors: Friendly, tolerant, trusting, team player, considerate, accepting
Negative descriptors: Syrupy, spineless, gullible, dependent, doormat, unprincipled, conflict averse

Conscientiousness Scale

	Flexible				Balanced			Focused			Conscientiousness Scale
20	25	30	35	40	45	50	55	60	65	70	75	80

Positive descriptors: Relaxed, spontaneous, open-ended, multitasking, experimental, roles not goals, accepts uncertainty
Negative descriptors: Lackadaisical, quitter, indecisive, chaotic, irresponsible, nonproductive, permissive, procrastinator

Positive descriptors: Industrious, dependable, will to achieve, productive, organized, decisive, persevering, driven
Negative descriptors: Overbearing, compulsive, workaholic, suppressed, meticulous, stubborn

Appendix E

Developing the Five Dimensions

Negative Emotionality

To Increase	To Decrease
Use structured exercise (such as force-field analysis and itemized response) to communicate negative feelings.	Perform aerobic exercise within four hours of an event in which calmness is particularly important.
Engage in competitive sports or other competitive activities (such as chess) with someone you have a reasonable chance of beating (or use an appropriate handicap).	Take aerobic exercise soon after a stressful episode to trigger parasympathetic arousal.
When you are aware of your body beginning to react internally to your thoughts and feelings (rapid heart rate, queasy stomach, perspiration, and so on), communicate these changes to a significant other or partner and identify their cause and meaning, or write a note or journal entry about them.	Plan to consume your daily allowance of fats and simple carbohydrates *after* particularly stressful episodes.
Use caffeine in some form as a way to increase general arousal.	Refer to the list of stress relievers in Topic 20.4.
Minimize the consumption of fats and simple carbohydrates for four hours before events in which the identification and expression of feelings is important.	Read from the wide literature available on the subject of mental self-control, such as Epictetus's *Enchiridion* and works by the Stoic philosophers and Norman Cousins.
Read novels, biographies, or poetry that express negative emotion and emulate appropriate models.	If necessary, reduce or eliminate sources of stress by examining bad Big Five fits in your marriage or job.
Join a drama or theater group.	Read Redford Williams's *Trusting Heart* (more technical) and *Anger Kills* (which he wrote with his wife, and which is more application-oriented, with specific suggestions on how to get a handle on your hostility). They also conduct a public workshop; he teaches at Duke University Medical School.
Participate in physical activities that emphasize expression, such as sports, music, dance, or landscaping.	Read Chapter Nineteen, which discusses the emotions.
Find and use support groups, either on the Internet or in the community, that explore a particular aspect of Negative Emotionality: how to express your anger, how to show your concern, and so on.	The combination of antidepressant drugs and psychotherapy works effectively to reduce depression.
Use a journal or diary as a means of identifying, describing, and exploring your internal feelings.	Katharina Dalton has found success in treating the mood swings of premenstrual tension by helping patients maintain optimum blood sugar levels by periodically snacking throughout the day.
Practice observing nonverbal behavior and other environmental cues to the negative emotions of others.	Try taking ten-minute "brief" walks as an antidote for various kinds of stress: sadness, anger, and anxiety.
Give explicit direction and permission to others so that they may encourage you to express feelings that they perceive you are holding back.	Try self-hypnosis or biofeedback.

Appendix F

Extraversion

To Increase	To Decrease
Take a training seminar on assertiveness skills (broken-record technique, smoke screens, I-messages).	Keep a journal or diary as a means of developing your writing habit.
Read from the assertiveness-training literature.	Develop the habit of writing letters to your family or customers or letters of recognition to employees.
Read and digest Martin Seligman's *Learned Optimism* as a way to use explanatory style as a tool for developing more positive emotional responses.	Schedule a daily time for reading and/or writing.
Read Maureen Guirdham's *Interpersonal Skills at Work* (1995); it is a bit more academic than some approaches but provides some helpful models for the more thoughtful reader.	Schedule a few hours daily (for example, from 8:00 to 10:00 A.M.) during which you take no calls or visits and essentially work "behind closed doors." Have a co-worker protect this time by fending off would-be invaders!
Read Stephen P. Robbins's *Training in Interpersonal Skills* (1996); it contains self-assessment exercises, key concepts, and skill development methods.	Get a laptop computer and start a computer-based project, such as writing a biography of a family member, developing a database on a particular topic, or organizing your memoirs.

Openness

To Increase	To Decrease
Read Chapters Twenty-Nine through Thirty-One (all deal with the nature of creativity and how to develop it).	Develop a reward system that discourages unfocused exploration and encourages people to increase knowledge and expertise in a more restricted area.
Attend one of the many creativity workshops available, such as Charleen Swansea's "MindWorks."	Develop short-term lists.
Become familiar with the works of E. Paul Torrance (for example, Torrance, 1974).	Prepare a feedback system for short-term projects.
Learn the Synectics problem-solving technique.	Do volunteer work with groups—for example, Habitat for Humanity—that include people who are more practical and down-to-earth than you.
Practice brainstorming with two or three others.	Attend Stephen Covey's seminars to bring reality into the planning.
Join groups or activities that have values different from yours.	Limit the number of projects or interests you have so that you can prioritize them and begin to reach a sense of closure.
Ask for special projects that focus on the future.	
Develop the habit of playing "What if . . . ?"	

Agreeableness

To Increase	To Decrease
Read books on negotiation skills, such as *Getting to Yes: Negotiating Agreement Without Giving In* (R. Fisher and W. Ury, 1991).	Read *Women's Ways of Knowing* (Belenky, Clinchy, Goldberger, and Tarule, 1997).
Find a role model to serve as your coach or mentor and give ongoing feedback.	Take assertiveness-training courses or read books on the subject.
Practice using neutral, open-ended questions rather than declarative statements.	Find a coach who is moderately less agreeable than you—that is, a negotiator.
Identify the more abrasive words that you use and practice substituting less abrasive ones.	Learn to recognize early on when you are losing control of the momentum, then reassert yourself and state what you need.
Resist "shooting the messenger."	Practice assertive behaviors in nonthreatening, safe situations—for example, around children or strangers.
Pull back; redirect your energy by "putting it in writing."	Read books such as R. Fisher and W. Ury's *Getting to Yes* (1991) or attend seminars on negotiation skills.
Develop the ability to read the body language of others; this will help you to detect when you've intimidated someone who is unable to respond verbally.	Read and discuss Sisela Bok's *Lying* (1979).
Find someone to give you feedback on how you affect others who are important to you.	Whenever you hear people tell you what's important to them, automatically think to yourself: "Well, what's important to me in this situation is . . ." When what's important to you is clear, express it to the others.
Practice listening without interrupting until the speaker has clearly finished. Read Tony Hillerman's novel *Coyote Waits* for the importance of not interrupting in Navajo culture.	Intentionally select partners you can beat, whether at sports, cards, or business. Gradually increase your skill level and your competition.
Learn and practice the "talking stick" listening exercise. The talking stick is a Native American tradition in which some object, such as a feather or a pipe, is designated as the talking stick, and only the person holding the stick may talk. Others cannot talk until they have the stick in hand.	

Conscientiousness

To Increase	To Decrease
Identify an appropriate time management system (also called a personal organizer), such as the Franklin/Covey or DayTimer, and learn how to use it and adhere to it.	Read Bryan Robinson's *Work Addiction* (1989).
Set attainable goals for yourself and establish a reward system for attaining those goals.	Have your child call you at the office once a day and have a good chat.
	Call a friend and chat with no specific agenda in mind.
Read Stephen Covey's *Seven Habits of Highly Effective People* and implement the suggestions; attend one of his workshops.	Reprioritize your values and activities to provide for greater balance between work and leisure.
Engage in competitive activities or sports with someone you have a reasonable chance of beating.	Set a time to go home and make the next day's "to-do" list before going home.
	Perform relaxation exercises fourteen minutes each day.
Ask a partner to regularly help you to set priorities and hold you accountable for sticking to them.	Increase the portion of your responsibilities that you can delegate both at home and at work.

Appendix G

Compensating for the Five Dimensions

Negative Emotionality

If You Think You're Too High	If You Think You're Too Low
Invite significant others or co-workers to sit down with you after an outburst and rethink the outcome of the outburst.	Schedule a time to offer feedback to people whose relationship with you is particularly important, so that they'll know better where they stand in relation to you.
Negotiate with your team or partner to legitimize the value of your giving constructive criticism that comes naturally.	Invite members of your team or family who are high in Negative Emotionality to play the role of moderate opposer.
If you feel you are too self-conscious, try going in disguise to settings in which you would otherwise be uncomfortable.	Solicit the observations and feedback of more reactive people who can provide an insight into your blind side.

Extraversion

If You Think You're Too High	If You Think You're Too Low
Use the round-robin technique and only say one thing per turn.	Delegate the responsibility for leading meetings to someone who is more extraverted than you.
Allow others to talk first.	Station yourself near food and drink.
Time yourself so that you talk no longer in a group than the total time divided by the number of people (for example, in a half-hour meeting of six people, talk no more than five minutes).	Think of specific things to say or questions to ask ahead of time.
	To get comfortable, find someone you know right away.
If it has been said, don't say it again.	Get with an Extravert, and keep the group small.
Don't expect everyone close to you to have your same need for stimulation; find appropriate partners.	Make it a point to speak with a minimum number of people.
	Don't speak first; get your thoughts organized and even prepare notes.
	Commit to having lunch with someone weekly.

Openness

If You Think You're Too High	If You Think You're Too Low
Frequently ask others to evaluate your current "to-do" list as an aid in focusing on the areas with maximum benefit to your goals.	Bounce ideas off a person who is high in Openness.
	Delegate idea generation to those who are higher in Openness.

Agreeableness

If You Think You're Too High	If You Think You're Too Low
Avoid surrounding yourself with Challengers; you'll end up either a doormat or a second-class citizen.	Practice asking others something like "What are three things you don't like about this plan?"
Delegate the leader role to others.	Occasionally eliminate yourself from decision making and abide by the group's decision.
Invite others to raise questions.	Choose Negotiators as leaders.

Conscientiousness

If You Think You're Too High	If You Think You're Too Low
Have a child call you at the office to remind you to go home.	Align yourself with a job or other setting that does not require ambition or responsibility.
Engage in planning to ensure maximum delegation: examine everything on your list and identify what others can or should do; then delegate tasks (or train or orient others and then delegate).	Find crutches for organizing, such as having a secretary, assistant, or computer remind you to focus on a schedule or other priorities.
Hire extra help for home or office.	Avoid being around too many people of either extreme in Conscientiousness.
Commit to regular (noncompetitive) aerobic exercise.	

Complete Listing of Rapport and Influence Strategies

Trait	Rapport and Influence Strategies That Tend to Be Most Effective with People with Specific Traits	
Resilient *(Low Negative Emotionality)*	Use a setting that is fresh, with appropriate background stimulation (for example, a park). Avoid excessive distances (for example, take the closer chair). Use logic and reasonableness.	Make your limits clear. Do not interrupt Resilients. Use a problem-solving method or structure. Ask how Resilients see the alternatives; build on mutual ones.
Reactive *(High Negative Emotionality)*	Minimize distractions (noise, music, activity). Maximize the distance between you; avoid the closer chair. Appeal to Reactives' pride in their organization or family. Take Reactives' stress seriously but not personally.	Minimize your reliance on logic and reasonableness. Emphasize what's in it for them. Show the appropriate emotion to support your position. Illustrate that what you want will minimize their worry.
Introvert *(Low Extraversion)*	Rely on memos, letters, and E-mail. Try to match Introverts when their energy level is lower than yours. Don't rush Introverts; give them time to readjust. Allow or even initiate a move toward greater privacy. Resist your urge to draw other people in. Use ample visual cues. Use nonphysical rewards (for example, an honorary degree).	Allow time for Introverts to read and have moments of silence. Don't get too close physically. Appeal to an Introvert's uniqueness as a person. Avoid sexual and aggressive humor; use subtlety. Remind Introverts of the names of things. Ensure that they don't become overstimulated. Give Introverts written material to review before meetings.
Extravert *(High Extraversion)*	Go out for a meal. Feel free to telephone. Meet with two or more people at a time. Don't assume that Extraverts want privacy (for example, don't assume that they would like to close their door during a conference). Hold frequent face-to-face meetings.	Enjoy small talk if Extraverts initiate it. Try to match Extraverts' high energy in a genuine way (if they stand, you stand; if they walk, you walk; and so on). Appeal to an Extravert's sense of responsibility. Use the promise of physical rewards, such as sports tickets or dinner certificates.
Preserver *(Low Openness)*	Emphasize the tried-and-true. Walk Preservers through your proposal or idea step-by-step (use flowcharts). Play up to the Preserver's need to compete and win. Don't waste a Preserver's time; be specific and give examples. Emphasize the simple and easy-to-use aspects of your proposal or idea. Refer to established companies who've used your product, service, or idea. Emphasize the positive impact on efficiency.	Use mainstream humor, but in general be serious. Avoid appealing to novelty and curiosity. Avoid a complex vocabulary that is not common to a Preserver's specialty. Appeal to established, traditional values. Emphasize conformity with policies and procedures. Appeal to a Preserver's distrust of newfangled notions. Emphasize immediate returns and the payoff.

Appendix H

Trait	Rapport and Influence Strategies That Tend to Be Most Effective with People with Specific Traits	
Explorer (*High Openness*)	Do not oversimplify. Refer to the individuals who developed the idea. Emphasize the uniqueness of the idea or product. Use metaphors to describe it. Take your time. Let Explorers take credit where possible. Appreciate an Explorer's unusual sense of humor.	Refer to the theory behind the application. Appeal to an Explorer's need to innovate. Avoid concentrating on details (give the big picture first). Ask questions about an Explorer's opinions and ideas. Get agreement on specifics, yet be prepared for Explorers to change their mind. Appeal to their curiosity; use reason and logic.
Challenger (*Low Agreeableness*)	Push for closure on the basis of bottom-line results. Emphasize the logical tightness of your position. Be sure to do what you say you will. Have alternatives drawn up with plans for each.	Encourage Challengers' criticisms and build on their skepticism. Build on their need to win and to be right. Avoid references to consideration for others. Don't take apparent belligerence personally; be flexible.
Adapter (*High Agreeableness*)	Emphasize how specific groups of people will react. Show how your agenda relates to human values. Push for closure on the basis of the impact on people. Inquire about an Adapter's family, hobbies, and so on. Emphasize your trustworthiness.	Emphasize the ethical rightness of your proposal. Take time to develop a relationship. Adapters tend to defer; hence, ask questions that draw them out. Emphasize how your proposal will help others. Elicit sympathy and empathy.
Flexible (*Low Conscientiousness*)	Help Flexibles identify what they need to make a decision. Emphasize your flexibility. Summarize the discussion frequently. Be patient if Flexibles make you wait or make you late. Permit yourself to be spontaneous; don't rush them.	Don't insist on your agenda when they want to veer from it. Help Flexibles to manage their time and priorities. Be willing to wander off in new and different directions. Emphasize the pleasurable aspects of your position. Appeal to a Flexible's role as a consultant and adviser.
Focused (*High Conscientiousness*)	Be sure to arrive on time or somewhat early. Give plenty of advance warning about changes of plan. Relate to Focused people's good health and record of achievement; identify with their exercise of choice. To avoid a premature decision against your position, agree on steps for follow-up or future meeting dates.	Set goals and a point-by-point agenda for the meeting. Notify a Focused person if you're going to be late. Emphasize good work ethics. Be sensitive to Focused people's need and respect for structure. Use logic, with clearly identified priorities and goals. Emphasize that they are in control.

Guide for Evaluating the Intelligence (Mental Self-Management) of Someone You Are Recruiting or Interviewing.

1. Does this person have the ability to administer a project from beginning to end in compliance with project requirements (cost, time, quality, and so on)?

    a. Interview evidence:

    b. Reference evidence:

2. Does this person have the ability to scan relevant resources and obtain accurate, current, relevant, and effective information to use in solving problems? Include habits and attitudes toward reading (using the library, periodicals, books, and so on), using Internet "search engines," and asking questions (particularly the habit of asking open-ended questions).

    a. Interview evidence:

    b. Reference evidence:

3. Does this person show flexibility in selecting problem-solving strategies? Through interviews or paper-and-pencil tests, determine the level of rigidity in choosing to alter self, others, or the situation in solving problems.

    a. Interview evidence:

    b. Reference evidence:

    c. Test evidence (Tacit Knowledge Inventory, Hersey-Blanchard Situational Leadership Inventory, or other measures of flexibility or rigidity found in multidimensional instruments):

4. Does this person have the ability to plan a sequence of events in a logical, effective manner?

    a. Interview evidence (ask about time management practices, use of tickler files, and use of various planning techniques; look at the individual's "calendars," such as daily agendas):

    b. Reference evidence:

    c. In-basket exercise (this shows the ability to prioritize a diverse set of documents):

Appendix I

5. Does this person have the ability to be appropriately creative?

   a. Interview evidence:

   b. Reference evidence:

   c. Test evidence (using multidimensional or single-dimension tests):

6. Does this person have the ability to execute through fluent use of words, numbers, and other tools?

   a. Test evidence (from the Wunderlich Personnel Test or some other similar test):

   b. Artifactual evidence (sample reports, drawings, and so on):

   c. Interview evidence (the ability to grasp complex patterns and concepts presented in organizational reports, charts, spread-sheets, and so on):

Personal Checklist for Intelligent Behaviors

This self-evaluation is based on Robert Sternberg's theory of intelligence presented in Chapter Twenty-Two. More intelligent people will answer affirmatively to many of the items in all of the sections. Consider increasing your "intelligent behavior" repertoire in any section in which you check few or no items.

1. Administrative Behaviors

_____ a. Do I keep a prioritized "to-do" list?

_____ b. Do I use a tickler file?

_____ c. Do I take time to evaluate my progress toward goals?

_____ d. Do I regularly solicit feedback from others on how I'm doing?

_____ e. Am I aware of my weaknesses, and do I delegate to compensate for them?

_____ f. Do I consciously devote resources to developing in areas that need improvement?

_____ g. Do I keep myself in good condition and full of energy?

2. Research Behaviors

_____ a. Do I regularly read periodicals that are relevant to my goals?

_____ b. Do I regularly read sections of the newspaper that are relevant to my goals?

_____ c. Do I scan the television schedules (especially of public or educational stations) for programs of value to my goals, and then either view them or tape them for future viewing?

_____ d. Do I visit and use one or more libraries regularly?

_____ e. Do I call reference librarians with my questions, and do I use the research capabilities of the Internet?

_____ f. Do I practice the art of asking open-ended questions to all the significant people in my life?

_____ g. Do I attend seminars and courses to update my knowledge and skills?

Appendix J

3. Problem-Solving Behaviors

Altering self

_____ a. Do I learn new skills or bodies of knowledge?

_____ b. Do I consciously try to improve old skills or bodies of knowledge?

_____ c. Do I discontinue ineffective habits?

_____ d. Do I consult a therapist or counselor when the need arises?

_____ e. Do I ask for feedback from the significant people in my life, then act on it by changing my behavior or habits when appropriate?

Altering others

_____ a. Am I a consistently good listener?

_____ b. Do I take the time to train others when they need training?

_____ c. Do I consciously make an effort to be a helper when others have problems?

_____ d. Do I offer sufficient praise and encouragement to others?

_____ e. Do I take the time to give nonblameful, constructive criticism when it is needed? Do I allow time to discuss corrective measures?

_____ f. When conflict arises, do I take the time to discuss its causes and to explore possible solutions?

Altering the situation

_____ a. Do I know when to call it quits?

_____ b. Can I let go of existing ways of doing things and explore new, improved designs or processes?

_____ c. Do I regularly observe others' ways of accomplishing tasks similar to mine with an eye out for how I might change my situation for the better?

4. Planning Behaviors

_____ a. Do I take the time to map out complex projects using tools such as timelines, PERT charts, or Gantt charts?

_____ b. Do I take the time to test my project design or outline before actually implementing it by using potential problem analysis (Kepner and Tregoe, 1981), visualization techniques, simulations, modeling, and other tools?

_____   c. Do I start a project with the end in mind and then determine the best way to get there?

5. Creativity Behaviors

_____   a. Do I practice the habit of seeing old patterns in new ways (for example, seeing the half-empty glass as half-full, or letting go of old perceptual sets)?

_____   b. Do I occasionally let go of old skills or ways of doing things and explore new, different, and possibly improved ways?

_____   c. Do I ask W. Edwards Deming's question: "What can I do to improve, today?"

_____   d. Do I tolerate ambiguity long enough to explore effective resolutions? (Or do I jump to find answers?)

_____   e. Do I enjoy trying to understand complex situations?

_____   f. Can I keep my options open long enough to find the best one?

_____   g. Can I suspend judgment while exploring ideas?

_____   h. Do I resist peer and social pressure to conform?

6. Execution Behaviors

_____   a. Do I look up words when I don't know them?

_____   b. Do I work puzzles such as crossword puzzles and math riddles?

_____   c. Do I take pride in having my presentations show careful crafting?

_____   d. Do I regularly edit my work for accuracy, completeness, and effectiveness?

_____   e. Do I watch for feedback during my presentations and alter my behavior according to the feedback?

_____   f. Do I ask for feedback after my presentations and incorporate suggestions into future presentations?

_____   g. In general, am I genuinely interested in improving myself in most facets of my being?

Checklist for the Self-Evaluation of Learning Practices

_____ 1. Do I design activities aimed at helping students remember what they are learning?

_____ 2. Do I periodically check with learners to see if they remember what they've learned in an earlier session?

_____ 3. Do I consciously assess my learning environment for stressors and attempt to keep it as stress-free as possible?

_____ 4. Do I provide learners with an opportunity to organize new learning into a form that is meaningful to them?

_____ 5. Do I provide learners with opportunities to rehearse or practice their newly acquired information as an aid in converting it to long-term memory?

_____ 6. Do I administer tests as a means to encourage learning?

_____ 7. Do I help learners to identify preexisting schemas that could help or hinder new learning?

_____ 8. Do I provide opportunities for learners to apply new learnings to situations that are meaningful to them?

_____ 9. Do I ensure that distractions are eliminated so learners can focus on the subject at hand?

_____ 10. Do I maintain appropriately high expectations for all my learners?

_____ 11. Do I expect and measure mastery on the part of all my learners?

_____ 12. Do I use a variety of methods and materials, resisting the temptation to use printed materials alone?

_____ 13. Do I communicate with learners ahead of time to prepare them for what they are about to learn?

_____ 14. Do I avoid trying to cover too many different lessons at one sitting by spacing lessons for maximum retention?

_____ 15. Do I allow and encourage both scheduled and spontaneous breaks?

_____ 16. Do I build follow-up for previous sessions into my lesson plans as well as pointing to follow-up for the current session?

Appendix K

_____ 17. Do I solicit learner feedback and respond appropriately?

_____ 18. Do I practice effective listening skills with learners?

_____ 19. Do I consciously do things to establish better rapport with learners?

_____ 20. Do I engage in specific activities at the beginning of each session that help learners feel at ease?

_____ 21. Do I vary my voice, posture, gestures, and location enough to prevent learners from habituating to me?

_____ 22. Do I consciously do things to enhance my prestige and respect with the learners?

_____ 23. Do I ensure that the learning environment has sufficient visual, tactile, and auditory stimulation to keep learners alert?

_____ 24. Do I provide opportunities for learners to get feedback from their peers?

_____ 25. Do I introduce new concepts with both an experiential-narrative approach and a rational-expository approach?

_____ 26. Do I assist my students in identifying how they can be more effective in their study strategies?

_____ 27. Do I allow students the opportunity to explain their answers?

_____ 28. After introducing new concepts or skills, do I allow time for them to settle in (with breaks, practice, review, and elaboration of familiar material) before introducing other new concepts or skills?

Brainstorming

Goals

1. To generate an extensive number of ideas or solutions to a problem by suspending criticism and evaluation

2. To develop skills in creative problem solving

Group Size

Any number of small groups composed of approximately six participants each

Materials

Newsprint and felt-tipped marker for each group

Procedure

1. The facilitator forms small groups of approximately six participants each. Each group selects a secretary.

2. The facilitator instructs each group to form a circle. He or she provides newsprint and a felt-tipped marker for each secretary and asks the secretary to record every idea generated by the group.

3. The facilitator states the following rules:
    a. There will be no criticism during the brainstorming phase.
    b. Farfetched ideas are encouraged because they may trigger more practical ideas.
    c. Many ideas are desirable. Go for quantity, not quality.
    d. Let others' ideas suggest new ideas to you; "piggyback" on their ideas.

4. The facilitator announces the topic, for example, "How could we reduce costs?" She or he tells the groups that they have five or ten minutes to generate ideas.

5. At the end of the generating phase, the facilitator tells the groups that the ban on criticism is over, then directs them to evaluate their ideas and to select the best ones.

Appendix L

Brainwriting

A procedure for generating ideas, brainwriting is a form of brainstorming. It is particularly useful in more introverted groups with less outward verbal energy.

Procedure

1. Each member of the group makes a list of ideas that address the issue at hand. The groups are directed to go for quantity, not quality, and to refrain from talking.

2. After five to ten minutes, the members pass their papers to the member on their left. They then read the items on their new list and allow these items to "suggest" new items, which are added to the list.

3. This continues until each member has had an opportunity to read and add ideas to each of the other lists.

4. The lists are circulated and some voting system is used to evaluate the ideas, for example, one to five stars. The scores are tallied and the top ten or so ideas are written on the board for everyone to see. The group continues to evaluate the ideas, either by consensus or by a rational decision analysis process, such as the Five-Step Rational Decision Analysis (Plunkett and Hale, 1982; Kepner and Tregoe, 1981) or the Precedence Chart (Saaty, 1982).

Appendix M

Definitions

Acetylcholine. A neurotransmitter released in the neuron that is essential to the health of the neuronal membrane itself and to learning and memory; it is derived from fat in the diet.

Action potential. An electrical charge in response to a stimulus that is strong enough to result in the release of neurotransmitters at the synapse; a basic measure of neural activity. See also Amplitude; Latency.

Adrenaline. See Epinephrine.

Agonist. A drug that mimics (that is, can occupy the same receptor sites as and send the same signals as) a particular neurotransmitter (for example, sumatriptan is an agonist for serotonin); the opposite of an antagonist.

Amino acids. This family of twenty major compounds (each containing one carboxyl molecule –COOH) comprises the alphabet of life. Various combinations of amino acids form "peptide chains." Chains of fewer than about one hundred amino acid molecules are peptides. Chains of more than one hundred but fewer than about two hundred are polypeptides. Proteins are peptide chains comprised of some two hundred or more amino acid molecules. The amino acid molecules are

Cystine	L-histidine	L-serine
DL-alanine	L-hydroxyprolin	L-tryptophan
Glycine	L-isoleucine	L-tyrosine
L-arginine	L-leucine	L-valine
L-asparagine	L-lysine	Methionine
L-aspartic acid	L-phenylalanine	Threonine
L-glutamic acid	L-proline	

Amplitude. The height of the wave resulting from measuring action potential; a measure of the amount of neural resources brought to bear on a particular stimulus. See also Latency.

Androgens. The family of male sex hormones (and drugs), the most familiar of which is testosterone; their level in the body is associated with degree of male gender characteristics, from body hair to aggression. It is present in both males and females but is usually higher in males.

Antagonist. A drug that blocks the receptor site for a particular neurotransmitter. The opposite of an agonist.

Antioxidant. A natural chemical with the capability for neutralizing free radicals, such as vitamins A, B-1, B-5, B-6, C, E, and beta-carotene; selenium and zinc; and uric acid.

Arousal. The level of activity of a bodily system: high limbic arousal indicates a rapid pulse, for example, and low limbic arousal suggests a far slower pulse. The absence of arousal is associated with sleep.

Attention. The capacity to focus the senses on a specific stimulus source; it is only possible to focus on one stimulus source at a time. When we appear to be focusing on two sources simultaneously (for example, using a car phone and driving), we are actually alternating attention. Attempting to focus on more than one stimulus source increases error-proneness, unless one of the perceptual activities is completely routinized (we can suck a mint and drive at the same time).

Attributional style. The manner in which an individual attributes the causes of success or failure; it is usually described as either external (the causes are outside the individual, such as luck or sour grapes) or internal (the causes are inside the individual, such as hard work or talent). Also called explanatory style and locus of control.

Automatic behavior. See Automatization.

Automation. See Automatization.

Automatization. The process by which a new learning becomes automatic or routine; it refers to a skill or behavior that requires intense attentional focus when it is first learned but eventually demands little or no attentional focus, as in learning to tie one's shoes. Also called automation and automization.

Automatizer. Said of a person who can perform routine and repetitive activities for long periods with relatively little fatigue; associated with higher levels of testosterone. Also called automizer.

Automization. See Automatization.

Automizer. See Automatizer.

Average evoked potential (AEP). The printed wave that represents the average of many actual waves; it is described in terms of its amplitude and latency.

Axon. The connective branch of a neuron that conveys messages through the synapse to other neurons.

Behaviorism. A school of psychology popular through the 1960s that maintained a monistic view of the mind-brain, saying that humans display no mental activity between stimulus and response. Behaviorism is associated with B. F. Skinner and J. B. Watson; it is also called stimulus-response psychology. It has generally been replaced today by cognitive psychology.

Binding. The process in which a ligand leaves its axonic terminal, enters its dedicated receptor, and remains long enough to send its chemical message on its way. Candace Pert calls it "sex on a molecular level."

Biofeedback. Information about a bodily function; it is used in biofeedback training to gain personal control over that function.

Blocker. Generally speaking, any chemical that prevents passage of a neurotransmitter at the synapse.

Blood-brain barrier. A kind of membrane that surrounds the brain through which blood vessels feeding the brain must pass. At the point of entry, unwanted chemicals are turned back physically, electrically, or chemically. Only a select few chemicals, such as oxygen and sugar, may enter the brain.

Brain attack. Another (and more current) name for stroke.

Calpain. A neurotransmitter associated with efficiency of synaptic transmission. It is a calcium-activated intracellular proteinase.

Catecholamine. A family of neurotransmitters that includes dopamine, norepinephrine, and epinephrine.

Cerebral cortex. The part of the brain associated with rational thought; the most recent to appear, evolution-wise. Also called the cerebrum.

Chemotaxis. The capacity of a cell with, for example, receptor "X," to detect the presence of chemical "X" at some distance and then move itself (chemotax) toward the concentration of that chemical. Along with synaptic transmission, chemotaxis is the complementary process for intercellular communication.

Cholecystokinin (CCK). A neurotransmitter influential in controlling appetite. It is found at lower levels in bulimia cases.

Chunk. A single element of learning or memory; chunks are pieced together to create memories.

Classical conditioning. The learning procedure in which a neutral stimulus (a stimulus that does not elicit any particular response, such as a ringing bell) precedes an unconditioned stimulus (a stimulus that elicits a predictable response, as when red meat causes a dog to salivate) and thereby becomes a conditioned response (the dog starts salivating after hearing the bell and before seeing meat); the meat is said to have been "associated to" the bell.

Cognitive dissonance. The situation that occurs when a person's behavior (for example, eating snails and enjoying them) conflicts with his or her attitude toward that behavior (the person believes that snails are disgusting).

Cognitive psychology. The study of how the mind performs its operations, such as perception, judgment, memory, and problem solving; the term is typically used in opposition to the term *behavioral psychology,* which, in its purest form, denies that the mind performs any operations, but rather only hooks stimuli together with their responses. See also Behaviorism.

Cognitive therapy. The practice of changing the way a person thinks about the world for the purpose of improving her or his mental health.

Commissurotomy. A surgical procedure in which the corpus callosum is severed.

Comorbid, comorbidity. The situation that occurs when two diseases or disorders tend to occur together in the same person; for example, coronary heart disease is often comorbid with depression.

Corpus callosum. A bundle of neurons that connects and permits communication between the two hemispheres of the brain.

Cortex. The outer layer of a bodily organ. From the Latin *cortex,* or bark (of a tree). See also Cerebral cortex.

Cortisol. A hormone produced by the adrenal gland that contributes to sympathetic arousal and the general adaptation syndrome. See also Hydrocortisol.

Dehydroepiandrosterone. See DHEA.

Dementia. A disease (also called senility) characterized by disinterest in life, disorientation, carelessness, and personality changes. It is often associated—wrongly—with aging, but it should be distinguished from age-related disorders.

Dendrite. The connective branching of the neuron that receives messages across the synapse from other neurons.

Deoxyribonucleic acid. See DNA.

DHEA (dehydroepiandrosterone). A steroid called the "mother steroid" because it metabolizes into estrogen, testosterone, and other steroids; the levels naturally produced at age eighty are about 10 percent of the levels at age twenty-five.

DNA (deoxyribonucleic acid). The molecular basis of heredity found in cell nuclei.

Dopamine. One of the neurotransmitters associated with mood and movement.

DSM-IV. *Diagnostic and Statistical Manual of Mental Disorders,* fourth edition, the book that is the American Psychiatric Association's authority for the diagnosis of mental disorders.

Dualism. The theory that the mind and brain are two separate entities that act independent of one another.

Dvorak keyboard. A redesigned keyboard in which the most frequently used keys are assigned to the strongest fingers, to increase speed and accuracy and reduce fatigue. See also Qwerty keyboard.

Electroencephalograph (EEG). An instrument that places the business end of electrodes at various locations on the scalp, with the other end attached to a moving graph. Electrical impulses at each electrode location are recorded in real time on the graph paper.

Endorphins. Neurotransmitters that are triggered by aerobic exercise, pain, and laughter and that result in a noticeably pleasurable sensation, as in "runner's high."

Epinephrine. A hormone and neurotransmitter produced by the adrenal gland that is associated with sympathetic arousal. Also called adrenaline.

Epistemology. The branch of philosophy that studies the structure of knowledge.

Estrogens. The family of female sex hormones that is responsible for the development of female sexual characteristics, from reproduction to calmness.

Evoked potential. An electroencephalographic measure of a neural impulse in response to a controlled stimulus; it may take the form of a light flash or an audible beep.

Explanatory style. See Attributional style.

Extrinsic motivation. The condition in which an activity is performed in expectation of rewards that are controlled by someone other than oneself, such as a teacher, boss, or parent. See also Intrinsic motivation.

Fight-or-flight syndrome. See General adaptation syndrome.

Free radicals. Molecules with an unpaired electron. They are unstable, seeking any other unpaired electron in their path, whether it is an element of DNA in the cell nucleus or antioxidants from your daily dose of broccoli. If an antioxidant is available, then the free radical will clutch it in an eternal embrace, leaving the DNA undisturbed.

GABA (gamma aminobutyric acid). An inhibiting neurotransmitter; low levels are associated with proneness to violence. Valium is a catalyst for GABA.

Gamma aminobutyric acid. See GABA.

GAS. See General adaptation syndrome.

General adaptation syndrome (GAS). The condition in which the body reacts to stress through activation of the sympathetic nervous system in preparation for having to fight, flee, or freeze. Also called the fight-or-flight syndrome.

Glial cells. Cells that support the networked structure of neurons; a kind of skeleton for the nervous system.

Gray matter. The outer covering of the brain.

Habituation. A loss of sensitivity resulting from a prolonged pattern of stimulation; for example, the steady blinking of a neon sign will soon become unnoticeable (we habituate to it), but a randomly blinking light will keep our attention.

Hard-wired. In computerese, said of a program that is built into the computer and can't be changed without major surgery. In brain lingo, the term refers to behaviors, traits, and instincts that we are born with.

Hemisphericity. The division of the cerebrum into two hemispheres, the right and the left. The right hemisphere is associated with more creative and holistic processes, such as painting and music; the left hemisphere is associated with more linear and rational processes, such as language and mathematics. See also Left-brained and Right-brained.

Homeostasis. A state that exists when all the body's elements and systems are present and operating in ideal amounts and balance. It is disturbed by stressors; chemicals such as glucocorticoids and adrenaline are released in order to permit restoration of homeostasis.

Hormones. Substances (typically peptides or steroids) made by one tissue that move to another tissue in order to perform a specific function.

Hydrocortisol. The pharmaceutical version of cortisol.

Hypothalamus. A part of the limbic system that is regarded as the body's main thermostat; it coordinates basic metabolism and related functions and the alternation between sympathetic and parasympathetic arousal.

Immunoglobulin A (IgA). A protective antibody; the immune system's first line of defense against all diseases.

Intrinsic motivation. The condition in which an activity is performed for its own enjoyment, with no expectation of rewards from other people. See also Extrinsic motivation.

Ischemia. A more technical name for stroke.

Latency. The width of the wave that measures action potential; a measure of the speed of response.

Left-brained. A figure of speech that refers to the more linear and logical processes associated with the left cerebral hemisphere. Acknowledging the left brain means paying attention to one's need for logic and reason. See also Hemisphericity.

Ligand. A substance (either natural or produced in a laboratory) that binds—for a brief time—to specific receptors on the surface of a cell and thereby transfers information. The three types of ligands are neurotransmitters, steroids, and peptides.

Limbic system. The portion of the midbrain (including the hippocampus, amygdala, hypothalamus, and olfactory area) that is associated with activating the general adaptation syndrome, or preparing the body for fight or flight. It is the main housing of emotional functions and has the densest concentration of endorphin receptors.

Linkage study. In genetics, a study designed to find chromosomal patterns that are common to all family members who exhibit a particular trait across the generations.

Locus of control. See Attributional style.

Massed learning. An approach to learning in which a single topic of instruction is executed without significant interruptions (or "spaces") between modules; it is the opposite of spaced learning.

Melatonin. A neurotransmitter originating in the pineal gland (a metabolite of serotonin) whose production is suppressed by natural light. It plays a key role in setting the body clock and in sleep onset and is available in pill form.

Mentation. A shorter expression than (but meaning the same thing as) mental activity.

Meta-analysis. A statistical technique in which a large number of separate studies on the same subject are analyzed for patterns.

Metabolite. In metabolism, something (the metabolite) that is the product of something else (the precursor). For example, serotonin is the precursor of melatonin and melatonin is the metabolite of serotonin. Serotonin comes first, then melatonin.

Microsleep. A brief period of loss of consciousness that is not restorative like a nap but is a signal of loss of control of consciousness; the result of sleep deprivation.

Modular perspective. See Molar perspective.

Molar perspective. A big-picture, or top-down, look at a subject, as in studying the behaviors associated with a personality trait; the opposite of molecular perspective. Also called modular perspective.

Molecular perspective. A microscopic, or bottom-up, look at a subject, as in studying the body chemistry associated with personality traits; the opposite of molar perspective.

Monism. The view that brain and mind are one and the same, or that spirit cannot exist independent of matter.

Monoamine oxidase (MAO). An enzyme that breaks down some neurotransmitters, including serotonin, norepinephrine, and dopamine. Two variants of MAO exist: MAO-A and MAO-B. MAO-A is found in serotonin- and norepinephrine-secreting cells, and MAO-B is found in dopamine-secreting cells.

Monoamine oxidase inhibitor (MAO-I). A drug that prevents MAO from breaking down neurotransmitters, with the effect of raising levels of those neurotransmitters; used as an antidepressant.

Monozygotic twins. Twins that develop from one single fertilized egg and possess an identical genetic structure.

Myelin sheath. The coating of the neural fiber; the thicker it is, the more efficient the neural transmission. Poor nutrition prevents normal myelin development.

Negative feedback. In neurophysiology, the tendency of a system that has changed to return to a normal state, as when a fire is doused; this happens with the general adaptation syndrome. See also Positive feedback.

Nerve growth factor (NGF). One of many trophic agents; it is released as a result of neural transmission and supports the growth of neural processes.

Neurolinguistic programming (NLP). The theory that people are programmed to communicate through one or more of three channels—visual, auditory, or kinesthetic—and can communicate more effectively by matching another person's preferred channel.

Neuron. A nerve cell; its major parts are the nucleus, axon, and dendrite.

Neuropeptide. Any of a large group of peptides that act as neurotransmitters; they are involved particularly in emotions, hunger (for example, cholecystokinin), pain (for example, endorphins), and sleep (for example, melatonin).

Neuropharmacology. The study of the effect of pharmaceuticals on the nervous system.

Neurotransmitter. The smallest of the ligands. Neurotransmitters are often a modification of an amino acid; several are composed of just one amino acid (for example, glycine). These tiny chemical molecules send specific messages across the synapse. Different combinations of neurotransmitters, each of which can exhibit different states (such as weak versus strong), result in different behaviors, thoughts, and emotions.

Neurotrophins. Proteins such as BDNF (brain-derived neurotrophic factor) that are essential to the growth, plasticity, and maintenance of the nervous system—fertilizers, as it were, for the brain.

NGF. See Nerve growth factor.

NLP. See Neurolinguistic programming.

NMDA (N-methyl-D-aspartate). A glutamate essential for neuronal transmission and growth.

N-methyl-D-aspartate. See NMDA.

Nootropics. A family of drugs that purportedly enhance brain structure and function.

Noradrenaline. See Norepinephrine.

Norepinephrine. Like epinephrine, a hormone and neurotransmitter from the adrenal gland that is associated with sympathetic arousal. Also called noradrenaline.

Ontogeny recapitulates phylogeny. This terse phrase states that the development of each individual organism (ontogeny) reproduces the development of its species (phylogeny) from its origins to the present. In other words, during a human embryo's time in the womb, one can trace the stages of development from lizard through ape to human: the reptilian brain is the first to be identified (hindbrain), followed by the mammalian brain (midbrain) and culminating with the human brain (forebrain).

Paradigm. A set of assumptions in a defined area of knowledge that guides both research and applications in that area, such as the assumption in pre-Copernican cosmology that the Earth was at the center of the universe.

Paradigmatic shift. A fundamental change in one or more assumptions in a defined area of knowledge, such as Copernicus's assertion that the Sun, not the Earth, occupies the center of our solar system.

Parasympathetic arousal. See Sympathetic arousal.

Peptide. A compound formed by so-called head-to-tail linkups of two or more amino acids. When about one hundred amino acids are linked, they are called polypeptides; chains of two hundred or more are called proteins. As of 1996, eighty-eight peptides had been identified with from two to over two hundred amino acid links; more await discovery.

Perisylvian region. The region of the brain surrounding the Sylvian fissure. Language activity occurs in this area.

Pharmacotherapy. The treatment of disease, especially mental disease, with drugs.

Phylogeny. See Ontogeny recapitulates phylogeny.

Plasticity. The capacity of the brain to learn, remember, reorganize, and recover from damage.

PNI. See Psychoneuroimmunology.

Polypeptide. A chain of somewhere between one hundred and two hundred amino acids; a polypeptide is larger than a peptide and smaller than a protein.

Positive feedback. In neurophysiology, the tendency of a change in a system to continue increasing in intensity, as in fanning a fire. See also Negative feedback.

Progesterone. A female sex hormone that is associated with preparation of the woman's body to care for a fertilized egg; levels increase at ovulation and decrease at menses.

Proteins. Complex molecules containing (at a minimum) carbon, hydrogen, nitrogen, oxygen, and a variety of amino acids that are connected by peptide bonds.

Proto-oncogenes. About one hundred genes that, when activated in certain combinations, cause cancer.

Psychoneuroimmunology (PNI). The study of how the body's immune system is affected by changes in mental and physical states. Its premise is that negative emotions lower resistance to disease antigens and positive emotions increase resistance.

Qwerty keyboard. The traditional keyboard in which the second row from the top begins, from the left side, "q-w-e-r-t-y." See also Dvorak keyboard.

Rapid eye movement (REM). The phase of the sleep cycle that consists of dreaming and motor neuron activity (but without physical movement other than eye movement); it is also called paradoxical sleep, since the motor neuron activity makes it appear on a brain scan that the sleeper is awake.

RAS. See Reticular activating system.

Rational drugs. Drugs based on genetic information about a specific condition.

RDA. Recommended Daily Allowance for specific nutritional categories.

Receptor. A protein on a dendritic terminal that receives a ligand from the axon connected at its synaptic gap; it serves as a kind of lock into which the ligand fits like a key.

Relaxation response. The body's response to an activity, such as meditation or aerobic exercise, that helps to return a stressed or sympathetically aroused person to a more relaxed state (parasympathetic arousal). See also Sympathetic arousal.

REM. See Rapid eye movement.

Reticular activating system (RAS). An area of the brain that acts like a kind of toggle switch, so that when the cerebral cortex is fully functional (relaxing, problem solving, planning, creating) the limbic system (stress response) is not, and vice versa. Under stress, the RAS shuts the cerebral cortex down; in the absence of stress it allows the cerebral cortex to be fully functional.

Reuptake inhibitor. Any chemical agent that prevents a neurotransmitter that has not reached the postsynaptic region from returning to the presynaptic region; it thus keeps the neurotransmitter from being retained for later use, leaving it available for maximum current use.

Ribonucleic acid. See RNA.

Ribosomes. Tiny manufacturing plants in the cell that produce peptides and proteins.

Right-brained. A figure of speech that refers to the more creative and holistic processes associated with the right cerebral hemisphere. Acknowledging the right brain means paying attention to one's creative needs. See also Hemisphericity.

RNA (ribonucleic acid). A copy of DNA in the cell nucleus made by the DNA. RNA migrates to the ribosomes and triggers the production of peptides and proteins. This is analogous to the process in which a computer operating system (like DOS) makes copies of its own key files (with human prompting, of course!).

Routinize. To practice a skill to the point of being able to do it without consciously thinking about it.

SD. See Standard deviation.

Serotonin. A neurotransmitter involved in depression (too little), relaxation and sleep (just right), and aggression (too much); it is associated with vasoconstriction and headache relief; when serotonin metabolizes, melatonin results.

Somatosensory system. The neural process that conveys messages that deal with the bodily sensations of touch and movement.

Spaced learning. An approach to learning in which a single topic of instruction is broken up into modules and scheduled over time with breaks (or "spaces") between modules; it is the opposite of massed learning.

Standard deviation (SD). A measure of the distance from the mean of the scores of members of a group; roughly one-third of a group will score within 1 SD above the mean, another one-third will score within 1 SD below the mean, and the rest will score higher or lower than 1 SD from the mean.

Steroid (also called steroidal hormone). A kind of ligand that starts out as cholesterol, then gets transformed (for example, by an enzyme) into a more specific kind of steroid, such as a hormone from the gonads or the adrenal cortex. Unlike the other two kinds of ligands, steroids engage receptors inside the cell rather than on the cell's surface.

Stimulus-response psychology. See Behaviorism.

Stroke. A brain disorder brought on by reduction of the oxygen supply (from blood flow) to the brain; also called brain attack or ischemia.

Sylvian fissure. The deep indentation, or split, between the temporal lobe and the remainder of the brain.

Sympathetic arousal. Mobilization by the body of its vast energy resources to fight off threat; parasympathetic arousal is the body's return to a more normal, relaxed state. See also General adaptation syndrome; Relaxation response.

Synapse. The point of connection between two neurons. The synapse is the area where a branch of an axon of one neuron has established a connection (they don't actually touch!) with the branch of a dendrite of another neuron. The synapse is the basic unit of learning. Knowledge can be measured by the number of existing synapses; effective use of knowledge is a reflection of their physical condition. The actual space through which neurotransmitters pass from one neuron to another is called the synaptic gap. As with the gap in a spark plug, the adjacent membranes of the axon and dendrite that form the synapse must be clean and healthy.

Synaptic gap. See Synapse.

Synesthesia. The tendency of one sensory system to become excited as a result of the excitation of another sensory system. A common example would be the elicitation of visual memories by listening to music.

Talking therapy. The practice of talking with a therapist for relief of psychological distress; it may be used instead of, or in addition to, drug therapy.

Testosterone. See Androgens.

Trophic. Contributing to growth; nutritional.

Type I, II error. Terms used in research to describe two related cases: when a difference in means is claimed when in fact no difference exists (Type I error) and when an equality of means is claimed when in fact the means are different (Type II error); that is, in Type I, an effect is claimed and none is present, and in Type II, no effect is claimed when one is in fact present.

Vasoconstriction. Shrinkage of the walls of a blood vessel; it is thought to be associated with headache relief. See also Vasodilation.

Vasodilation. Stretching, dilation, or relaxation of the walls of a blood vessel; vasodilation of blood vessels in the brain is associated with the onset of headaches. See also Vasoconstriction.

Visualization. The process of using the mind to review a series of bodily movements such as a downhill ski run or to prepare for an activity such as delivering a speech by giving it without actually going through the bodily movements. Visualization may be accompanied by either a running verbal commentary, some limited physical movement (such as so-called body English), or both. It is usually performed with the eyes closed.

White matter. The inner portion of the brain, covered by the outer gray matter.

Bibliography

Ackerman, D. (1990). *A Natural History of the Senses.* New York: Random House.

Adams, J. L. (1980). *Conceptual Blockbusting: A Guide to Better Ideas* (2nd ed.). New York: Norton.

Adams, J. L. (1986). *The Care and Feeding of Ideas: A Guide to Encouraging Creativity.* Reading, Mass.: Addison-Wesley.

Agor, W. H. (n.d.). "The Use of Hypnosis to Induce Creative Problem Solving." Unpublished manuscript, University of Texas at El Paso.

Agor, W. H. (Ed.). (1989). *Intuition in Organizations: Leading and Managing Productively.* Thousand Oaks, Calif.: Sage.

Albrecht, K. (n.d.). *Mind Mapping: A Tool for Clear Thinking.* San Diego, Calif.: Shamrock. Videotape, 10 minutes.

Alkon, D. L. (1992). *Memory's Voice: Deciphering the Brain-Mind Code.* New York: HarperCollins.

Allison, M. (1991, October). "Stopping the Brain Drain." *Harvard Health Letter, 16,* 6 ff.

Allport, G. W., and Odbert, H. S. (1936). "Trait Names: A Psycho-Lexical Study." *Psychological Monographs, 47*(1, whole no. 211).

Amabile, T. M. (1983). *The Social Psychology of Creativity.* New York: Springer-Verlag.

American Psychiatric Association. (1994). *Diagnostic and Statistical Manual of Mental Disorders* (4th ed.). Washington, D.C.: American Psychiatric Association.

American Psychological Association. (1992). "Ethical Principles of Psychologists and Code of Conduct." *American Psychologist, 47,* 1597–1611.

Anderson, J. R. (1993, January). "Problem Solving and Learning." *American Psychologist, 48*(1), 35–44.

Arkin, A. M., Antrobus, J. S., and Ellman, S. J. (Eds.). (1978). *The Mind in Sleep.* Hillsdale, N.J.: Erlbaum.

Armstrong, T. (1993). *Seven Kinds of Smart: Identifying and Developing Your Many Intelligences.* New York: Plume.

Arnow, B. (1996). "Cognitive-Behavioral Therapy for Bulimia Nervosa." In J. Werne (Ed.), *Treating Eating Disorders.* San Francisco: Jossey-Bass.

Atkins, S. (1978). *LIFO Training: Discovery Workbook.* Beverly Hills, Calif.: Stuart Atkins.

Axel, R. (1995, October). "The Molecular Logic of Smell." *Scientific American,* pp. 154–159.

Bailey, C. (1991). *The New Fit or Fat.* Boston: Houghton Mifflin.

Baker, J. G., Zevon, M. A., and Rounds, J. B. (1994). "Differences in Positive and Negative Affect Dimensions: Latent Trait Analysis." *Personality and Individual Differences, 17*(2), 161–167.

Baldwin, T. T., and Ford, K. (1988). "Transfer of Training: A Review and Directions for Future Research." *Personnel Psychology, 41,* 63–105.

Bales, J. (1991, November). "Work Stress Grows, but Services Decline." *APA Monitor,* p. 32.

Bandler, R., and Grinder, J. (1982). *ReFraming: Neuro-Linguistic Programming and the Transformation of Meaning.* Moab, Utah: Real People Press.

Barker, J. (n.d.). *Discovering the Future.* Burnsville, Minn.: Charthouse International. Videotape.

Bar-On, R. (1996). *Bar-On Emotional Quotient Inventory.* North Tonawanda, N.Y.: Multi-Health Systems.

Barron, F., and Harrington, D. M. (1981). "Creativity, Intelligence, and Personality." *Annual Review of Psychology, 32,* 439–476.

Bartlett, F. C. (1932). *Remembering.* Cambridge: Cambridge University Press.

Basadur, M., Graen, G., and Wakabayashi, M. (1990). "Identifying Differences in Creative Problem Solving Style." *Journal of Creative Behavior, 24*(2), 111–131.

Behn, R. D., and Vaupel, J. W. (1982). *Quick Analysis for Busy Decision Makers.* New York: Basic Books.

Belenky, M. F., Clinchy, B. M., Goldberger, N. R., and Tarule, J. M. (1997). *Women's Ways of Knowing: The Development of Self, Voice, and Mind* (10th anniversary edition). New York: Basic Books.

Bem, D. J. (1996, April). "Exotic Becomes Erotic: A Developmental Theory of Sexual Orientation." *Psychological Review, 103*(2), 320–321.

Bem, S. L. (1993). *The Lenses of Gender: Transforming the Debate on Sexual Inequality.* New Haven: Yale University Press.

Bennett, W. (1991, October). "Obesity Is Not an Eating Disorder." *Harvard Mental Health Letter, 8*(4).

Benson, H., with Klipper, M. Z. (1990). *The Relaxation Response.* New York: Avon.

Biederman, J., and Faraone, S. (1996, Winter). "Attention Deficit Hyperactivity Disorder." *On the Brain* (Harvard Mahoney Neuroscience Institute Letter), pp. 4–7.

Birdwhistell, R. L. (1970). *Kinesics and Context: Essays on Body Motion Communication.* Philadelphia: University of Pennsylvania Press.

Birren, F. (1978a). *Color and Human Response.* New York: Van Nostrand Reinhold.

Birren, F. (1978b). *Color in Your World.* New York: Collier Books.

Bjork, R. (1994). "Memory and Metamemory Considerations in the Training of Human Beings." In J. Metcalfe and A. P. Shimamura (Eds.), *Metacognition: Knowing About Knowing* (pp. 185–206). Cambridge Mass.: MIT Press.

Black, I. B. (1991). *Information in the Brain: A Molecular Perspective.* Cambridge, Mass.: MIT Press.

Blakeslee, S. (1991, September 15). "Study Ties Dyslexia to Brain Flaw Affecting Vision and Other Senses." *New York Times,* Current Events edition, p. 11.

Block, P. (1987). *The Empowered Manager: Positive Political Skills at Work.* San Francisco: Jossey-Bass.

Boden, M. A. (1990). *The Creative Mind: Myths and Mechanisms.* New York: Basic Books.

Bois, J. S. (1966). *The Art of Awareness: A Textbook on General Semantics.* Dubuque, Iowa: W. C. Brown.

Bok, S. (1979). *Lying: Moral Choice in Public and Private Life.* New York: Vintage Books.

Bolles, E. B. (1988). *Remembering and Forgetting: An Inquiry into the Nature of Memory.* New York: Walker.

Bond, J. T., Galinsky, E., and Swanberg, J. E. (1998). *The 1997 National Study of the Changing Workforce.* New York: Families and Work Institute. (See also www.familiesandwork.org.)

Borod, J. (1999). *The Neuropsychology of Emotion.* Oxford: Oxford University Press.

Borysenko, J. (1987). *Minding the Body, Mending the Body.* Reading, Mass.: Addison-Wesley.

Bouchard, C., and Bray, G. A. (Eds.). (1996). *Regulation of Body Weight: Biological and Behavioral Mechanisms.* New York: Wiley.

Bradley, R. H., and Caldwell, B. M. (1984). "The Relation of Infants' Home Environment to Achievement Test Performance in First Grade: A Follow-Up Study." *Child Development, 52,* 708–710.

Bransford, J. D., and Stein, B. S. (1984). *The Ideal Problem Solver.* New York: Freeman.

Brink, S. (1995, May 15). "Smart Moves." *U.S. News & World Report,* pp. 76–85.

Broad, M. L. (Ed.). (1997). *In Action: Transferring Learning to the Workplace.* Alexandria, Va.: American Society for Training and Development.

Broad, M. L., and Newstrom, J. W. (1992). *Transfer of Training: Action-Packed Strategies to Ensure High Payoff from Training Investments.* Reading, Mass.: Addison-Wesley.

Brody, N. (1992). *Intelligence* (2nd ed.). Orlando: Academic Press.

Brown, D. E. (1991). *Human Universals.* New York: McGraw-Hill.

Brown, J. L., and Pollitt, E. (1996, February). "Malnutrition, Poverty and Intellectual Development." *Scientific American,* pp. 38–43.

Brown, W. A. (1998, January). "The Placebo Effect." *Scientific American,* pp. 90–95.

Brownell, K. D., and Rodin, J. (1994, September). "The Dieting Maelstrom: Is It Possible and Advisable to Lose Weight?" *American Psychologist, 49*(9), 781–791.

Brutus, S., Fleenor, J., and London, M. (1998). "Does 360-Degree Feedback Work in Different Industries? A Between-Industry Comparison of the Reliability and Validity of Multi-Source Ratings." *Journal of Management Development, 17,* 177–190.

Bush, B. J. (1986, June). *A Study of Innovative Training Techniques at the Defense Language Institute Foreign Language Center.* Research Report 1426. Alexandria, Va.: U.S. Army Research Institute for the Behavioral and Social Sciences. 25 pp.

Buss, A. H. (1989). "Personality as Traits." *American Psychologist, 44*(11), 1378–1388.

Buss, D. M. (1991). "Evolutionary Personality Psychology." *Annual Review of Psychology, 42,* 459–491.

Buss, D. M. (1994). *The Evolution of Desire.* New York: Basic Books.

Buss, D. M. (Ed.). (1990, March). "Biological Foundations of Personality: Evolution, Behavioral Genetics, and Psychophysiology" [Special Issue]. *Journal of Personality, 58*(1).

Buzan, T. (1991). *Use Your Perfect Memory* (3rd ed.). New York: Penguin Books.

Buzan, T. (1996). *The Mind Map Book.* New York: Plume.

Cacioppo, J. T., and Berntson, G. G. (1992, August). "Social Psychological Contributions to the Decade of the Brain: Doctrine of Multilevel Analysis." *American Psychologist, 47*(8), 1019–1028.

Cacioppo, J. T., and Tassinary, L. G. (Eds.). (1990). *Principles of Psychophysiology: Physical, Social, and Inferential Elements.* Cambridge: Cambridge University Press.

Caine, R. N., and Caine, G. (1991). *Making Connections: Teaching and the Human Brain.* Alexandria, Va.: Association for Supervision and Curriculum Development.

Calvin, W. H. (1996). *How Brains Think: Evolving Intelligence, Then and Now.* New York: Basic Books.

Campbell, B. (1994). *The Multiple Intelligences Handbook: Lesson Plans and More.* Marysville, Wash.: Campbell and Associates.

Campbell, D. (1997). *The Mozart Effect.* New York: Avon.

Campbell, L., Campbell, B., and Dickinson, D. (1996). *Teaching and Learning Through Multiple Intelligences.* Needham Heights, Mass.: Allyn & Bacon.

Campbell, R. J. (1989). *Psychiatric Dictionary* (6th ed.). New York: Oxford University Press.

Caplan, P. J., Crawford, M., Hyde, J. S., and Richardson, J.T.E. (1997). *Gender Differences in Human Cognition.* New York: Oxford University Press.

Caplan, T., and Caplan, F. (1982). *The Second Twelve Months of Life.* New York: Bantam Books.

Caplan, T., and Caplan, F. (1984). *The Early Childhood Years: The Two to Six Year Old.* New York: Bantam Books.

Caplan, T., and Caplan, F. (1995). *The First Twelve Months of Life* (rev. ed.). New York: Bantam Books.

Cappon, D. (1994a). *Intuition and Management: Research and Application.* Westport, Conn.: Quorum Books.

Cappon, D. (1994b). "A New Approach to Intuition: IQ2." *Omni, 16*(12), 34 ff.

Capra, F. (1984). *The Tao of Physics* (2nd ed.). New York: Bantam Books.

Carver, R. (1990). *Reading Rate: A Review of Research and Theory.* Orlando: Academic Press.

Cassandro, V. (1998, October). "Explaining Premature Mortality Across Fields of Creative Endeavor." *Journal of Personality, 66*(5), 805–833.

Cavett, D. (1992, August 3). "Goodbye, Darkness." *People Weekly, 38,* 88 ff.

Chalmers, D. J. (1995, December). "The Puzzle of Conscious Experience." *Scientific American,* pp. 80–86.

Changeux, J.-P. (1997). *Neuronal Man: The Biology of Mind.* (L. Garey, Trans.). Princeton, N.J.: Princeton University Press.

Chi, M., de Leeuw, N., Chiu, M. H., and LaVancher, C. (1994). "Eliciting Self-Explanations Improves Understanding." *Cognitive Science, 18,* 439–477.

Clarke, W. V. (1956). "The Construction of an Industrial Selection Personality Test." *Journal of Psychology, 41,* 379–394.

Claude-Pierre, P. (1999). *The Secret Language of Eating Disorders: The Revolutionary New Approach to Understanding and Curing Anorexia and Bulimia.* New York: Vintage Books.

Collin, F. (1992, May). "Sarah Leibowitz (Interview)." *Omni, 14*(8), 73 ff.

"Combatting Stress at Work" [Special Issue]. (1993, January). *Conditions of Work Digest, 12*(1).

Coop, R. H. (1993). *Mind over Golf: Play Your Best by Thinking Smart.* Old Tappan, N.J.: Macmillan.

Cooper, K. (1968). *Aerobics.* New York: Evans.

Cooper, R. (1991). *The Performance Edge.* Boston: Houghton Mifflin.

Cooper, R., and Sawaf, A. (1997). *Executive EQ: Emotional Intelligence and Leadership in Organizations.* New York: Grosset & Dunlap.

Cooperrider, D. L., and Dutton, J. E. (1998). *Organizational Dimensions of Global Change.* Thousand Oaks, Calif.: Sage.

Coren, S. (1992). *The Left-Hander Syndrome: The Causes and Consequences of Left-Handedness.* New York: Free Press.

Coren, S. (1996). *Sleep Thieves.* New York: Free Press.

Costa, P. T., Jr., and McCrae, R. R. (1992). *NEO PI-R Professional Manual.* Odessa, Fla: Psychological Assessment Resources.

Cousins, N. (1979). *Anatomy of an Illness.* New York: Norton.

Cousins, N. (1989). *Head First: The Biology of Hope.* New York: NAL/Dutton.

Covey, S. R. (1990). *The Seven Habits of Highly Effective People.* New York: Simon & Schuster.

Crawford, H. J., and Strapp, C. H. (1994, February). "Effects of Vocal and Instrumental Music on Visuospatial and Verbal Performance as Moderated by Studying Preference and Personality." *Personality and Individual Differences, 16*(2), 237–245.

Crawford, M. (1995). *Talking Difference: On Gender and Language.* Thousand Oaks, Calif.: Sage.

Crawford, M., and Gentry, M. (Eds.). (1989). *Gender and Thought.* New York: Springer-Verlag.

Crichton, M. (1990). *Jurassic Park: A Novel.* New York: Knopf.

Crick, F. (1994). *The Astonishing Hypothesis: The Scientific Search for the Soul.* New York: Scribner.

Csikszentmihalyi, M. (1990). *Flow: The Psychology of Optimal Experience.* New York: HarperCollins.

Csikszentmihalyi, M. (1996). *Creativity: Flow and the Psychology of Discovery and Invention.* New York: HarperCollins.

Cummings, T. G., and Worley, C. G. (1997). *Organization Development and Change* (6th ed.). Cincinnati: South-Western.

Cytowic, R. E. (1993). *The Man Who Tasted Shapes.* Los Angeles: Tarcher.

Dahlitz, M., and others. (1991, May 11). "Delayed Sleep Phase Syndrome Response to Melatonin." *Lancet, 337,* 1121 ff.

Dalton, K. (1987). *Once a Month* (4th ed.). Glasgow, Scotland: Fontana Original.

Damasio, A. R. (1994). *Descartes' Error: Emotion, Reason and the Human Brain.* New York: Grosset & Dunlap.

Dawkins, R. (1989). *The Selfish Gene* (2nd ed.). Oxford: Oxford University Press.

De Bono, E. (1967). *New Think.* New York: Basic Books.

De Bono, E. (1970). *Lateral Thinking: Creativity Step by Step.* New York: HarperCollins.

De Bono, E. (1994). *De Bono's Thinking Course.* New York: Facts on File.

Dean, W., and Morgenthaler, J. (1990). *Smart Drugs and Nutrients.* Santa Cruz, Calif.: B & J Publications.

DeAngelis, T. (1992, February). "Cutting Cholesterol: Feeling Feisty?" *APA Monitor,* pp. 8–9.

DeAngelis, T. (1995, April). "New Threat Associated with Child Abuse." *APA Monitor, 26*(4), 1, 38.

Deming, W. E. (1986). *Out of the Crisis.* Cambridge, Mass.: MIT Center for Advanced Engineering Study.

Dennett, D. C. (1995). *Darwin's Dangerous Idea: Evolution and the Meanings of Life.* New York: Simon & Schuster.

Dennett, D. C. (1996). *Kinds of Minds: Toward an Understanding of Consciousness.* New York: Basic Books.

Detterman, D. K., and Sternberg, R. J. (1993). *Transfer on Trial: Intelligence, Cognition, and Instruction.* Norwood, N.J.: Ablex.

Diamond, J. (1992). *The Third Chimpanzee: The Evolution and Future of the Human Animal.* New York: HarperCollins.

Diamond, J. (1997a). *Guns, Germs, and Steel: The Fates of Human Societies.* New York: Norton.

Diamond, J. (1997b). *Why Is Sex Fun? The Evolution of Human Sexuality.* New York: Basic Books.

Diamond, M. (1988). *Enriching Heredity: The Impact of the Environment on the Anatomy of the Brain.* New York: Free Press.

Dietz, W. H., and Stern, L. (1999). *Guide to Your Child's Nutrition.* Elk Grove Village, Ill.: American Academy of Pediatrics.

Digman, J. M., and Inouye, J. (1986). "Further Specification of the Five Robust Factors of Personality." *Journal of Personality and Social Psychology, 50,* 116–123.

Dinges, D. F., and Broughton, R. J. (1989). *Sleep and Alertness: Chronobiological, Behavioral, and Medical Aspects of Napping.* New York: Raven Press.

Dossey, L. (1996). *Healing Words: The Power of Prayer and the Power of Medicine.* San Francisco: Harper San Francisco.

Dotto, L. (1990). *Losing Sleep: How Your Sleeping Habits Affect Your Life.* New York: Morrow.

Dreikurs, R., and Cassel, P. (1972). *Discipline Without Tears* (rev. ed.). New York: Hawthorne Books.

Dreikurs, R., and Gray, L. (1993). *Logical Consequences.* New York: Meredith Press.

Druckman, D., and Bjork, R. A. (Eds.). (1991). *In the Mind's Eye: Enhancing Human Performance.* Washington, D.C.: National Academy Press.

Druckman, D., and Swets, J. A. (Eds.). (1988). *Enhancing Human Performance: Issues, Theories, and Techniques.* Washington, D.C.: National Academy Press.

Dunbar, R. (1996). *Grooming, Gossip, and the Evolution of Language.* Cambridge, Mass.: Harvard University Press.

Dunn, R., and Dunn, K. (1978). *Teaching Students Through Their Individual Learning Styles.* Englewood Cliffs, N.J.: Prentice Hall.

Eagly, A. (1995, March). "The Science and Politics of Comparing Women and Men." *American Psychologist, 50*(3), 145–158.

Eaves, L. J., Eysenck, H. J., and Martin, N. G. (1989). *Genes, Culture and Personality.* London: Academic Press.

Eckles, R. W., Carmichael, R. L., and Sarchet, B. R. (1981). *Supervisory Management.* New York: Wiley.

Edelman, G. M. (1987). *Neural Darwinism: The Theory of Neuronal Group Selection.* New York: Basic Books.

Edelman, G. M. (1992). *Bright Air, Brilliant Fire: On the Matter of the Mind.* New York: Basic Books.

Education Research. (1987). *Problem Solving.* New York: Education Research.

Education Research. (1988). *Decision Making.* New York: Education Research.

Edwards, B. (1989). *Drawing on the Right Side of the Brain* (rev. ed.). Los Angeles: Tarcher.

Eisenberger, R., and Cameron, J. (1996). "Detrimental Effects of Reward: Reality or Myth?" *American Psychologist, 51*(11), 1153–1166.

Ekman, P. (1985). *Telling Lies.* New York: Norton.

Elman, J. L., and others. (1996). *Rethinking Innateness: A Connectionist Perspective on Development.* Cambridge, Mass.: MIT Press.

Epstein, R. (1996, July–August). "Capturing Creativity." *Psychology Today, 29*(4), 41 ff.

Epstein, S. (1994, August). "Integration of the Cognitive and the Psychodynamic Unconscious." *American Psychologist, 49*(8), 709–724.

Epstein, S. (1997, March). "This I Have Learned from over Forty Years of Personality Research." *Journal of Personality, 65*(1), 3–32.

Epstein, S., and Meier, P. (1989). "Constructive Thinking: A Broad Coping Variable with Specific Components." *Journal of Personality and Social Psychology, 57*(2), 332–350.

Escher, M. C. (1983). *M. C. Escher: Twenty-Nine Master Prints.* New York: Abrams.

Eysenck, H. J. (1967). *The Biological Basis of Personality.* Springfield, Ill.: Thomas.

Eysenck, H. J. (1970). *The Structure of Human Personality* (rev. ed.). London: Methuen.

Eysenck, H. J. (Ed.). (1981). *A Model for Personality.* Berlin: Springer-Verlag.

Eysenck, H. J., and Eysenck, M. W. (1985). *Personality and Individual Differences: A Natural Science Approach.* New York: Plenum.

Eysenck, H. J., and Kamin, L. (1981). *The Intelligence Controversy.* New York: Wiley.

Ezzo, G., and Bucknam, R. (1998). *On Becoming Baby Wise.* Sisters, Oreg.: Multnomah.

Falletta, N. (1983). *The Paradoxicon.* New York: Doubleday.

Fausto-Sterling, A. (1992). *Myths of Gender: Biological Theories About Women and Men* (2nd ed.). New York: Basic Books.

Fausto-Sterling, A. (1993, March–April). "The Five Sexes: Why Male and Female Are Not Enough." *The Sciences, 33*(2), 20–25.

Fausto-Sterling, A., and Rose, H. (1994). *Love, Power, and Knowledge.* Bloomington: Indiana University Press.

Fernald, R. D. (1993, July–August). "Cichlids in Love." *The Sciences, 33*(4), 27–31.

Festinger, L. (1953). *A Theory of Cognitive Dissonance.* Stanford, Calif.: Stanford University Press.

Field, T. (1998, December). "Massage Therapy Effects." *American Psychologist, 53*(12), 1270–1281.

Fisher, H. E. (1982). *The Sex Contract.* New York: Morrow.

Fisher, H. E. (1995). *Anatomy of Love: A Natural History of Mating, Marriage, and Why We Stray.* New York: Fawcett.

Fisher, M. (1981). *Intuition: How to Use It for Success and Happiness.* New York: NAL/Dutton.

Fisher, R., and Ury, W. (1991). *Getting to Yes: Negotiating Agreement Without Giving In* (2nd ed.). New York: Penguin Books.

Flanders, N. A. (1970). *Analyzing Teacher Behavior.* Reading, Mass.: Addison-Wesley.

Fleenor, J., and Prince, J. (1997). *Using 360–Degree Feedback in Organizations: An Annotated Bibliography.* Greensboro, N.C.: Center for Creative Leadership.

Fluegelman, A. (Ed.). (1976). *The New Games Book.* New York: Dolphin/Doubleday.

Flynn, J. R. (1999). "Searching for Justice: The Discovery of IQ Gains over Time." *American Psychologist, 54*(1), 5–20.

Folkins, C. H., and Sime, W. E. (1981, April). "Physical Fitness Training and Mental Health." *American Psychologist, 36*(4), 373–389.

Forabosco, G., and Ruch, W. (1994). "Sensation Seeking, Social Attitudes and Humor Appreciation in Italy." *Personality and Individual Differences, 16*(4), 515–528.

Ford, C. M. (1995). *Lies!, Lies!!, Lies!!!: The Psychology of Deceit.* Washington, D.C.: American Psychiatric Press.

Foreman, J. (1996, December 17). "Anxiety: It's Not Just a State of Mind." *Boston Globe,* p. C1.

Fossel, M. (1996). *Reversing Human Aging.* New York: Morrow.

Fowler, J. W. (1982). *Stages of Faith: The Psychology of Human Development and the Quest for Meaning.* New York: HarperCollins.

Fox, N. A. (1991). "If It's Not Left, It's Right: Electroencephalograph Asymmetry and the Development of Emotion." *American Psychologist, 46,* 863–872.

Franklin, J. (1987). *Molecules of the Mind: The Brave New Science of Molecular Psychology.* New York: Atheneum.

Fredrickson, B. L., and others. (1998, July). "That Swimsuit Becomes You: Sex Differences in Self-Objectification, Restrained Eating, and Math Performance." *Journal of Personality and Social Psychology, 75*(1), 269–284.

Friedan, B. (1993). *The Fountain of Age.* New York: Simon & Schuster.

Gallagher, R. M. (Ed.). (1990). *Drug Therapy for Headache.* New York: Dekker.

Gardner, H. (1983). *Frames of Mind: The Theory of Multiple Intelligences.* New York: Basic Books.

Gardner, H. (1985). *The Mind's New Science: A History of the Cognitive Revolution.* New York: Basic Books.

Gardner, H. (1991). *The Unschooled Mind: How Schools Should Teach.* New York: Basic Books.

Gardner, H. (1993). *Creating Minds.* New York: Basic Books.

Gardner, M. (1979). *The Ambidextrous Universe: Mirror Asymmetry and Time-Reversed Worlds* (2nd ed.). New York: Scribner.

Garfield, C. A. (1984). *Peak Performance: Mental Training Techniques of the World's Greatest Athletes.* Los Angeles: Tarcher.

Gavin, J. (1992). *The Exercise Habit.* Champaign, Ill.: Human Kinetics.

Gawain, S. (1978). *Creative Visualization.* Berkeley, Calif.: New World Library.

Gazzaniga, M. S. (1985). *The Social Brain.* New York: Basic Books.

Gazzaniga, M. S. (1988). *Mind Matters: How Mind and Brain Interact to Create Our Conscious Lives.* Boston: Houghton Mifflin.

Geen, R. G., Beatty, W. W., and Arkin, R. M. (1984). *Human Motivation: Physiological, Behavioral, and Social Approaches.* Needham Heights, Mass.: Allyn & Bacon.

Gibbs, W. W. (1996, August). "Gaining on Fat." *Scientific American,* pp. 88–94.

Gitlow, H., Gitlow, S., Oppenheim, A., and Oppenheim, R. (1989). *Tools and Methods for the Improvement of Quality.* Burr Ridge, Ill.: Irwin.

Glasser, W. (1990). *The Quality School: Managing Students Without Coercion.* New York: HarperCollins.

Gleick, J. (1987). *Chaos: Making a New Science.* New York: Viking Penguin.

Goldberg, J. (1988). *Anatomy of a Scientific Discovery.* New York: Bantam Books.

Goldberg, L. R. (1993, January). "The Structure of Phenotypic Personality Traits." *American Psychologist, 48*(1), 26–34.

Goldberg, P. (1983). *The Intuitive Edge.* Los Angeles: Tarcher.

Goleman, D. (1995). *Emotional Intelligence.* New York: Bantam Books.

Goleman, D. (1996, August 13). "Brain Images of Addiction in Action Show Its Neural Basis." *New York Times,* p. C1.

Goleman, D. (1998). *Working with Emotional Intelligence.* New York: Bantam Books.

Goleman, D., Kaufman, P., and Ray, M. (1992). *The Creative Spirit.* New York: NAL/Dutton.

Golembiewski, R. T. (1988). *Phases of Burnout.* New York: Praeger.

Gordon, B. (1995). *Memory: Remembering and Forgetting in Everyday Life.* New York: MasterMedia.

Gould, S. J. (1996). *Full House: The Spread of Excellence from Plato to Darwin.* New York: Three Rivers Press.

Gray, J. A. (1971). *The Psychology of Fear and Stress.* New York: McGraw-Hill.

Greenfield, S. A. (Ed.). (1996). *The Human Mind Explained.* New York: Henry Holt.

Gregorc, A. F. (1982). *Gregorc Style Delineator.* Maynard, Mass.: Gabriel Systems.

Gregory, R. L. (Ed.). (1987). *The Oxford Companion to the Mind.* New York: Oxford University Press.

Guirdham, M. (1995). *Interpersonal Skills at Work* (2nd ed.). Englewood Cliffs, N.J.: Prentice Hall.

Haas, R. (1994). *Eat Smart, Think Smart.* New York: HarperCollins.

Hafen, B. Q., Karren, K. J., Frandsen, K. J., and Smith, N. L. (1996). *Mind/Body Health: The Effects of Attitudes, Emotions, and Relationships.* Needham Heights, Mass.: Allyn & Bacon.

Hallowell, E. M. (1997). *Worry: Controlling It and Using It Wisely.* New York: Pantheon Books.

Halverson, C. F., Jr., Kohnstamm, G. A., and Martin, R. P. (Eds.). (1994). *The Developing Structure of Temperament and Personality from Infancy to Adulthood.* Hillsdale, N.J.: Erlbaum.

Hammond, S. A. (1996). *The Thin Book of Appreciative Inquiry.* Plano, Tex.: Thin Book Publishing.

Harris, J. R. (1998). *The Nurture Assumption.* New York: Free Press.

Hart, B., and Risley, T. (1995). *Meaningful Differences in the Everyday Experiences of Young American Children.* Baltimore: P. H. Brookes.

Hart, L. A. (1983). *Human Brain and Human Learning.* White Plains, N.Y.: Longman.

Hatfield, E., and Rapson, R. L. (1993). *Love, Sex, and Intimacy: Their Psychology, Biology, and History.* Reading, Mass.: Addison-Wesley.

Hayes, J. R. (1989). *The Complete Problem Solver* (2nd ed.). Hillsdale, N.J.: Erlbaum.

Healy, J. (1990). *Endangered Minds: Why Our Children Don't Think.* New York: Simon & Schuster.

Hedges, L. V., and Nowell, A. (1995, July 7). "Sex Differences in Mental Test Scores, Variability, and Numbers of High-Scoring Individuals." *Science, 269*(5220), 41.

Heisenberg, W. (1962). *Physics and Philosophy: The Revolution in Modern Science.* New York: Harper-Collins.

Heller, W. (1993). "Neuropsychological Mechanism of Individual Differences in Emotion, Personality, and Arousal." *Neuropsychology, 7*(4), 476–489.

Henson, K. T., and Borthwick, P. (1984). "Matching Styles: A Historical Look." *Theory into Practice, 23,* 3–9.

Herber, H. (1978). *Teaching Reading in Content Areas* (2nd ed.). Englewood Cliffs, N.J.: Prentice Hall.

Herrmann, D. J. (1991). *Super Memory: A Quick-Action Program for Memory Improvement.* Emmaus, Pa.: Rodale.

Herrmann, N. (1989). *The Creative Brain.* Lake Lure, N.C.: Brain Books.

Herrnstein, R. J., and Murray, C. (1994). *The Bell Curve.* New York: Free Press.

Hersey, P., and Blanchard, K. H. (1976). *Management of Organizational Behavior: Utilizing Human Resources* (3rd ed.). Englewood Cliffs, N.J.: Prentice Hall.

Hirsh, R. (1990). "Modulatory Integration: A Concept Capable of Explaining Cognitive Learning and Purposive Behavior in Physiological Terms." *Psychobiology, 18*(1), 3–15.

Hobson, J. A. (1988). *The Dreaming Brain.* New York: Basic Books.

Hobson, J. A. (1994). *The Chemistry of Conscious States.* New York: Little, Brown.

Hobson, J. A. (1995). *Sleep.* New York: Freeman.

Hoffmann, R. (1995). *The Same and Not the Same.* New York: Columbia University Press.

Hofstadter, D. R. (1979). *Gödel, Escher, Bach: An Eternal Golden Braid.* New York: Basic Books.

Holland, J. L. (1985). *Making Vocational Choices: A Theory of Vocational Personalities and Work Environments.* Englewood Cliffs, N.J.: Prentice Hall.

Holt, J. (1995). *How Children Fail.* Reading, Mass.: Perseus Press.

Honey, P., and Mumford, A. (1982). *The Manual of Learning Styles.* Maidenhead, England: Honey Press.

Hooper, J., and Teresi, D. (1986). *The Three-Pound Universe.* Old Tappan, N.J.: Macmillan.

Horgan, J. (1994, July). "Can Science Explain Consciousness?" *Scientific American,* pp. 88–94.

Horgan, J. (1996, December). "Why Freud Isn't Dead." *Scientific American,* pp. 106–111.

Horney, K. (1945). *Our Inner Conflicts.* New York: Norton.

Howard, P. J. (1972). "The Nonverbal Communication of Teacher Expectations." Unpublished doctoral dissertation, University of North Carolina at Chapel Hill.

Howard, P. J., and Howard, J. M. (1993). *The Big Five Workbook: A Roadmap for Individual and Team Interpretation for Scores on the Five-Factor Model of Personality.* Charlotte, N.C.: Center for Applied Cognitive Studies.

Hrushesky, W.J.M. (1994, July–August). "Timing Is Everything." *The Sciences,* pp. 32–37.

Huff, D. (1954). *How to Lie with Statistics.* New York: Norton.

Hughes, J. R., Daaboul, Y., Fino, J. J., and Shaw, G. L. (1998). "The 'Mozart Effect' on Epileptiform Activity." *Clinical Electroencephalography, 29,* 109–119.

Hunt, M. (1982). *The Universe Within: A New Science Explores the Human Mind.* New York: Simon & Schuster.

Hyerle, D. (1996). *Visual Tools for Constructing Knowledge.* Alexandria, Va.: Association for Supervision and Curriculum Development.

"Hypnosis." (1991). *Harvard Mental Health Letter, 7*(10), 1–4.

Ingelfinger, F. (1980). "Arrogance." *New England Journal of Medicine, 303,* 1506–1511.

Ironson, G., and others. (1992, August). "Effects of Anger on Left Ventricular Ejection Fraction in Coronary Artery Disease." *American Journal of Cardiology, 70,* 281–285.

Izard, C. E., Kagan, J., and Zajonc, R. B. (Eds.). (1984). *Emotions, Cognition, and Behavior.* Cambridge: Cambridge University Press.

Jaffe, C. L., Jr. (1991). "Using 'Practical Knowledge' Versus Cognitive Ability to Predict Job Performance for Personnel in Customer Oriented Jobs." Unpublished doctoral dissertation, University of South Florida, Tampa.

Jaques, E. (1994). *Human Capability.* Falls Church, Va.: Cason Hall.

John, O. P., Angleitner, A., and Ostendorf, F. (1988). "The Lexical Approach to Personality: A Historical Review of Trait Taxonomic Research." *European Journal of Personality, 2,* 171–203.

Johnson-Laird, P. (1988). *The Computer and the Mind: An Introduction to Cognitive Science.* Cambridge, Mass.: Harvard University Press.

Jones, S. (1994). *The Language of Genes: Unraveling the Mysteries of Human Genetics.* New York: Anchor Books.

Jourdain, R. (1997). *Music, the Brain, and Ecstasy: How Music Captures Our Imagination.* New York: Morrow.

Joyce, B. R., and Hodges, R. E. (1966). "Instructional Flexibility Training." *Journal of Teacher Education, 17,* 409–416.

Jung, C. G. (1971). *Psychological Types.* Princeton, N.J.: Princeton University Press.

Kagan, J. (1966). "Reflection: Impulsivity and Reading Ability in Primary Grade Children." *Child Development, 36,* 609–628.

Kallan, C. (1991, October). "Probing the Power of Common Scents." *Prevention, 43*(10), 39–43.

Kassirer, J. P., and Angell, M. (1998, January 1). "Losing Weight: An Ill-Fated New Year's Resolution." *New England Journal of Medicine, 338*(1), 52–56.

Katahn, M. (1991). *One Meal at a Time.* New York: Norton.

Keeton, K. (1992). *Longevity: The Science of Staying Young.* New York: Viking Penguin.

Keirsey, D., and Bates, M. (1978). *Please Understand Me.* Del Mar, Calif.: Prometheus Nemesis.

Kelley, H. H., and Thibaut, J. W. (1978). *Interpersonal Relations: A Theory of Interdependence.* New York: Wiley.

Kepner, C. H., and Tregoe, B. B. (1981). *The New Rational Manager.* Princeton, N.J.: Princeton Research Press.

Kiecolt-Glaser, J. K., and Glaser, R. (1992). "Psychoneuroimmunology: Can Psychological Interventions Modulate Immunity?" *Journal of Consulting and Clinical Psychology, 60*(4), 569–575.

Kiesler, D. J. (1996). *Contemporary Interpersonal Theory and Research: Personality, Psychopathology, and Psychotherapy.* New York: Wiley.

Kimble, J. (1992). "Plain English: A Charter for Clear Writing." *Thomas M. Cooley Law Review, 9*(1), 1–58.

Kimura, D. (1994). "Body Asymmetry and Intellectual Pattern." *Personality and Individual Differences, 17*(1), 53–60.

Kimura, D., and Carson, M. W. (1995). "Dermatoglyphic Asymmetry: Relation to Sex, Handedness, and Cognitive Pattern." *Personality and Individual Differences, 19*(4), 471–478.

Kimura, D., and Hampson, E. (1990, April). *Neural and Hormonal Mechanisms Mediating Sex Differences in Cognition.* Research Bulletin No. 689. London, Ontario, Canada: Department of Psychology, University of Western Ontario.

Kinlaw, D. C. (1990). *Developing Superior Work Teams.* New York: Free Press.

Kintsch, W. (1994). "Text Comprehension, Memory, and Learning." *American Psychologist, 49*(4), 294–303.

Kirsch, I., and Lynn, S. J. (1995, October). "The Altered State of Hypnosis: Changes in the Theoretical Landscape." *American Psychologist, 50*(10), 846–858.

Kirton, M. J. (1977). *Research Edition: Kirton Adaption-Innovation Inventory.* London: National Federation for Educational Research.

Kline, M. (1953). *Mathematics in Western Culture.* New York: Oxford University Press.

Koestler, A. (1964). *The Act of Creation.* Old Tappan, N.J.: Macmillan.

Kogan, Z. (1956). *Essentials in Problem Solving.* New York: Arco.

Kohlberg, L. (1984). *The Psychology of Moral Development: The Nature and Validity of Moral Stages.* New York: HarperCollins.

Kolata, G. B. (1976). "Brain Biochemistry: Effects of Diet." *Science, 192,* 41–42.

Kolata, G. B. (1979). "Mental Disorders: A New Approach to Treatment?" *Science, 203,* 36–38.

Kolb, D. A. (1978). *Learning Styles Inventory Technical Manual.* Boston: McBer.

Kolbe, K. (1990). *The Conative Connection.* Reading, Mass.: Addison-Wesley.

Kolodnor, J. (1997, January). "Educational Implications of Analogy: A View from Case-Based Reasoning." *American Psychologist, 52*(1), 57–66.

Korzybski, A. (1948). *Science and Sanity: An Introduction to Non-Aristotelian Systems and General Semantics* (3rd ed.). Lakeville, Conn.: International Non-Aristotelian Library.

Kosslyn, S. M. (1994). *Image and Brain: The Resolution of the Imagery Debate.* Cambridge, Mass.: MIT Press.

Kuhn, T. S. (1970). *The Structure of Scientific Revolutions* (2nd ed.). Chicago: University of Chicago Press.

Laborde, G. Z. (1983). *Influencing with Integrity.* Palo Alto, Calif.: Syntony.

Laborde, G. Z. (1988). *Fine Tune Your Brain.* Palo Alto, Calif.: Syntony.

Labov, W. (1969). "The Logic of Nonstandard English." *Georgetown Monographs on Language and Linguistics, 22,* 1–31.

Lagatree, K. M. (1996). *Feng Shui.* New York: Villard.

Lakoff, G. (1987). *Women, Fire, and Dangerous Things: What Categories Reveal About the Mind.* Chicago: University of Chicago Press.

Langer, E. (1989). *Mindfulness.* Reading, Mass.: Addison-Wesley.

Langer, E. (1997). *The Power of Mindful Learning.* Reading, Mass.: Addison-Wesley.

Latané, B., and Darley, J. (1970). *The Unresponsive Bystander: Why Doesn't He Help?* Englewood Cliffs, N.J.: Appleton-Century-Crofts.

Lazarus, R. S. (1991a). *Emotion and Adaptation.* New York: Oxford University Press.

Lazarus, R. S. (1991b, August). "Progress on a Cognitive-Motivational-Relational Theory of Emotion." *American Psychologist, 46,* 819–834.

Leach, P. (1997). *Your Baby and Child: From Birth to Age Five* (rev. ed.). New York: Knopf.

Lecanuet, J. P. (1995). *Fetal Development: A Psychobiological Perspective.* Hillsdale, N.J.: Erlbaum.

LeDoux, J. (1996). *The Emotional Brain: The Mysterious Underpinnings of Emotional Life.* New York: Simon & Schuster.

Lee, C. (1987, September). "Mindmapping: Brainstorming on Paper." *Training, 24*(9), 71–76.

Lefton, R. E., Buzzotta, V., and Sherberg, M. (1985). *Improving Productivity Through People Skills.* New York: Ballinger.

Lemieux, M., and Bordage, G. (1992, April–June). "Propositional Versus Semantic Analysis of Medical Diagnostic Thinking." *Cognitive Science, 16*(2), 185–204.

Lenneberg, E. H. (1967). *Biological Foundations of Language.* New York: Wiley.

LeShan, L. (1989). *Cancer as a Turning Point.* New York: NAL/Dutton.

Leslie, J., and Fleenor, J. (1998). *Feedback to Managers: A Review and Comparison of Multi-Rater Instruments for Management Development* (3rd ed.). Greensboro, N.C.: Center for Creative Leadership.

Lester, B. (1998, October 23). "Cocaine Exposure and Children: The Meaning of Subtle Effects." *Science, 282*(5389), 633–634.

LeVay, S. (1996). *Queer Science: The Use and Abuse of Research into Homosexuality.* Cambridge, Mass.: MIT Press.

Livingstone, M. S., Rosen, G. D., Drislane, F. W., and Galaburda, A. M. (1991). "Physiological and Anatomical Evidence for a Magnocellular Defect in Developmental Dyslexia." *Proceedings of the National Academy of Science, 88,* 7943–7947.

Loehlin, J. C. (1992). *Genes and Environment in Personality Development.* Thousand Oaks, Calif.: Sage.

Loftus, E. (1997, September). "Creating False Memories." *Scientific American, 277*(3), 70–75.

Loftus, E., and Ketcham, K. (1994). *The Myth of Repressed Memory.* New York: St. Martin's Press.

Long, M. E. (1987, December). "What Is This Thing Called Sleep?" *National Geographic, 172*(6), 787–821.

Lorayne, H., and Lucas, J. (1974). *The Memory Book.* New York: Stein & Day.

Louis, D. N. (1995, Spring). "The Brain's 'Other Cells' Go Awry." *On the Brain* (Harvard Mahoney Neuroscience Institute Letter), pp. 1–3, 7.

MacLean, P. D. (1990). *The Triune Brain in Evolution.* New York: Plenum.

Mallandain, I., and Davies, M. F. (1994). "The Colours of Love: Personality Correlates of Love Styles." *PAID, 17*(4), 557–560.

Marston, W. M. (1987). *The Emotions of Normal People.* Minneapolis: Carlson Learning.

Maslow, A. H. (1943). "A Theory of Human Motivation." *Psychological Review, 50,* 370–396.

Masten, A. S., and Coatsworth, J. D. (1998, February). "The Development of Competence in Favorable and Unfavorable Environments." *American Psychologist, 53*(2), 205–220. [Special issue: "Applications of Developmental Science"].

McClelland, D. C. (1986). "Some Reflections on the Two Psychologies of Love." *Journal of Personality, 54,* 334–353.

McClelland, D. C., and Kirshnit, C. (1988). "The Effect of Motivational Arousal Through Films on Immunoglobulin A." *Psychology and Health, 2,* 31–52.

McCrae, R. M., and Costa, P. T. (1989). "Reinterpreting the Myers-Briggs Type Indicator from the Perspective of the Five-Factor Model of Personality." *Journal of Personality, 57*(1), 17–40.

McCrae, R. M., and Costa, P. T. (1990). *Personality in Adulthood.* New York: Guilford Press.

McDaniel, R. N. (1992). "The Relationship Between Personality and Perceived Success of Organizational Change." Doctoral dissertation, The Fielding Institute. *Dissertation Abstracts International, 53*(06), 3196B.

McEwan, B. S., and Schmeck, H. M., Jr. (1996). *The Hostage Brain.* New York: Rockefeller University Press.

McGuire, C. B., and Radner, R. (Eds.). (1972). *Decision and Organization.* Amsterdam: North-Holland.

McKay, M., Davis, M., and Fanning, P. (1995). *Messages: The Communication Skills Book* (2nd ed.). Oakland, Calif.: New Harbinger.

McNair, D. M., Lorr, M., and Droppleman, L. F. (1971). *Profile of Mood States Manual.* San Diego, Calif.: Educational and Industrial Testing Service.

McNamee, P., and Celona, J. (1987). *Decision Analysis for the Professional with Supertree.* Redwood City, Calif.: Scientific Press.

Medina, J. J. (1996). *The Clock of Ages.* Cambridge: Cambridge University Press.

Mehrabian, A. (1971). *Silent Messages.* Belmont, Calif.: Wadsworth.

"Mental Health: Does Therapy Help?" (1995, November). *Consumer Reports,* pp. 734–739.

Merrill, D. W., and Reid, H. H. (1981). *Personal Style and Effective Performance.* Radnor, Pa.: Chilton.

Merzbacher, C. F. (1979, April). "A Diet and Exercise Regimen: Its Effect upon Mental Acuity and Personality. A Pilot Study." *Perceptual and Motor Skills, 48*(2), 367–371.

Metcalfe, J., and Shimamura, A. P. (Eds.). (1994). *Metacognition: Knowing About Knowing.* Cambridge, Mass.: MIT Press.

Michalko, M. (1991). *Thinkertoys: A Handbook of Business Creativity for the '90s.* Berkeley, Calif.: Ten Speed Press.

Miller, E. M. (1994). "Intelligence and Brain Myelination: A Hypothesis." *Personality and Individual Differences, 17*(6), 803–832.

Miller, G. A. (1956). "The Magical Number Seven, Plus or Minus Two: Some Limits on Our Capacity for Processing Information." *Psychological Review, 63,* 81–97.

Minninger, J. (1984). *Total Recall: How to Boost Your Memory Power.* Emmaus, Pa.: Rodale.

Mischel, W. (1968). *Personality and Assessment.* New York: Wiley.

Moir, A., and Jessel, D. (1991). *Brain Sex: The Real Difference Between Men and Women.* New York: Carol.

Moody, P. E. (1983). *Decision Making: Proven Methods for Better Decisions.* New York: McGraw-Hill.

Moore-Ede, M. (1993). *The Twenty-Four-Hour Society: Understanding Human Limits in a World That Never Stops.* Reading, Mass.: Addison-Wesley.

Morgan, W. P. (Ed.). (1997). *Physical Activity and Mental Health.* Washington, D.C.: Taylor & Francis.

Morier, D., and Seroy, C. (1994, October). "The Effect of Interpersonal Expectancies on Men's Self-Presentation of Gender Role Attitudes to Women." *Sex Roles, 31*(7–8), 493–504.

Mukerjee, M. (1995, October). "Hidden Scars." *Scientific American,* pp. 14, 20.

Murray, H. A. (1938). *Explorations in Personality.* New York: Oxford University Press.

Myers, I. B., and McCaulley, M. H. (1985). *Manual: A Guide to the Development and Use of the Myers-Briggs Type Indicator.* Palo Alto, Calif.: Consulting Psychologists Press.

Nadler, G., and Hibino, S. (1990). *Breakthrough Thinking.* Rocklin, Calif.: Prima.

National Research Council, Committee on Diet and Health. (1989). *Diet and Health: Implications for Reducing Chronic Disease Risk.* Washington, D.C.: National Academy Press.

Neeper, S. A., Gomez-Pinilla, F., Choi, J., and Cotman, C. W. (1995). "Exercise Raises Brain Neuro-trophins." *Nature, 373,* 109.

Nelson, H. D., Nevitt, M. C., and Scott, J. C. (1994). "Smoking, Alcohol, and Neuromuscular and Physical Function of Older Women." *Journal of the American Medical Association, 272,* 1825–1831.

Nemeroff, C. B. (1998, June). "The Neurobiology of Depression." *Scientific American,* pp. 42–49.

Neubauer, P. B., and Neubauer, A. (1990). *Nature's Thumbprint: The New Genetics of Personality.* Reading, Mass.: Addison-Wesley.

Nicholson, N. (1998, July–August). "How Hardwired Is Human Behavior?" *Harvard Business Review,* pp. 135–147.

Nierenberg, G. I. (1985). *The Idea Generator.* Berkeley, Calif.: Experience in Software.

Norman, D. A. (1993). *Things That Make Us Smart: Cognitive Artifacts as Tools for Thought.* Reading, Mass.: Perseus Press.

Norman, W. T. (1963). "Toward an Adequate Taxonomy of Personality Attributes: Replicated Factor Structure in Peer Nomination Personality Ratings." *Journal of Abnormal and Social Psychology, 66,* 574–583.

Northrop, F.S.C. (1946). *The Meeting of East and West: An Inquiry Concerning World Understanding.* Old Tappan, N.J.: Macmillan.

Northrop, F.S.C. (1947). *The Logic of the Sciences and the Humanities.* Cleveland: World.

Okogbaa, O. G., and Shell, R. L. (1986, December). "The Measurement of Knowledge Worker Fatigue." *IEEE Transactions, 18*(4), 335–342.

Ornstein, R. (1986). *Multimind: A New Way of Looking at Human Behavior.* New York: Anchor Books.

Ornstein, R. (1993). *The Roots of the Self: Unraveling the Mystery of Who We Are.* San Francisco: Harper San Francisco.

Ornstein, R., and Sobel, D. (1987). *The Healing Brain.* New York: Simon & Schuster.

Ortiz, J. M. (1997). *The Tao of Music: Sound Psychology.* York Beach, Maine: Samuel Weiser.

Peck, M. S. (1987). *The Different Drum: Community-Making and Peace.* New York: Simon & Schuster.

Pemberton, W. H. (1989). *Sanity for Survival: A Semantic Approach to Conflict Resolution.* San Francisco: Graphic Guides.

Pennington, B. F. (1991). *Diagnosing Learning Disorders: A Neuropsychological Framework.* New York: Guilford Press.

Pert, C. B. (1997). *Molecules of Emotion: Why You Feel the Way You Feel.* New York: Scribner.

Petri, H. L. (1991). *Motivation: Theory, Research, and Applications* (3rd ed.). Belmont, Calif.: Wadsworth.

Piaget, J. (1977). *The Essential Piaget.* (H. E. Guber and J. J. Vaneche, eds.). New York: Basic Books.

Pidikiti, R. D., and others. (1996, June). "A New Technique for Improving Rehabilitation of Movement After Stroke: A Pilot Study." *Journal of Rehabilitation Research and Development, 33,* 108 ff.

Pierpaoli, W., Regelson, W., and Coleman, C. (1996). *The Melatonin Miracle.* New York: G. K. Hall.

Pinker, S. (1994). *The Language Instinct.* New York: Morrow.

Pinker, S. (1997). *How the Mind Works.* New York: Norton.

Pirsig, R. M. (1974). *Zen and the Art of Motorcycle Maintenance: An Inquiry into Values.* New York: Morrow.

Plunkett, L. C., and Hale, G. A. (1982). *The Proactive Manager: The Complete Book of Problem Solving and Decision Making.* New York: Wiley.

Plutchik, R., and Kellerman, H. (Eds.). (1989). *The Measurement of Emotions.* Vol. 4 of *Emotion: Theory, Research, and Experience.* Orlando: Academic Press.

Pollitt, E., Leibel, R. L., and Greenfield, D. (1981). "Brief Fasting, Stress, and Cognition in Children." *American Journal of Clinical Nutrition, 34,* 1526–1533.

Polya, G. C. (1971). *How to Solve It: A New Aspect of Mathematical Method* (2nd ed.). Princeton, N.J.: Princeton University Press.

Pope, K. S. (1996, September). "Memory, Abuse, and Science: Questioning Claims About the False Memory Syndrome Epidemic." *American Psychologist, 51*(9), 957–974.

Poundstone, W. (1988). *Labyrinths of Reason: Paradox, Puzzles, and the Frailty of Knowledge.* New York: Anchor Books.

Prince, G. M. (1970). *The Practice of Creativity.* New York: Collier Books.

Raloff, J. (1991, October 5). "Searching Out How a Severe Diet Slows Aging." *Science News, 140*(14), 215.

Real, T. (1997). *I Don't Want to Talk About It: Overcoming the Secret Legacy of Male Depression.* New York: Scribner.

Reid, D. P. (1989). *The Tao of Health, Sex, and Longevity: A Modern Guide to the Ancient Way.* New York: Simon & Schuster.

Renzulli, J. S., and Smith, L. H. (1978). *The Learning Styles Inventory: A Measure of Student Preference for Instructional Techniques.* Mansfield Center, Conn.: Creative Learning Press.

Restak, R. M. (1984). *The Brain.* New York: Bantam Books.

Restak, R. M. (1988). *The Mind.* New York: Bantam Books.

Restak, R. M. (1991). *The Brain Has a Mind of Its Own.* New York: Harmony.

Restak, R. M. (1994). *The Modular Brain.* New York: Scribner.

Restak, R. M. (1997). *Older and Wiser.* New York: Simon & Schuster.

Rickards, T. (1974). *Problem-Solving Through Creative Analysis.* Epping, England: Gower.

Ricklefs, R. E., and Finch, C. E. (1995). *Aging: A Natural History.* New York: Scientific American Library.

Riskind, P. (1996, Fall). "Multiple Sclerosis: The Immune System's Terrible Mistake." *On the Brain* (Harvard Mahoney Neuroscience Institute Letter), 1–4.

Robbins, S. P. (1996). *Training in Interpersonal Skills: Tips for Managing People at Work* (2nd ed.). Englewood Cliffs, N.J.: Prentice Hall.

Robinson, B. E. (1989). *Work Addiction: Hidden Legacies of Adult Children.* Deerfield Beach, Fla.: Health Communications.

Rogers, K. B. (1986). "Do the Gifted Think and Learn Differently? A Review of Recent Research and Its Implications for Instruction." *Journal for the Education of the Gifted, 10,* 17–39.

Rogers, R. (Ed.). (1997). *Clinical Assessment of Malingering and Deception* (2nd ed.). New York: Guilford Press.

Rose, R. J. (1998). "A Developmental Behavior–Genetic Perspective on Alcoholism Risk." *Alcohol Health and Research World, 22*(2), 131–143.

Rosenfield, I. (1988). *The Invention of Memory: A New View of the Brain.* New York: Basic Books.

Rosenthal, R., Hall, J. A., DiMatteo, M. R., and Rogers, P. L. (1979). *Sensitivity to Nonverbal Communication: The PONS Test.* Baltimore: Johns Hopkins University Press.

Rosenthal, R., and Jacobson, L. (1968). *Pygmalion in the Classroom.* Austin, Tex.: Holt, Rinehart and Winston.

Rossi, E. L., and Nimmons, D. (1991). *The 20-Minute Break: Using the New Science of Ultradian Rhythms.* Los Angeles: Tarcher.

Rowan, R. (1986). *The Intuitive Manager.* New York: Little, Brown.

Rozin, P. (1997). "Disgust Faces, Basal Ganglia and Obsessive-Compulsive Disorder: Some Strange Brainfellows." *Trends in Cognitive Sciences, 1*(9), 321–325. (Includes response.)

Ruch, W. (1988). "Sensation Seeking and the Enjoyment of Structure and Content of Humour: Stability of Findings Across Four Samples." *Personality and Individual Differences, 9,* 861–871.

Saaty, T. L. (1982). *Decision Making for Leaders: The Analytical Hierarchy Process for Decisions in a Complex World.* Belmont, Calif.: Lifetime Learning.

Sagan, C. (1995). *The Demon-Haunted World.* New York: Random House.

Sahelian, R. (1997). *Melatonin: Nature's Sleeping Pill* (2nd ed.). Garden City Park, N.Y.: Avery Publishing Group.

Salovey, P., and Mayer, J. D. (1990). "Emotional Intelligence." *Imagination, Cognition, and Personality, 9,* 185–211.

Saper, C. (1996, Summer). "Why We Sleep (or Can't)." *On the Brain* (Harvard Mahoney Neuroscience Institute Letter), *5*(3), 1–3.

Sapolsky, R. M. (1994). *Why Zebras Don't Get Ulcers: A Guide to Stress, Stress-Related Diseases, and Coping.* New York: Freeman.

Schacter, D. (1996). *Searching for Memory.* New York: Basic Books.

Schachter, S., and Singer, J. E. (1962). "Cognitive, Social, and Physiological Determinants of Emotional States." *Psychological Review, 69,* 379–399.

Schaie, K. W. (1994, April). "The Course of Adult Intellectual Development." *American Psychologist, 49*(4), 304–313.

Schlosberg, H. S. (1954). "Three Dimensions of Emotion." *Psychological Review, 61,* 81–88.

Schmeck, R. R. (1983). "Learning Style of College Students." In R. F. Dillon and R. R. Schmeck (Eds.), *Individual Differences in Cognition* (vol. 1, pp. 233–279). Orlando: Academic Press.

Schmidt, D. E., and Keating, J. P. (1979). "Human Crowding and Personal Control: An Integration of the Research." *Psychological Bulletin, 86,* 680–700.

Schoenthaler, S. (1983). "Diet and Crime: An Empirical Examination of the Value of Nutrition in the Control and Treatment of Incarcerated Juvenile Offenders." *International Journal of Biosocial Research, 14,* 25–39.

Schutte, N., and others. (1998, August). "Development and Validation of a Measure of Emotional Intelligence." *Personality and Individual Differences, 25*(2), 167–177.

Searle, J. R. (Ed.). (1992). *The Rediscovery of the Mind.* Cambridge, Mass.: MIT Press.

Sears, W., and Sears, M. (1993). *The Baby Book.* New York: Little, Brown.

Seligman, M.E.P. (1984). *Seligman Attributional Style Questionnaire.* (Available by calling Martin Seligman or Peter Schulman at 215-898-2748.)

Seligman, M.E.P. (1991). *Learned Optimism.* New York: Knopf.

Seligman, M.E.P. (1994). *What You Can Change and What You Can't.* New York: Knopf.

Seligman, M.E.P. (1996, October). "Science as an Ally of Practice." *American Psychologist, 51*(10), 1072–1079. [Special issue: "Outcome Assessment of Psychotherapy"].

Seligman, M.E.P., Reivich, K., Jaycox, L., and Gillham, J. (1995). *The Optimistic Child.* Boston: Houghton Mifflin.

Selye, H. (1952). *The Story of the Adaptation Syndrome.* Montreal: Acta.

Senge, P. (1990). *The Fifth Discipline.* New York: Doubleday/Currency.

Shapiro, L. (1997). *How to Raise a Child with a High EQ.* New York: HarperCollins.

Shaywitz, S. E. (1996, November). "Dyslexia." *Scientific American,* pp. 98–104.

Shaywitz, S. E., and others. (1992). "Evidence That Dyslexia May Represent the Lower Tail of a Normal Distribution of Reading Ability." *New England Journal of Medicine, 326*(3), 145–150.

Shelov, S. P. (1998). *Caring for Your Baby and Young Child* (rev. ed.). New York: Bantam Books.

Shute, N. (1998, March 30). "The Ten-Minute Test for Strokes: New Breakthroughs in What MRIs Can See." *U.S. News & World Report,* pp. 69–72.

Siegel, B. (1987). *Love, Medicine and Miracles.* New York: HarperCollins.

Siegler, R. (1996). *Emerging Minds: The Process of Change in Children's Thinking.* New York: Oxford University Press.

Simon, H. (1969). *Sciences of the Artificial.* Cambridge, Mass.: MIT Press.

Simonton, O. C., Simonton, S., and Creighton, J. (1980). *Getting Well Again.* New York: Bantam Books.

Singer, R. B., Murphey, M., and Tennant, L. K. (Eds.). (1993). *Handbook of Research on Sport Psychology.* Old Tappan, N.J.: Macmillan.

Slon, S. (1997, June). "Night Moves." *Prevention,* pp. 106–113.

Somer, E. (1995). *Food and Mood.* New York: Henry Holt.

"Spinal Cord Injury: Treatment and Outlook" [Special issue]. (1997, March–April). *BrainWork: The Neuroscience Newsletter* (Charles A. Dana Foundation), *7*(2).

Staso, W. (1995). *What Stimulation Your Baby Needs to Become Smart.* Orcutt, Calif.: Great Beginnings Press.

Steele, C. M. (1997, June). "A Threat in the Air: How Stereotypes Shape Intellectual Identity and Performance." *American Psychologist, 52*(6), 613–629.

Sternberg, R. J. (1986). *Intelligence Applied: Understanding and Increasing Your Intellectual Skills.* Orlando: Harcourt Brace.

Sternberg, R. J. (1988). *The Triarchic Mind: A New Theory of Human Intelligence.* New York: Viking Penguin.

Sternberg, R. J. (1997a). "Does the Graduate Record Examination Predict Meaningful Success in the Graduate Training of Psychologists? A Case Study." *American Psychologist, 52*(6), 630–641.

Sternberg, R. J. (1997b). *Successful Intelligence.* New York: Plume.

Sternberg, R. J. (1997c). *Thinking Styles.* New York: Cambridge University Press.

Sternberg, R. J., and Davidson, J. E. (Eds.). (1995). *The Nature of Insight.* Cambridge, Mass.: MIT Press.

Sternberg, R. J., and Grigorenko, E. L. (1997, July). "Are Cognitive Styles Still in Style?" *American Psychologist, 52*(7), 700–712.

Sternberg, R. J., and Lubart, T. I. (1996, July). "Investing in Creativity." *American Psychologist, 51*(7), 677–688.

Sternberg, R. J., and Wagner, R. K. (1991). "MSG Thinking Styles Inventory Manual." Unpublished test manual, Yale University Department of Psychology, New Haven, Conn.

Stevens, W. (1967a). *The Collected Poems of Wallace Stevens.* New York: Knopf.

Stevens, W. (1967b). *The Necessary Angel.* New York: Knopf.

Stickgold, R. (1998). "Sleep: Off-Line Memory Reprocessing." *Trends in Cognitive Science, 2*(12), 484–492.

Strunk, W., Jr., and White, E. B. (1979). *The Elements of Style* (3rd ed.). Old Tappan, N.J.: Macmillan.

Stumpf, H., and Jackson, D. N. (1994). "Gender-Related Differences in Cognitive Abilities: Evidence from a Medical School Admissions Testing Program." *Personality and Individual Differences, 17*(3), 335–344.

Sylwester, R. (1995). *A Celebration of Neurons: An Educator's Guide to the Human Brain.* Alexandria, Va.: Association for Supervision and Curriculum Development.

Sylwester, R., and Hasegawa, C. (1989, January). "How to Explain Drugs to Your Students." *Middle School,* pp. 8–11.

Tellagen, A., and others. (1988). "Personality Similarity in Twins Reared Apart and Together." *Journal of Personality and Social Psychology, 54*(6), 1031–1039.

Tesser, A., and Crelia, R. (1994). "Attitude Heritability and Attitude Reinforcement: A Test of the Niche Building Hypothesis." *Personality and Individual Differences, 16*(4), 571–577.

Thagard, P. (1992). "Adversarial Problem Solving: Modeling an Opponent Using Explanatory Coherence." *Cognitive Science, 16,* 123–149.

Thayer, R. E. (1989). *Biopsychology of Mood and Arousal.* New York: Oxford University Press.

Thayer, R. E. (1996). *The Origin of Everyday Moods: Managing Energy, Tension, and Stress.* New York: Oxford University Press.

Thomas, M. C., and Thomas, T. S. (1990). *Getting Commitment at Work: A Guide for Managers and Employees.* Chapel Hill, N.C.: Commitment Press.

Thomas, P. R. (Ed.). (1995). *Weighing the Options: Criteria for Evaluating Weight-Management Programs.* Washington, D.C.: National Academy of Sciences Press.

Thompson, C. (1992). *What a Great Idea! The Key Steps Creative People Take.* New York: HarperCollins.

Thompson, H. (1995, June). "Walk, Don't Run." *Texas Monthly,* pp. 114, 116–117, 136.

Thompson, J. G. (1988). *The Psychobiology of Emotions.* New York: Plenum.

Toates, F. (1986). *The Biological Foundations of Behavior.* Bristol, Pa.: Open University Press.

Tomatis, A. (1991). *The Conscious Ear.* Barrytown, N.Y.: Station Hill Press.

Tornow, W., and London, M. (Eds.). (1998). *Maximizing the Value of 360–Degree Feedback: A Process for Successful Individual and Organizational Development.* San Francisco: Jossey-Bass.

Torrance, E. P. (1974). *Torrance Tests of Creative Thinking.* Bensenville, Ill.: Scholastic Testing Service.

Toufexis, A. (1989, March 13). "The Latest Word on What to Eat." *Time, 133*(11), 51–52.

Veggeberg, S. K. (1997, September–October). "The Big Story in Depression: What Isn't Happening." *BrainWork: The Neuroscience Newsletter* (Charles A. Dana Foundation), 7(4), 1–3.

Vernon, P. A. (Ed.). (1987). *Speed of Information-Processing and Intelligence.* Norwood, N.J.: Ablex.

von Bertalanffy, L. (1967). *Robots, Men and Minds: Psychology in the Modern World.* New York: Braziller.

von Oech, R. (1983). *A Whack on the Side of the Head: How to Unlock Your Mind for Innovation.* New York: Warner Books.

Vroon, P. (1997). *Smell: The Secret Seducer.* New York: Farrar, Straus & Giroux.

Wagner, M. J., and Tilney, G. (1983, March 17). "The Effect of 'Superlearning' Techniques on the Vocabulary Acquisition and Alpha Brainwave Production of Language Learners." *TESOL Quarterly,* 7(1), 5–17.

Wallas, G. (1926). *The Art of Thought.* London: J. Cape.

Walsh, A. (1996). *The Science of Love: Understanding Love and Its Effects on Mind and Body.* Amherst, N.Y.: Prometheus.

Walsh, C. A. (1997, Winter). "Epilepsy: Genes May Build the Road to Treatment." *On the Brain* (Harvard Mahoney Neuroscience Institute Letter), pp. 1–3.

Walton, M. (1986). *The Deming Management Method.* New York: Dodd, Mead.

Watson, J. B. (1925). *Behaviorism.* New York: Norton.

Watzlawick, P., Weakland, J. H., and Fisch, R. (1974). *Change: Principles of Problem Formation and Problem Resolution.* New York: Norton.

Weatherall, D. (1987, September). "New Light on Light." *Management Services, 31*(9), 38–39.

Webb, W. B. (1992). *Sleep: The Gentle Tyrant* (2nd ed.). Bolton, Mass.: Anker.

Webb, W. B. (Ed.). (1982). *Biological Rhythms, Sleep, and Performance.* Chichester, England: Wiley.

Weingardt, K. R., Leonesio, R. J., and Loftus, E. F. (1994). "On Eyewitness Metacognition." In J. Metcalfe and A. P. Shimamura (Eds.), *Metacognition: Knowing About Knowing* (pp. 155–184). Cambridge, Mass.: MIT Press.

Weston, D. C., and Weston, M. S. (1996). *Playwise: 365 Fun-Filled Activities for Building Character, Conscience, and Emotional Intelligence in Children.* Los Angeles: Tarcher.

Wetter, D. W., and others. (1998, June). "The Agency for Health Care Policy and Research Smoking Cessation Clinical Practice Guideline: Findings and Implications for Psychologists." *American Psychologist, 53*(6), 657–669.

Wheatley, M. J. (1994). *Leadership and the New Science.* San Francisco: Berrett-Koehler.

Whetten, D., and Cameron, K. (1984). *Development Management Skills.* London: Scott, Foresman.

Whybrow, P. C. (1997). *A Mood Apart: Depression, Mania, and Other Afflictions of Self.* New York: Basic Books.

Wiertelak, E., Meier, S. F., and Watkins, L. R. (1992, May 8). "Cholecystokinin Antianalgesia: Safety Cues Abolish Morphine Analgesia." *Science, 256,* 830 ff.

Wilcox, S. M., Himmelstein, D. U., and Woolhandler, S. (1994, July 27). "Inappropriate Drug Prescribing for the Community-Dwelling Elderly." *Journal of the American Medical Association, 272*(4), 292–296.

Williams, C. L., and others. (1985). *The Negotiable Environment: People, White Collar Work, and the Office.* Ann Arbor, Mich.: Miller, Herman.

Williams, J. M. (1990). *Style: Toward Clarity and Grace.* Chicago: University of Chicago Press.

Williams, R. (1989). *The Trusting Heart: Great News About Type A Behavior.* New York: Times Books.

Williams, R., and Williams, V. (1994). *Anger Kills.* New York: HarperPerennial.

Williams, W., and Ceci, S. (1997, November). "Are Americans Becoming More or Less Alike?" *American Psychologist, 52*(11), 1226–1235.

Wilson, E. O. (1975). *Sociobiology: The New Synthesis.* Cambridge, Mass.: Harvard University Press.

Wilson, G. D. (1994). *Psychology for Performing Artists: Butterflies and Bouquets.* London: Jessica Kingsley.

Winner, E. (1996). *Gifted Children: Myths and Realities.* New York: Basic Books.

Winner, E. (1997, October). "Exceptionally High Intelligence and Schooling." *American Psychologist, 52*(10), 1070–1081.

Winter, A., and Winter, R. (1988). *Eat Right, Be Bright.* New York: St. Martin's Press.

Winter, R. (1995). *A Consumer's Guide to Medicines in Food.* New York: Crown Trade Paperbacks.

Witkin, H. A., and Goodenough, D. R. (1981). *Cognitive Styles: Essence and Origins.* Madison, Conn.: International Universities Press.

Wolfe, D. A., McMahon, R. J., and Peters, R. D. (1997). *Child Abuse: New Directions in Prevention and Treatment Across the Lifespan.* Thousand Oaks, Calif.: Sage.

Wolfson, A., and Carskadon, M. (1996). "Early School Start Times Affect Sleep and Daytime Functioning in Adolescents." *Sleep Research, 25,* 117.

Woteki, C. E., and Thomas, P. R. (Eds.). (1992). *Eat for Life: The Food and Nutrition Board's Guide to Reducing Your Risk of Chronic Disease.* Washington, D.C.: National Academy Press.

Wrangham, R., and Peterson, D. (1996). *Demonic Males: Apes and the Origins of Human Violence.* Boston: Houghton Mifflin.

Wright, R. (1994). *The Moral Animal: The New Science of Evolutionary Psychology.* New York: Vintage Books.

Wright, W. (1998). *Born That Way: Genes, Behavior, Personality.* New York: Knopf.

Wyatt, R. J., and Henter, I. D. (1997, May–June). "Schizophrenia: An Introduction." *BrainWork: The Neuroscience Newsletter* (Charles A. Dana Foundation), 7(3), 1–3, 8.

Wydick, R. C. (1994). *Plain English for Lawyers* (3rd ed.). Durham, N.C.: Carolina Academic Press.

Yepsen, R. B., Jr. (1987). *How to Boost Your Brain Power: Achieving Peak Intelligence, Memory and Creativity.* Emmaus, Pa.: Rodale.

Zanna, M., and Pack, S. (1975). "On the Self-Fulfilling Nature of Apparent Sex Differences in Behavior." *Journal of Experimental Social Psychology, 11,* 583–591.

Zatorre, R. J. (1998, March 17). "Functional Anatomy of Musical Processing in Listeners with Absolute Pitch and Relative Pitch." *Proceedings of the National Academy of Sciences of the United States of America, 95*(6), 3172–3177.

Zdenek, M. (1985). *The Right-Brain Experience.* New York: McGraw-Hill.

Zeskind, P. S., Marshall, T. R., and Goss, D. M. (1992). "Rhythmic Organization of Heart Rate in Breast Fed and Bottle Fed Newborn Infants." *Early Development and Parenting, 1*(2), 79–87.

Zuckerman, M. (1991). *The Psychobiology of Personality.* New York: Cambridge University Press.

Free Resources

The Brain in the News. Published by The Dana Alliance for Brain Initiatives; 1001 G. Street, NW, Suite 1025; Washington, D.C. 20001. A monthly collection of reprints from U.S. newspapers.

BrainWork: The Neuroscience Newsletter. Published by the Charles A. Dana Foundation; 745 Fifth Avenue, Suite 700; New York, N.Y. 10151. A bimonthly newsletter with feature articles and brief news reports.

Mind-Body Health News. Newsletter of the Mind-Body Health Study Group Network; 444 North Capitol Street, NW, Suite 428; Washington, D.C. 20001; phone: 202-393-2210.

Resources with a Charge

The Brain Based Education/Learning Styles Networker. $15/year. Publisher: The Institute for Learning and Teaching; CARE; Rockhurst College; 1100 Rockhurst Road; Kansas City, Mo. 64110; phone: 703-599-9110.

Brain/Mind Bulletin. $45/year. Publisher: Marilyn Ferguson; Box 42211; Los Angeles, Calif. 90042; phone: 213-223-2500.

Consortium for Whole Brain Learning. $9/year. Publisher: Launa Ellison; 3348 47th Avenue South; Minneapolis, Minn. 55406.

Mental Medicine Update (The Mind/Body Health Newsletter). $9.95/year. Edited by David Sobel and Robert Ornstein. Published by The Center for Health Sciences; Cambridge, Mass.; phone: 800-222-4745.

Internet Resources

Web Sites

The following list includes every web site mentioned in the text of this book, and possibly a few more. Each web address is preceded by the prefix "http://" without the quotation marks. Addresses were accurate at the time of writing but may have changed by the time you try them. If they don't work, try a keyword search on the agency of interest and you should be able to get the current web site address. Happy surfing!

General

American Academy of Child and Adolescent Psychiatry:
  www.psych.med.umich.edu/web/aacap

American Psychological Association's PsychNET site:
  www.apa.org

Brain Lab:
  www.newhorizons.org/blab.html

Cognitive and Linguistic Sciences Department of Brown University:
  www.cog.brown.edu/

Cognitive and Psychological Sciences Index (in Europe):
  dawww.essex.ac.uk/~roehl/PsycIndex

Cognitive and Psychological Sciences Index (in the United States):
  www.psych.stanford.edu/cogsci/

COGSCI discussion list:
  www.mailbase.ac.uk/lists/cogsci/

Evolutionary Psychology: A Primer (J. Tooby and L. Cosmides):
  www.clark.net/pub/ogas/evolution/EVPSYCH primer.htm

Hampshire College cognitive science program (oldest of its kind in North America):
  www.hampshire.edu/academics/cs/CS.shtml

Healthfinder (government-maintained, with links to over 500 documents and over 550 web sites):
  www.healthfinder.gov

Healthgate (for-pay and free health information):
  www.healthgate.com

help! A Consumer's Guide to Mental Health Information:
  www.io.org/madmagic/help/help.html

Internet Mental Health:
  www.mentalhealth.com

Journal of the American Medical Association:
www.ama-assn.org/public/journals/jama

Mediconsult (a "virtual medical clinic"):
www.mediconsult.com

Medline medical database:
www.nlm.nih.gov

Mental Health InfoSource:
www.mhsource.com

Mental Health Library:
melhlp.netusa.mntlhlth.htm

Mental Health Net (John Grohol):
www.cmhc.com

Multiple intelligence theory (Howard Gardner's theory):
education.twsu.edu/faculty/gladhart/mihtml

National Alliance for the Mentally Ill:
www.cais.net/vikings/nami

National Institute of Mental Health:
gopher.nimh.nih.gov

National Institutes of Health:
www.nih.gov

National Mental Health Association:
www.worldcorp.com/dc-online/nmha

New England Journal of Medicine:
www.nejm.org

Online Psych:
www.onlinepsych.com

Psych Central (John Grohol's site with all on-line resources for mental health):
www.coil.com/grohol

PsycSite (Science of psychology; Nipissing University)
www.stange.simplenet.com/psycsite/

Scientific American magazine:
www.sciam.com

Shape Up America (C. Everett Koop):
www2.shapeup.org

Society for Applied Research in Memory and Cognition:
www.atkinson.yorku.ca/~sarmac/index.htm

University of Arizona's Interdisciplinary Dialogues on Consciousness:
www.consciousness.arizona.edu/dialogs

Virtual Psychology Lab:
www.cardiff.ac.uk/uwcc/psych/stevensonwc/vp-lab

Part One: Forming a Foundation

National Center for Biotechnology Information (Human Genome Project information):
www.ncbi.nlm.nih.gov

Part Two: Wellness

American Council for Drug Education referral service:
www.drughelp.org

American Music Therapy Association home page:
www.musictherapy.org

Carnegie Corporation early childhood development site (*The Early Brain*):
www.carnegie.org

Centers for Disease Control and Prevention, report on survey on vitamin and mineral supplements:
www.cdc.gov

Environmental Protection Agency report on passive smoke:
www.oehha.org

Humor profile based on Lee Berk's SMILE software:
www.touchstarpro.com/smile-software.html

Mozart Effect Resource Center:
www.mozarteffect.com

Music and mind site, with a variety of links, including the *International Journal of Arts Medicine* and the Mozart Effect Resource Center:
www.mmbmusic.com

Music Intelligence Neural Development project:
www.mindinst.org

National Association for Music Therapy home page:
www.namt.com

National Clearinghouse for Alcohol and Drug Information, Research and Statistics page:
www.health.org/survey.htm

National Council on Alcoholism and Drug Dependence:
www.ncadd.com

National Sleep Foundation:
www.sleepfoundation.org

National Sleep Foundation site on women and sleep:
206.215.227.10/nsf/publications/women.html

School Start Time Study: Final Report Summary:
www.coled.umn.edu/CAREIwww/General/sstbiblio.htm

Searle healthNet: sleep:
www.searlehealthnet.com/sleep/dateline

Staleness and sports psychology information (John Raglin's site):
www.indiana.edu/~kines/raglin.htm

USDA Center for Nutrition Policy and Promotion home page:
www.usda.gov/fcs/cnpp

Part Four: Illness and Injury

Allied Products site on EEG neurofeedback and ADHD:
www.biof.com/neuroarticles.html

ALS site (Doug Jacobson's site):
www.phoenix.net/~jacobson/beatals.html

Alzheimer's disease:
www.alzheimers.com

American Brain Tumor Association:
neurosurgery.mgh.harvard.edu/abta/

American Neurological Association neuro-oncology site:
www.aneuroa.org/nlinkst97.html

Anorexia Nervosa and Related Eating Disorders, Inc.:
www.anred.com

Brain tumor site (Al Musella):
www.lanminds.com/local/brain/trial.html

BrainWork: The Neuroscience Newsletter (full text copies):
www.dana.org/dana/brainwrk.html

Brookhaven National Laboratories' GVG (gammavinyl-GABA) trials for cocaine addiction:
www.pet.bnl.gov

Children's learning disabilities:
www.ldonline.org

Dana Alliance for Brain Initiatives:
www.dana.org

Eating disorders site:
www.eating-disorder.com

Epilepsy Foundation of America:
www.efa.org/index/htm

Huntington's disease site:
www.interlog.com/~rlaycock/what.html

International Federation for Multiple Sclerosis:
www.ifmss.org.uk/

Mental retardation site:
www.healthanswers.com/database/ami/converted/001523.html

National Alliance for Research on Schizophrenia and Depression:
www.mhsource.com/narsad.html

National Institute of Mental Health site on anxiety disorders:
www.nimh.nih.gov/anxiety

National Institute of Neural Disorders and Stroke:
www.ninds.nih.gov/healinfo/disorder

Obsessive-compulsive disorder site:
www.ocdresource.com

Paralysis site for information and support:
neurosurgery.mgh.harvard.edu/paral-r.htm

Parkinson's disease:
www.santel.lu/SANTEL/diseases/parkins.html

Scientific Learning Principles, company with CD-ROM for working with dyslexia
(Paula Tallal and Michael Merzenich's site):
www.scilearn.com

Secret Language of Eating Disorders (Peggy Claude-Pierre):
www.randomhouse.com

Trauma and Abuse Support Forum by OurPlace:
ourworld.compuserve.com/homepages/Arael_Et_Al/TRMA-RX.htm

Traumatic brain injury site:
www.tbidoc.com

U.S. Office of Disease Prevention and Health Promotion:
www.healthfinder.gov

University of Alabama–Birmingham's "Comprehensive Stroke Center":
www.uab.edu/neurol/stroke.htm

University of Washington's neuro-oncology site:
weber.u.washington.edu/~chudler/disorders.html

Part Five: Being in Control

Bar-On Emotional Quotient Inventory (EQ-i), published by Multi-Health Systems Inc.:
www.mhs.com

Executive EQ instrument (Salovey and Mayer):
www.virtent.com/ei

Part Six: Individual Differences

Big Five information:
www.centacs.com

Center for Applied Cognitive Studies:
www.centacs.com

New Horizons site on Gardner and multiple intelligences:
www.newhorizons.org/trm_gardner.html

Part Seven: Learning

Critical Thinking presentation:
www.centacs.com

Gifted Resources home page:
www.eskimo.com/~user/kids.html

H & H Publishing Company's LASSI site:
www.hhpublishing.com

Learning Styles site:
www.geocities.com/CollegePark/Library/3543/learnstyle.html

Plain English law information (U.K.):
www.wordcentre.co.uk

Plain English law information (U.S.):
www.plainlanguage.gov

Part Eight: Creativity and Problem Solving

Brain Store site (Eric and Diane Jensen's catalog):
www.thebrainstore.com

Computer Assisted Qualitative Data Analysis Software site (Inspiration plus links to other tools and sites):
www.soc.surrey.ac.uk/cagdas

De Bono site:
   www.edwdebono.com
Decision Explorer software:
   www.banxia.com

Part Nine: Working Smarter

Families and Work Institute *1997 National Study of the Changing Workforce:*
   www.familiesandwork.org
Mediappraise: On-line 360° feedback:
   www.mediappraise.com
Paradigm Mastery videotapes by StarThrower:
   www.starthrower.com
Thin Book Publishing Company (Sue Hammond):
   www.thinbook.com
Vita-Lite:
   www.backbenimble.com/office/vitalite.htm

Part Ten: Schemas, Reality, and Spirituality

allCLEAR 4.5 flowcharting software:
   www.clearsoft.com
Critical Thinking Presentation:
   www.centacs.com
Decide Right 1.2 for Windows 95:
   www.avantos.com
Institute for Professional Education problem-solving seminars:
   www.theIPE.com
Laban symbol system, software for notating movement:
   www.dance.ohio-state.edu/files/LabanWriter/index.html
Mind map software:
   www.mindman.com
STELLA system process flow software:
   www.hps-inc.com
SureFire Decisions for Windows 95, decision matrix:
   www.beaconrock.com

E-Mail Addresses

Ruediger Oehlmann (COGSCI editor, European address):
   oehlmann@essex.ac.uk
Ruediger Oehlmann (COGSCI editor, U.S. address):
   oehlmann@psych.stanford.edu

Newsgroups and Bulletin Boards

alt.bio.minority	alt. support.shyness
alt.brain	alt. support.sleep-disorder
alt.drugs.caffeine	alt. support.stuttering
alt.education.research	bionet.neuroscience
alt.fan.hofstadter	cbiz.ergonomic-sciences
alt.handed	clari.news.aging
alt.human-brain	clari.tw.health
alt.left	clari.tw.science
alt.lefthanders	comp.ai
alt.psychology.personality	comp.ai.fuzzy
alt.recovery.aa	comp.ai.genetic
alt.support.attn-deficit	comp.ai.neural-nets
alt.support.cerebral-palsy	comp.ai.philosophy
alt. support.depression	comp.ai.vision
alt. support.dev-delays	misc.creativity
alt. support.diet	rec.org.mensa
alt. support.eating-disord	sci.anthropology
alt. support.epilepsy	sci.cognitive
alt. support.ex-cult	sci.med.psychobiology
alt. support.grief	sci.psychology.research
alt. support.learning-disab	uw.neural-nets
alt. support.menopause	

Listservers

Name	*Address to Subscribe*	*Message*
Cognitive Science	mailbase@mailbase.ac.uk	join COGSCI <firstname lastname>
De Bono	LISTSERV@SJUVM.STJOHNS.EDU	Subscribe DEBONO <firstname lastname>
Depression Forum	mailbase@mailbase.ac.uk	join depression <firstname lastname>
Tacit Knowledge	listproc@scu.edu.au	subscribe tacit-l <your E-mail address>

Index

Reader Participation Card

The Center for Applied Cognitive Studies continually scans the research literature to find new topics with practical applications. We plan to publish an updated edition of *The Owner's Manual for the Brain* every several years. If you know of Topics you would like to see included in the next edition, or if you know of an Application idea for one of the Topics included in this edition, please list them below and mail or fax them to us for inclusion in the next edition. Of course, we will credit you as the contributor. Items that you send in may also be printed in our quarterly newsletter.

Topics I'd like to see included in the next edition:

_____

_____

_____

Application ideas for Topics in this edition:

Topic number _____ : _____

Topic number _____ : _____

Topic number _____ : _____

Topic number _____ : _____

Topic number _____ : _____
(Add continuation page for additional contributions)

Other comments:

Fax to 704-331-9408, send to Internet E-mail address pjhoward@centacs.com, or send by regular mail to *Cent*ACS, 1100 Harding Place, Charlotte, NC 28204-2825.

Submitted by:

Name _____

Street address _____

City _____ State/Province _____ Country _____ Zip code _____

Phone: Work ( ) ____-_____ Fax ( ) ____-_____ Home ( ) ____-_____

E-mail address _____